GRAY'S ATLAS
OF ANATOMY

SECOND EDITION

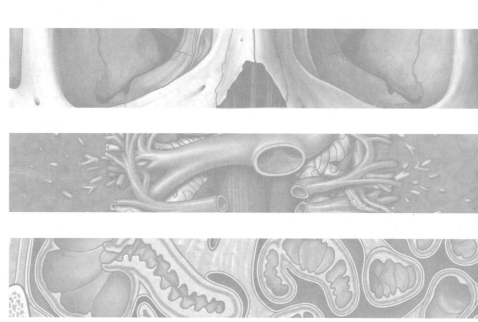

Richard L. Drake, PhD, FAAA

Director of Anatomy
Professor of Surgery
Cleveland Clinic Lerner College of Medicine
Case Western Reserve University
Cleveland, Ohio, USA

A. Wayne Vogl, PhD, FAAA

Professor of Anatomy and Cell Biology
Department of Cellular and Physiological Sciences
Faculty of Medicine
University of British Columbia
Vancouver, British Columbia, Canada

Adam W. M. Mitchell, MBBS, FRCS, FRCR

Consultant Radiologist and Senior Lecturer Imperial College
Chelsea and Westminster Hospital
London, UK

Illustrated by

Richard M. Tibbitts

Saffron Walden, UK

Paul E. Richardson

Cambridge, UK

Photographs by

Ansell Horn

GRAY'S
ATLAS
OF ANATOMY
SECOND EDITION

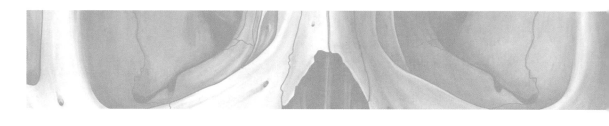
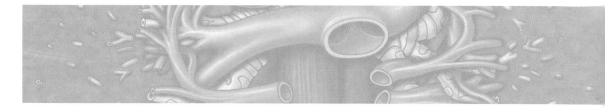
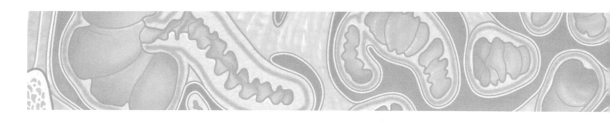

Richard L. Drake   A. Wayne Vogl   Adam W. M. Mitchell

Richard M. Tibbitts   Paul E. Richardson

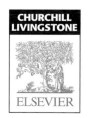

CHURCHILL
LIVINGSTONE

ELSEVIER

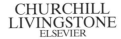

1600 John F. Kennedy Blvd.
Ste 1800
Philadelphia, PA 19103-2899

GRAY'S ATLAS OF ANATOMY, SECOND EDITION
INTERNATIONAL EDITION

ISBN: 978-1-4557-4802-0
ISBN: 978-0-7020-5237-8

Notices

Knowledge and best practice in this field are constantly changing. As new research and experience broaden our understanding, changes in research methods, professional practices, or medical treatment may become necessary.

Practitioners and researchers must always rely on their own experience and knowledge in evaluating and using any information, methods, compounds, or experiments described herein. In using such information or methods they should be mindful of their own safety and the safety of others, including parties for whom they have a professional responsibility.

With respect to any drug or pharmaceutical products identified, readers are advised to check the most current information provided (i) on procedures featured or (ii) by the manufacturer of each product to be administered, to verify the recommended dose or formula, the method and duration of administration, and contraindications. It is the responsibility of practitioners, relying on their own experience and knowledge of their patients, to make diagnoses, to determine dosages and the best treatment for each individual patient, and to take all appropriate safety precautions.

To the fullest extent of the law, neither the Publisher nor the authors, contributors, or editors, assume any liability for any injury and/or damage to persons or property as a matter of products liability, negligence or otherwise, or from any use or operation of any methods, products, instructions, or ideas contained in the material herein.

The Publisher

ISBN: 978-1-4557-4802-0

VP Global Medical Education Content: Madelene Hyde
Senior Manager, Content Development: Rebecca Gruliow
Publishing Services Manager: Patricia Tannian
Senior Project Manager: John Casey
Design and Art Direction: Antbits Ltd.

Working together to grow
libraries in developing countries

www.elsevier.com | www.bookaid.org | www.sabre.org

ELSEVIER   BOOK AID International   Sabre Foundation

Printed in Canada
Last digit is the print number: 9 8 7 6 5 4 3 2 1

To my wife who supports me and to my parents who are always with me.
Richard L. Drake

To my family, to my professional colleagues and role models, and to my students.
Wayne Vogl

Thanks, to Cathy, Max and Elsa
Adam W. M. Mitchell

To my family – my inspiration, Evi, Zoë, and Nicholas x
Richard M. Tibbitts

To Lesley and in memory of AMR and JER
Paul Richardson

ACKNOWLEDGMENTS

The following reviewers helped enormously with their detailed critiques and suggestions for every chapter. Their assistance was invaluable.

Mark Hankin, PhD, University of Toledo College of Medicine, Toledo, Ohio

Marios Loukas, MD, PhD, St. George's University School of Medicine, Grenada

James J. Rechtien, DO, PhD, Michigan State University School of Medicine, East Lansing, Michigan

William A. Roy, PT, PhD, Touro University, Henderson, Nevada

Susan Standring, PhD, DSc, Professor of Experimental Neurobiology and Head, Division of Anatomy, Cell and Human Biology, Guy's, King's and St Thomas' School of Biomedical Sciences, King's College London, London

William Swartz, PhD, Louisiana State University Health Sciences Center, Baton Rouge, Louisiana

Mark F. Teaford, PhD, Johns Hopkins University School of Medicine, Baltimore, Maryland

We want to thank Dr. Bruce Crawford for a radiograph of the head and neck and Dr. Murray Morrison for laryngoscopic images of the larynx; Dr. Jerry Healy for three images in the Abdomen section: the celiac artery, the bile duct system, and a three-dimensional view of abdominal vessels; and Siemens Medical Solutions USA and the following individuals with that company: Mollie Beaver, Director, CT Clinical Solutions, and Dr. Louise McKenna, Global Clinical Marketing Manager, CT Oncology, who supplied a *syngo* Multi-modality Workplace, which was used to acquire the majority of the clinical images.

Stuart Morrison, MD, helped with all aspects of coordinating the collection of the radiographic material. Radiological assistance and images were contributed in each of the following areas:

Back	Mark Kayanja, MD, PhD
	Jeffrey S. Ross, MD
Thorax	Mario Garcia, MD
	A. Michael Lincoff, MD
Abdomen	Namita Gandhi, MD
	Michelle Inkster, MD, PhD
	Brian R. Lane, MD
	Anand Rao, MD
	James S. Wu, MD
Pelvis	Matthew Barber, MD, MHS
	Tommaso Falcone, MD
	J. Stephen Jones, MD
	Eunice Moon, MD
	James S. Newman, MD, PhD
Extremities	Hakan Ilaslan, MD
	Bradford J. Richmond, MD
	Joshua Polster, MD
Head and Neck	Todd W. Stultz, DDS, MD
	J. Martin Paloma, DDS, MSD
	Cindy McConnaughy
	Ronald Lemmo, DDS

A working knowledge of anatomy is not an "optional extra" for health care professionals – it is fundamental. Acquiring that knowledge has always challenged even the most motivated students. Over many generations, learning materials that aid the process effectively have been warmly welcomed by students and their teachers (and by patients, who are the ultimate beneficiaries of that knowledge). I remember my own students' response when I first included illustrations from *Gray's Anatomy for Students* in a lecture—afterward, I was asked repeatedly for the source of the marvelous pictures. Looking beyond the "wow" factor that leapt from the pages of the book, it was clear that an enormous amount of thought and skill had gone into producing the artwork.

This atlas contains a series of additional outstanding pieces of anatomical art from the illustrative team of Richard Tibbitts and Paul Richardson that will complement those in *Gray's Anatomy for Students*, combined with relevant clinical pictures, surface anatomy, and images from a range of modern imaging procedures. Of course, anatomy cannot be learned from books and interactive DVDs alone, no matter how excellent they may be. Anatomy is a practical subject, best learned by gaining hands-on experience of the body. Students should spend as much time as they can examining cadaveric dissections (if they do not have the opportunity to dissect themselves) and should always read from screen or page with the appropriate bones in front of them. They need to combine and correlate information from a wide variety of sources in order to gain the working knowledge mentioned earlier.

This atlas will provide a valuable companion to their studies, and I am confident that it will remain in their libraries long after they have completed the early stages of their training.

Susan Standring, PhD, DSc, FKC, Hon FRCS
Emeritus Professor of Anatomy
King's College, London

FOREWORD

We began working on *Gray's Atlas of Anatomy* in 2005 following the publication of our textbook, *Gray's Anatomy for Students*. We wanted to produce an atlas that would build on themes and concepts established in the textbook and that would couple artistic renderings of "internal" gross anatomy with actual "living" anatomy, as visualized with modern imaging techniques and with surface anatomy. We believe that the final atlas presents a fresh and integrated approach to anatomy that is accessible to entry-level students in anatomy, as well as to students at more advanced levels.

Because an atlas is used in a much different way than a textbook, we could not simply repackage figures used in *Gray's Anatomy for Students* and put them in the atlas. Consequently, most of the figures in the atlas are new and were designed to present structures in a more complete context than in the textbook, even though the color palette and overall look of the figures in both the atlas and textbook are similar. Also, figures in the atlas provide additional detail not included in the textbook and directly correlate artistic representations of anatomy with computed tomography (CT) and magnetic resonance imaging (MRI). Where appropriate, we have included endoscopic, laryngoscopic, and laparoscopic views of the anatomy and have included examples of ultrasound images. In a number of regions, we also have reconstructed the internal anatomy of patients by abstracting specific information from multiple MR or CT images, and we present these reconstructions together with artwork of the same anatomy. Although the artwork was done independently of the reconstructed images, the two types of representations are strikingly similar.

Each page of this atlas was planned prior to beginning work on the figures, and all of the artwork was generated digitally. Most of the figures were created from an extensive digital database created for the textbook. Each figure was reviewed for accuracy and revised accordingly.

We hope that the textbook and atlas used together will provide new and powerful learning tools for students of human gross anatomy.

The Authors

The 2nd edition of *Gray's Atlas of Anatomy* continues in the tradition of the 1st edition, coupling artistic rendering with actual living anatomy as visualized with modern imaging techniques and surface anatomy. The combination of modern illustrations, imaging, and surface anatomy is unique among atlases available today.

We have also added additional study aids that should enhance the learning experience. At the end of every chapter tables and schematic drawings have been added for quick review of subject matter. These include major nerves plexuses throughout the body, branching patterns of major arteries, summaries of muscles organized into compartments or regions, and other helpful information. This material is designed to provide the reader quick access to information.

It's our hope that the 2nd edition of *Gray's Atlas of Anatomy* will become a valuable learning aid for students encountering anatomy for the first time or for the individual seeking to review information critical to their daily experiences.

The Authors

CONTENTS

CONTENTS

CONTENTS

CONTENTS

7 UPPER LIMB

CONTENTS

8 HEAD AND NECK

CONTENTS

THE BODY

1

CONTENTS

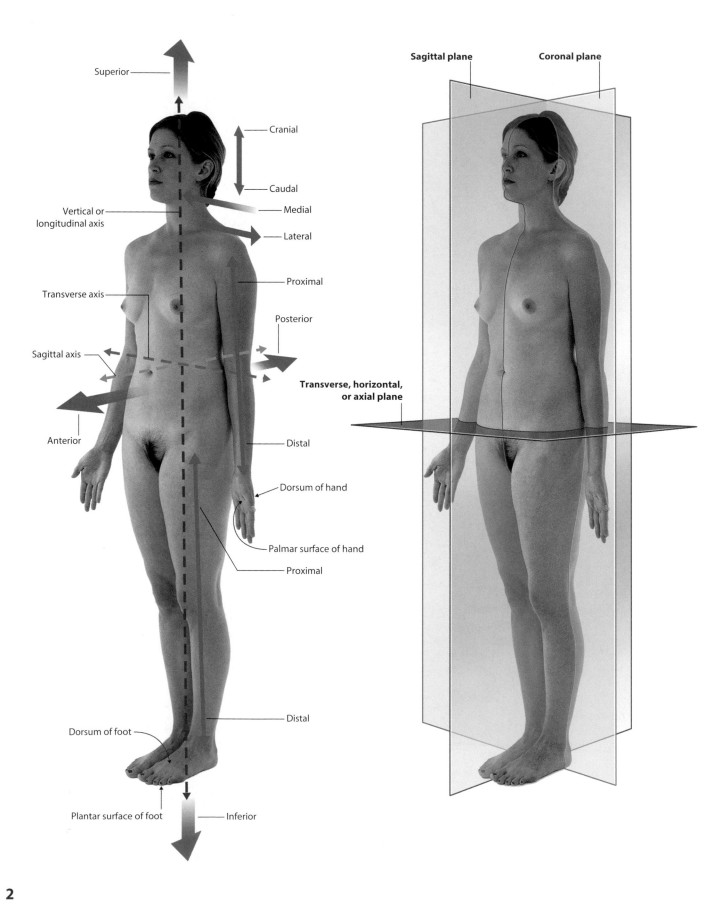

Superior

Cranial

Caudal

Medial

Vertical or longitudinal axis

Lateral

Proximal

Transverse axis

Posterior

Sagittal axis

Anterior

Distal

Dorsum of hand

Palmar surface of hand

Proximal

Distal

Dorsum of foot

Plantar surface of foot

Inferior

Sagittal plane

Coronal plane

Transverse, horizontal, or axial plane

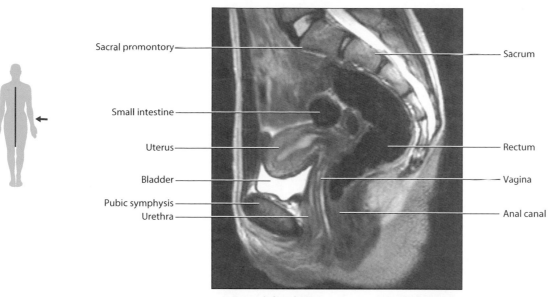

Sacral promontory — — Sacrum

Small intestine —

Uterus — — Rectum

Bladder — — Vagina

Pubic symphysis — — Anal canal

Urethra —

T2-weighted MR image, in sagittal plane

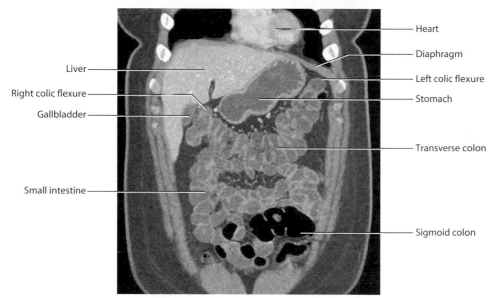

— Heart

— Diaphragm

Liver — — Left colic flexure

Right colic flexure — — Stomach

Gallbladder —

— Transverse colon

Small intestine —

— Sigmoid colon

CT image, with contrast, in coronal plane

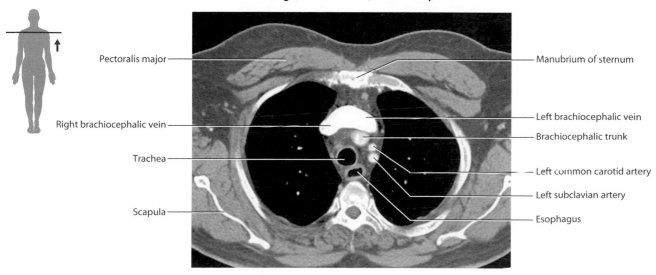

Pectoralis major — — Manubrium of sternum

Right brachiocephalic vein — — Left brachiocephalic vein

— Brachiocephalic trunk

Trachea —

— Left common carotid artery

— Left subclavian artery

Scapula —

— Esophagus

CT image, with contrast, in axial plane

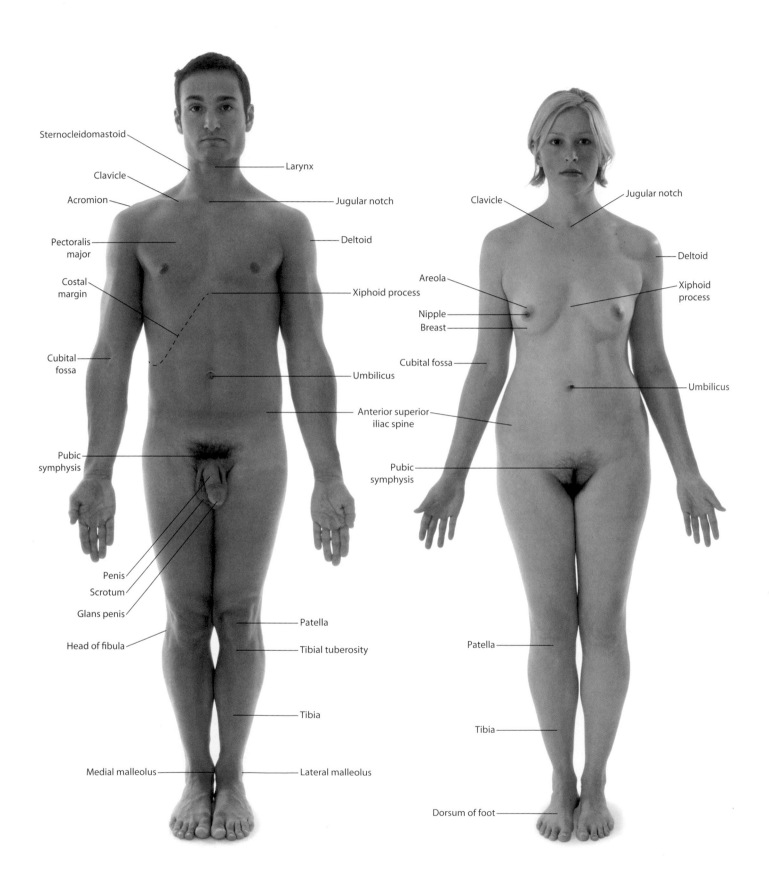

Sternocleidomastoid

Clavicle

Acromion

Pectoralis major

Costal margin

Cubital fossa

Pubic symphysis

Penis

Scrotum

Glans penis

Head of fibula

Medial malleolus

Larynx

Jugular notch

Deltoid

Xiphoid process

Umbilicus

Anterior superior iliac spine

Patella

Tibial tuberosity

Tibia

Lateral malleolus

Clavicle

Areola

Nipple

Breast

Cubital fossa

Pubic symphysis

Patella

Tibia

Dorsum of foot

Jugular notch

Deltoid

Xiphoid process

Umbilicus

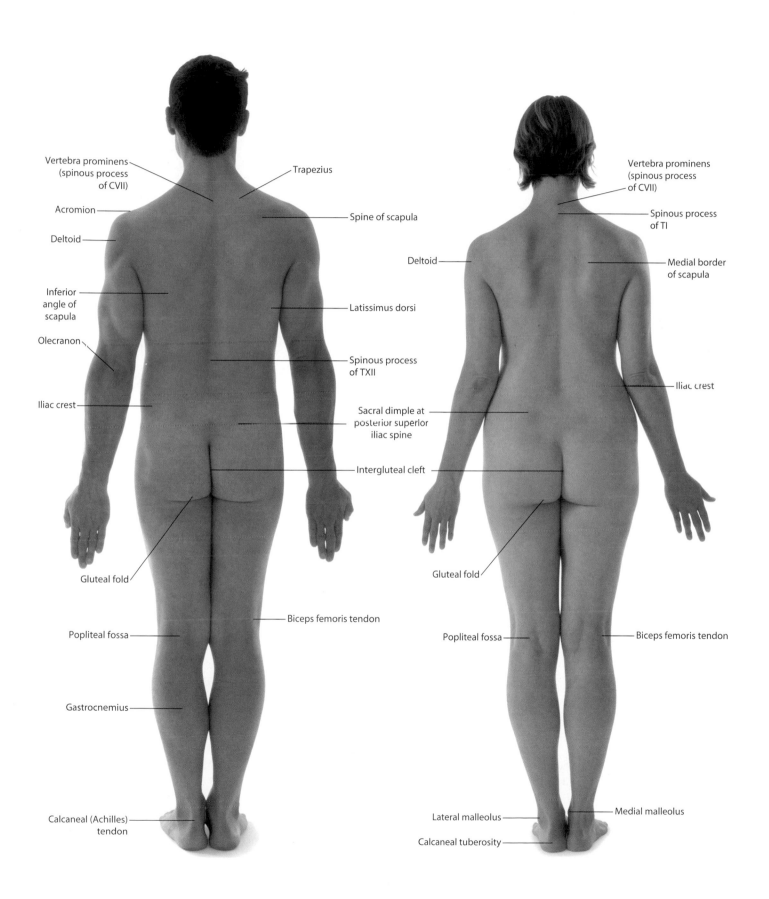

Vertebra prominens (spinous process of CVII)

Trapezius

Acromion

Spine of scapula

Deltoid

Inferior angle of scapula

Latissimus dorsi

Olecranon

Spinous process of TXII

Iliac crest

Sacral dimple at posterior superior iliac spine

Intergluteal cleft

Gluteal fold

Biceps femoris tendon

Popliteal fossa

Gastrocnemius

Calcaneal (Achilles) tendon

Vertebra prominens (spinous process of CVII)

Spinous process of TI

Deltoid

Medial border of scapula

Iliac crest

Gluteal fold

Popliteal fossa

Biceps femoris tendon

Lateral malleolus

Medial malleolus

Calcaneal tuberosity

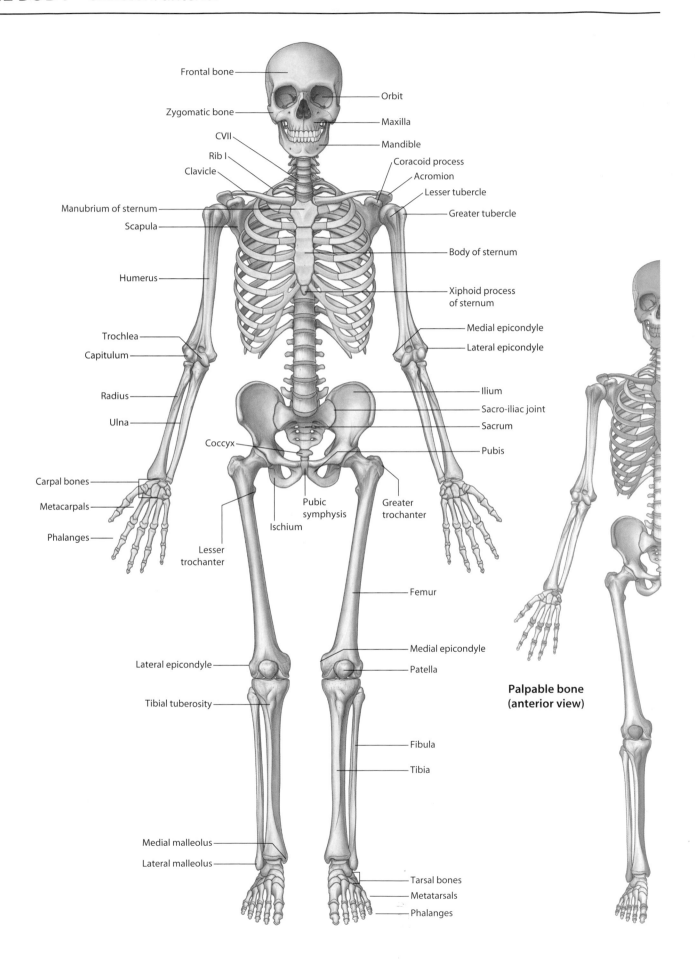

Frontal bone

Orbit

Zygomatic bone

Maxilla

CVII

Mandible

Rib I

Coracoid process

Clavicle

Acromion

Lesser tubercle

Manubrium of sternum

Greater tubercle

Scapula

Body of sternum

Humerus

Xiphoid process
of sternum

Trochlea

Medial epicondyle

Capitulum

Lateral epicondyle

Radius

Ilium

Ulna

Sacro-iliac joint

Sacrum

Coccyx

Pubis

Carpal bones

Metacarpals

Phalanges

Pubic
symphysis

Greater
trochanter

Ischium

Lesser
trochanter

Femur

Lateral epicondyle

Medial epicondyle

Patella

Tibial tuberosity

Fibula

Tibia

Medial malleolus

Lateral malleolus

Tarsal bones

Metatarsals

Phalanges

**Palpable bone
(anterior view)**

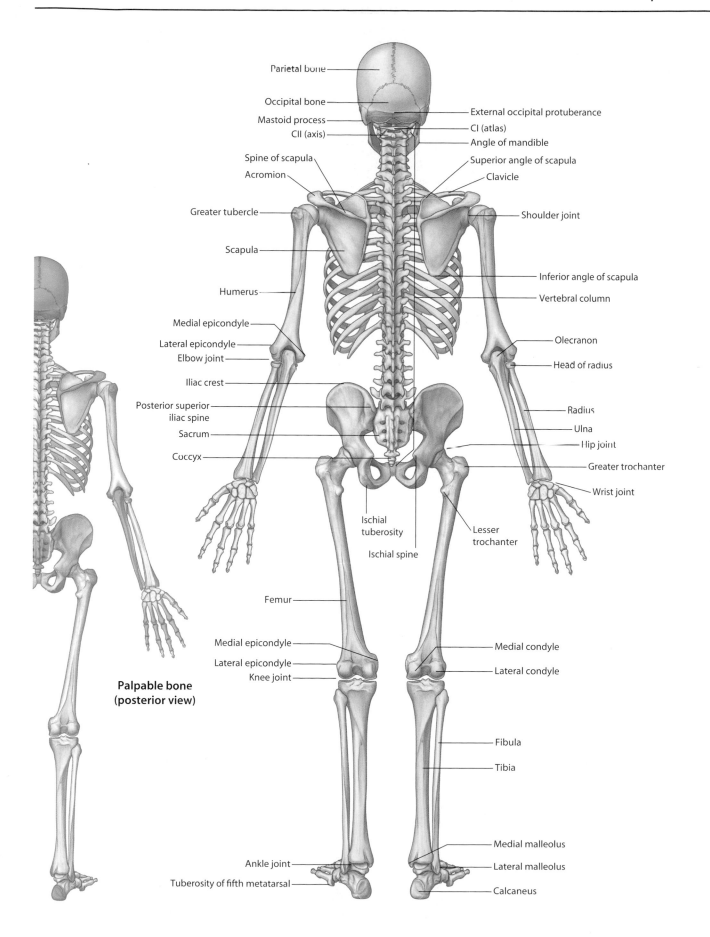

Parietal bone

Occipital bone

Mastoid process

CII (axis)

External occipital protuberance

CI (atlas)

Angle of mandible

Spine of scapula

Acromion

Superior angle of scapula

Clavicle

Greater tubercle

Shoulder joint

Scapula

Inferior angle of scapula

Humerus

Vertebral column

Medial epicondyle

Lateral epicondyle

Elbow joint

Olecranon

Head of radius

Iliac crest

Posterior superior
iliac spine

Sacrum

Coccyx

Radius

Ulna

Hip joint

Greater trochanter

Wrist joint

Ischial
tuberosity

Lesser
trochanter

Ischial spine

Femur

Medial epicondyle

Lateral epicondyle

Knee joint

Medial condyle

Lateral condyle

**Palpable bone
(posterior view)**

Fibula

Tibia

Medial malleolus

Ankle joint

Lateral malleolus

Tuberosity of fifth metatarsal

Calcaneus

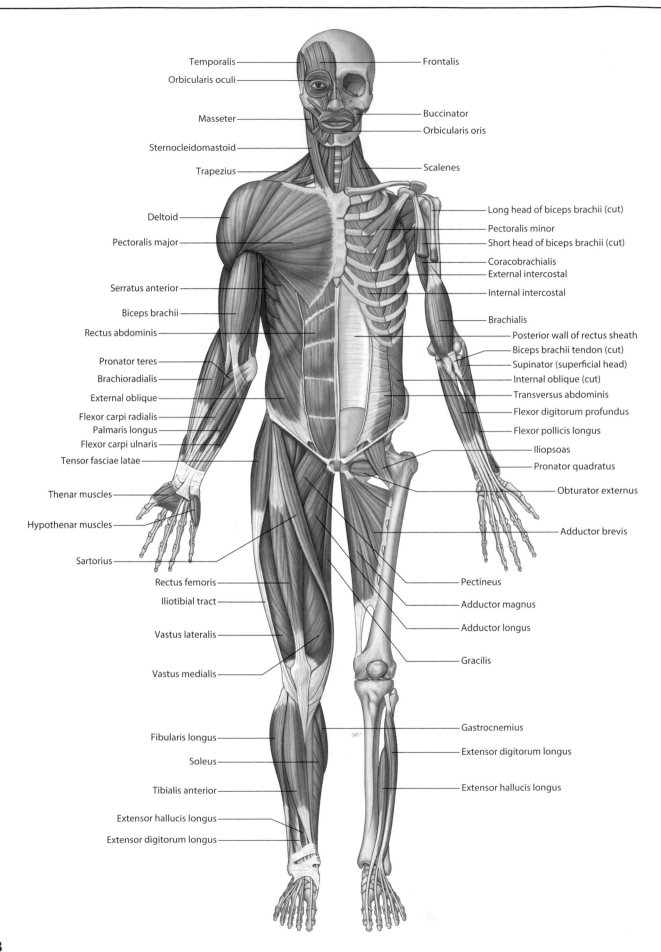

Temporalis
Orbicularis oculi
Masseter
Sternocleidomastoid
Trapezius
Deltoid
Pectoralis major
Serratus anterior
Biceps brachii
Rectus abdominis
Pronator teres
Brachioradialis
External oblique
Flexor carpi radialis
Palmaris longus
Flexor carpi ulnaris
Tensor fasciae latae
Thenar muscles
Hypothenar muscles
Sartorius
Rectus femoris
Iliotibial tract
Vastus lateralis
Vastus medialis
Fibularis longus
Soleus
Tibialis anterior
Extensor hallucis longus
Extensor digitorum longus

Frontalis
Buccinator
Orbicularis oris
Scalenes
Long head of biceps brachii (cut)
Pectoralis minor
Short head of biceps brachii (cut)
Coracobrachialis
External intercostal
Internal intercostal
Brachialis
Posterior wall of rectus sheath
Biceps brachii tendon (cut)
Supinator (superficial head)
Internal oblique (cut)
Transversus abdominis
Flexor digitorum profundus
Flexor pollicis longus
Iliopsoas
Pronator quadratus
Obturator externus
Adductor brevis
Pectineus
Adductor magnus
Adductor longus
Gracilis
Gastrocnemius
Extensor digitorum longus
Extensor hallucis longus

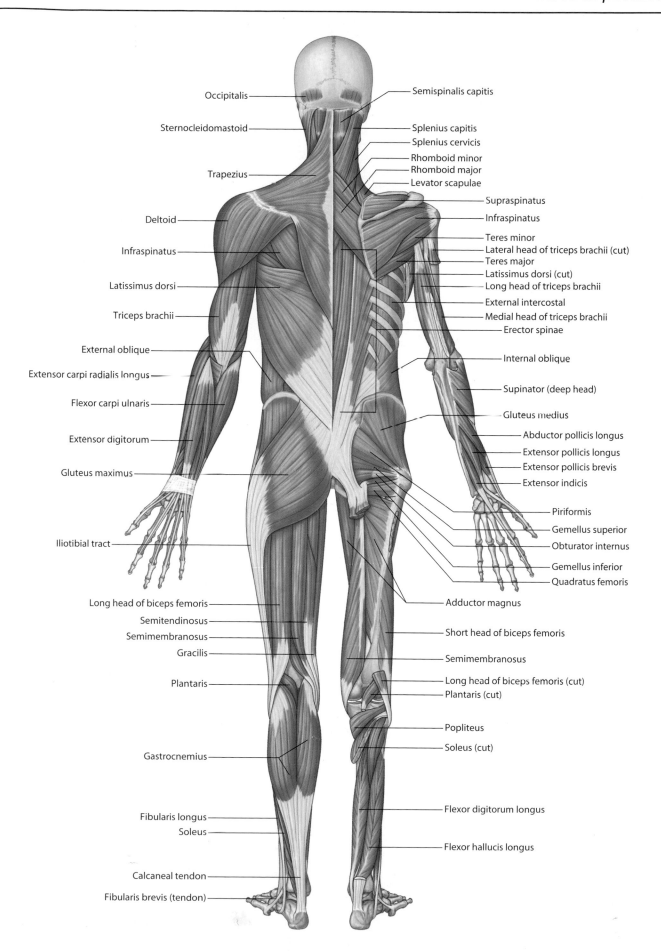

Occipitalis
Sternocleidomastoid
Trapezius
Deltoid
Infraspinatus
Latissimus dorsi
Triceps brachii
External oblique
Extensor carpi radialis longus
Flexor carpi ulnaris
Extensor digitorum
Gluteus maximus
Iliotibial tract
Long head of biceps femoris
Semitendinosus
Semimembranosus
Gracilis
Plantaris
Gastrocnemius
Fibularis longus
Soleus
Calcaneal tendon
Fibularis brevis (tendon)

Semispinalis capitis
Splenius capitis
Splenius cervicis
Rhomboid minor
Rhomboid major
Levator scapulae
Supraspinatus
Infraspinatus
Teres minor
Lateral head of triceps brachii (cut)
Teres major
Latissimus dorsi (cut)
Long head of triceps brachii
External intercostal
Medial head of triceps brachii
Erector spinae
Internal oblique
Supinator (deep head)
Gluteus medius
Abductor pollicis longus
Extensor pollicis longus
Extensor pollicis brevis
Extensor indicis
Piriformis
Gemellus superior
Obturator internus
Gemellus inferior
Quadratus femoris
Adductor magnus
Short head of biceps femoris
Semimembranosus
Long head of biceps femoris (cut)
Plantaris (cut)
Popliteus
Soleus (cut)
Flexor digitorum longus
Flexor hallucis longus

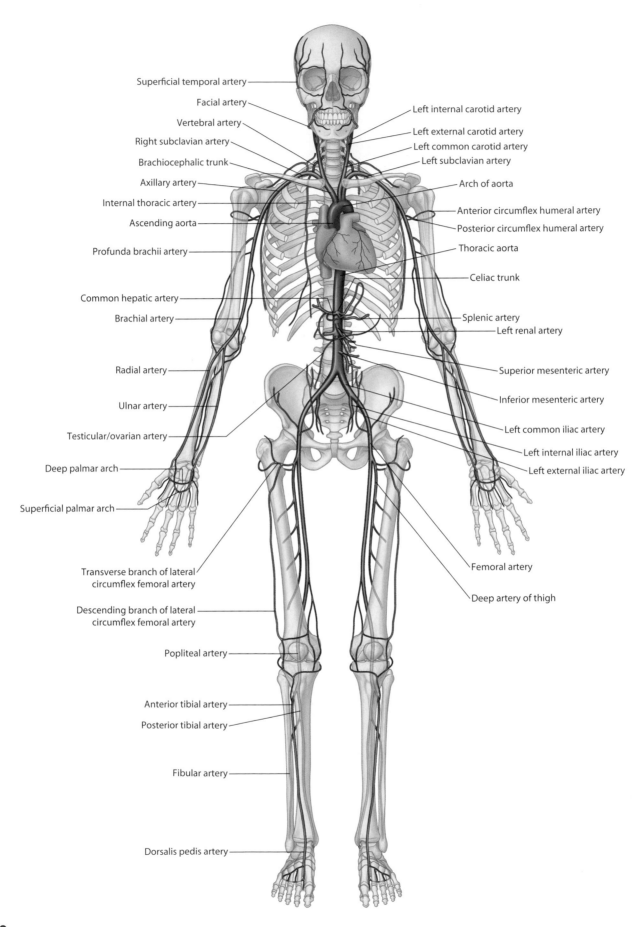

Superficial temporal artery

Facial artery

Vertebral artery

Right subclavian artery

Brachiocephalic trunk

Axillary artery

Internal thoracic artery

Ascending aorta

Profunda brachii artery

Common hepatic artery

Brachial artery

Radial artery

Ulnar artery

Testicular/ovarian artery

Deep palmar arch

Superficial palmar arch

Transverse branch of lateral circumflex femoral artery

Descending branch of lateral circumflex femoral artery

Popliteal artery

Anterior tibial artery

Posterior tibial artery

Fibular artery

Dorsalis pedis artery

Left internal carotid artery

Left external carotid artery

Left common carotid artery

Left subclavian artery

Arch of aorta

Anterior circumflex humeral artery

Posterior circumflex humeral artery

Thoracic aorta

Celiac trunk

Splenic artery

Left renal artery

Superior mesenteric artery

Inferior mesenteric artery

Left common iliac artery

Left internal iliac artery

Left external iliac artery

Femoral artery

Deep artery of thigh

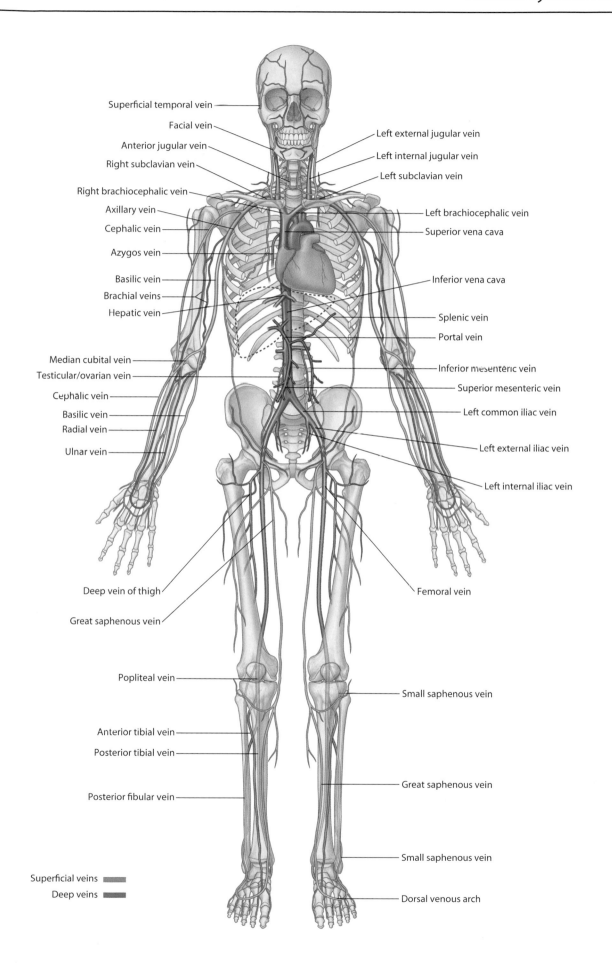

Superficial temporal vein
Facial vein
Anterior jugular vein
Right subclavian vein
Right brachiocephalic vein
Axillary vein
Cephalic vein
Azygos vein
Basilic vein
Brachial veins
Hepatic vein
Median cubital vein
Testicular/ovarian vein
Cephalic vein
Basilic vein
Radial vein
Ulnar vein
Deep vein of thigh
Great saphenous vein
Popliteal vein
Anterior tibial vein
Posterior tibial vein
Posterior fibular vein

Left external jugular vein
Left internal jugular vein
Left subclavian vein
Left brachiocephalic vein
Superior vena cava
Inferior vena cava
Splenic vein
Portal vein
Inferior mesenteric vein
Superior mesenteric vein
Left common iliac vein
Left external iliac vein
Left internal iliac vein
Femoral vein
Small saphenous vein
Great saphenous vein
Small saphenous vein
Dorsal venous arch

Superficial veins
Deep veins

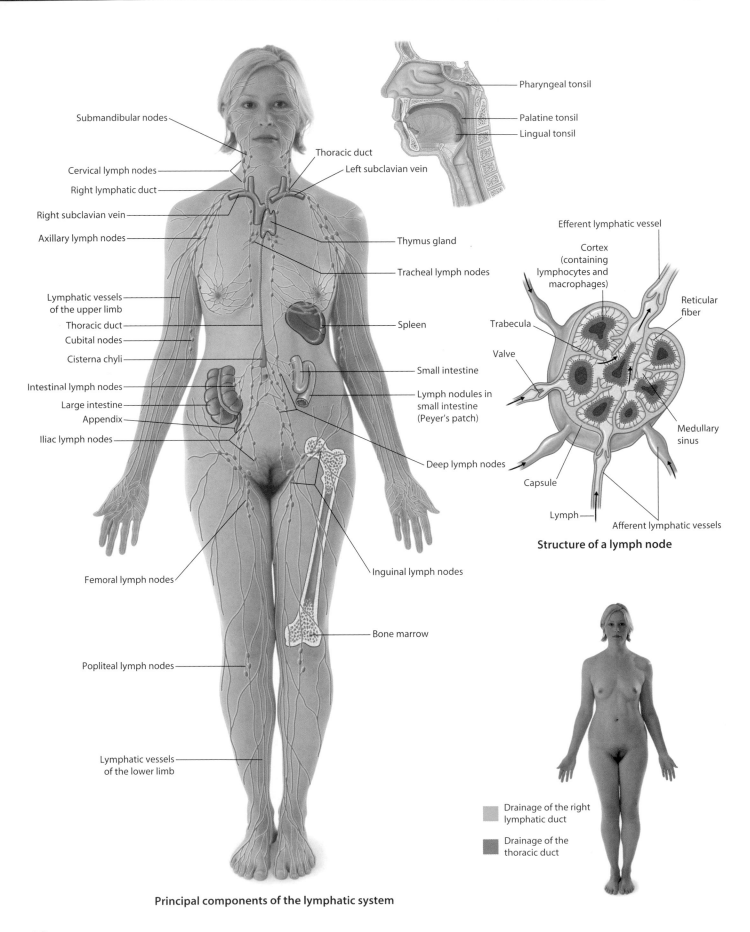

Submandibular nodes

Cervical lymph nodes

Right lymphatic duct

Right subclavian vein

Axillary lymph nodes

Lymphatic vessels of the upper limb

Thoracic duct

Cubital nodes

Cisterna chyli

Intestinal lymph nodes

Large intestine

Appendix

Iliac lymph nodes

Femoral lymph nodes

Popliteal lymph nodes

Lymphatic vessels of the lower limb

Thoracic duct

Left subclavian vein

Thymus gland

Tracheal lymph nodes

Spleen

Small intestine

Lymph nodules in small intestine (Peyer's patch)

Deep lymph nodes

Inguinal lymph nodes

Bone marrow

Pharyngeal tonsil

Palatine tonsil

Lingual tonsil

Efferent lymphatic vessel

Cortex (containing lymphocytes and macrophages)

Reticular fiber

Trabecula

Valve

Medullary sinus

Capsule

Lymph

Afferent lymphatic vessels

Structure of a lymph node

Drainage of the right lymphatic duct

Drainage of the thoracic duct

Principal components of the lymphatic system

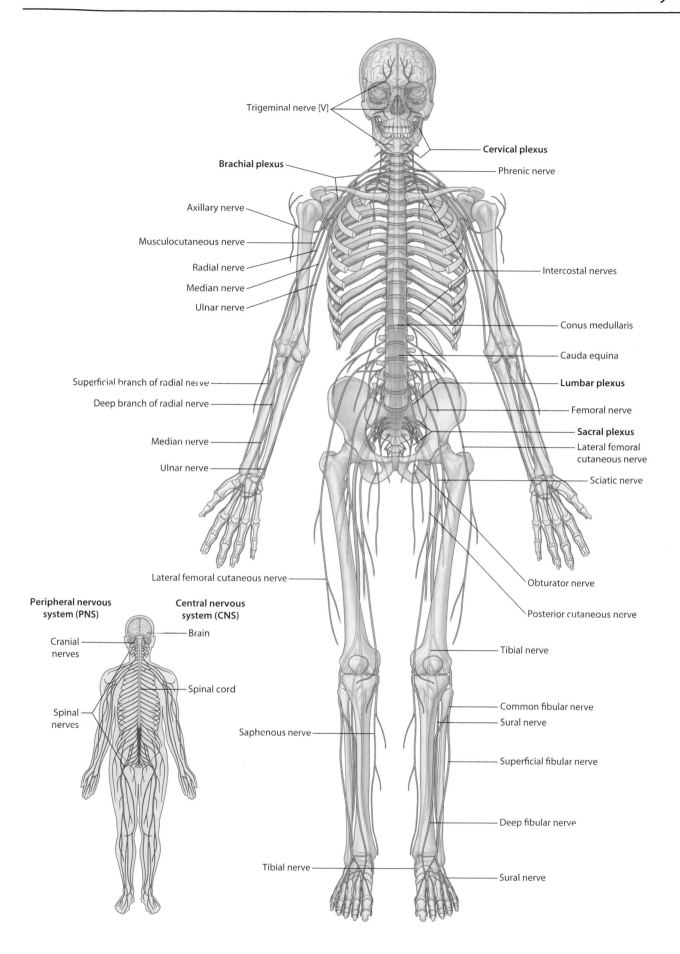

Trigeminal nerve [V]

Cervical plexus

Brachial plexus

Phrenic nerve

Axillary nerve

Musculocutaneous nerve

Radial nerve

Median nerve

Ulnar nerve

Intercostal nerves

Conus medullaris

Cauda equina

Superficial branch of radial nerve

Deep branch of radial nerve

Lumbar plexus

Femoral nerve

Median nerve

Sacral plexus

Ulnar nerve

Lateral femoral cutaneous nerve

Sciatic nerve

Lateral femoral cutaneous nerve

Obturator nerve

Posterior cutaneous nerve

Peripheral nervous system (PNS)

Central nervous system (CNS)

Cranial nerves

Brain

Spinal cord

Spinal nerves

Tibial nerve

Common fibular nerve

Sural nerve

Saphenous nerve

Superficial fibular nerve

Deep fibular nerve

Tibial nerve

Sural nerve

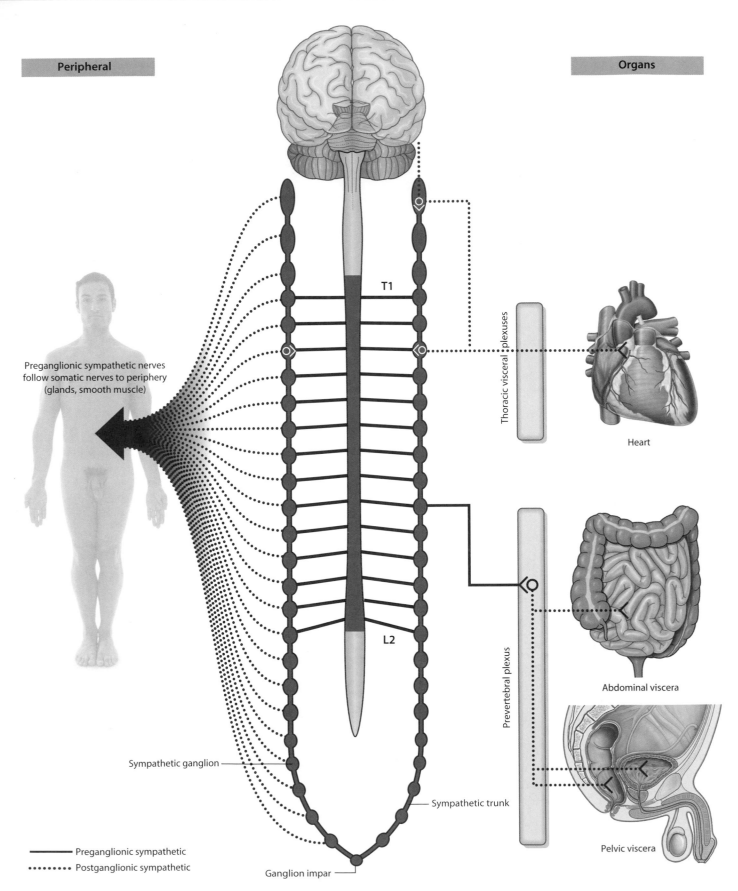

Peripheral

Organs

Preganglionic sympathetic nerves follow somatic nerves to periphery (glands, smooth muscle)

T1

L2

Thoracic visceral plexuses

Prevertebral plexus

Heart

Abdominal viscera

Pelvic viscera

Sympathetic ganglion

Sympathetic trunk

Ganglion impar

—— Preganglionic sympathetic

•••••••• Postganglionic sympathetic

All sympathetic visceral efferent (motor) nerves originate from spinal levels T1–L2 and pass into the associated spinal nerves

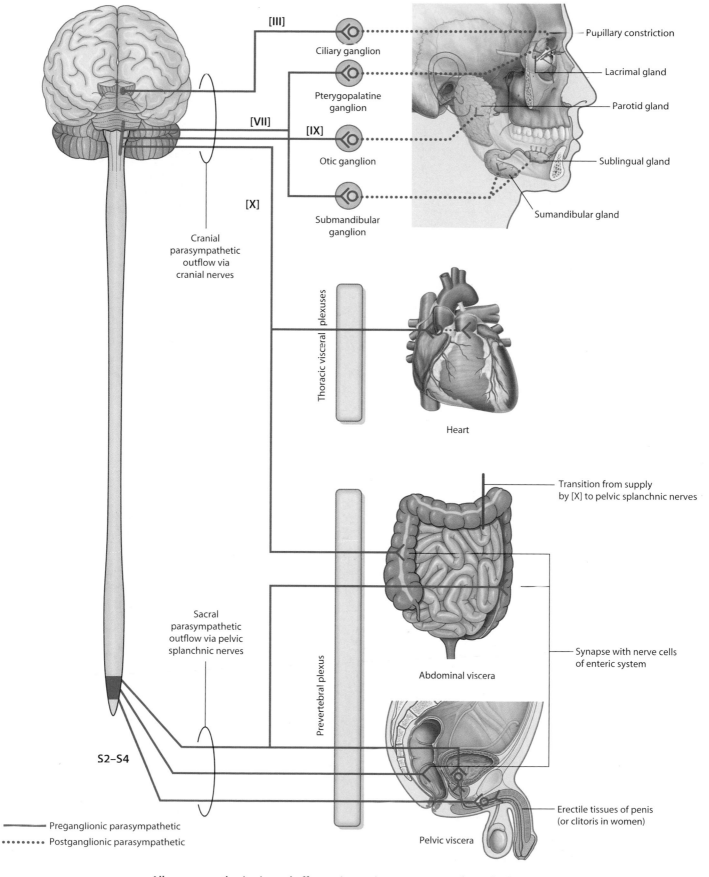

[III]

Ciliary ganglion

Pupillary constriction

Pterygopalatine ganglion

Lacrimal gland

Parotid gland

[VII]

[IX]

Otic ganglion

Sublingual gland

[X]

Submandibular ganglion

Sumandibular gland

Cranial parasympathetic outflow via cranial nerves

Thoracic visceral plexuses

Heart

Transition from supply by [X] to pelvic splanchnic nerves

Sacral parasympathetic outflow via pelvic splanchnic nerves

Prevertebral plexus

Synapse with nerve cells of enteric system

Abdominal viscera

S2–S4

Erectile tissues of penis (or clitoris in women)

Pelvic viscera

——— Preganglionic parasympathetic

·········· Postganglionic parasympathetic

All paraympathetic visceral efferent (motor) nerves emerge from the brain in cranial nerves III, VII, IX, and X and from spinal levels S2–S4

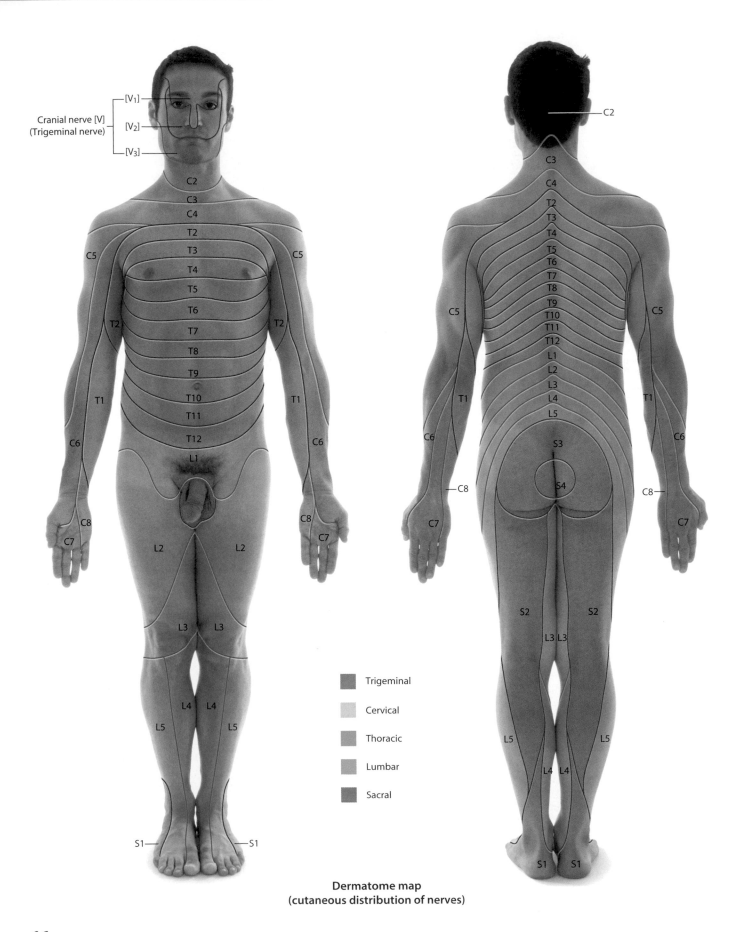

Cranial nerve [V]
(Trigeminal nerve)

[V₁]
[V₂]
[V₃]

Trigeminal
Cervical
Thoracic
Lumbar
Sacral

Dermatome map
(cutaneous distribution of nerves)

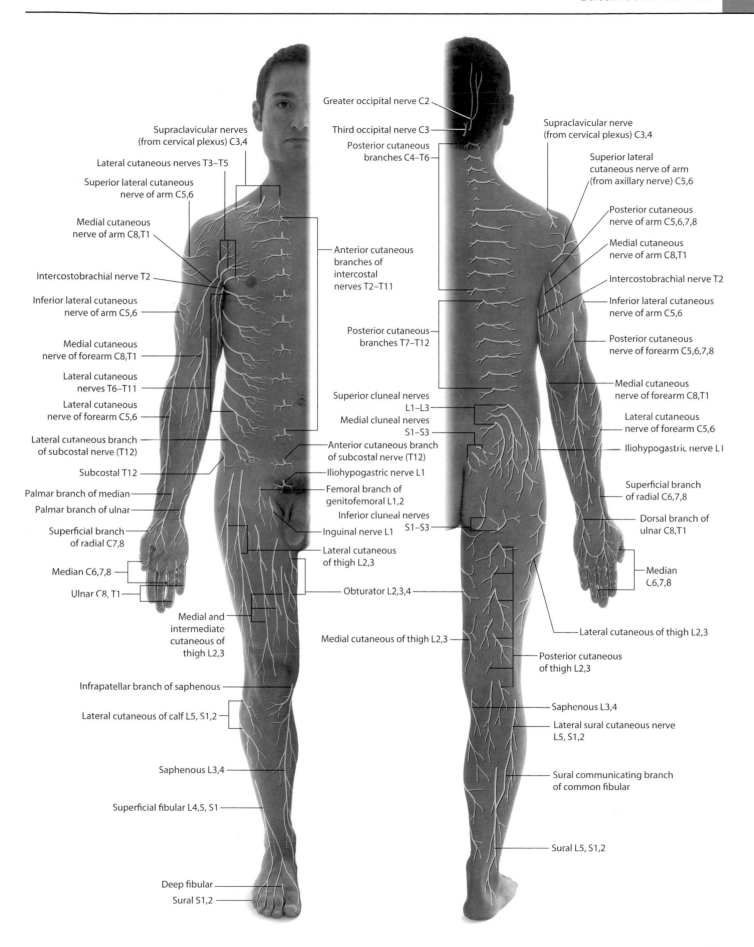

Greater occipital nerve C2

Third occipital nerve C3

Posterior cutaneous branches C4–T6

Supraclavicular nerves (from cervical plexus) C3,4

Lateral cutaneous nerves T3–T5

Superior lateral cutaneous nerve of arm C5,6

Medial cutaneous nerve of arm C8,T1

Intercostobrachial nerve T2

Inferior lateral cutaneous nerve of arm C5,6

Medial cutaneous nerve of forearm C8,T1

Lateral cutaneous nerves T6–T11

Lateral cutaneous nerve of forearm C5,6

Lateral cutaneous branch of subcostal nerve (T12)

Subcostal T12

Palmar branch of median

Palmar branch of ulnar

Superficial branch of radial C7,8

Median C6,7,8

Ulnar C8, T1

Medial and intermediate cutaneous of thigh L2,3

Infrapatellar branch of saphenous

Lateral cutaneous of calf L5, S1,2

Saphenous L3,4

Superficial fibular L4,5, S1

Deep fibular

Sural S1,2

Anterior cutaneous branches of intercostal nerves T2–T11

Posterior cutaneous branches T7–T12

Superior cluneal nerves L1–L3

Medial cluneal nerves S1–S3

Anterior cutaneous branch of subcostal nerve (T12)

Iliohypogastric nerve L1

Femoral branch of genitofemoral L1,2

Inferior cluneal nerves S1–S3

Inguinal nerve L1

Lateral cutaneous of thigh L2,3

Obturator L2,3,4

Medial cutaneous of thigh L2,3

Posterior cutaneous of thigh L2,3

Supraclavicular nerve (from cervical plexus) C3,4

Superior lateral cutaneous nerve of arm (from axillary nerve) C5,6

Posterior cutaneous nerve of arm C5,6,7,8

Medial cutaneous nerve of arm C8,T1

Intercostobrachial nerve T2

Inferior lateral cutaneous nerve of arm C5,6

Posterior cutaneous nerve of forearm C5,6,7,8

Medial cutaneous nerve of forearm C8,T1

Lateral cutaneous nerve of forearm C5,6

Iliohypogastric nerve L1

Superficial branch of radial C6,7,8

Dorsal branch of ulnar C8,T1

Median C6,7,8

Lateral cutaneous of thigh L2,3

Saphenous L3,4

Lateral sural cutaneous nerve L5, S1,2

Sural communicating branch of common fibular

Sural L5, S1,2

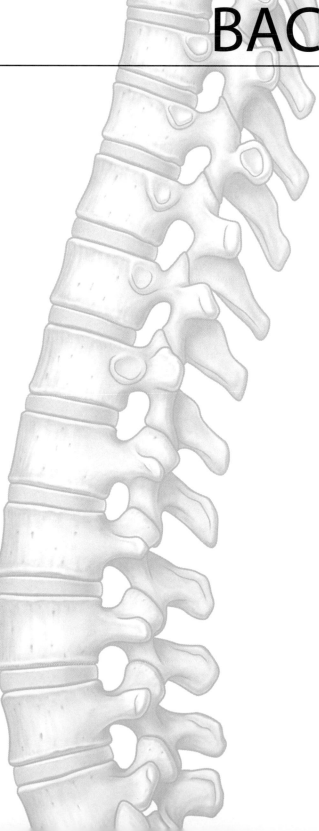

CONTENTS

2
BACK

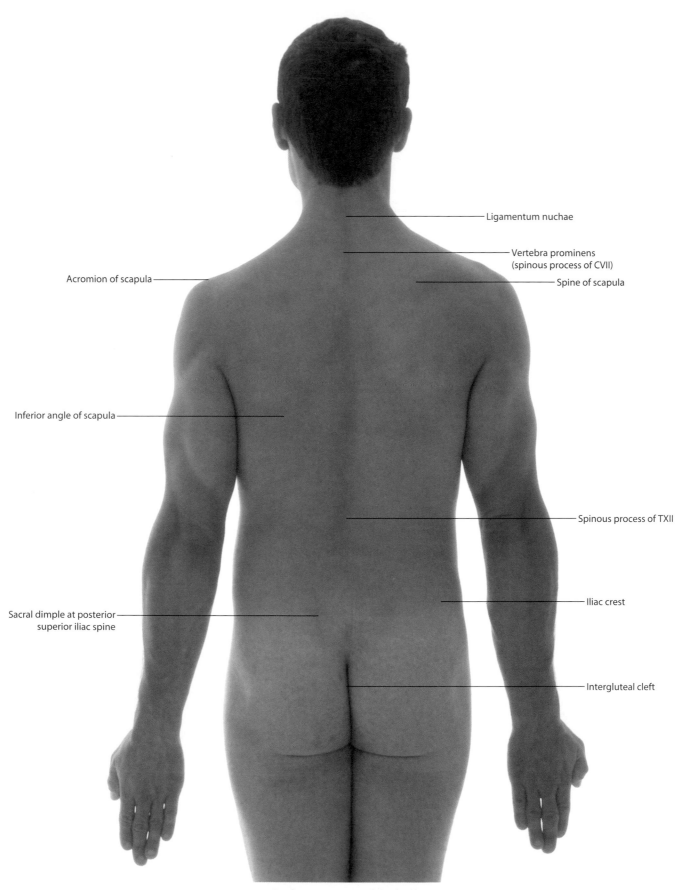

Ligamentum nuchae

Vertebra prominens
(spinous process of CVII)

Spine of scapula

Acromion of scapula

Inferior angle of scapula

Spinous process of TXII

Iliac crest

Sacral dimple at posterior
superior iliac spine

Intergluteal cleft

Surface anatomy of the back

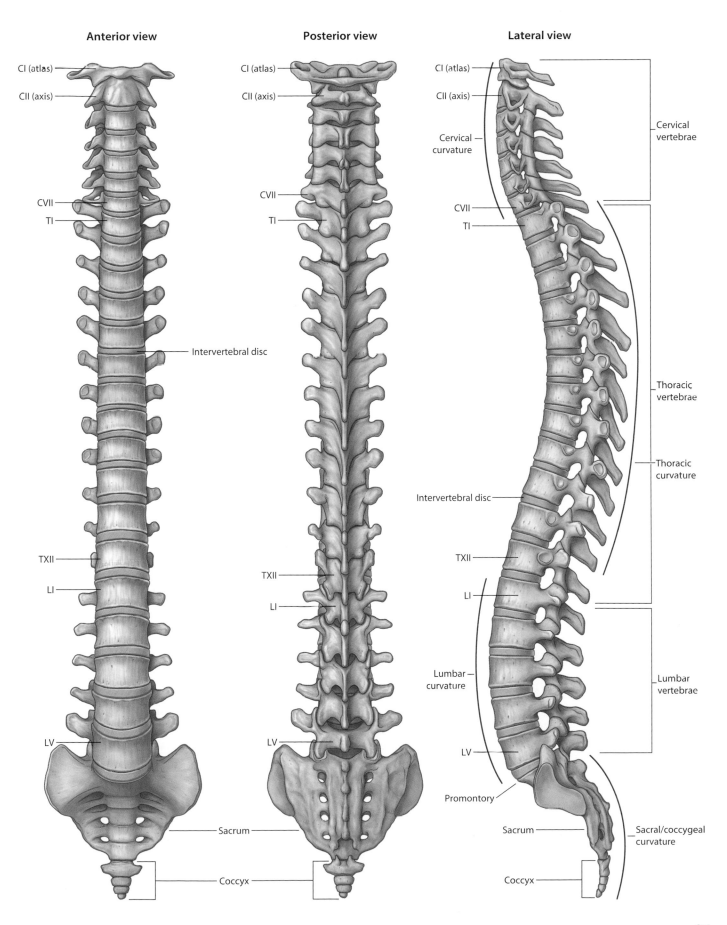

Anterior view

CI (atlas)
CII (axis)
CVII
TI
Intervertebral disc
TXII
LI
LV
Sacrum
Coccyx

Posterior view

CI (atlas)
CII (axis)
CVII
TI
TXII
LI
LV
Sacrum
Coccyx

Lateral view

CI (atlas)
CII (axis)
Cervical curvature
CVII
TI
Intervertebral disc
TXII
LI
Lumbar curvature
LV
Promontory
Sacrum
Coccyx
Cervical vertebrae
Thoracic vertebrae
Thoracic curvature
Lumbar vertebrae
Sacral/coccygeal curvature

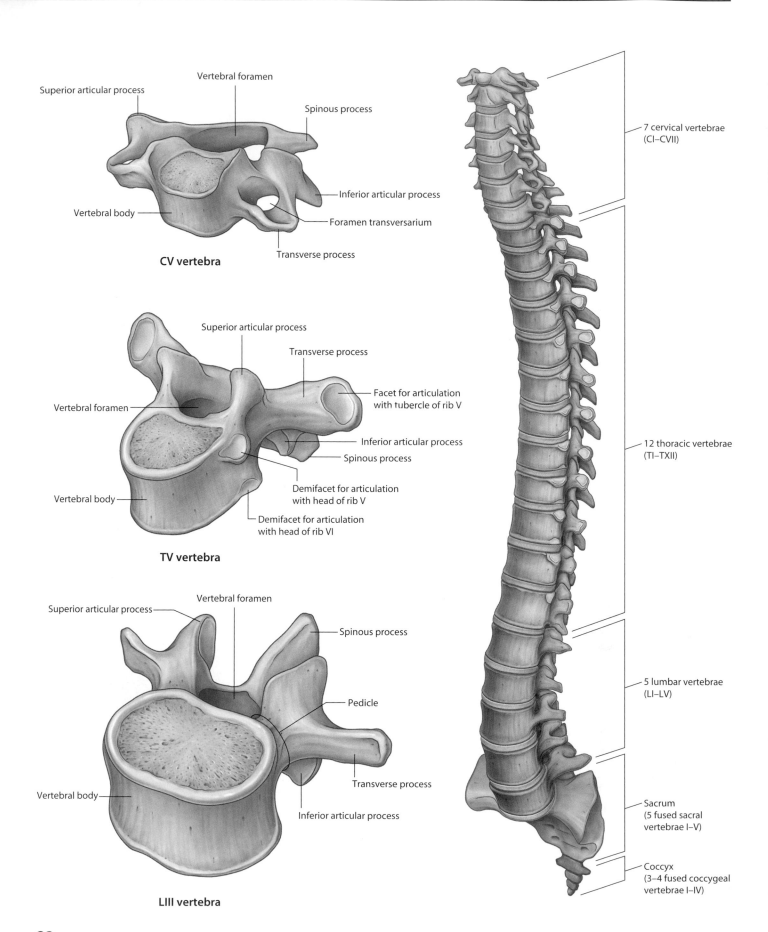

Superior articular process

Vertebral foramen

Spinous process

Inferior articular process

Foramen transversarium

Vertebral body

Transverse process

CV vertebra

Superior articular process

Transverse process

Facet for articulation with tubercle of rib V

Vertebral foramen

Inferior articular process

Spinous process

Demifacet for articulation with head of rib V

Vertebral body

Demifacet for articulation with head of rib VI

TV vertebra

Superior articular process

Vertebral foramen

Spinous process

Pedicle

Transverse process

Vertebral body

Inferior articular process

LIII vertebra

7 cervical vertebrae (CI–CVII)

12 thoracic vertebrae (TI–TXII)

5 lumbar vertebrae (LI–LV)

Sacrum (5 fused sacral vertebrae I–V)

Coccyx (3–4 fused coccygeal vertebrae I–IV)

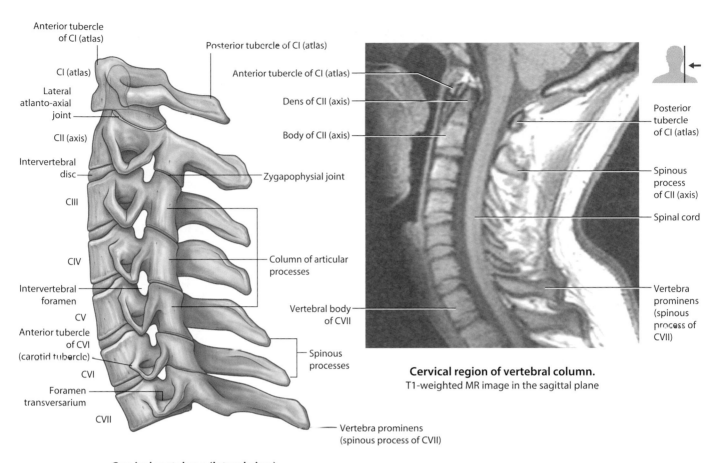

Anterior tubercle
of CI (atlas)

CI (atlas)

Lateral
atlanto-axial
joint

CII (axis)

Intervertebral
disc

CIII

CIV

Intervertebral
foramen

CV

Anterior tubercle
of CVI
(carotid tubercle)

CVI

Foramen
transversarium

CVII

Posterior tubercle of CI (atlas)

Anterior tubercle of CI (atlas)

Dens of CII (axis)

Body of CII (axis)

Zygapophysial joint

Column of articular
processes

Spinous
processes

Vertebra prominens
(spinous process of CVII)

Cervical vertebrae (lateral view)

Posterior
tubercle
of CI (atlas)

Spinous
process
of CII (axis)

Spinal cord

Vertebra
prominens
(spinous
process of
CVII)

Vertebral body
of CVII

Cervical region of vertebral column.
T1-weighted MR image in the sagittal plane

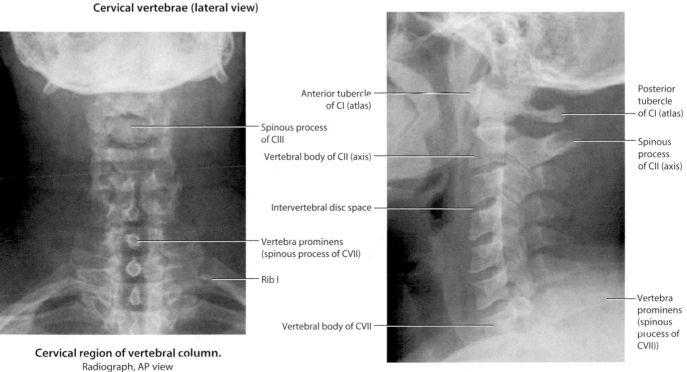

Spinous process
of CIII

Vertebra prominens
(spinous process of CVII)

Rib I

Cervical region of vertebral column.
Radiograph, AP view

Anterior tubercle
of CI (atlas)

Vertebral body of CII (axis)

Intervertebral disc space

Vertebral body of CVII

Posterior
tubercle
of CI (atlas)

Spinous
process
of CII (axis)

Vertebra
prominens
(spinous
process of
CVII))

Cervical region of vertebral column.
Radiograph, lateral view

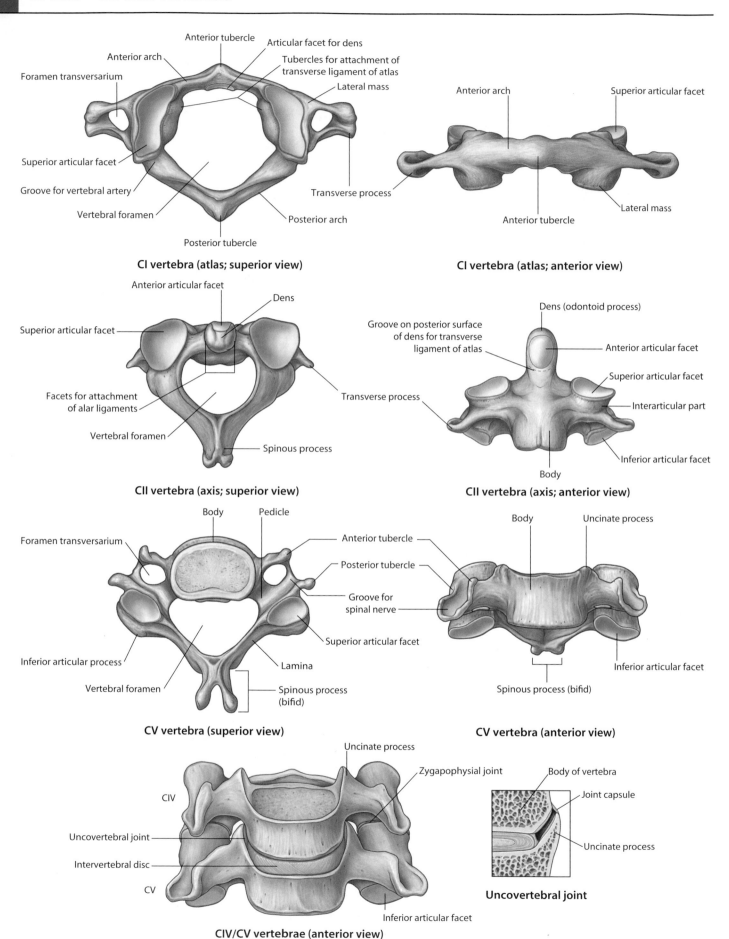

Anterior tubercle
Articular facet for dens
Anterior arch
Tubercles for attachment of
transverse ligament of atlas
Foramen transversarium
Lateral mass
Superior articular facet
Groove for vertebral artery
Vertebral foramen
Transverse process
Posterior arch
Posterior tubercle

CI vertebra (atlas; superior view)

Anterior arch
Superior articular facet
Lateral mass
Anterior tubercle

CI vertebra (atlas; anterior view)

Anterior articular facet
Dens
Superior articular facet
Facets for attachment
of alar ligaments
Vertebral foramen
Transverse process
Spinous process

CII vertebra (axis; superior view)

Dens (odontoid process)
Groove on posterior surface
of dens for transverse
ligament of atlas
Anterior articular facet
Superior articular facet
Interarticular part
Inferior articular facet
Body

CII vertebra (axis; anterior view)

Body
Pedicle
Foramen transversarium
Anterior tubercle
Posterior tubercle
Groove for
spinal nerve
Superior articular facet
Inferior articular process
Lamina
Vertebral foramen
Spinous process
(bifid)

CV vertebra (superior view)

Body
Uncinate process
Inferior articular facet
Spinous process (bifid)

CV vertebra (anterior view)

Uncinate process
Zygapophysial joint
Body of vertebra
Joint capsule
CIV
Uncovertebral joint
Intervertebral disc
CV
Uncinate process
Inferior articular facet

Uncovertebral joint

CIV/CV vertebrae (anterior view)

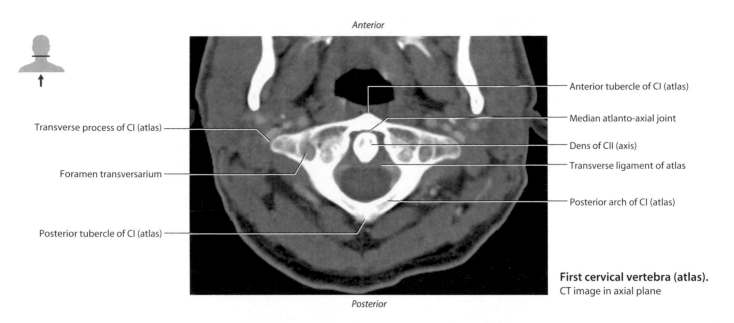

Anterior

Transverse process of CI (atlas)

Foramen transversarium

Posterior tubercle of CI (atlas)

Anterior tubercle of CI (atlas)

Median atlanto-axial joint

Dens of CII (axis)

Transverse ligament of atlas

Posterior arch of CI (atlas)

First cervical vertebra (atlas).
CT image in axial plane

Posterior

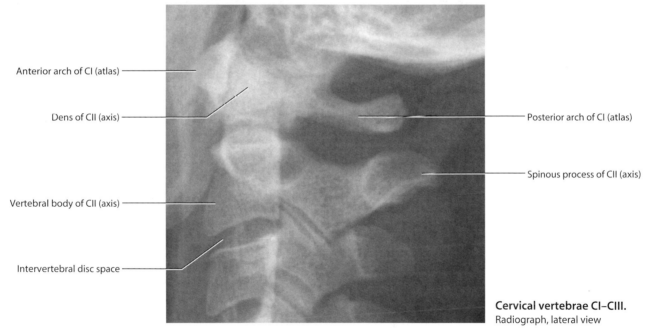

Anterior arch of CI (atlas)

Dens of CII (axis)

Vertebral body of CII (axis)

Intervertebral disc space

Posterior arch of CI (atlas)

Spinous process of CII (axis)

Cervical vertebrae CI–CIII.
Radiograph, lateral view

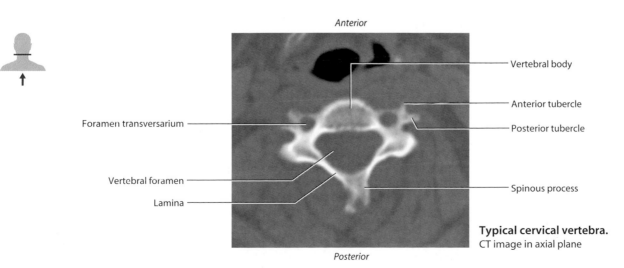

Anterior

Foramen transversarium

Vertebral foramen

Lamina

Vertebral body

Anterior tubercle

Posterior tubercle

Spinous process

Typical cervical vertebra.
CT image in axial plane

Posterior

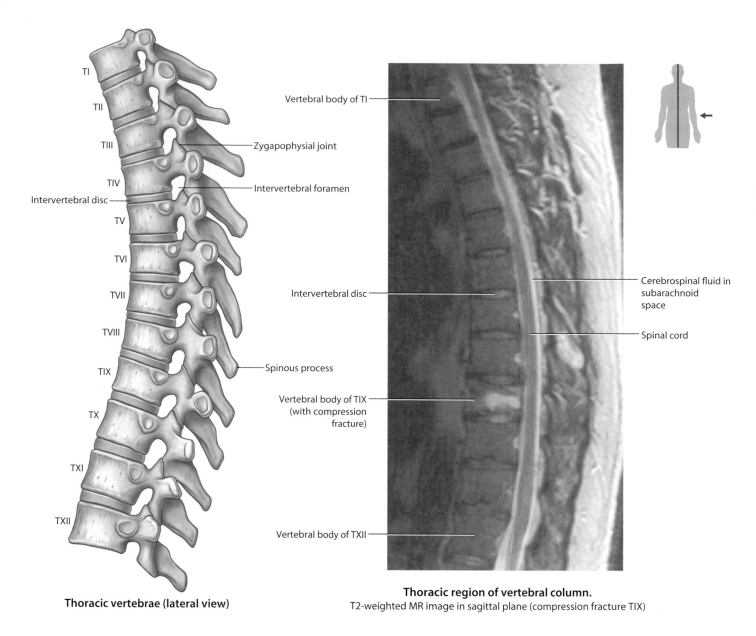

TI

TII

TIII — Zygapophysial joint

TIV — Intervertebral foramen

Intervertebral disc — TV

TVI

TVII

TVIII

TIX — Spinous process

TX

TXI

TXII

Thoracic vertebrae (lateral view)

Vertebral body of TI

Intervertebral disc

Vertebral body of TIX (with compression fracture)

Vertebral body of TXII

Cerebrospinal fluid in subarachnoid space

Spinal cord

Thoracic region of vertebral column.
T2-weighted MR image in sagittal plane (compression fracture TIX)

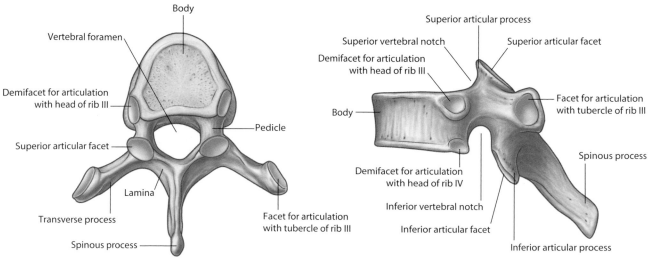

Body

Vertebral foramen

Demifacet for articulation with head of rib III

Superior articular facet

Pedicle

Transverse process

Lamina

Spinous process

TIII vertebra (superior view)

Superior articular process

Superior vertebral notch

Demifacet for articulation with head of rib III

Body

Superior articular facet

Facet for articulation with tubercle of rib III

Demifacet for articulation with head of rib IV

Inferior vertebral notch

Inferior articular facet

Inferior articular process

Spinous process

TIII vertebra (lateral view)

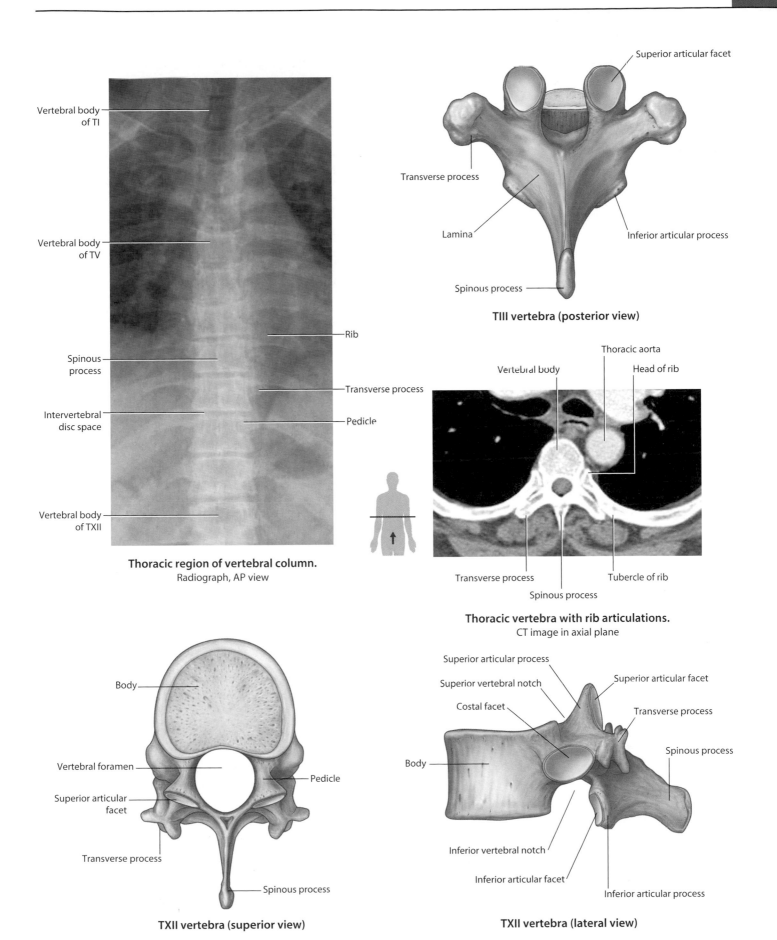

Vertebral body of TI

Vertebral body of TV

Spinous process

Intervertebral disc space

Vertebral body of TXII

Thoracic region of vertebral column.
Radiograph, AP view

Rib

Transverse process

Pedicle

Superior articular facet

Transverse process

Lamina

Inferior articular process

Spinous process

TIII vertebra (posterior view)

Thoracic aorta

Vertebral body

Head of rib

Transverse process

Spinous process

Tubercle of rib

Thoracic vertebra with rib articulations.
CT image in axial plane

Body

Vertebral foramen

Superior articular facet

Transverse process

Pedicle

Spinous process

TXII vertebra (superior view)

Superior articular process

Superior vertebral notch

Costal facet

Body

Superior articular facet

Transverse process

Spinous process

Inferior vertebral notch

Inferior articular facet

Inferior articular process

TXII vertebra (lateral view)

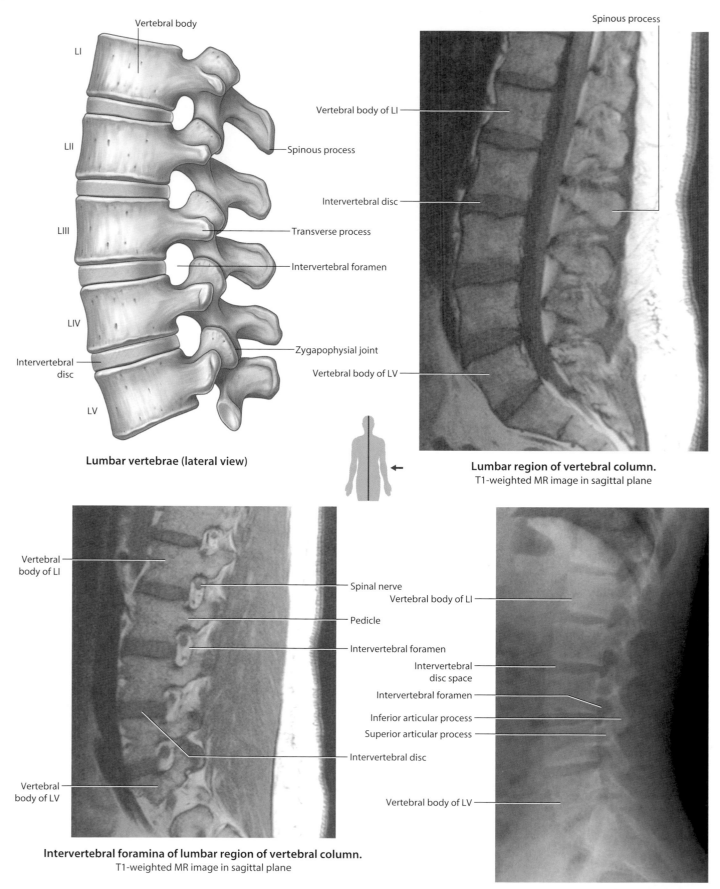

Vertebral body

LI

Spinous process

LII

LIII

Transverse process

Intervertebral foramen

LIV

Intervertebral disc

Zygapophysial joint

LV

Lumbar vertebrae (lateral view)

Spinous process

Vertebral body of LI

Intervertebral disc

Vertebral body of LV

Lumbar region of vertebral column.
T1-weighted MR image in sagittal plane

Vertebral body of LI

Spinal nerve

Pedicle

Intervertebral foramen

Intervertebral disc

Vertebral body of LV

Intervertebral foramina of lumbar region of vertebral column.
T1-weighted MR image in sagittal plane

Vertebral body of LI

Intervertebral disc space

Intervertebral foramen

Inferior articular process

Superior articular process

Vertebral body of LV

Lumbar region of vertebral column.
Radiograph, lateral view

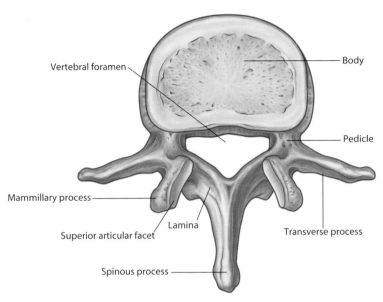

LIV vertebra (superior view)

Vertebral foramen

Body

Pedicle

Mammillary process

Lamina

Superior articular facet

Transverse process

Spinous process

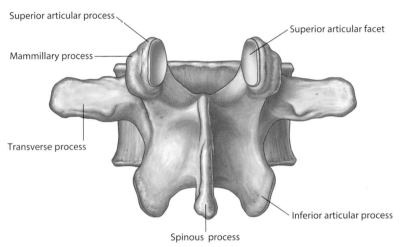

LIV vertebra (posterior view)

Superior articular process

Mammillary process

Transverse process

Superior articular facet

Inferior articular process

Spinous process

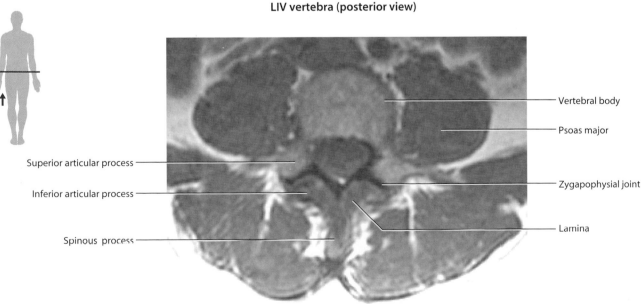

Superior articular process

Inferior articular process

Spinous process

Vertebral body

Psoas major

Zygapophysial joint

Lamina

Articulation of lumbar vertebrae.
T1-weighted MR image in axial plane

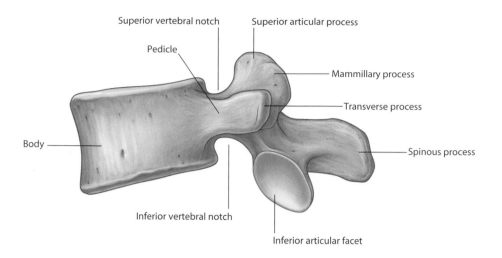

Superior vertebral notch

Pedicle

Superior articular process

Mammillary process

Transverse process

Body

Spinous process

Inferior vertebral notch

Inferior articular facet

LIV vertebra (lateral view)

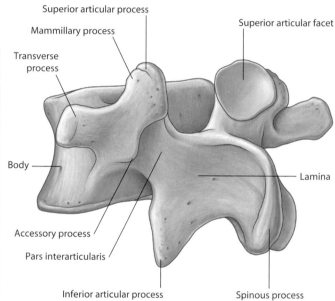

Superior articular process

Mammillary process

Transverse process

Superior articular facet

Body

Lamina

Accessory process

Pars interarticularis

Inferior articular process

Spinous process

LIV vertebra (oblique view)

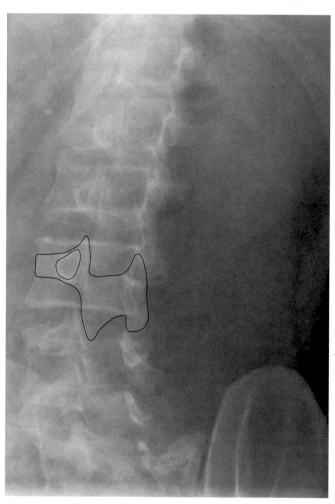

Lumbar region of vertebral column ("Scottie dog").
Radiograph, oblique view

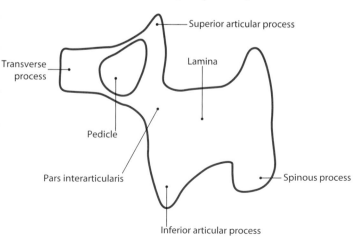

Transverse process

Superior articular process

Lamina

Pedicle

Pars interarticularis

Inferior articular process

Spinous process

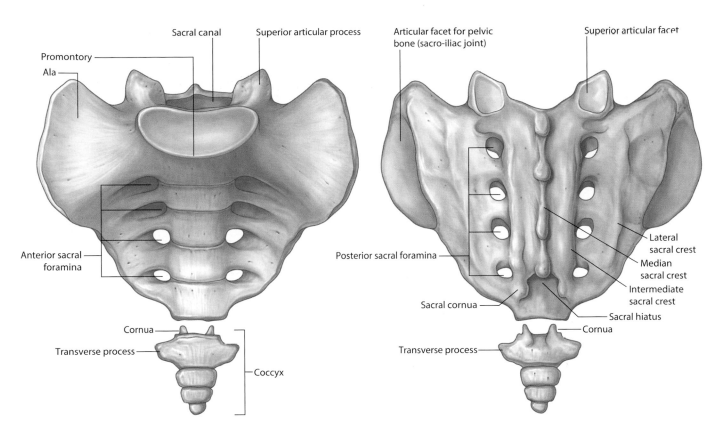

Sacrum and coccyx (anterior view)

Sacrum and coccyx (posterior view)

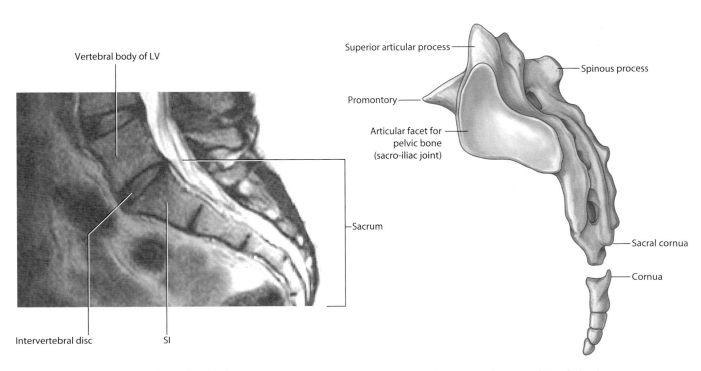

Sacral region of vertebral column.
T2-weighted MR image in sagittal plane

Sacrum and coccyx (lateral view)

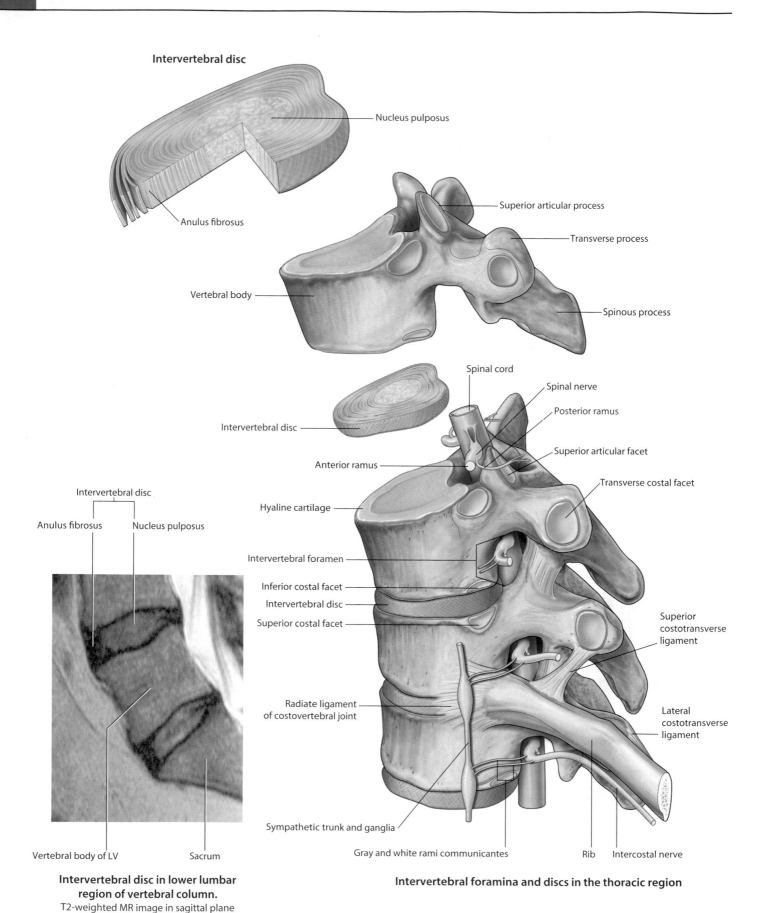

Intervertebral disc

Nucleus pulposus

Anulus fibrosus

Superior articular process

Transverse process

Vertebral body

Spinous process

Spinal cord

Spinal nerve

Posterior ramus

Intervertebral disc

Superior articular facet

Anterior ramus

Transverse costal facet

Hyaline cartilage

Intervertebral foramen

Inferior costal facet

Intervertebral disc

Superior costal facet

Superior costotransverse ligament

Intervertebral disc

Anulus fibrosus

Nucleus pulposus

Radiate ligament of costovertebral joint

Lateral costotransverse ligament

Sympathetic trunk and ganglia

Vertebral body of LV

Sacrum

Gray and white rami communicantes

Rib

Intercostal nerve

Intervertebral disc in lower lumbar region of vertebral column.
T2-weighted MR image in sagittal plane

Intervertebral foramina and discs in the thoracic region

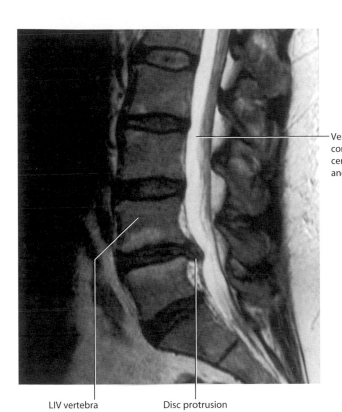

LIV vertebra   Disc protrusion

Vertebral canal containing cerebrospinal fluid and cauda equina

Intervertebral disc protrusion in lower lumbar region of vertebral column.
T2-weighted MR image in sagittal plane

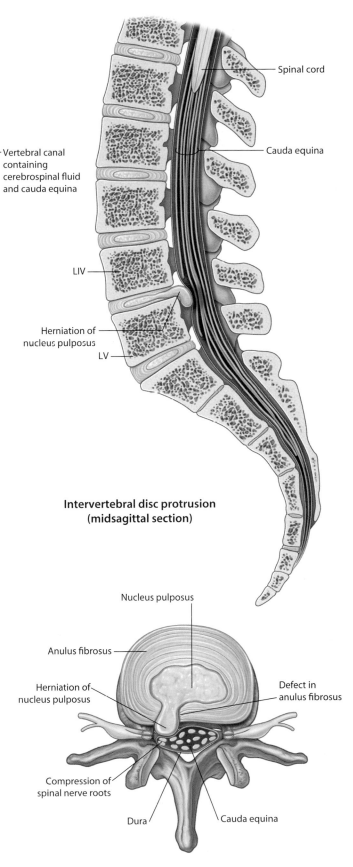

Spinal cord

Cauda equina

Vertebral canal containing cerebrospinal fluid and cauda equina

LIV

Herniation of nucleus pulposus

LV

Intervertebral disc protrusion (midsagittal section)

Nucleus pulposus

Anulus fibrosus

Herniation of nucleus pulposus

Defect in anulus fibrosus

Compression of spinal nerve roots

Dura

Cauda equina

Intervertebral disc protrusion (superior view)

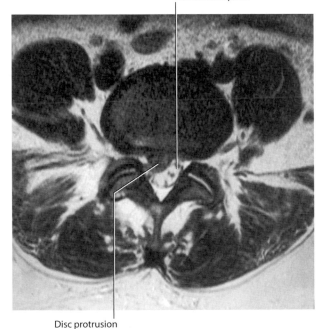

Vertebral canal containing cerebrospinal fluid and cauda equina

Disc protrusion

Intervertebral disc protrusion in lower lumbar region of vertebral column.
T2-weighted MR image in axial plane

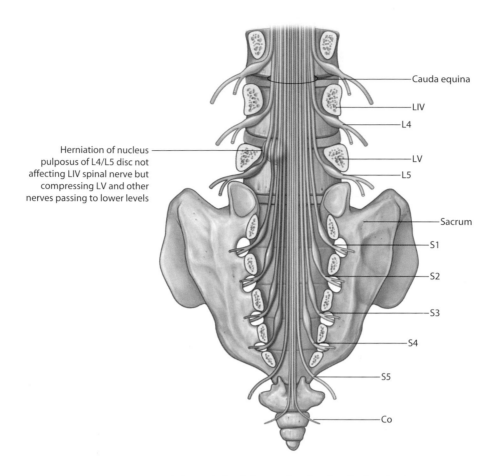

Herniation of nucleus pulposus of L4/L5 disc not affecting LIV spinal nerve but compressing LV and other nerves passing to lower levels

Cauda equina

LIV

L4

LV

L5

Sacrum

S1

S2

S3

S4

S5

Co

Intervertebral disc protrusion (posterior view)

Nerve root	Main weakness	Reflex decreased	Area of sensory decrease	Disc involved
C5	Deltoid (biceps)	(biceps, pectoralis)	Shoulder, upper lateral arm	C4–C5
C6	Wrist extension	(biceps, brachioradialis)	1st and 2nd digits (lateral forearm)	C5–C6
C7	Triceps	Triceps	Third finger	C6–C7
C8	Intrinsic hand muscles		4th and 5th digits (medial forearm)	C7–T1

Clinically important nerve roots in the upper limb

Nerve root	Main weakness	Reflex decreased	Area of sensory decrease	Disc involved
L4	Iliopsoas and quadriceps	Patellar tendon (knee jerk)	Knee, medial lower leg	L3–L4
L5	Dorsiflexion of foot at ankle (big toe extension, foot eversion and inversion)		Dorsum of foot, big toe	L4–L5
S1	Plantar flexion of foot at ankle	Achilles tendon (ankle jerk)	Lateral foot, small toe, sole	L5–S1

Clinically important nerve roots in the lower limb

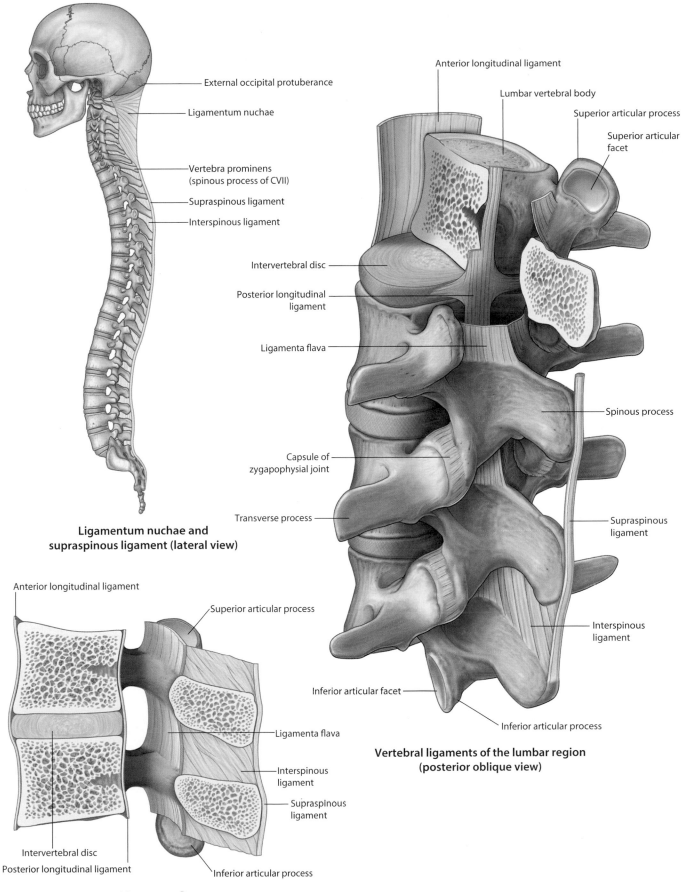

External occipital protuberance

Ligamentum nuchae

Vertebra prominens
(spinous process of CVII)

Supraspinous ligament

Interspinous ligament

**Ligamentum nuchae and
supraspinous ligament (lateral view)**

Anterior longitudinal ligament

Lumbar vertebral body

Superior articular process

Superior articular facet

Intervertebral disc

Posterior longitudinal ligament

Ligamenta flava

Spinous process

Capsule of zygapophysial joint

Transverse process

Supraspinous ligament

Interspinous ligament

Inferior articular facet

Inferior articular process

**Vertebral ligaments of the lumbar region
(posterior oblique view)**

Anterior longitudinal ligament

Superior articular process

Ligamenta flava

Interspinous ligament

Supraspinous ligament

Intervertebral disc

Posterior longitudinal ligament

Inferior articular process

Ligamenta flava

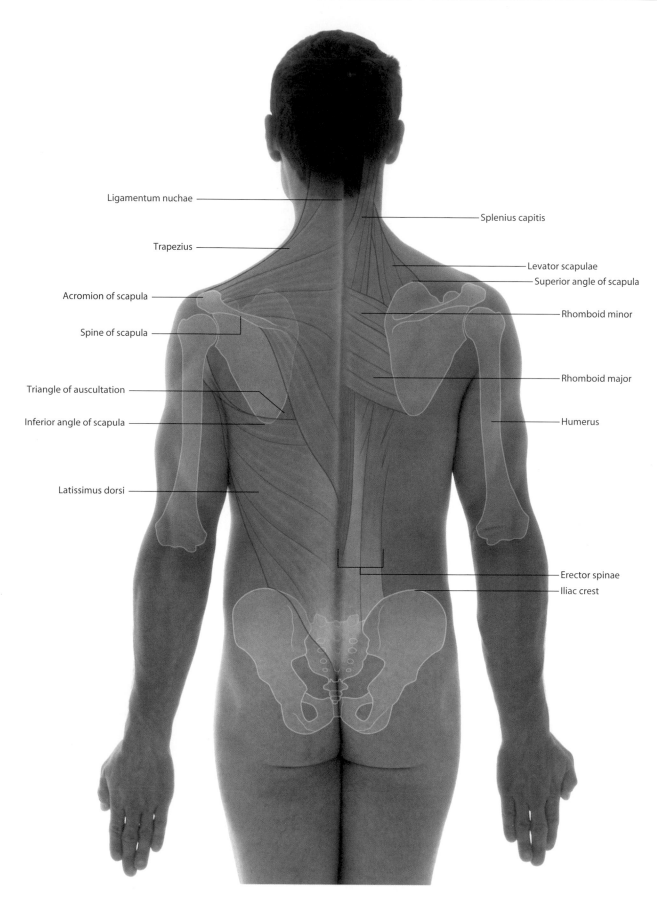

Ligamentum nuchae

Trapezius

Acromion of scapula

Spine of scapula

Triangle of auscultation

Inferior angle of scapula

Latissimus dorsi

Splenius capitis

Levator scapulae

Superior angle of scapula

Rhomboid minor

Rhomboid major

Humerus

Erector spinae

Iliac crest

Posterior view of male showing surface projections of back muscles

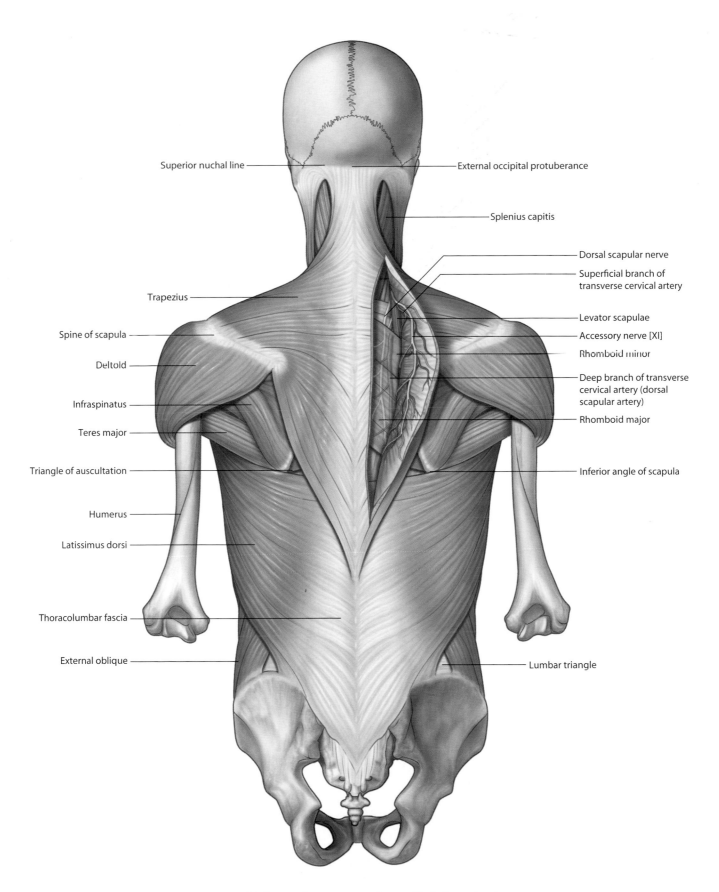

Superior nuchal line

External occipital protuberance

Splenius capitis

Dorsal scapular nerve

Superficial branch of transverse cervical artery

Trapezius

Levator scapulae

Spine of scapula

Accessory nerve [XI]

Deltold

Rhomboid minor

Infraspinatus

Deep branch of transverse cervical artery (dorsal scapular artery)

Teres major

Rhomboid major

Triangle of auscultation

Inferior angle of scapula

Humerus

Latissimus dorsi

Thoracolumbar fascia

External oblique

Lumbar triangle

Superficial musculature – trapezius and latissimus dorsi

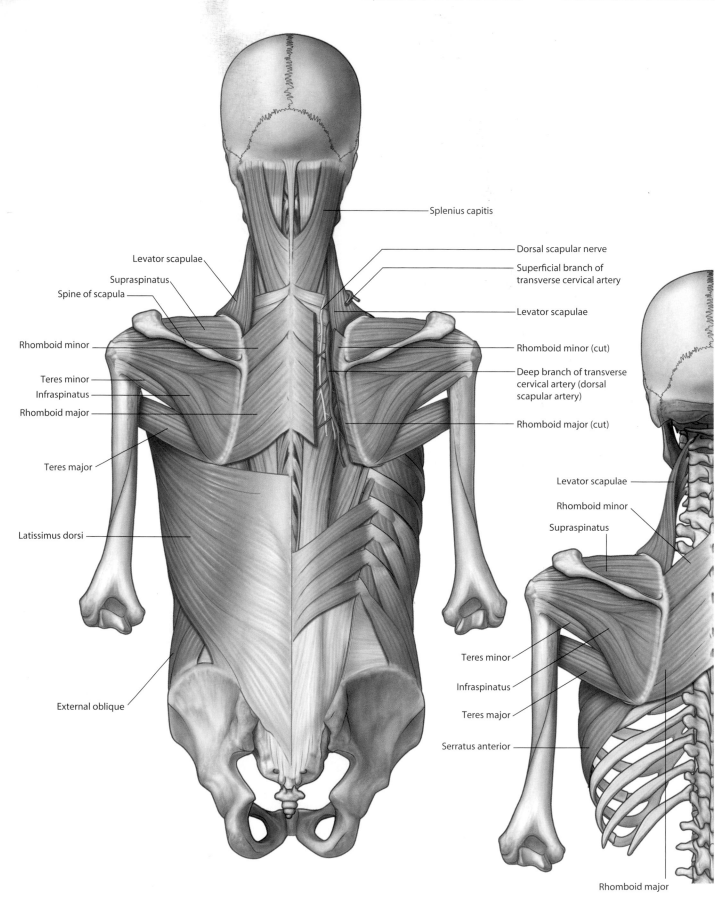

Splenius capitis

Dorsal scapular nerve

Superficial branch of
transverse cervical artery

Levator scapulae

Levator scapulae

Supraspinatus

Spine of scapula

Rhomboid minor (cut)

Rhomboid minor

Deep branch of transverse
cervical artery (dorsal
scapular artery)

Teres minor

Infraspinatus

Rhomboid major

Rhomboid major (cut)

Teres major

Levator scapulae

Rhomboid minor

Supraspinatus

Latissimus dorsi

Teres minor

Infraspinatus

Teres major

Serratus anterior

External oblique

Rhomboid major

Superficial musculature – levator scapulae and rhomboid major and minor

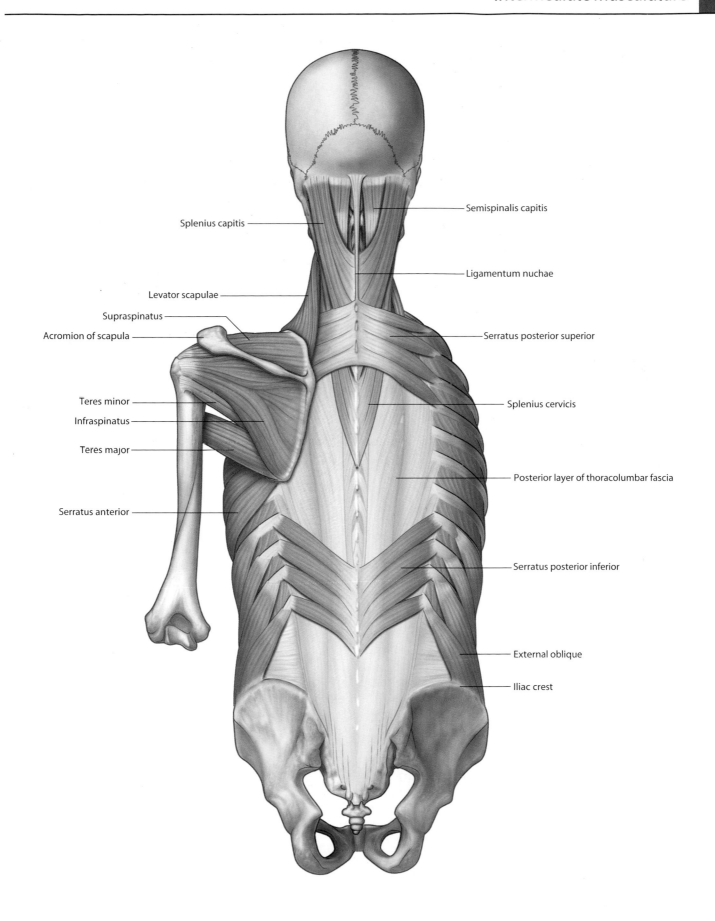

Splenius capitis

Levator scapulae

Supraspinatus

Acromion of scapula

Teres minor

Infraspinatus

Teres major

Serratus anterior

Semispinalis capitis

Ligamentum nuchae

Serratus posterior superior

Splenius cervicis

Posterior layer of thoracolumbar fascia

Serratus posterior inferior

External oblique

Iliac crest

Intermediate musculature

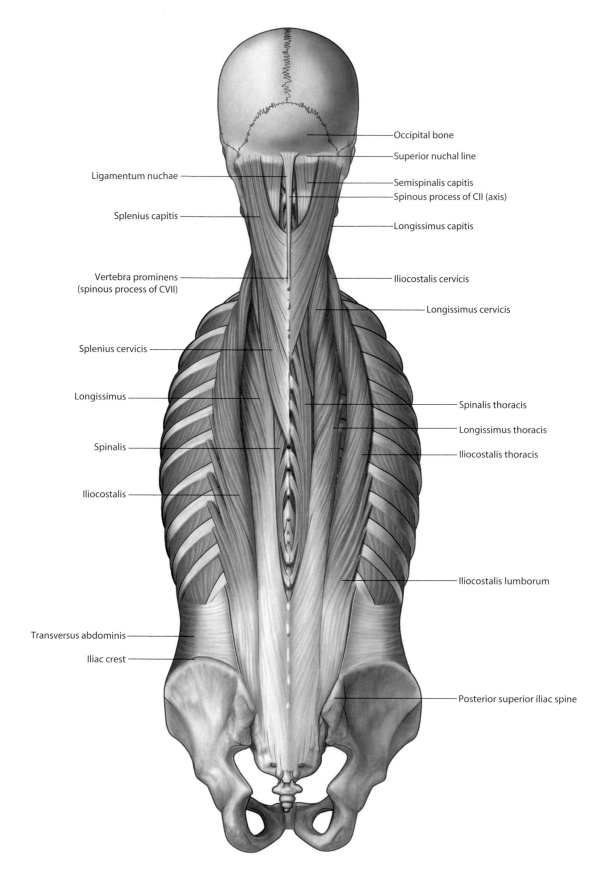

Occipital bone
Superior nuchal line
Ligamentum nuchae
Semispinalis capitis
Spinous process of CII (axis)
Splenius capitis
Longissimus capitis
Vertebra prominens
(spinous process of CVII)
Iliocostalis cervicis
Longissimus cervicis
Splenius cervicis
Longissimus
Spinalis thoracis
Longissimus thoracis
Spinalis
Iliocostalis thoracis
Iliocostalis
Iliocostalis lumborum
Transversus abdominis
Iliac crest
Posterior superior iliac spine

Deep group of back muscles – erector spinae muscles

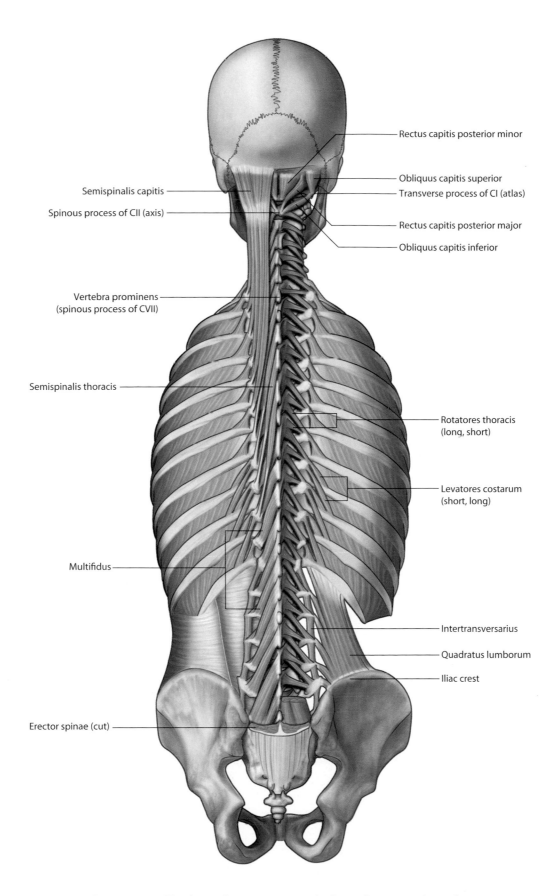

Rectus capitis posterior minor

Obliquus capitis superior

Transverse process of CI (atlas)

Semispinalis capitis

Spinous process of CII (axis)

Rectus capitis posterior major

Obliquus capitis inferior

Vertebra prominens
(spinous process of CVII)

Semispinalis thoracis

Rotatores thoracis
(long, short)

Levatores costarum
(short, long)

Multifidus

Intertransversarius

Quadratus lumborum

Iliac crest

Erector spinae (cut)

Deep group of back muscles – transversospinales and segmental muscles

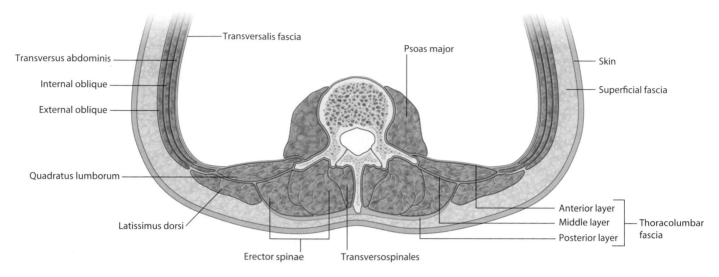

Transversalis fascia

Psoas major

Transversus abdominis

Internal oblique

External oblique

Skin

Superficial fascia

Quadratus lumborum

Latissimus dorsi

Anterior layer

Middle layer

Posterior layer

Thoracolumbar fascia

Erector spinae

Transversospinales

**Thoracolumbar fascia and the deep back muscles
(transverse section – lumbar region)**

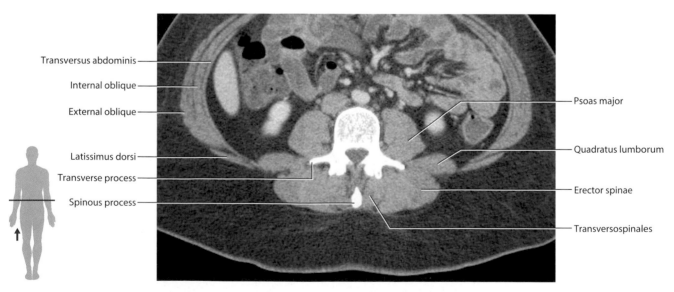

Transversus abdominis

Internal oblique

External oblique

Psoas major

Quadratus lumborum

Latissimus dorsi

Transverse process

Spinous process

Erector spinae

Transversospinales

Lumbar region (LIII) showing back musculature.
CT image in axial plane

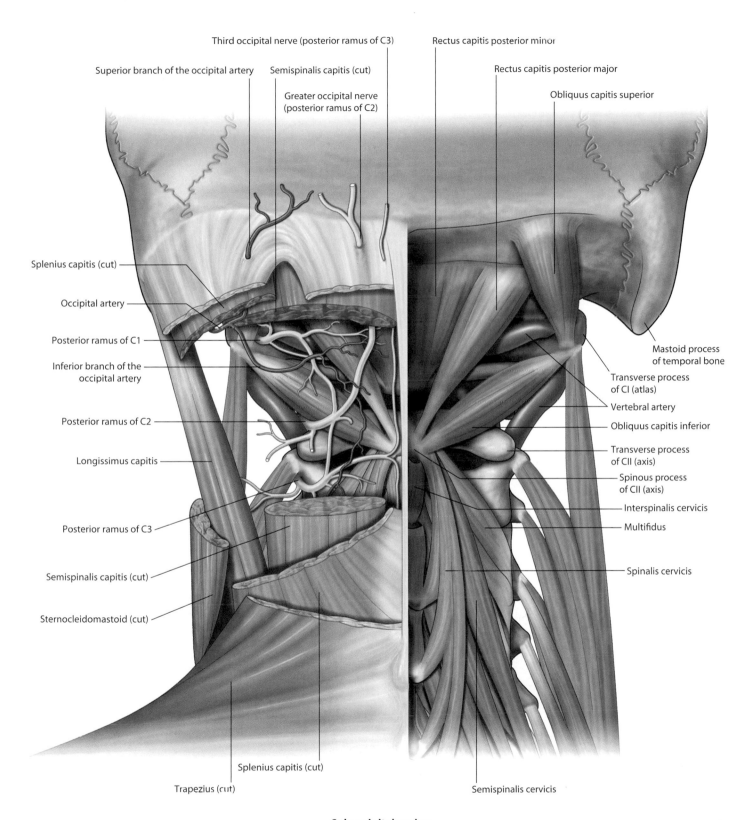

Third occipital nerve (posterior ramus of C3)

Rectus capitis posterior minor

Superior branch of the occipital artery

Semispinalis capitis (cut)

Rectus capitis posterior major

Greater occipital nerve (posterior ramus of C2)

Obliquus capitis superior

Splenius capitis (cut)

Occipital artery

Posterior ramus of C1

Inferior branch of the occipital artery

Posterior ramus of C2

Longissimus capitis

Posterior ramus of C3

Semispinalis capitis (cut)

Sternocleidomastoid (cut)

Mastoid process of temporal bone

Transverse process of CI (atlas)

Vertebral artery

Obliquus capitis inferior

Transverse process of CII (axis)

Spinous process of CII (axis)

Interspinalis cervicis

Multifidus

Spinalis cervicis

Splenius capitis (cut)

Trapezius (cut)

Semispinalis cervicis

Suboccipital region

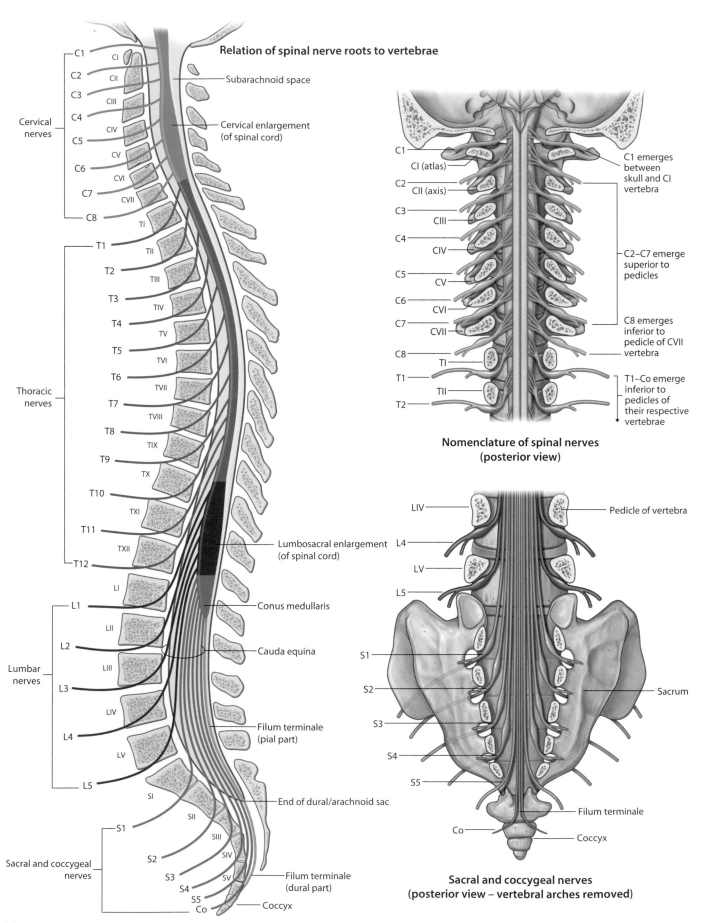

Relation of spinal nerve roots to vertebrae

Cervical nerves

C1 — CI
C2 — CII
C3 — CIII
C4 — CIV
C5 — CV
C6 — CVI
C7 — CVII
C8

Subarachnoid space

Cervical enlargement (of spinal cord)

Thoracic nerves

T1 — TI
T2 — TII
T3 — TIII
T4 — TIV
T5 — TV
T6 — TVI
T7 — TVII
T8 — TVIII
T9 — TIX
T10 — TX
T11 — TXI
T12 — TXII

Lumbar nerves

L1 — LI
L2 — LII
L3 — LIII
L4 — LIV
L5 — LV

Lumbosacral enlargement (of spinal cord)

Conus medullaris

Cauda equina

Filum terminale (pial part)

End of dural/arachnoid sac

Sacral and coccygeal nerves

S1 — SI
S2 — SII
S3 — SIII
S4 — SIV
S5 — SV
Co

Filum terminale (dural part)

Coccyx

Nomenclature of spinal nerves (posterior view)

C1 — CI (atlas)
C2 — CII (axis)
C3 — CIII
C4 — CIV
C5 — CV
C6 — CVI
C7 — CVII
C8 — TI
T1 — TII
T2

C1 emerges between skull and CI vertebra

C2–C7 emerge superior to pedicles

C8 emerges inferior to pedicle of CVII vertebra

T1–Co emerge inferior to pedicles of their respective vertebrae

Sacral and coccygeal nerves (posterior view – vertebral arches removed)

LIV
L4
LV
L5

S1
S2
S3
S4
S5
Co

Pedicle of vertebra

Sacrum

Filum terminale

Coccyx

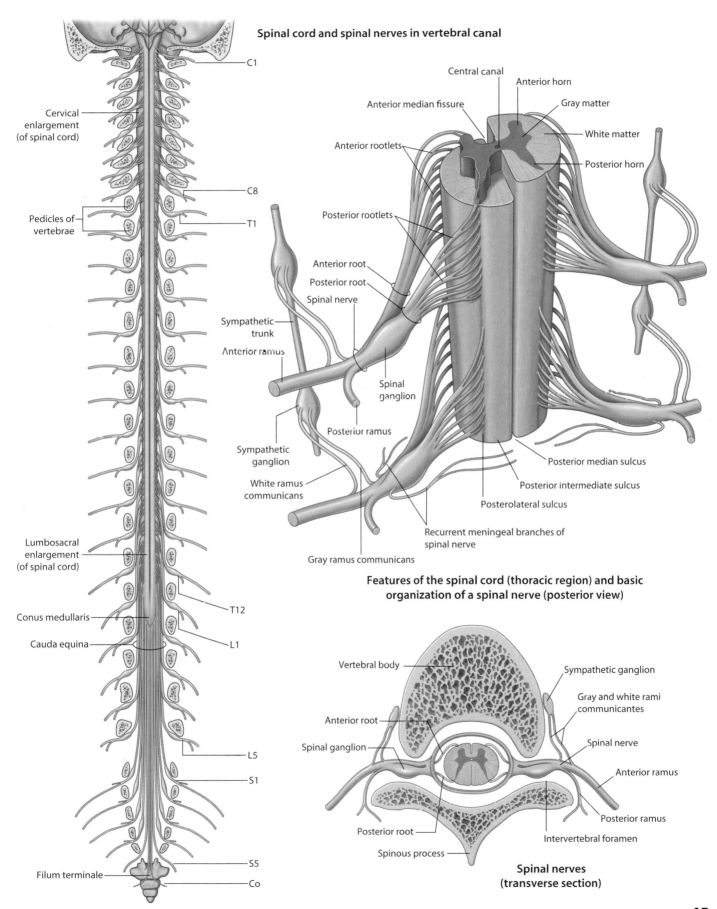

Spinal cord and spinal nerves in vertebral canal

C1

Cervical enlargement (of spinal cord)

Pedicles of vertebrae

C8

T1

Central canal

Anterior median fissure

Anterior horn

Gray matter

White matter

Anterior rootlets

Posterior horn

Posterior rootlets

Anterior root

Posterior root

Spinal nerve

Sympathetic trunk

Anterior ramus

Spinal ganglion

Posterior ramus

Sympathetic ganglion

White ramus communicans

Posterior median sulcus

Posterior intermediate sulcus

Posterolateral sulcus

Recurrent meningeal branches of spinal nerve

Gray ramus communicans

Features of the spinal cord (thoracic region) and basic organization of a spinal nerve (posterior view)

Lumbosacral enlargement (of spinal cord)

Conus medullaris

Cauda equina

T12

L1

L5

S1

S5

Filum terminale

Co

Vertebral body

Sympathetic ganglion

Gray and white rami communicantes

Spinal nerve

Anterior root

Spinal ganglion

Anterior ramus

Posterior ramus

Intervertebral foramen

Posterior root

Spinous process

Spinal nerves (transverse section)

45

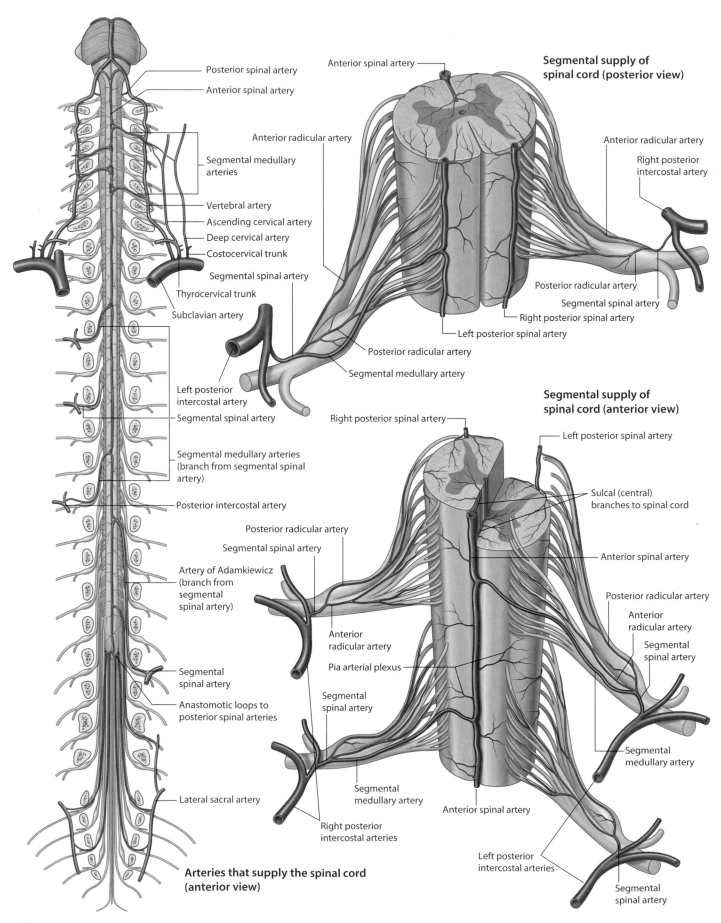

Posterior spinal artery

Anterior spinal artery

Anterior radicular artery

Segmental medullary arteries

Vertebral artery

Ascending cervical artery

Deep cervical artery

Costocervical trunk

Segmental spinal artery

Thyrocervical trunk

Subclavian artery

Left posterior intercostal artery

Segmental spinal artery

Segmental medullary arteries (branch from segmental spinal artery)

Posterior intercostal artery

Artery of Adamkiewicz (branch from segmental spinal artery)

Segmental spinal artery

Anastomotic loops to posterior spinal arteries

Lateral sacral artery

Arteries that supply the spinal cord (anterior view)

Anterior spinal artery

Segmental supply of spinal cord (posterior view)

Anterior radicular artery

Right posterior intercostal artery

Posterior radicular artery

Segmental spinal artery

Right posterior spinal artery

Left posterior spinal artery

Posterior radicular artery

Segmental medullary artery

Segmental supply of spinal cord (anterior view)

Right posterior spinal artery

Left posterior spinal artery

Sulcal (central) branches to spinal cord

Anterior spinal artery

Posterior radicular artery

Anterior radicular artery

Segmental spinal artery

Posterior radicular artery

Segmental spinal artery

Anterior radicular artery

Pia arterial plexus

Segmental spinal artery

Segmental medullary artery

Segmental medullary artery

Anterior spinal artery

Right posterior intercostal arteries

Left posterior intercostal arteries

Segmental spinal artery

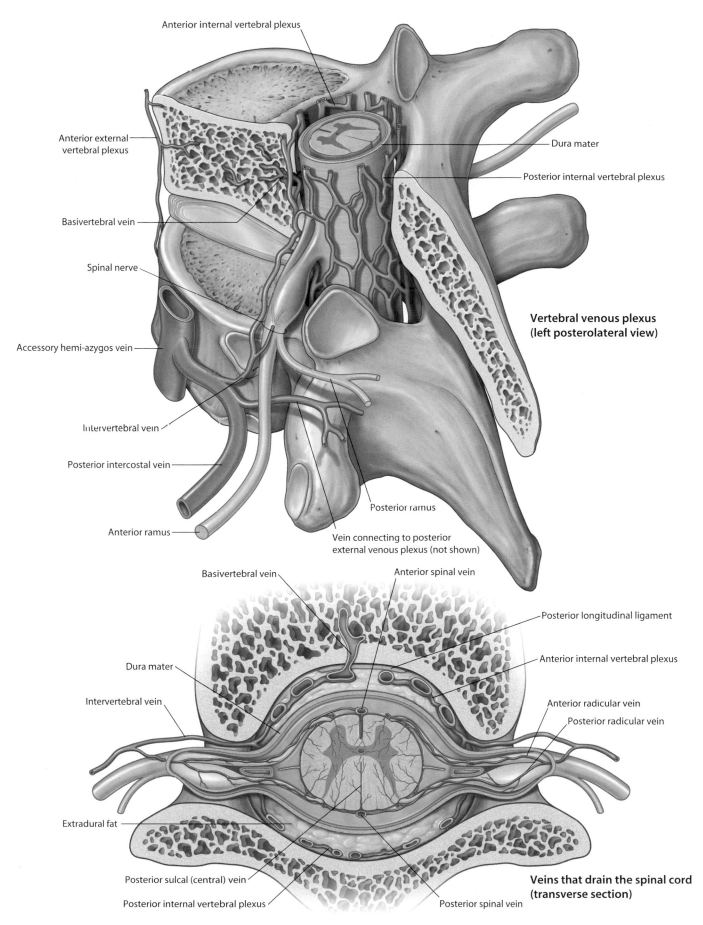

Anterior internal vertebral plexus

Anterior external vertebral plexus

Basivertebral vein

Spinal nerve

Accessory hemi-azygos vein

Intervertebral vein

Posterior intercostal vein

Anterior ramus

Dura mater

Posterior internal vertebral plexus

Vertebral venous plexus (left posterolateral view)

Posterior ramus

Vein connecting to posterior external venous plexus (not shown)

Basivertebral vein

Anterior spinal vein

Posterior longitudinal ligament

Dura mater

Anterior internal vertebral plexus

Intervertebral vein

Anterior radicular vein

Posterior radicular vein

Extradural fat

Posterior sulcal (central) vein

Posterior internal vertebral plexus

Posterior spinal vein

Veins that drain the spinal cord (transverse section)

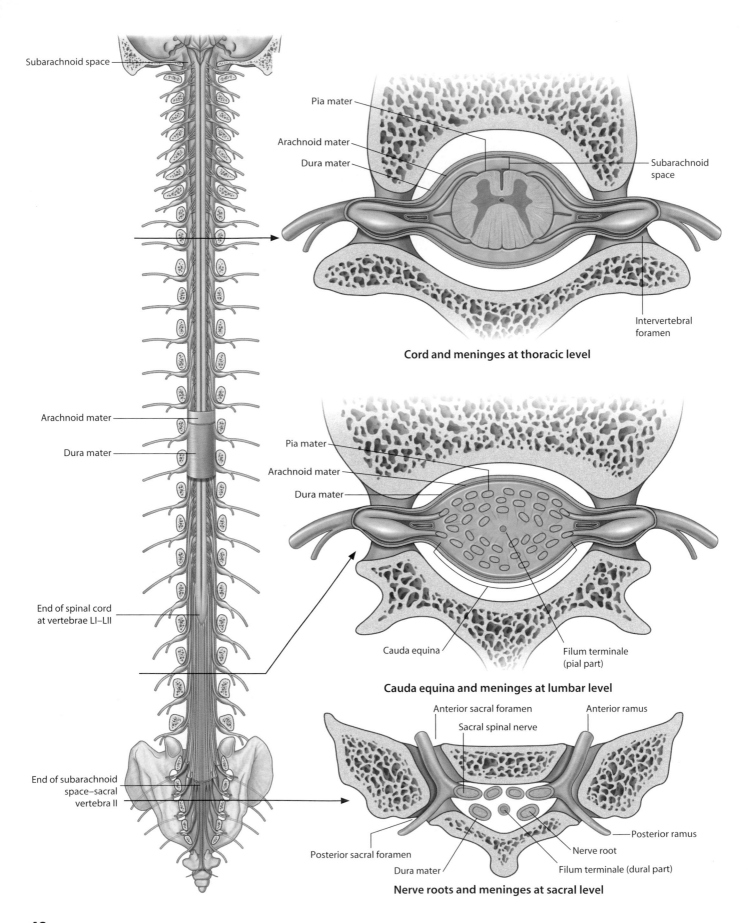

Subarachnoid space

Pia mater

Arachnoid mater

Dura mater

Subarachnoid space

Intervertebral foramen

Cord and meninges at thoracic level

Arachnoid mater

Dura mater

Pia mater

Arachnoid mater

Dura mater

Cauda equina

Filum terminale (pial part)

Cauda equina and meninges at lumbar level

End of spinal cord at vertebrae LI–LII

End of subarachnoid space–sacral vertebra II

Anterior sacral foramen

Sacral spinal nerve

Anterior ramus

Posterior ramus

Posterior sacral foramen

Dura mater

Nerve root

Filum terminale (dural part)

Nerve roots and meninges at sacral level

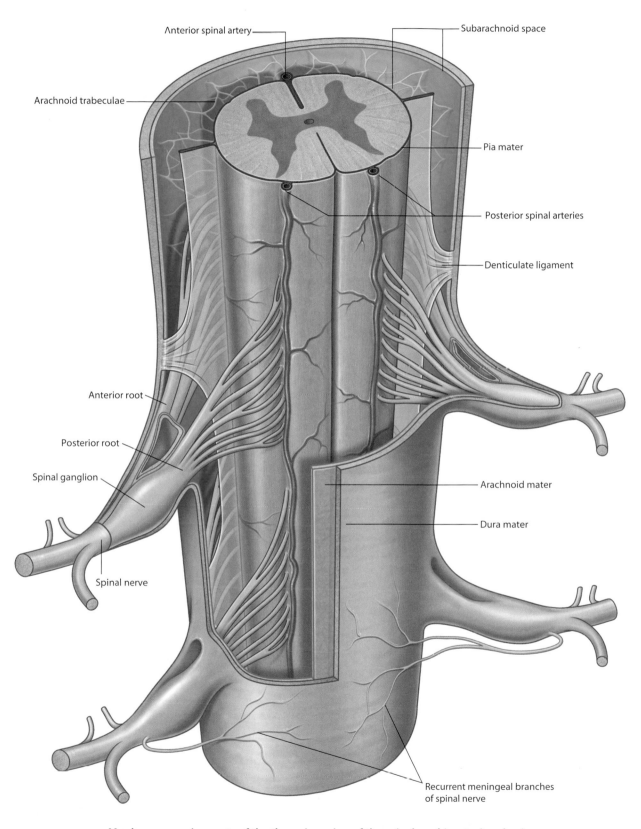

Anterior spinal artery

Subarachnoid space

Arachnoid trabeculae

Pia mater

Posterior spinal arteries

Denticulate ligament

Anterior root

Posterior root

Spinal ganglion

Arachnoid mater

Dura mater

Spinal nerve

Recurrent meningeal branches
of spinal nerve

Meninges covering parts of the thoracic region of the spinal cord (posterior view)

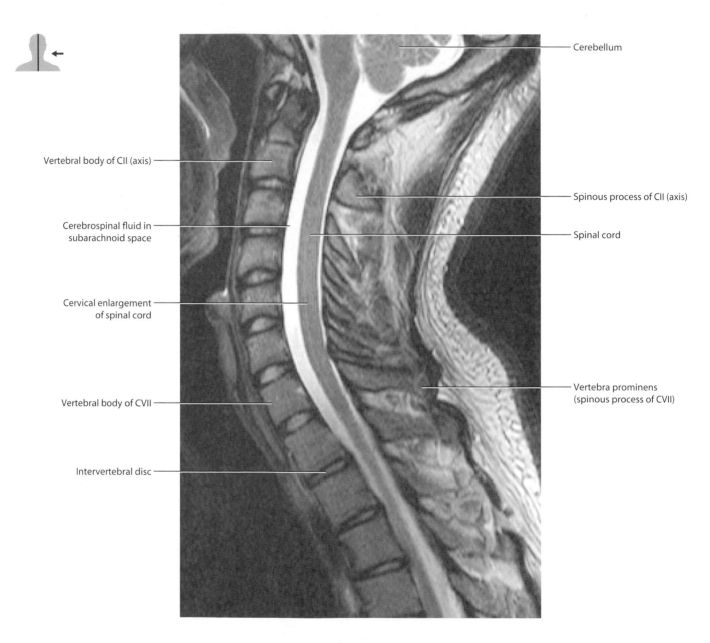

Cerebellum

Vertebral body of CII (axis)

Spinous process of CII (axis)

Cerebrospinal fluid in
subarachnoid space

Spinal cord

Cervical enlargement
of spinal cord

Vertebral body of CVII

Vertebra prominens
(spinous process of CVII)

Intervertebral disc

**Cervical and upper thoracic vertebral column showing
upper and middle portions of spinal cord.**
T2-weighted MR image in sagittal plane

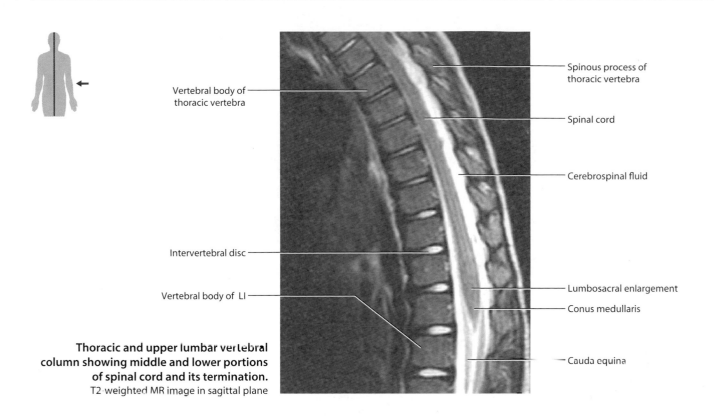

Spinous process of thoracic vertebra

Vertebral body of thoracic vertebra

Spinal cord

Cerebrospinal fluid

Intervertebral disc

Lumbosacral enlargement

Vertebral body of LI

Conus medullaris

Thoracic and upper lumbar vertebral column showing middle and lower portions of spinal cord and its termination.
T2-weighted MR image in sagittal plane

Cauda equina

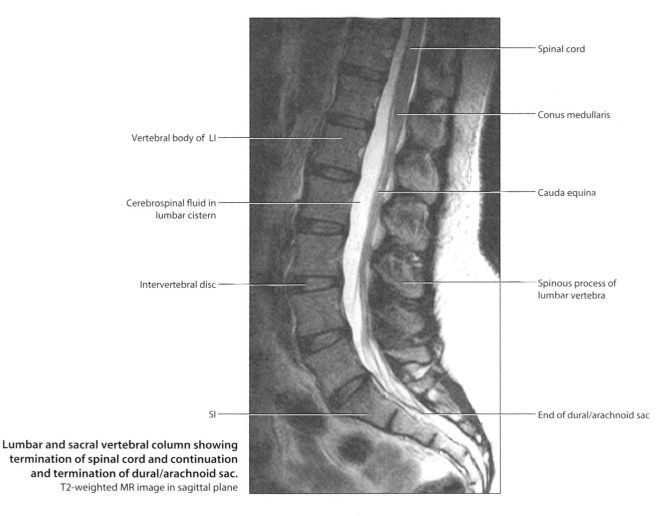

Spinal cord

Vertebral body of LI

Conus medullaris

Cerebrospinal fluid in lumbar cistern

Cauda equina

Intervertebral disc

Spinous process of lumbar vertebra

SI

End of dural/arachnoid sac

Lumbar and sacral vertebral column showing termination of spinal cord and continuation and termination of dural/arachnoid sac.
T2-weighted MR image in sagittal plane

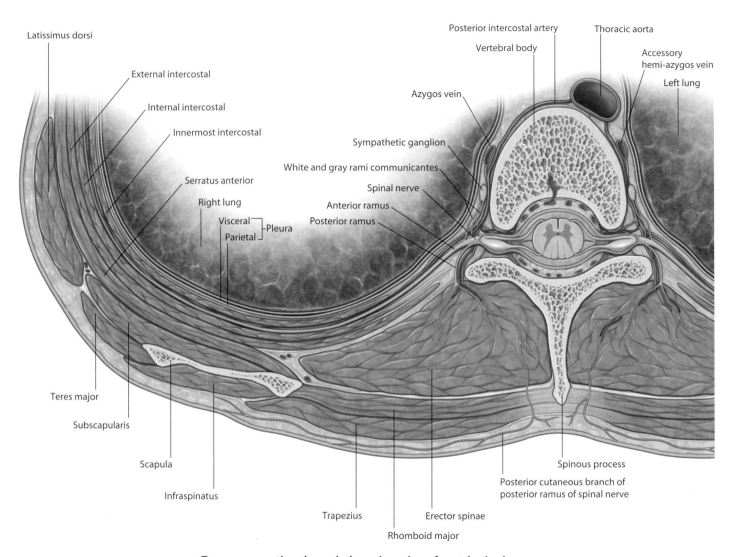

Latissimus dorsi

External intercostal

Internal intercostal

Innermost intercostal

Serratus anterior

Right lung

Visceral
Parietal ⎱ Pleura

Teres major

Subscapularis

Scapula

Infraspinatus

Trapezius

Rhomboid major

Erector spinae

Posterior cutaneous branch of
posterior ramus of spinal nerve

Spinous process

Posterior ramus

Anterior ramus

Spinal nerve

White and gray rami communicantes

Sympathetic ganglion

Azygos vein

Posterior intercostal artery

Vertebral body

Thoracic aorta

Accessory
hemi-azygos vein

Left lung

Transverse section through thoracic region of vertebral column

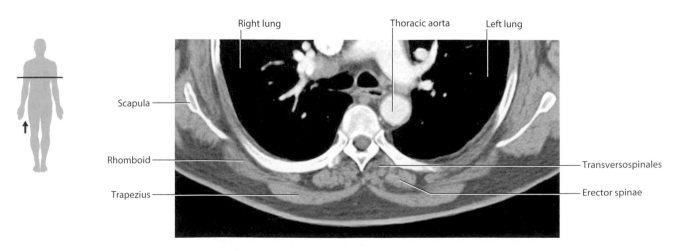

Right lung

Thoracic aorta

Left lung

Scapula

Rhomboid

Trapezius

Transversospinales

Erector spinae

Thoracic region of back.
CT image in axial plane

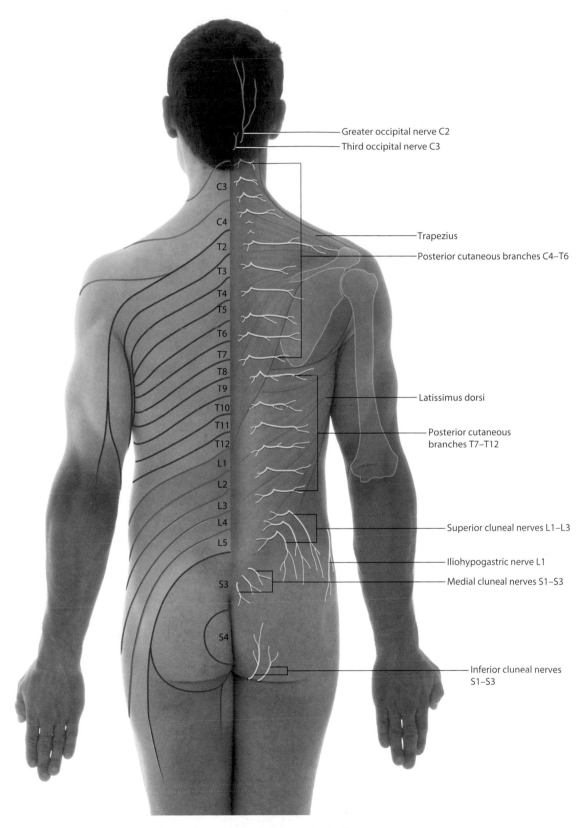

Greater occipital nerve C2

Third occipital nerve C3

Trapezius

Posterior cutaneous branches C4–T6

Latissimus dorsi

Posterior cutaneous branches T7–T12

Superior cluneal nerves L1–L3

Iliohypogastric nerve L1

Medial cluneal nerves S1–S3

Inferior cluneal nerves S1–S3

C3
C4
T2
T3
T4
T5
T6
T7
T8
T9
T10
T11
T12
L1
L2
L3
L4
L5
S3
S4

Dermatomes and cutaneous nerves of the back

Superficial (appendicular) group of back muscles

Muscle		Origin	Insertion	Innervation	Function
Trapezius	1	Superior nuchal line, external occipital protuberance, ligamentum nuchae, spinous processes of CVII to TXII	Lateral one third of clavicle, acromion, spine of scapula	Motor—accessory nerve [XI]; proprioception—C3 and C4	Assists in rotating the scapula during abduction of humerus above horizontal; upper fibers elevate, middle fibers adduct, and lower fibers depress scapula
Latissimus dorsi	2	Spinous processes of TVII to LV and sacrum, iliac crest, ribs X to XII	Floor of intertubercular sulcus of humerus	Thoracodorsal nerve (C6 to C8)	Extends, adducts, and medially rotates humerus
Levator scapulae	3	Transverse processes of CI to CIV	Upper portion of medial border of scapula	C3 to C4 and dorsal scapular nerve (C4, C5)	Elevates scapula
Rhomboid major	4	Spinous processes of TII to TV	Medial border of scapula between spine and inferior angle	Dorsal scapular nerve (C4, C5)	Retracts (adducts) and elevates scapula
Rhomboid minor	5	Lower portion of ligamentum nuchae, spinous processes of CVII and TI	Medial border of scapula at the spine of scapula	Dorsal scapular nerve (C4, C5)	Retracts (adducts) and elevates scapula

Intermediate (respiratory) group of back muscles

Muscle		Origin	Insertion	Innervation	Function
Serratus posterior superior	6	Lower portion of ligamentum nuchae, spinous processes of CVII to TIII and supraspinous ligaments	Mastoid process, skull below lateral one third of superior nuchal line	Anterior rami of upper thoracic nerves (T2 to T5)	Elevates ribs II to V
Serratus posterior inferior	7	Spinous processes of TXI to LIII and supraspinous ligaments	Lower border of ribs IX to XII just lateral to their angles	Anterior rami of lower thoracic nerves (T9 to T12)	Depresses ribs IX to XII and may prevent lower ribs from being elevated when the diaphragm contracts

Spinotransversales muscles

Muscle		Origin	Insertion	Innervation	Function
Splenius capitis	8	Lower half of ligamentum nuchae, spinous processes of CVII to TIV	Mastoid process, skull below lateral one third of superior nuchal line	Posterior rami middle cervical nerves	Together—draw head backward, extending neck; individually—draw and rotate head to one side (turn face to same side)
Splenius cervicis	9	Spinous processes of TIII to TVI	Transverse processes of CI to CIII	Posterior rami lower cervical nerves	Together—extend neck; individually—draw and rotate head to one side (turn face to same side)

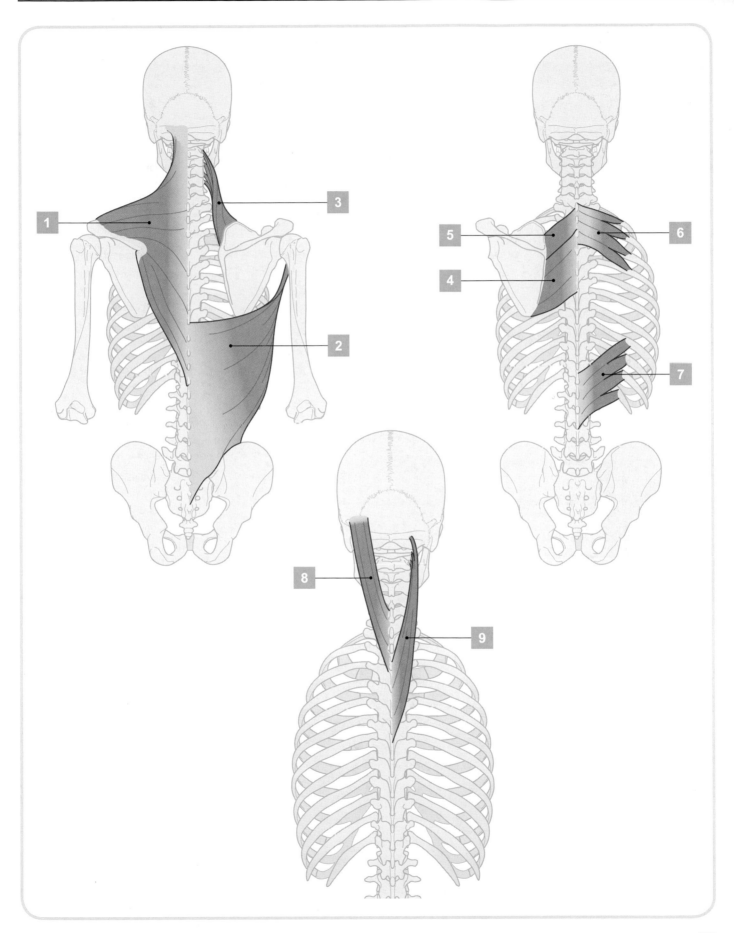

Erector spinae group of back muscles

Muscle		Origin	Insertion
Iliocostalis lumborum	1	Sacrum, spinous processes of lumbar and lower two thoracic vertebrae and their supraspinous ligaments, and the iliac crest	Angles of the lower six or seven ribs
Iliocostalis thoracis	2	Angles of the lower six ribs	Angles of the upper six ribs and the transverse process of CVII
Iliocostalis cervicis	3	Angles of ribs III to VI	Transverse processes of CIV to CVI
Longissimus thoracis	4	Blends with iliocostalis in lumbar region and is attached to transverse processes of lumbar vertebrae	Transverse processes of all thoracic vertebrae and just lateral to the tubercles of the lower nine or ten ribs
Longissimus cervicis	5	Transverse processes of upper four or five thoracic vertebrae	Transverse processes of CII to CVI
Longissimus capitis	6	Blends with iliocostalis in lumbar region and is attached to transverse processes of lumbar vertebrae	Transverse processes of all thoracic vertebrae and just lateral to the tubercles of the lower nine or ten ribs
Spinalis thoracis	7	Spinous processes of TX or TXI to LII	Spinous processes of TI to TVIII (varies)
Spinalis cervicis	8	Lower part of ligamentum nuchae and spinous process of CVII (sometimes TI to TII)	Spinous process of CII (axis)
Spinalis capitis	9	Usually blends with semispinalis capitis	With semispinalis capitis

Transversospinales group of back muscles

Muscle		Origin	Insertion
Semispinalis thoracis	10	Transverse processes of TVI to TX	Spinous processes of upper four thoracic and lower two cervical vertebrae
Semispinalis cervicis	11	Transverse processes of upper five or six thoracic vertebrae	Spinous processes of CII (axis) to CV
Semispinalis capitis	12	Transverse processes of TI to TVI (or TVII) and CVII and articular processes of CIV to CVI	Medial area between the superior and inferior nuchal lines of occipital bone
Multifidus	13	Sacrum, origin of erector spinae, posterior superior iliac spine, mammillary processes of lumbar vertebrae, transverse processes of thoracic vertebrae, and articular processes of lower four cervical vertebrae	Base of spinous processes of all vertebrae from LV to CII (axis)
Rotatores lumborum	14	Mammillary processes of lumbar vertebrae	Spinous processes of lumbar vertebrae
Rotatores thoracis	15	Transverse processes of thoracic vertebrae	Spinous processes of thoracic vertebrae
Rotatores cervicis	16	Articular processes of cervical vertebrae	Spinous processes of cervical vertebrae

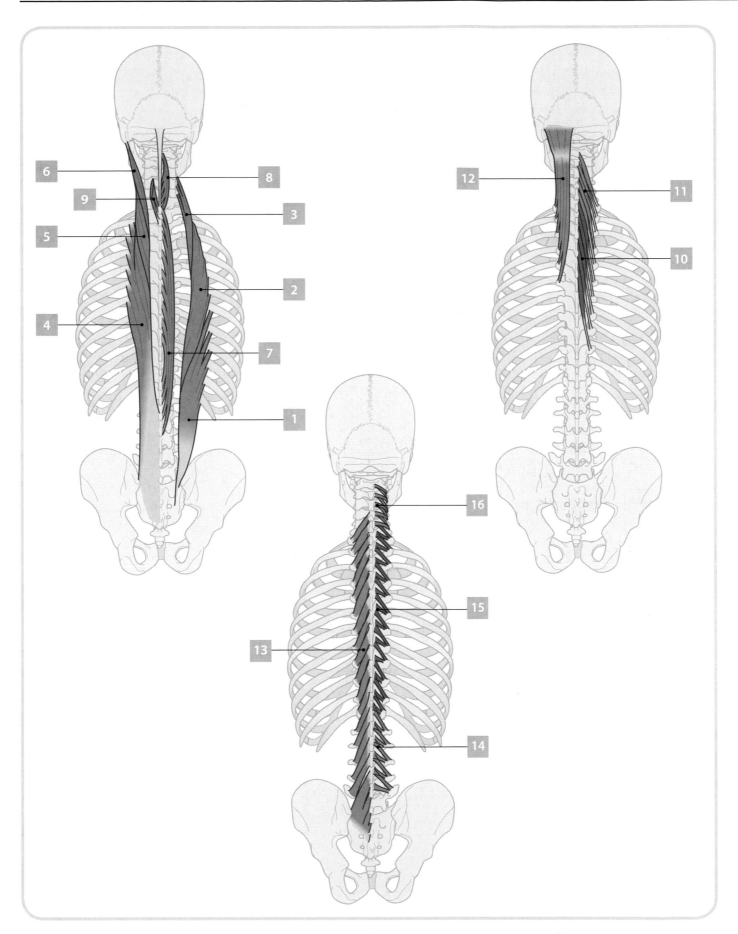

Segmental back muscles

Muscle		Origin	Insertion	Function
Levatores costarum	1	Short paired muscles arising from transverse processes of CVII to TXI	The rib below vertebra of origin near tubercle	Contraction elevates rib
Interspinales	2	Short paired muscles attached to the spinous processes of contiguous vertebrae, one on each side of the interspinous ligament		Postural muscles that stabilize adjoining vertebra during movements of vertebral column
Intertransversarii	3	Small muscles between the transverse processes of contiguous vertebrae		Postural muscles that stabilize adjoining vertebra during movements of vertebral column

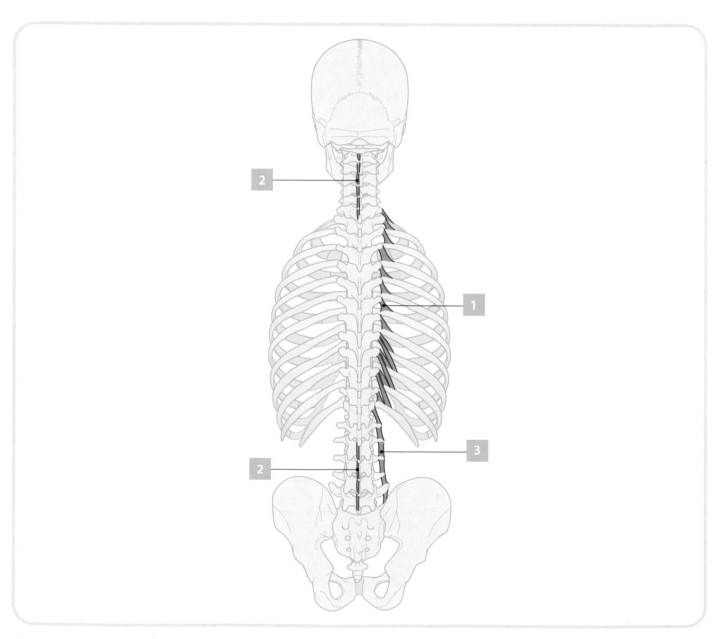

Suboccipital group of back muscles

Muscle		Origin	Insertion	Innervation	Function
Rectus capitis posterior major	1	Spinous process of axis (CII)	Lateral portion of occipital bone below inferior nuchal line	Posterior ramus of C1	Extension of head; rotation of face to same side as muscle
Rectus capitis posterior minor	2	Posterior tubercle of atlas (CI)	Medial portion of occipital bone below inferior nuchal line	Posterior ramus of C1	Extension of head
Obliquus capitis superior	3	Transverse process of atlas (CI)	Occipital bone between superior and inferior nuchal lines	Posterior ramus of C1	Extension of head and bends it to same side
Obliquus capitis inferior	4	Spinous process of axis (CII)	Transverse process of atlas (CI)	Posterior ramus of C1	Rotation of face to same side

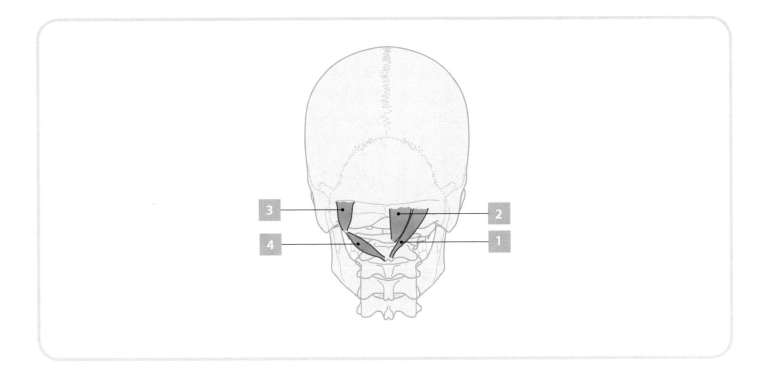

3

THORAX

CONTENTS

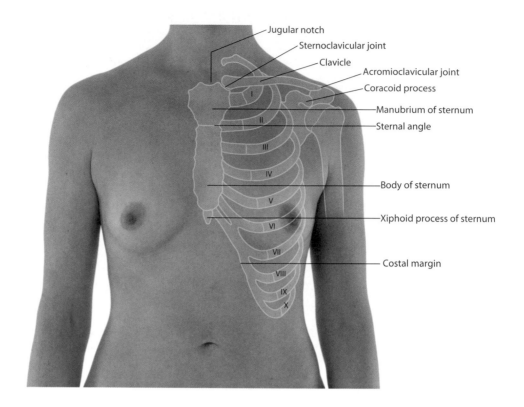

Jugular notch
Sternoclavicular joint
Clavicle
Acromioclavicular joint
Coracoid process
Manubrium of sternum
Sternal angle

I
II
III
IV
V
VI
VII
VIII
IX
X

Body of sternum

Xiphoid process of sternum

Costal margin

Anterior chest wall in a woman

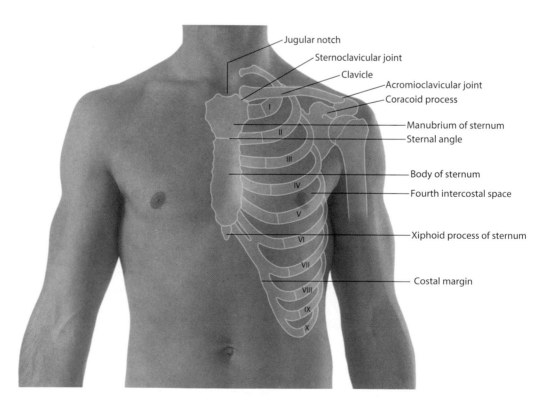

Jugular notch
Sternoclavicular joint
Clavicle
Acromioclavicular joint
Coracoid process
Manubrium of sternum
Sternal angle

I
II
III
IV
V
VI
VII
VIII
IX
X

Body of sternum

Fourth intercostal space

Xiphoid process of sternum

Costal margin

Anterior chest wall in a man

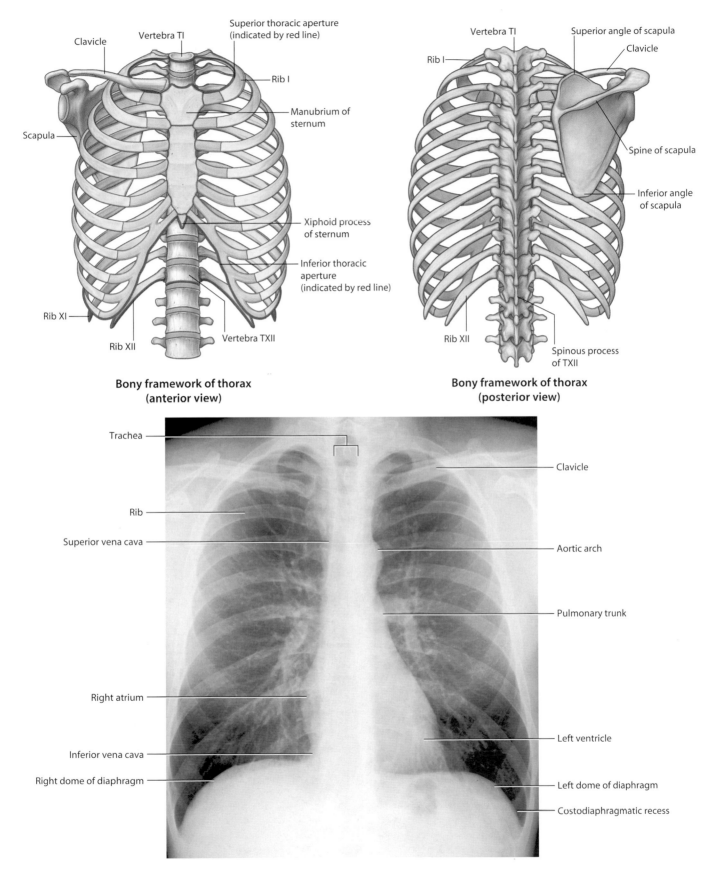

Clavicle

Vertebra TI

Superior thoracic aperture
(indicated by red line)

Rib I

Manubrium of
sternum

Scapula

Xiphoid process
of sternum

Inferior thoracic
aperture
(indicated by red line)

Rib XI

Rib XII

Vertebra TXII

**Bony framework of thorax
(anterior view)**

Vertebra TI

Rib I

Superior angle of scapula

Clavicle

Spine of scapula

Inferior angle
of scapula

Rib XII

Spinous process
of TXII

**Bony framework of thorax
(posterior view)**

Trachea

Rib

Superior vena cava

Right atrium

Inferior vena cava

Right dome of diaphragm

Clavicle

Aortic arch

Pulmonary trunk

Left ventricle

Left dome of diaphragm

Costodiaphragmatic recess

Positioning of structures in chest.
Radiograph, AP view

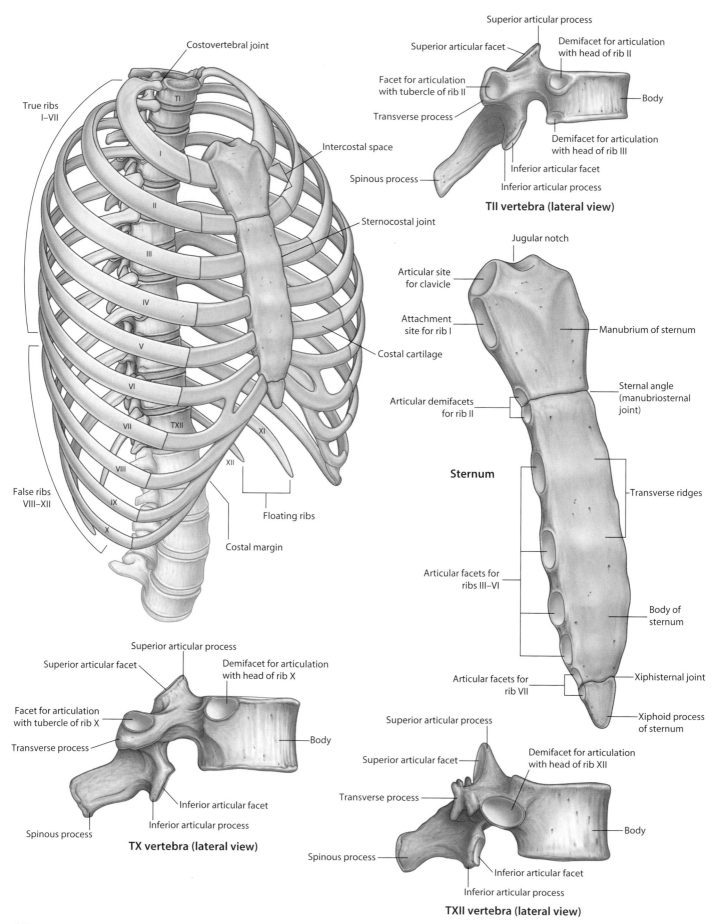

Costovertebral joint

True ribs I–VII

Intercostal space

Sternocostal joint

Costal cartilage

TXII

XI

XII

VII

VIII

IX

X

False ribs VIII–XII

Floating ribs

Costal margin

Superior articular process

Superior articular facet

Demifacet for articulation with head of rib II

Facet for articulation with tubercle of rib II

Transverse process

Body

Demifacet for articulation with head of rib III

Spinous process

Inferior articular facet

Inferior articular process

TII vertebra (lateral view)

Jugular notch

Articular site for clavicle

Attachment site for rib I

Manubrium of sternum

Articular demifacets for rib II

Sternal angle (manubriosternal joint)

Sternum

Transverse ridges

Articular facets for ribs III–VI

Body of sternum

Articular facets for rib VII

Xiphisternal joint

Xiphoid process of sternum

Superior articular process

Superior articular facet

Demifacet for articulation with head of rib X

Facet for articulation with tubercle of rib X

Transverse process

Body

Inferior articular facet

Inferior articular process

Spinous process

TX vertebra (lateral view)

Superior articular process

Superior articular facet

Demifacet for articulation with head of rib XII

Transverse process

Body

Spinous process

Inferior articular facet

Inferior articular process

TXII vertebra (lateral view)

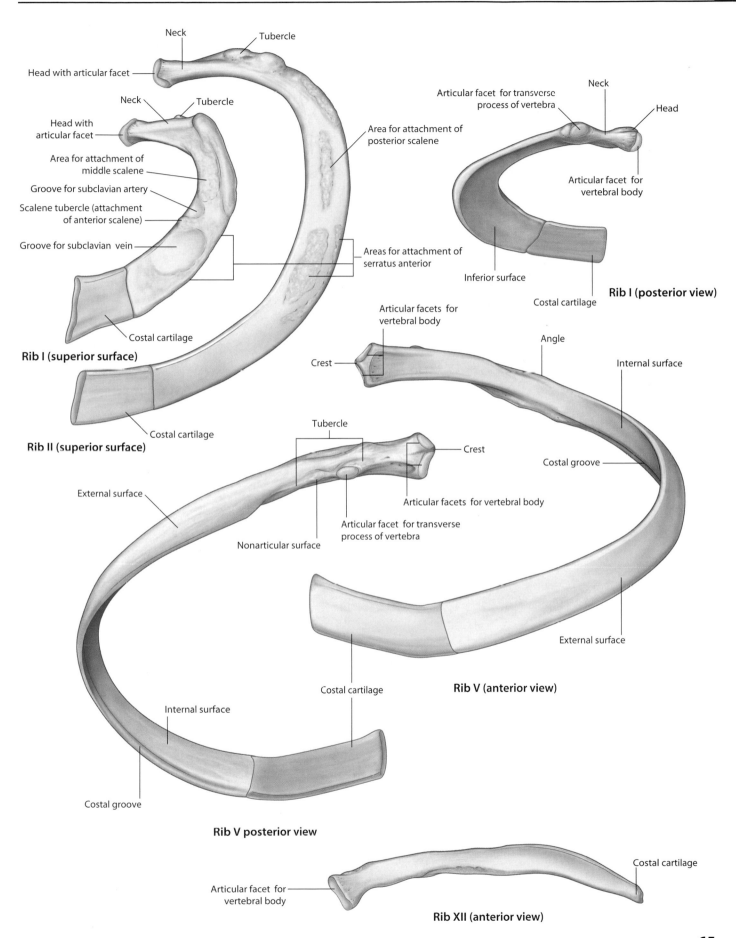

Neck
Tubercle
Head with articular facet
Neck
Tubercle
Head with articular facet
Area for attachment of middle scalene
Groove for subclavian artery
Scalene tubercle (attachment of anterior scalene)
Groove for subclavian vein
Area for attachment of posterior scalene
Areas for attachment of serratus anterior
Costal cartilage

Rib I (superior surface)

Costal cartilage

Rib II (superior surface)

Articular facet for transverse process of vertebra
Neck
Head
Articular facet for vertebral body
Inferior surface
Costal cartilage

Rib I (posterior view)

Articular facets for vertebral body
Crest
Angle
Internal surface
Costal groove

Tubercle
Crest
Articular facets for vertebral body
Articular facet for transverse process of vertebra
Nonarticular surface
External surface
Costal cartilage
External surface

Rib V (anterior view)

Internal surface
Costal cartilage
Costal groove

Rib V posterior view

Articular facet for vertebral body
Costal cartilage

Rib XII (anterior view)

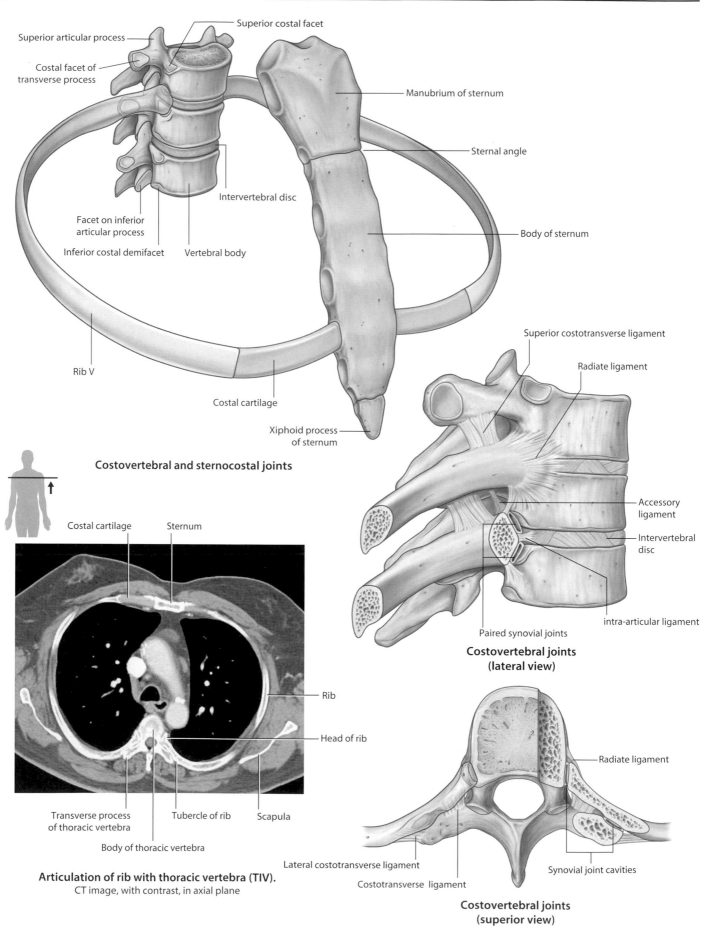

Superior articular process

Superior costal facet

Costal facet of transverse process

Manubrium of sternum

Sternal angle

Intervertebral disc

Body of sternum

Facet on inferior articular process

Inferior costal demifacet

Vertebral body

Rib V

Costal cartilage

Xiphoid process of sternum

Costovertebral and sternocostal joints

Superior costotransverse ligament

Radiate ligament

Accessory ligament

Intervertebral disc

intra-articular ligament

Paired synovial joints

Costovertebral joints (lateral view)

Costal cartilage

Sternum

Rib

Head of rib

Transverse process of thoracic vertebra

Tubercle of rib

Scapula

Body of thoracic vertebra

Articulation of rib with thoracic vertebra (TIV).
CT image, with contrast, in axial plane

Radiate ligament

Lateral costotransverse ligament

Costotransverse ligament

Synovial joint cavities

Costovertebral joints (superior view)

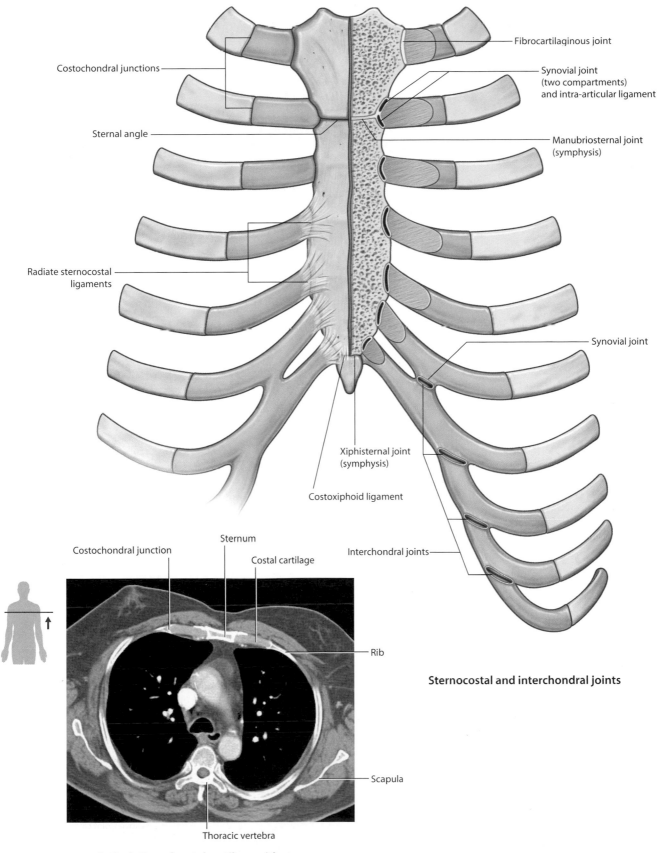

Costochondral junctions

Sternal angle

Radiate sternocostal ligaments

Fibrocartilaginous joint

Synovial joint (two compartments) and intra-articular ligament

Manubriosternal joint (symphysis)

Synovial joint

Xiphisternal joint (symphysis)

Costoxiphoid ligament

Interchondral joints

Sternocostal and interchondral joints

Costochondral junction

Sternum

Costal cartilage

Rib

Scapula

Thoracic vertebra

Articulation of costal cartilage with sternum.
CT image, with contrast, in axial plane

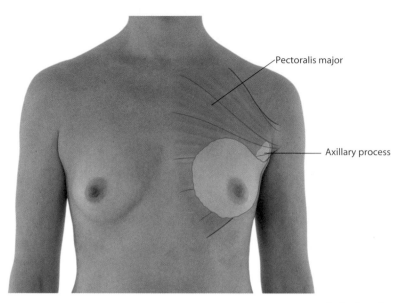

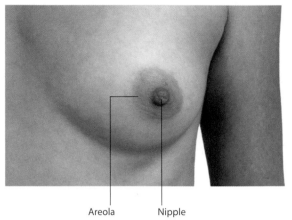

Pectoralis major

Axillary process

Areola   Nipple

Anterior view

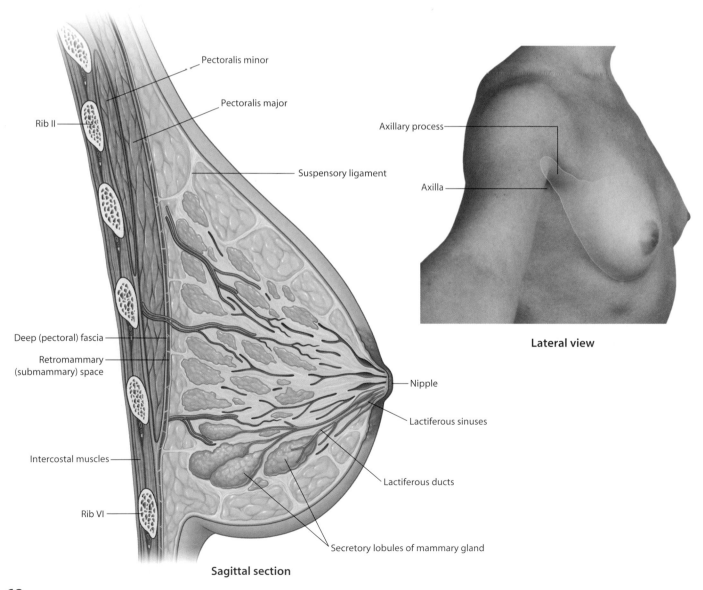

Pectoralis minor

Pectoralis major

Rib II

Suspensory ligament

Deep (pectoral) fascia

Retromammary
(submammary) space

Intercostal muscles

Rib VI

Nipple

Lactiferous sinuses

Lactiferous ducts

Secretory lobules of mammary gland

Sagittal section

Axillary process

Axilla

Lateral view

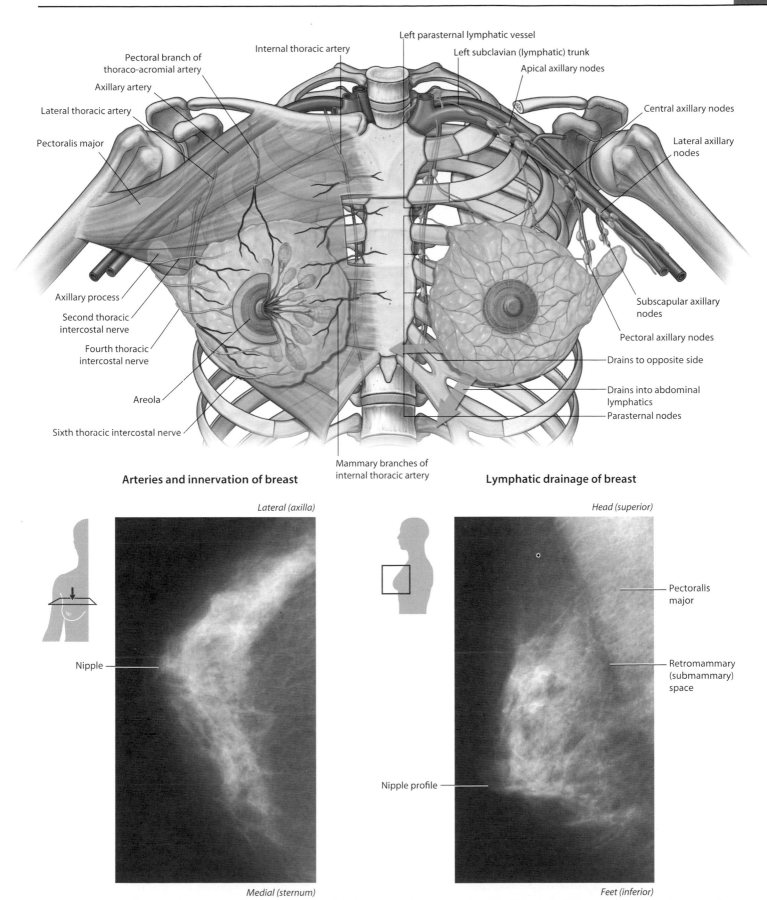

Arteries and innervation of breast

Left parasternal lymphatic vessel
Left subclavian (lymphatic) trunk
Apical axillary nodes
Central axillary nodes
Lateral axillary nodes
Subscapular axillary nodes
Pectoral axillary nodes
Drains to opposite side
Drains into abdominal lymphatics
Parasternal nodes

Lymphatic drainage of breast

Internal thoracic artery
Pectoral branch of thoraco-acromial artery
Axillary artery
Lateral thoracic artery
Pectoralis major
Axillary process
Second thoracic intercostal nerve
Fourth thoracic intercostal nerve
Areola
Sixth thoracic intercostal nerve
Mammary branches of internal thoracic artery

Lateral (axilla)
Nipple
Medial (sternum)

Mammography. Craniocaudal (CC) view of a normal right breast showing a heterogeneously dense appearance

Head (superior)
Pectoralis major
Retromammary (submammary) space
Nipple profile
Feet (inferior)

Mammography. Mediolateral oblique (MLO) view of a normal right breast showing a heterogeneously dense appearance

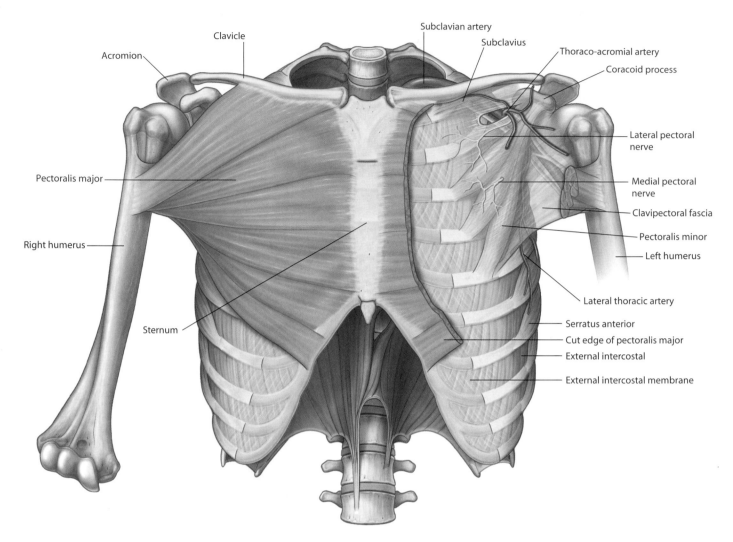

Acromion

Clavicle

Subclavian artery

Subclavius

Thoraco-acromial artery

Coracoid process

Lateral pectoral nerve

Pectoralis major

Medial pectoral nerve

Clavipectoral fascia

Pectoralis minor

Left humerus

Right humerus

Lateral thoracic artery

Sternum

Serratus anterior

Cut edge of pectoralis major

External intercostal

External intercostal membrane

Pectoralis major muscle and related deep structures

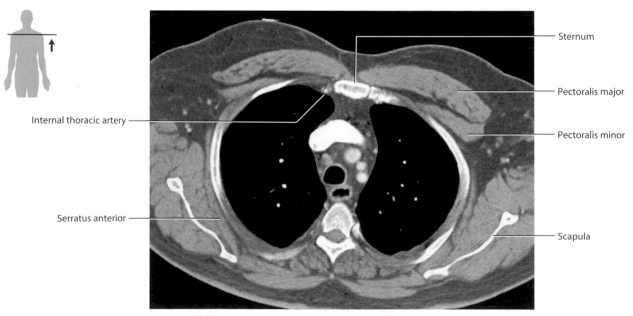

Sternum

Pectoralis major

Internal thoracic artery

Pectoralis minor

Serratus anterior

Scapula

Pectoralis major and minor muscles on anterior thoracic wall.
CT image, with contrast, in axial plane

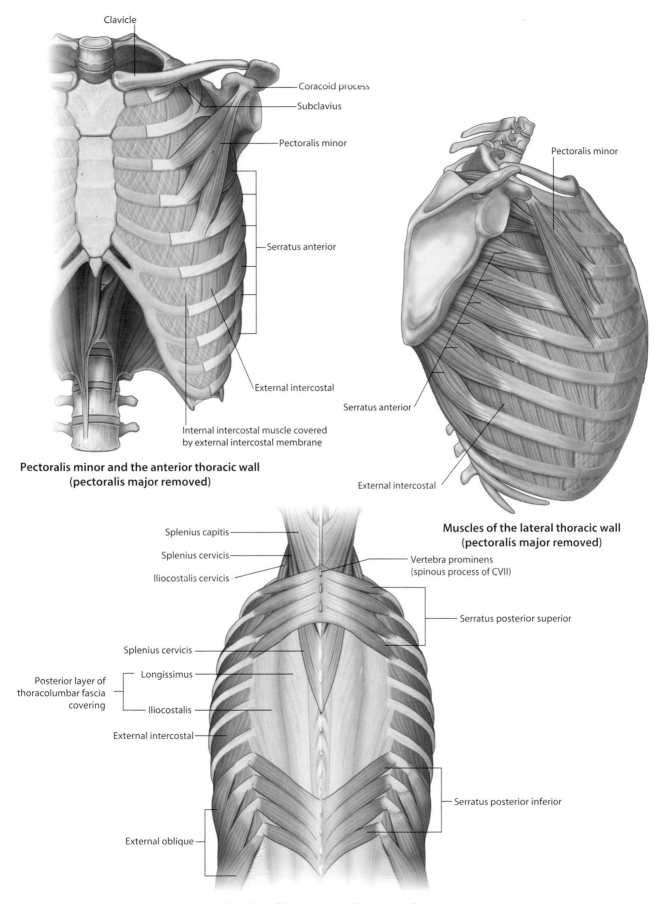

Clavicle

Coracoid process

Subclavius

Pectoralis minor

Serratus anterior

External intercostal

Internal intercostal muscle covered
by external intercostal membrane

**Pectoralis minor and the anterior thoracic wall
(pectoralis major removed)**

Pectoralis minor

Serratus anterior

External intercostal

**Muscles of the lateral thoracic wall
(pectoralis major removed)**

Splenius capitis

Splenius cervicis

Iliocostalis cervicis

Vertebra prominens
(spinous process of CVII)

Serratus posterior superior

Splenius cervicis

Longissimus

Posterior layer of
thoracolumbar fascia
covering

Iliocostalis

External intercostal

Serratus posterior inferior

External oblique

Muscles of the posterior thoracic wall

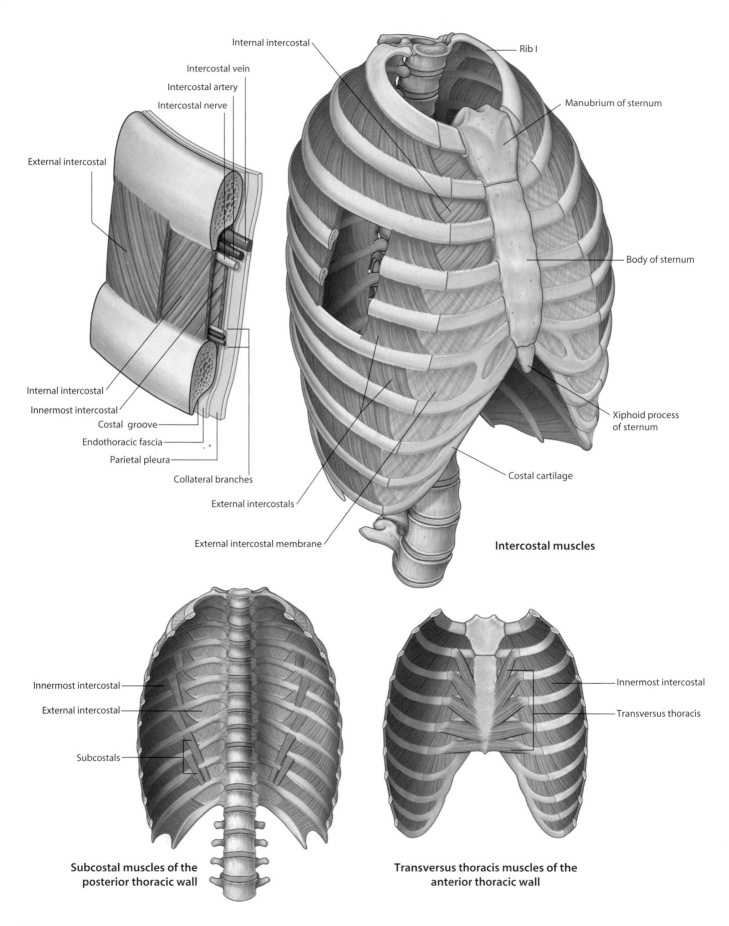

Internal intercostal

Intercostal vein

Intercostal artery

Intercostal nerve

External intercostal

Internal intercostal

Innermost intercostal

Costal groove

Endothoracic fascia

Parietal pleura

Collateral branches

External intercostals

External intercostal membrane

Rib I

Manubrium of sternum

Body of sternum

Xiphoid process of sternum

Costal cartilage

Intercostal muscles

Innermost intercostal

External intercostal

Subcostals

Subcostal muscles of the posterior thoracic wall

Innermost intercostal

Transversus thoracis

Transversus thoracis muscles of the anterior thoracic wall

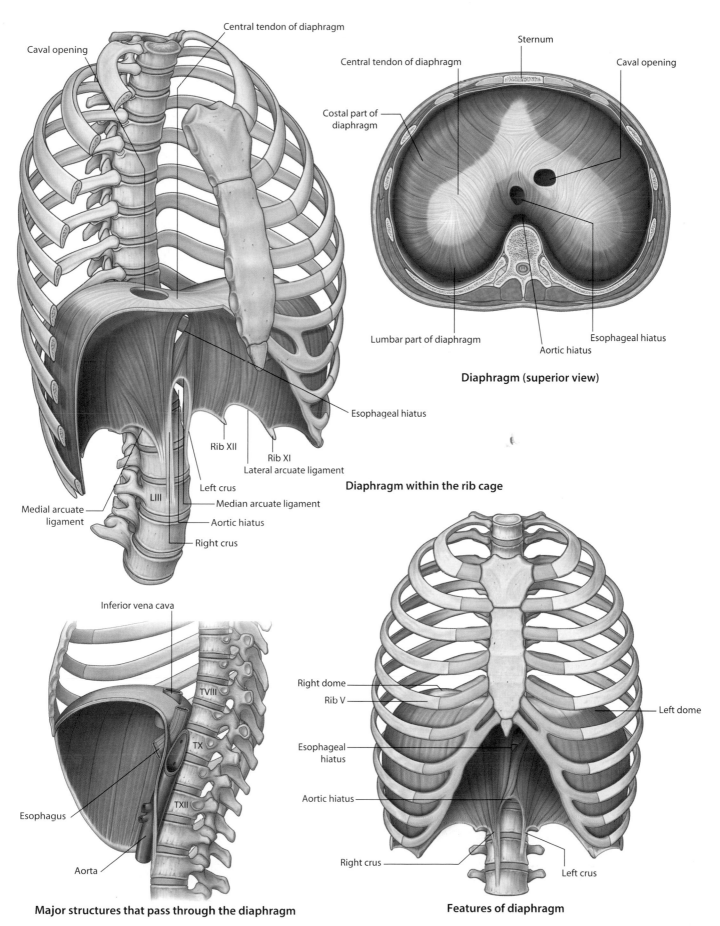

Caval opening

Central tendon of diaphragm

Sternum

Central tendon of diaphragm

Caval opening

Costal part of diaphragm

Esophageal hiatus

Lumbar part of diaphragm

Aortic hiatus

Diaphragm (superior view)

Esophageal hiatus

Rib XII

Rib XI

Lateral arcuate ligament

Left crus

Median arcuate ligament

Aortic hiatus

Right crus

Medial arcuate ligament

LIII

Diaphragm within the rib cage

Inferior vena cava

TVIII

TX

TXII

Esophagus

Aorta

Major structures that pass through the diaphragm

Right dome

Rib V

Esophageal hiatus

Aortic hiatus

Right crus

Left dome

Left crus

Features of diaphragm

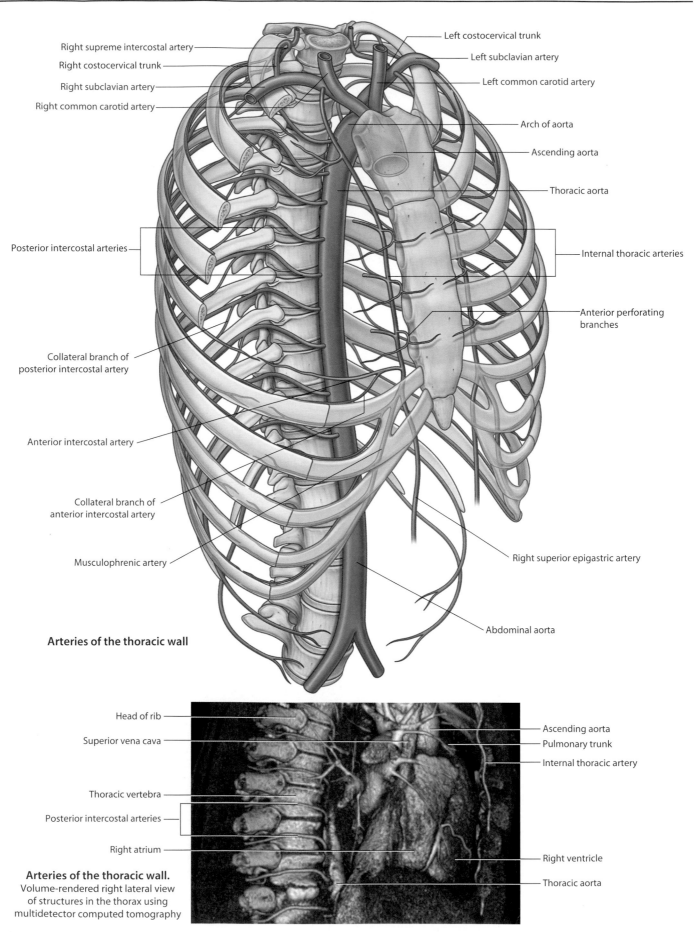

Right supreme intercostal artery

Right costocervical trunk

Right subclavian artery

Right common carotid artery

Left costocervical trunk

Left subclavian artery

Left common carotid artery

Arch of aorta

Ascending aorta

Thoracic aorta

Posterior intercostal arteries

Internal thoracic arteries

Anterior perforating branches

Collateral branch of posterior intercostal artery

Anterior intercostal artery

Collateral branch of anterior intercostal artery

Musculophrenic artery

Right superior epigastric artery

Abdominal aorta

Arteries of the thoracic wall

Head of rib

Superior vena cava

Ascending aorta

Pulmonary trunk

Internal thoracic artery

Thoracic vertebra

Posterior intercostal arteries

Right atrium

Right ventricle

Thoracic aorta

Arteries of the thoracic wall.
Volume-rendered right lateral view
of structures in the thorax using
multidetector computed tomography

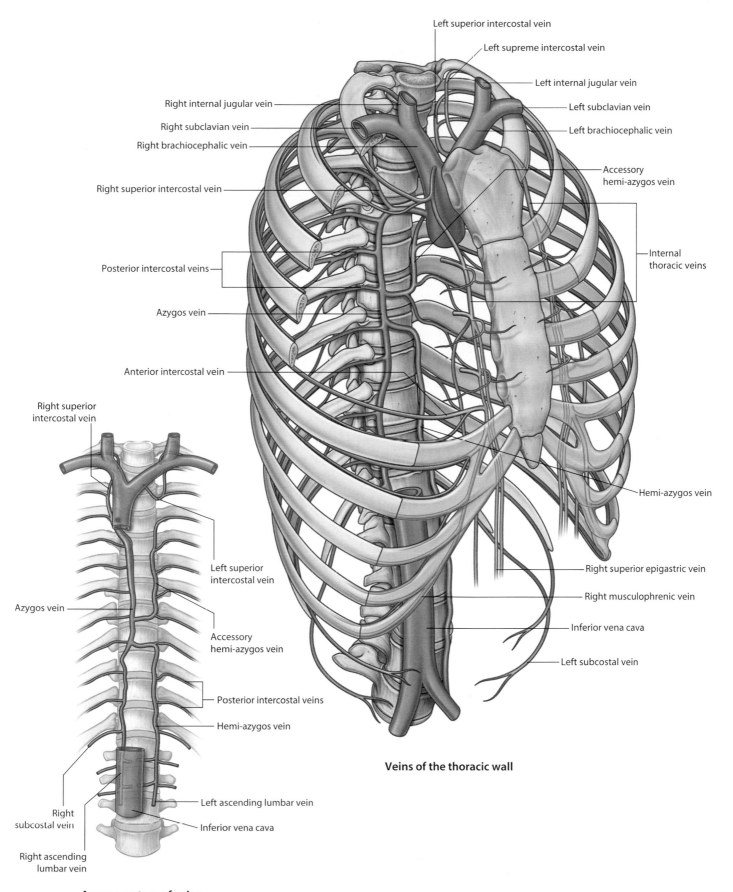

Left superior intercostal vein

Left supreme intercostal vein

Left internal jugular vein

Left subclavian vein

Left brachiocephalic vein

Accessory hemi-azygos vein

Internal thoracic veins

Hemi-azygos vein

Right superior epigastric vein

Right musculophrenic vein

Inferior vena cava

Left subcostal vein

Right internal jugular vein

Right subclavian vein

Right brachiocephalic vein

Right superior intercostal vein

Posterior intercostal veins

Azygos vein

Anterior intercostal vein

Veins of the thoracic wall

Right superior intercostal vein

Left superior intercostal vein

Azygos vein

Accessory hemi-azygos vein

Posterior intercostal veins

Hemi-azygos vein

Left ascending lumbar vein

Inferior vena cava

Right subcostal vein

Right ascending lumbar vein

Azygos system of veins

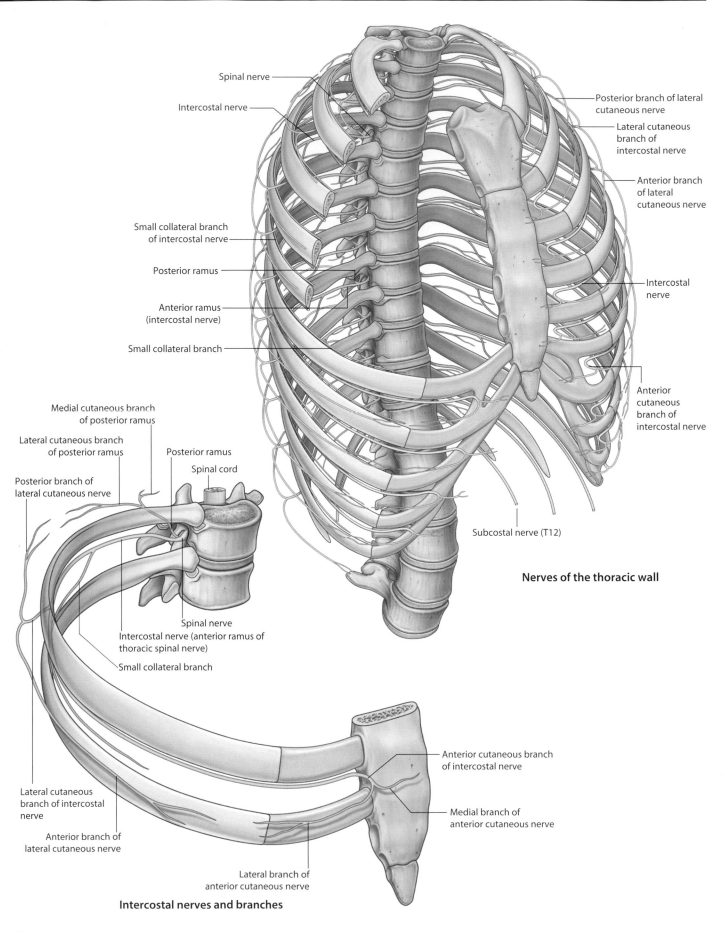

Spinal nerve

Intercostal nerve

Posterior branch of lateral cutaneous nerve

Lateral cutaneous branch of intercostal nerve

Anterior branch of lateral cutaneous nerve

Small collateral branch of intercostal nerve

Posterior ramus

Anterior ramus (intercostal nerve)

Small collateral branch

Intercostal nerve

Anterior cutaneous branch of intercostal nerve

Subcostal nerve (T12)

Nerves of the thoracic wall

Medial cutaneous branch of posterior ramus

Lateral cutaneous branch of posterior ramus

Posterior ramus

Posterior branch of lateral cutaneous nerve

Spinal cord

Spinal nerve

Intercostal nerve (anterior ramus of thoracic spinal nerve)

Small collateral branch

Anterior cutaneous branch of intercostal nerve

Medial branch of anterior cutaneous nerve

Lateral cutaneous branch of intercostal nerve

Anterior branch of lateral cutaneous nerve

Lateral branch of anterior cutaneous nerve

Intercostal nerves and branches

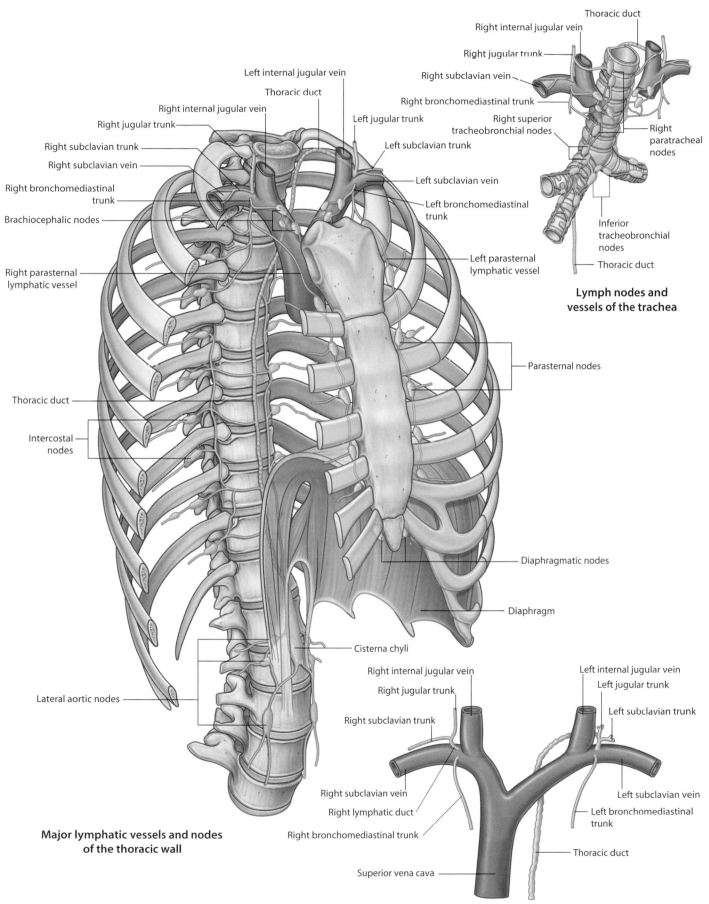

Thoracic duct
Right internal jugular vein
Right jugular trunk
Right subclavian vein
Right bronchomediastinal trunk
Right superior tracheobronchial nodes
Right paratracheal nodes
Inferior tracheobronchial nodes
Thoracic duct

Lymph nodes and vessels of the trachea

Left internal jugular vein
Thoracic duct
Right internal jugular vein
Right jugular trunk
Right subclavian trunk
Right subclavian vein
Right bronchomediastinal trunk
Brachiocephalic nodes
Right parasternal lymphatic vessel
Left jugular trunk
Left subclavian trunk
Left subclavian vein
Left bronchomediastinal trunk
Left parasternal lymphatic vessel
Parasternal nodes
Thoracic duct
Intercostal nodes
Diaphragmatic nodes
Diaphragm
Lateral aortic nodes
Cisterna chyli

Major lymphatic vessels and nodes of the thoracic wall

Right internal jugular vein
Right jugular trunk
Right subclavian trunk
Right subclavian vein
Right lymphatic duct
Right bronchomediastinal trunk
Superior vena cava
Left internal jugular vein
Left jugular trunk
Left subclavian trunk
Left subclavian vein
Left bronchomediastinal trunk
Thoracic duct

Termination of the lymphatic trunks

77

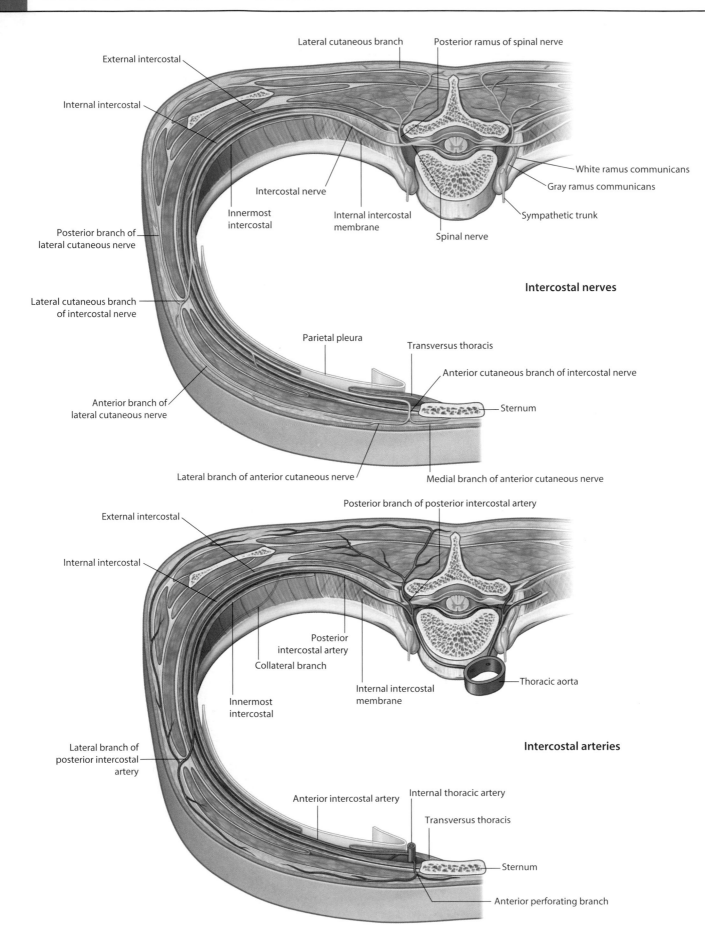

External intercostal

Internal intercostal

Lateral cutaneous branch

Posterior ramus of spinal nerve

White ramus communicans

Gray ramus communicans

Sympathetic trunk

Intercostal nerve

Innermost intercostal

Internal intercostal membrane

Spinal nerve

Intercostal nerves

Posterior branch of lateral cutaneous nerve

Lateral cutaneous branch of intercostal nerve

Anterior branch of lateral cutaneous nerve

Parietal pleura

Transversus thoracis

Anterior cutaneous branch of intercostal nerve

Sternum

Lateral branch of anterior cutaneous nerve

Medial branch of anterior cutaneous nerve

External intercostal

Internal intercostal

Posterior branch of posterior intercostal artery

Posterior intercostal artery

Collateral branch

Internal intercostal membrane

Thoracic aorta

Innermost intercostal

Intercostal arteries

Lateral branch of posterior intercostal artery

Anterior intercostal artery

Internal thoracic artery

Transversus thoracis

Sternum

Anterior perforating branch

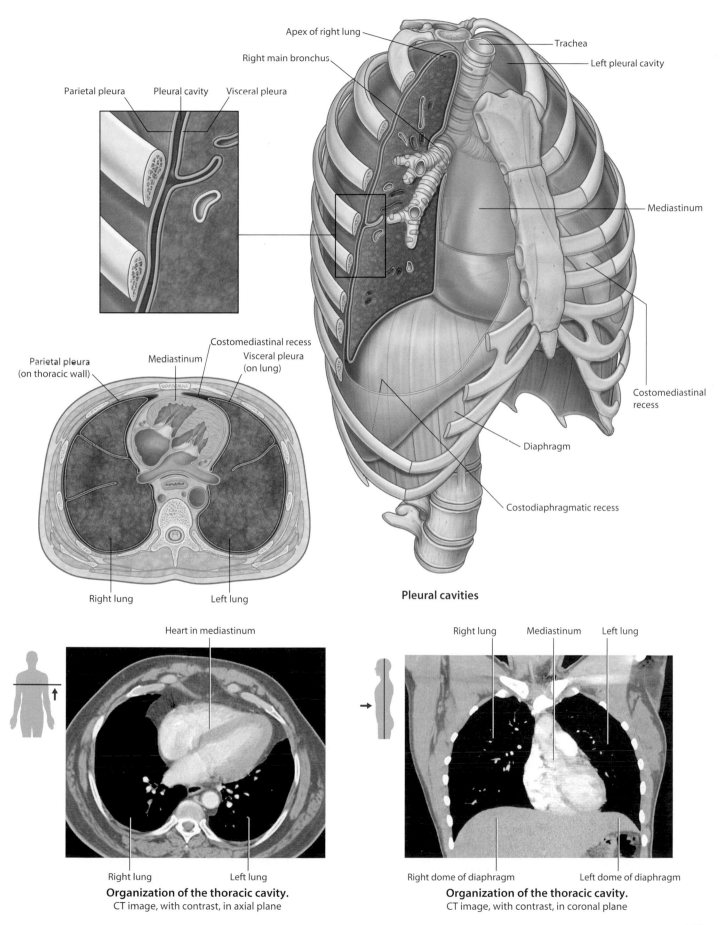

Apex of right lung

Right main bronchus

Trachea

Left pleural cavity

Parietal pleura

Pleural cavity

Visceral pleura

Mediastinum

Costomediastinal recess

Parietal pleura (on thoracic wall)

Mediastinum

Costomediastinal recess

Visceral pleura (on lung)

Diaphragm

Costodiaphragmatic recess

Right lung

Left lung

Pleural cavities

Heart in mediastinum

Right lung

Mediastinum

Left lung

Right lung

Left lung

Right dome of diaphragm

Left dome of diaphragm

Organization of the thoracic cavity.
CT image, with contrast, in axial plane

Organization of the thoracic cavity.
CT image, with contrast, in coronal plane

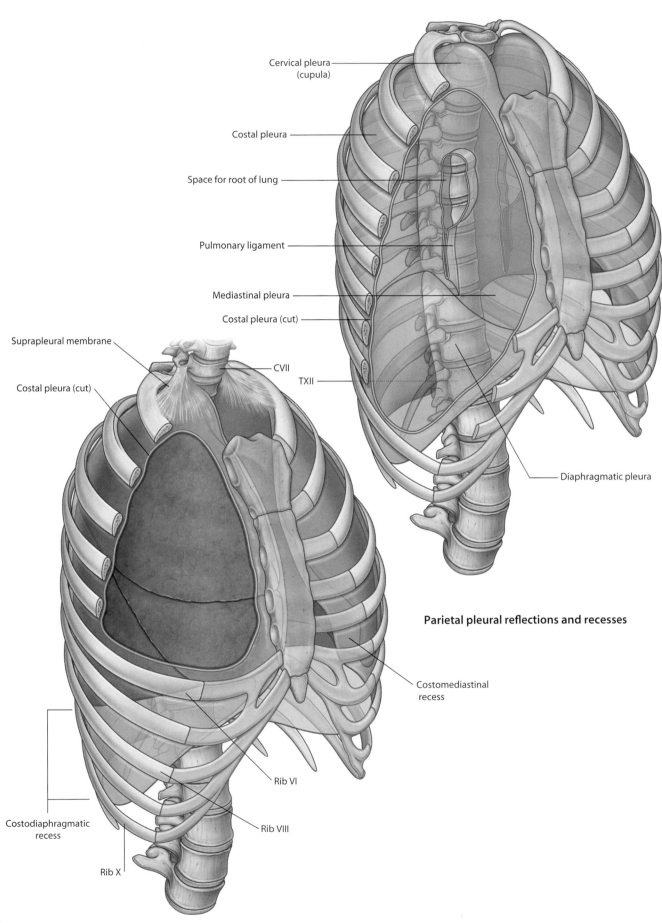

Cervical pleura
(cupula)

Costal pleura

Space for root of lung

Pulmonary ligament

Mediastinal pleura

Costal pleura (cut)

Suprapleural membrane

Costal pleura (cut)

CVII

TXII

Diaphragmatic pleura

Parietal pleural reflections and recesses

Costomediastinal
recess

Costodiaphragmatic
recess

Rib VI

Rib VIII

Rib X

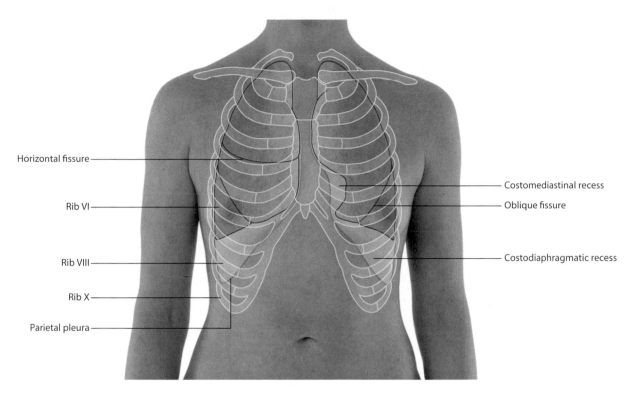

Horizontal fissure

Rib VI

Rib VIII

Rib X

Parietal pleura

Costomediastinal recess

Oblique fissure

Costodiaphragmatic recess

Surface projections of the pleura and lungs (anterior view)

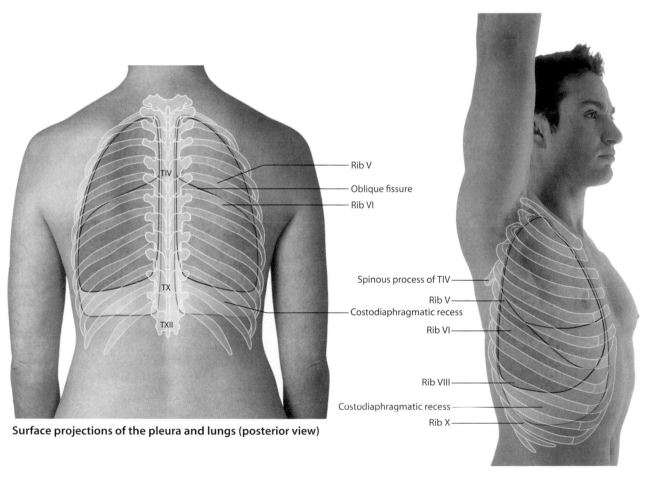

TIV

TX

TXII

Rib V

Oblique fissure

Rib VI

Surface projections of the pleura and lungs (posterior view)

Spinous process of TIV

Rib V

Costodiaphragmatic recess

Rib VI

Rib VIII

Costodiaphragmatic recess

Rib X

**Surface projections of the
pleura and right lung (lateral view)**

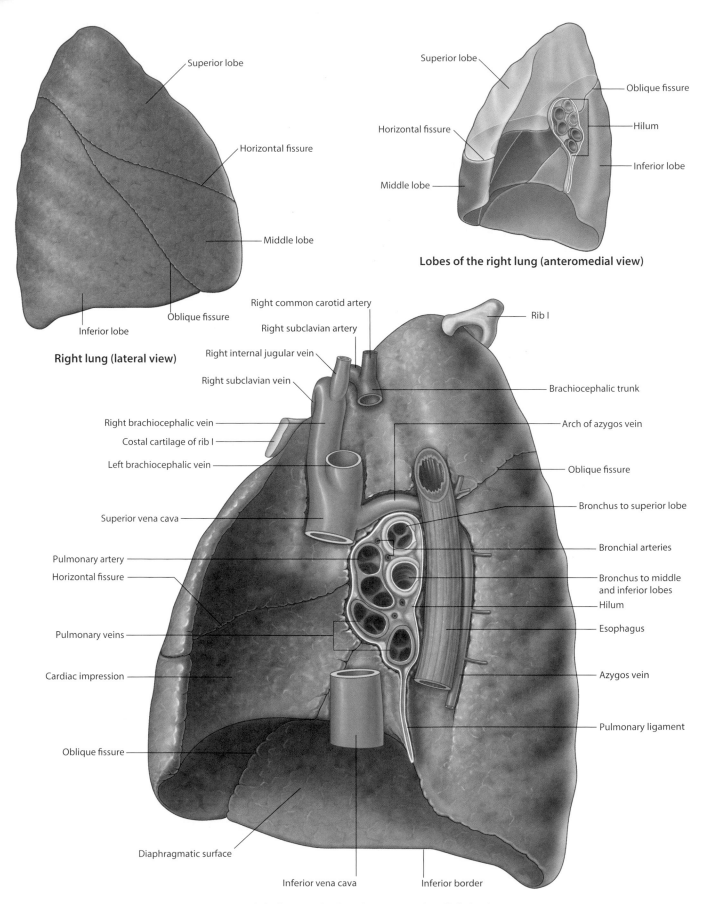

Superior lobe

Horizontal fissure

Middle lobe

Inferior lobe

Oblique fissure

Right lung (lateral view)

Superior lobe

Oblique fissure

Horizontal fissure

Hilum

Middle lobe

Inferior lobe

Lobes of the right lung (anteromedial view)

Right common carotid artery

Right subclavian artery

Right internal jugular vein

Right subclavian vein

Right brachiocephalic vein

Costal cartilage of rib I

Left brachiocephalic vein

Superior vena cava

Pulmonary artery

Horizontal fissure

Pulmonary veins

Cardiac impression

Oblique fissure

Diaphragmatic surface

Inferior vena cava

Inferior border

Rib I

Brachiocephalic trunk

Arch of azygos vein

Oblique fissure

Bronchus to superior lobe

Bronchial arteries

Bronchus to middle and inferior lobes

Hilum

Esophagus

Azygos vein

Pulmonary ligament

Right lung and related structures (medial view)

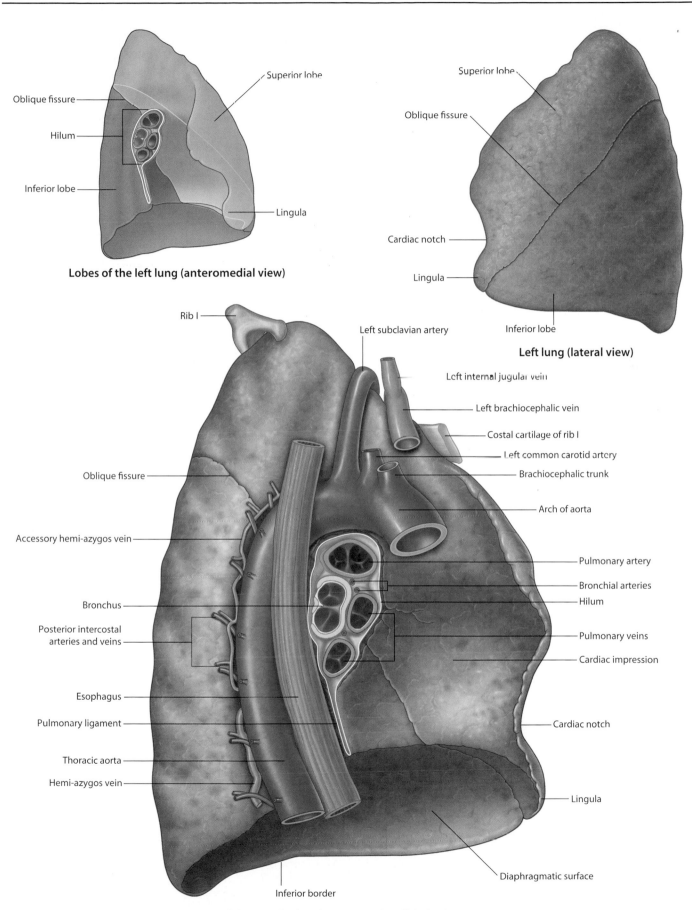

Oblique fissure

Hilum

Inferior lobe

Superior lobe

Lingula

Lobes of the left lung (anteromedial view)

Superior lobe

Oblique fissure

Cardiac notch

Lingula

Inferior lobe

Left lung (lateral view)

Rib I

Left subclavian artery

Left internal jugular vein

Left brachiocephalic vein

Costal cartilage of rib I

Left common carotid artery

Brachiocephalic trunk

Oblique fissure

Arch of aorta

Accessory hemi-azygos vein

Pulmonary artery

Bronchial arteries

Hilum

Bronchus

Posterior intercostal
arteries and veins

Pulmonary veins

Cardiac impression

Esophagus

Pulmonary ligament

Cardiac notch

Thoracic aorta

Hemi-azygos vein

Lingula

Diaphragmatic surface

Inferior border

Left lung and related structures (medial view)

83

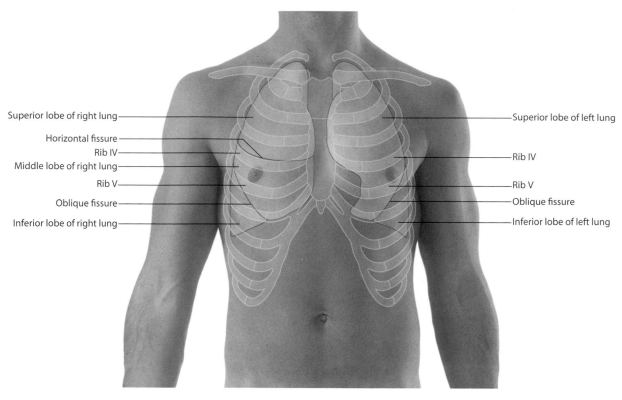

Superior lobe of right lung

Horizontal fissure

Rib IV

Middle lobe of right lung

Rib V

Oblique fissure

Inferior lobe of right lung

Superior lobe of left lung

Rib IV

Rib V

Oblique fissure

Inferior lobe of left lung

Surface projections of the lobes and fissures of the lungs (anterior view)

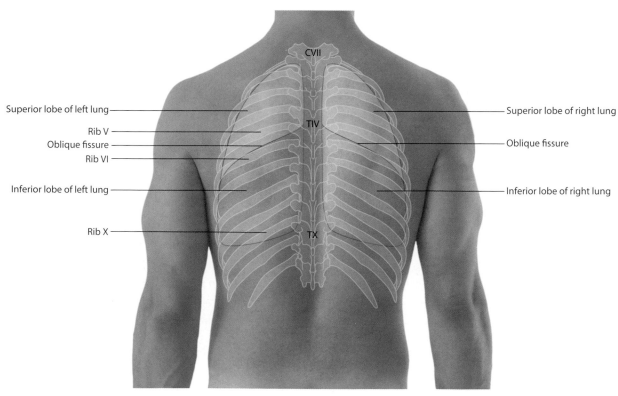

CVII

Superior lobe of left lung

Rib V

Oblique fissure

Rib VI

Inferior lobe of left lung

Rib X

TIV

TX

Superior lobe of right lung

Oblique fissure

Inferior lobe of right lung

Surface projections of the lobes and fissures of the lungs (posterior view)

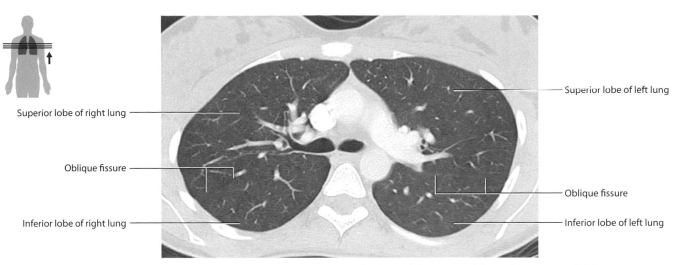

Superior lobe of right lung

Oblique fissure

Inferior lobe of right lung

Superior lobe of left lung

Oblique fissure

Inferior lobe of left lung

Right lung and left lung demonstrating superior and inferior lobes. The oblique fissures are visible.
CT image, with contrast, in axial plane

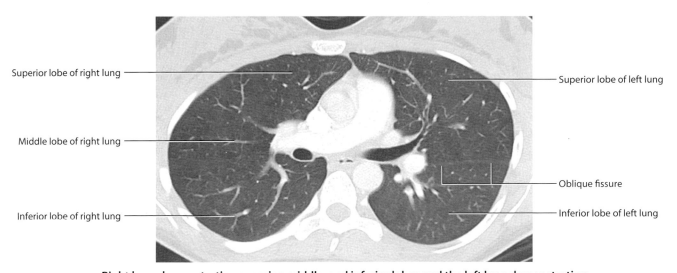

Superior lobe of right lung

Middle lobe of right lung

Inferior lobe of right lung

Superior lobe of left lung

Oblique fissure

Inferior lobe of left lung

Right lung demonstrating superior, middle, and inferior lobes and the left lung demonstrating superior and inferior lobes. The oblique fissure associated with the left lung is visible.
CT image, with contrast, in axial plane

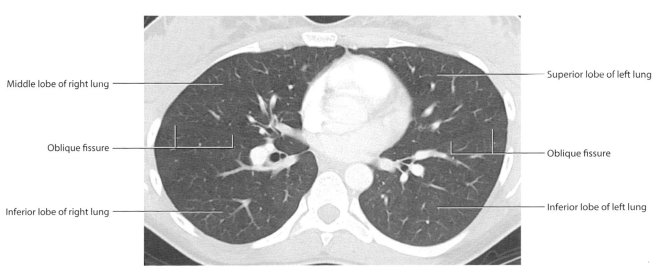

Middle lobe of right lung

Oblique fissure

Inferior lobe of right lung

Superior lobe of left lung

Oblique fissure

Inferior lobe of left lung

Right lung demonstrating middle and inferior lobes and the left lung demonstrating superior and inferior lobes. The oblique fissures are visible.
CT image, with contrast, in axial plane

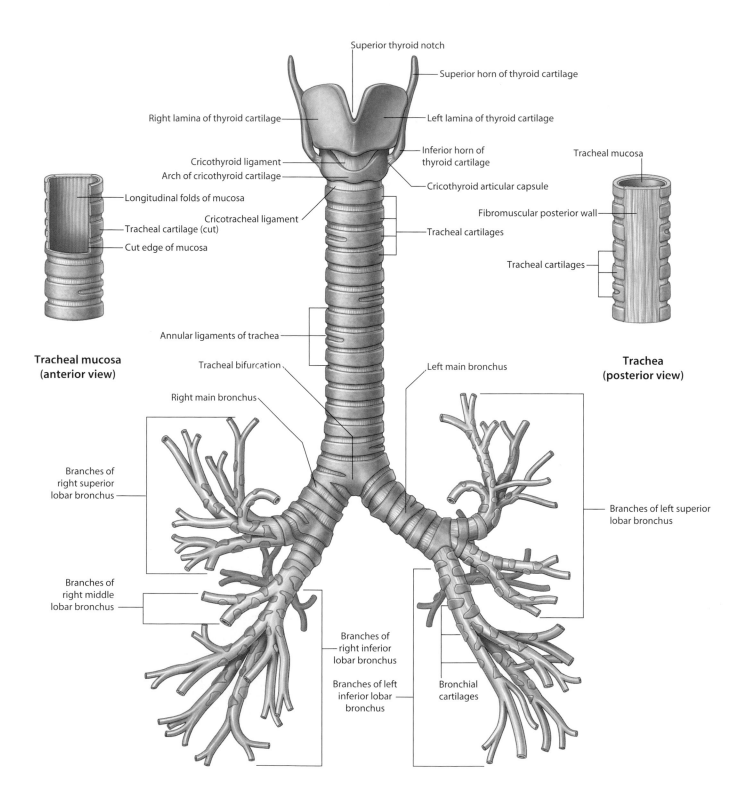

Superior thyroid notch

Superior horn of thyroid cartilage

Right lamina of thyroid cartilage

Left lamina of thyroid cartilage

Cricothyroid ligament

Inferior horn of thyroid cartilage

Arch of cricothyroid cartilage

Cricothyroid articular capsule

Tracheal mucosa

Longitudinal folds of mucosa

Cricotracheal ligament

Fibromuscular posterior wall

Tracheal cartilage (cut)

Tracheal cartilages

Cut edge of mucosa

Tracheal cartilages

**Tracheal mucosa
(anterior view)**

Annular ligaments of trachea

Left main bronchus

**Trachea
(posterior view)**

Tracheal bifurcation

Right main bronchus

Branches of
right superior
lobar bronchus

Branches of left superior
lobar bronchus

Branches of
right middle
lobar bronchus

Branches of
right inferior
lobar bronchus

Branches of left
inferior lobar
bronchus

Bronchial
cartilages

Trachea and bronchial tree

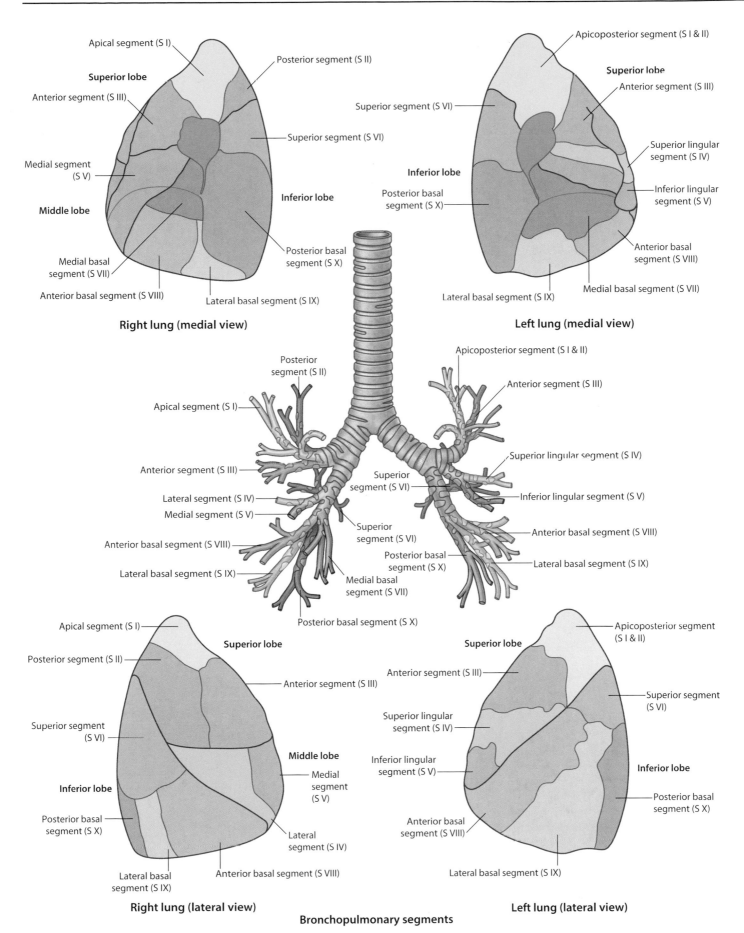

Apical segment (S I)

Superior lobe

Anterior segment (S III)

Posterior segment (S II)

Superior segment (S VI)

Medial segment (S V)

Middle lobe

Medial basal segment (S VII)

Anterior basal segment (S VIII)

Lateral basal segment (S IX)

Inferior lobe

Posterior basal segment (S X)

Right lung (medial view)

Apicoposterior segment (S I & II)

Superior lobe

Anterior segment (S III)

Superior segment (S VI)

Superior lingular segment (S IV)

Inferior lobe

Posterior basal segment (S X)

Inferior lingular segment (S V)

Anterior basal segment (S VIII)

Lateral basal segment (S IX)

Medial basal segment (S VII)

Left lung (medial view)

Posterior segment (S II)

Apical segment (S I)

Anterior segment (S III)

Lateral segment (S IV)

Medial segment (S V)

Anterior basal segment (S VIII)

Lateral basal segment (S IX)

Posterior basal segment (S X)

Medial basal segment (S VII)

Superior segment (S VI)

Superior segment (S VI)

Apicoposterior segment (S I & II)

Anterior segment (S III)

Superior lingular segment (S IV)

Inferior lingular segment (S V)

Anterior basal segment (S VIII)

Lateral basal segment (S IX)

Apical segment (S I)

Posterior segment (S II)

Superior segment (S VI)

Inferior lobe

Posterior basal segment (S X)

Lateral basal segment (S IX)

Anterior basal segment (S VIII)

Superior lobe

Anterior segment (S III)

Middle lobe

Medial segment (S V)

Lateral segment (S IV)

Right lung (lateral view)

Superior lobe

Anterior segment (S III)

Superior lingular segment (S IV)

Inferior lingular segment (S V)

Anterior basal segment (S VIII)

Apicoposterior segment (S I & II)

Superior segment (S VI)

Inferior lobe

Posterior basal segment (S X)

Lateral basal segment (S IX)

Left lung (lateral view)

Bronchopulmonary segments

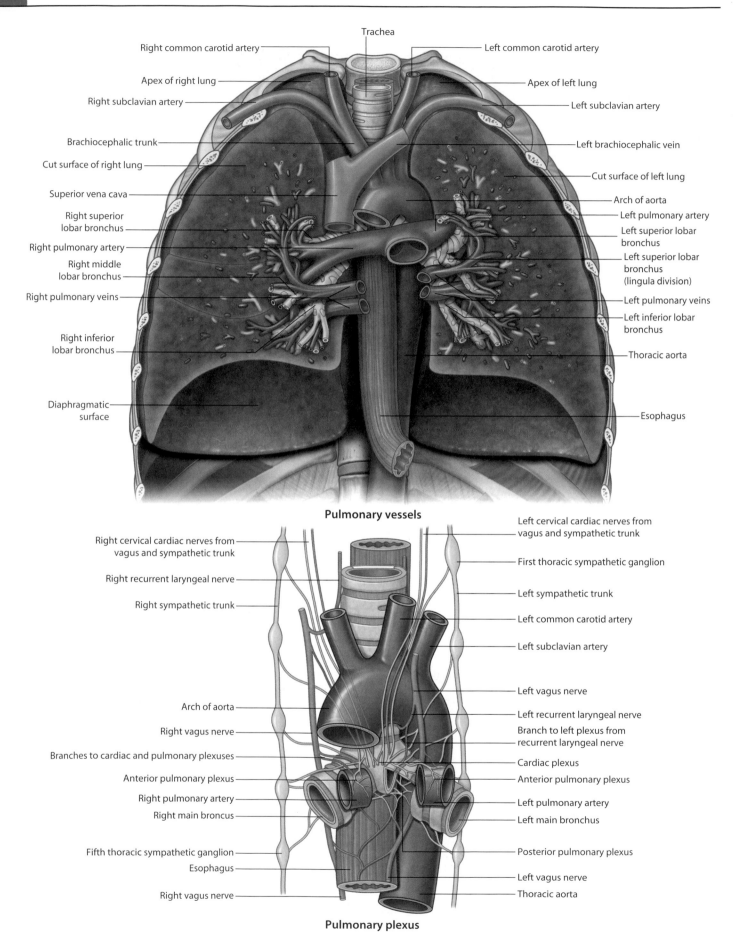

Trachea

Right common carotid artery

Left common carotid artery

Apex of right lung

Apex of left lung

Right subclavian artery

Left subclavian artery

Brachiocephalic trunk

Left brachiocephalic vein

Cut surface of right lung

Cut surface of left lung

Superior vena cava

Arch of aorta

Right superior lobar bronchus

Left pulmonary artery

Right pulmonary artery

Left superior lobar bronchus

Right middle lobar bronchus

Left superior lobar bronchus (lingula division)

Right pulmonary veins

Left pulmonary veins

Left inferior lobar bronchus

Right inferior lobar bronchus

Thoracic aorta

Diaphragmatic surface

Esophagus

Pulmonary vessels

Right cervical cardiac nerves from vagus and sympathetic trunk

Left cervical cardiac nerves from vagus and sympathetic trunk

First thoracic sympathetic ganglion

Right recurrent laryngeal nerve

Left sympathetic trunk

Right sympathetic trunk

Left common carotid artery

Left subclavian artery

Left vagus nerve

Arch of aorta

Left recurrent laryngeal nerve

Right vagus nerve

Branch to left plexus from recurrent laryngeal nerve

Branches to cardiac and pulmonary plexuses

Cardiac plexus

Anterior pulmonary plexus

Anterior pulmonary plexus

Right pulmonary artery

Left pulmonary artery

Right main broncus

Left main bronchus

Fifth thoracic sympathetic ganglion

Posterior pulmonary plexus

Esophagus

Left vagus nerve

Right vagus nerve

Thoracic aorta

Pulmonary plexus

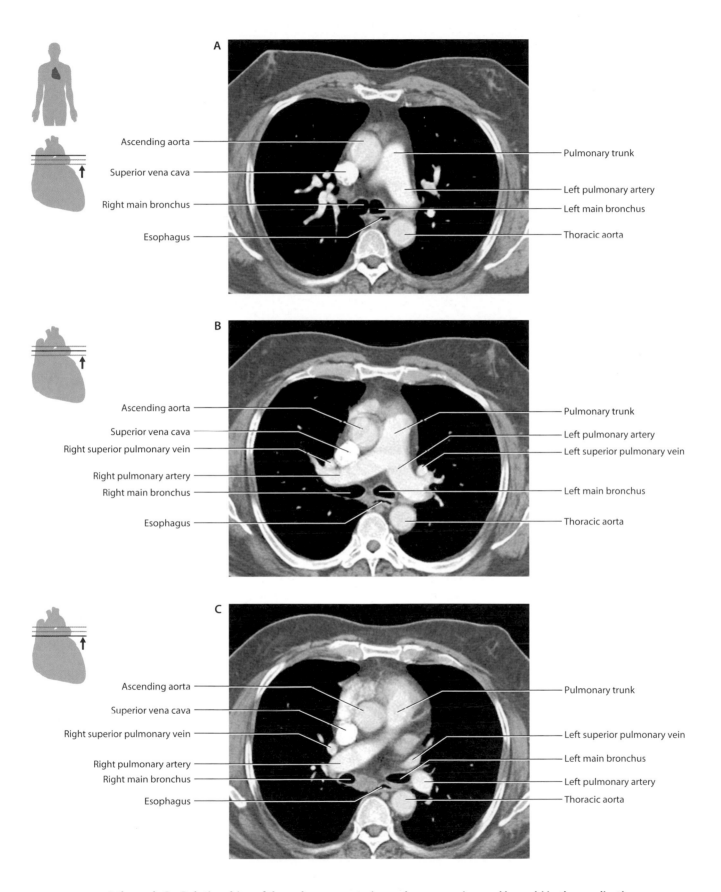

A — Ascending aorta, Superior vena cava, Right main bronchus, Esophagus, Pulmonary trunk, Left pulmonary artery, Left main bronchus, Thoracic aorta

B — Ascending aorta, Superior vena cava, Right superior pulmonary vein, Right pulmonary artery, Right main bronchus, Esophagus, Pulmonary trunk, Left pulmonary artery, Left superior pulmonary vein, Left main bronchus, Thoracic aorta

C — Ascending aorta, Superior vena cava, Right superior pulmonary vein, Right pulmonary artery, Right main bronchus, Esophagus, Pulmonary trunk, Left superior pulmonary vein, Left main bronchus, Left pulmonary artery, Thoracic aorta

A through C – Relationships of the pulmonary arteries, pulmonary veins, and bronchi in the mediastinum.
CT images, with contrast, in axial plane

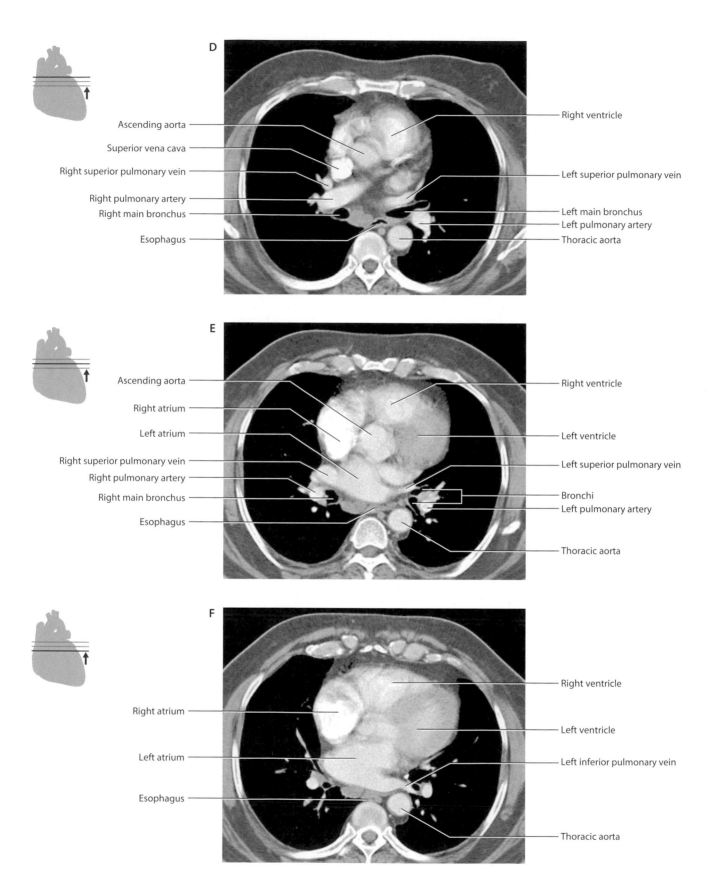

D

Ascending aorta
Superior vena cava
Right superior pulmonary vein
Right pulmonary artery
Right main bronchus
Esophagus

Right ventricle

Left superior pulmonary vein

Left main bronchus
Left pulmonary artery
Thoracic aorta

E

Ascending aorta
Right atrium
Left atrium
Right superior pulmonary vein
Right pulmonary artery
Right main bronchus
Esophagus

Right ventricle

Left ventricle

Left superior pulmonary vein

Bronchi
Left pulmonary artery
Thoracic aorta

F

Right atrium
Left atrium
Esophagus

Right ventricle

Left ventricle

Left inferior pulmonary vein

Thoracic aorta

D through F – Relationships of the pulmonary arteries, pulmonary veins, and bronchi in the mediastinum.
CT images, with contrast, in axial plane

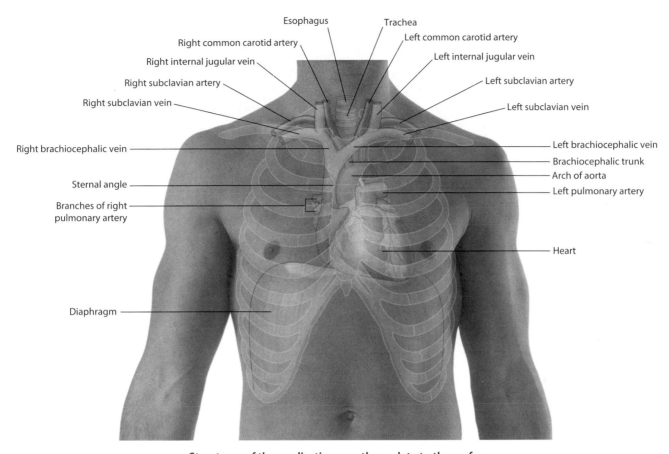

Structures of the mediastinum as they relate to the surface

- Esophagus
- Trachea
- Right common carotid artery
- Left common carotid artery
- Right internal jugular vein
- Left internal jugular vein
- Right subclavian artery
- Left subclavian artery
- Right subclavian vein
- Left subclavian vein
- Right brachiocephalic vein
- Left brachiocephalic vein
- Brachiocephalic trunk
- Sternal angle
- Arch of aorta
- Branches of right pulmonary artery
- Left pulmonary artery
- Heart
- Diaphragm

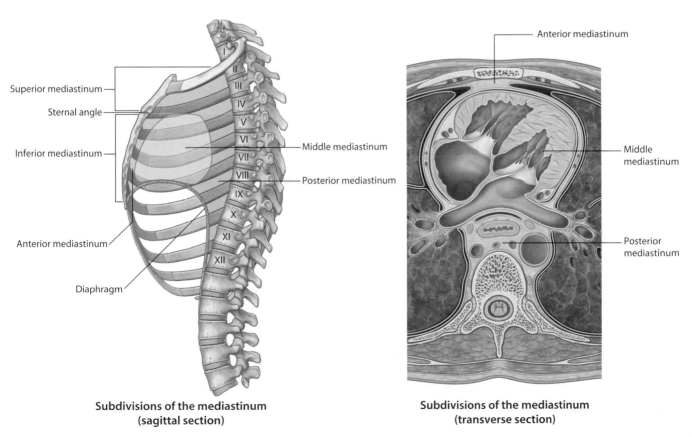

- Superior mediastinum
- Sternal angle
- Inferior mediastinum
- Middle mediastinum
- Posterior mediastinum
- Anterior mediastinum
- Diaphragm

Subdivisions of the mediastinum (sagittal section)

- Anterior mediastinum
- Middle mediastinum
- Posterior mediastinum

Subdivisions of the mediastinum (transverse section)

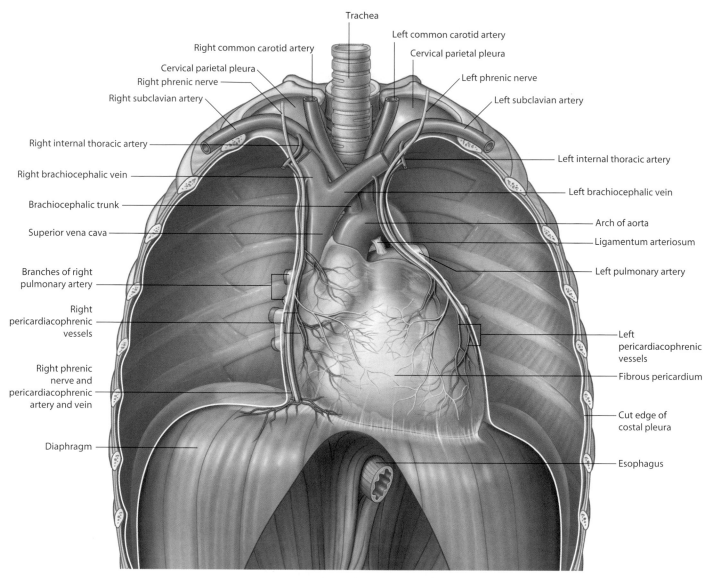

Trachea

Right common carotid artery

Cervical parietal pleura

Right phrenic nerve

Right subclavian artery

Left common carotid artery

Cervical parietal pleura

Left phrenic nerve

Left subclavian artery

Right internal thoracic artery

Right brachiocephalic vein

Brachiocephalic trunk

Superior vena cava

Branches of right pulmonary artery

Right pericardiacophrenic vessels

Right phrenic nerve and pericardiacophrenic artery and vein

Diaphragm

Left internal thoracic artery

Left brachiocephalic vein

Arch of aorta

Ligamentum arteriosum

Left pulmonary artery

Left pericardiacophrenic vessels

Fibrous pericardium

Cut edge of costal pleura

Esophagus

Pericardium with nerves and vessels

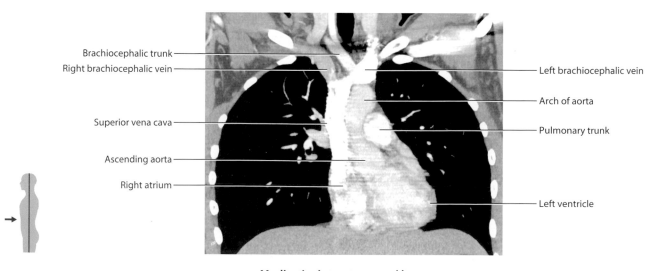

Brachiocephalic trunk

Right brachiocephalic vein

Superior vena cava

Ascending aorta

Right atrium

Left brachiocephalic vein

Arch of aorta

Pulmonary trunk

Left ventricle

Mediastinal structures and lungs.
CT image, with contrast, in coronal plane

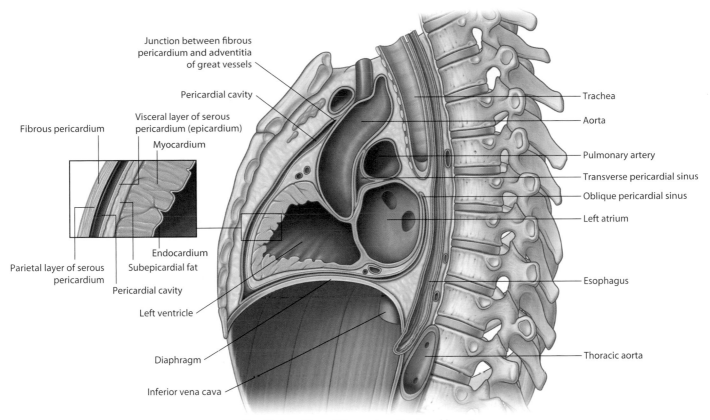

Junction between fibrous pericardium and adventitia of great vessels

Pericardial cavity

Visceral layer of serous pericardium (epicardium)

Myocardium

Fibrous pericardium

Parietal layer of serous pericardium

Subepicardial fat

Pericardial cavity

Endocardium

Left ventricle

Diaphragm

Inferior vena cava

Trachea

Aorta

Pulmonary artery

Transverse pericardial sinus

Oblique pericardial sinus

Left atrium

Esophagus

Thoracic aorta

Sagittal section of the pericardium and heart

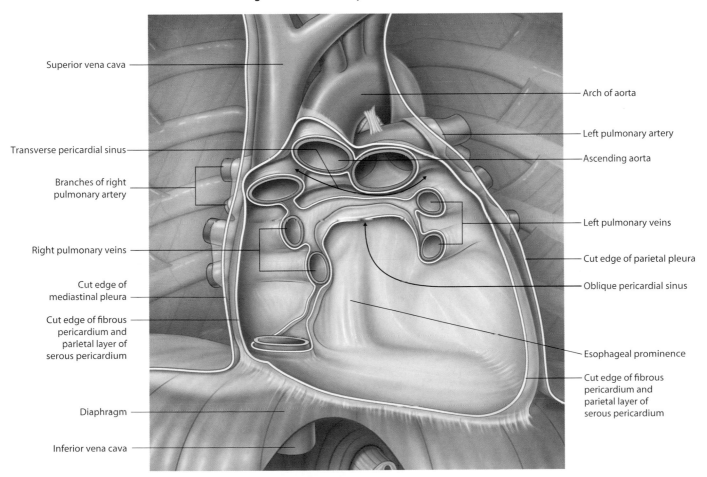

Superior vena cava

Transverse pericardial sinus

Branches of right pulmonary artery

Right pulmonary veins

Cut edge of mediastinal pleura

Cut edge of fibrous pericardium and parietal layer of serous pericardium

Diaphragm

Inferior vena cava

Arch of aorta

Left pulmonary artery

Ascending aorta

Left pulmonary veins

Cut edge of parietal pleura

Oblique pericardial sinus

Esophageal prominence

Cut edge of fibrous pericardium and parietal layer of serous pericardium

Pericardial sac with heart removed

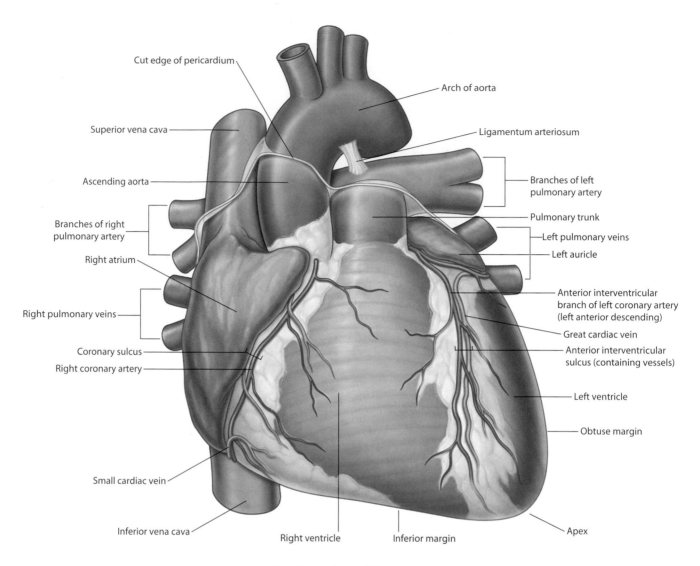

Cut edge of pericardium

Arch of aorta

Superior vena cava

Ligamentum arteriosum

Ascending aorta

Branches of left pulmonary artery

Branches of right pulmonary artery

Pulmonary trunk

Left pulmonary veins

Left auricle

Right atrium

Anterior interventricular branch of left coronary artery (left anterior descending)

Right pulmonary veins

Great cardiac vein

Anterior interventricular sulcus (containing vessels)

Coronary sulcus

Left ventricle

Right coronary artery

Obtuse margin

Small cardiac vein

Left ventricle

Inferior vena cava

Right ventricle

Inferior margin

Apex

Anterior surface of the heart

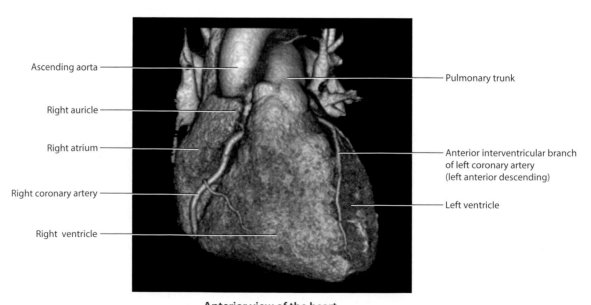

Ascending aorta

Pulmonary trunk

Right auricle

Right atrium

Anterior interventricular branch of left coronary artery (left anterior descending)

Right coronary artery

Left ventricle

Right ventricle

Anterior view of the heart.
Volume-rendered anterior view using multidetector computed tomography

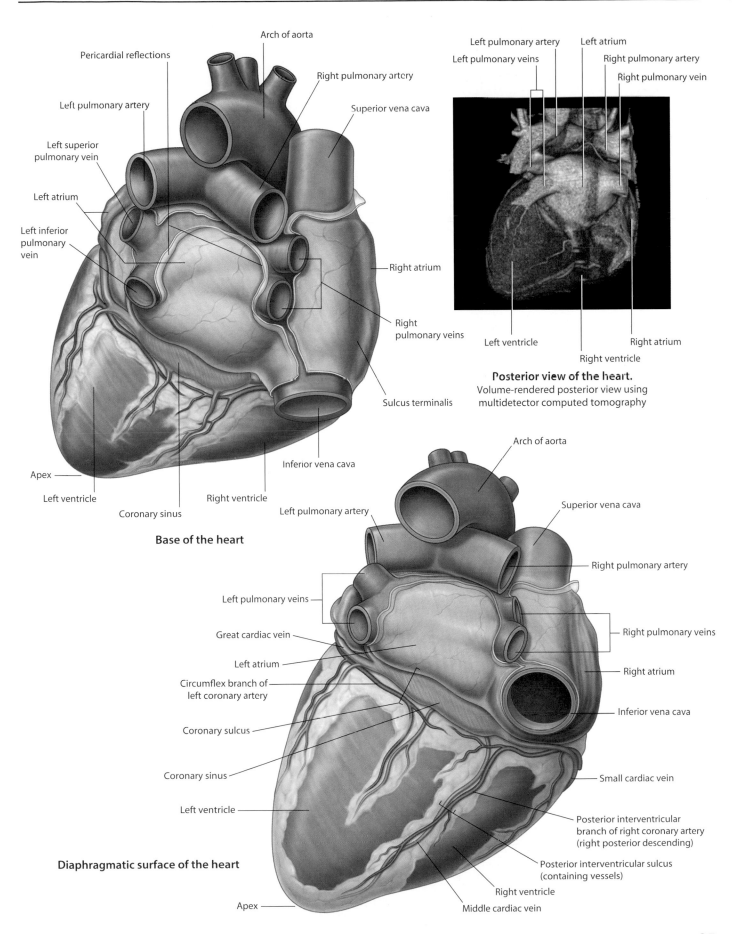

Base of the heart

Posterior view of the heart.
Volume-rendered posterior view using
multidetector computed tomography

Diaphragmatic surface of the heart

95

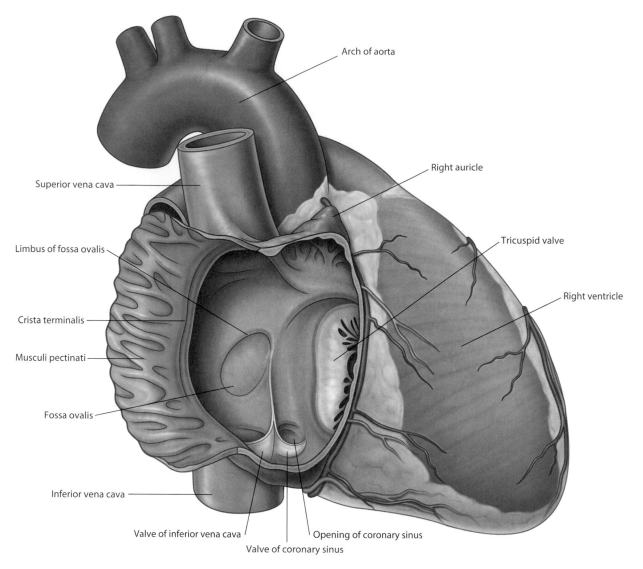

Arch of aorta

Superior vena cava

Right auricle

Limbus of fossa ovalis

Tricuspid valve

Crista terminalis

Right ventricle

Musculi pectinati

Fossa ovalis

Inferior vena cava

Valve of inferior vena cava

Opening of coronary sinus

Valve of coronary sinus

Internal view of right atrium

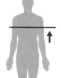

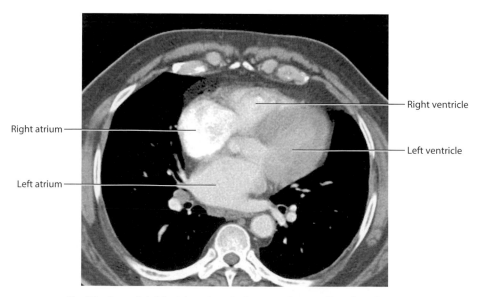

Right ventricle

Right atrium

Left ventricle

Left atrium

Positioning of right atrium in relation to other cardiac chambers.
CT image, with contrast, in axial plane

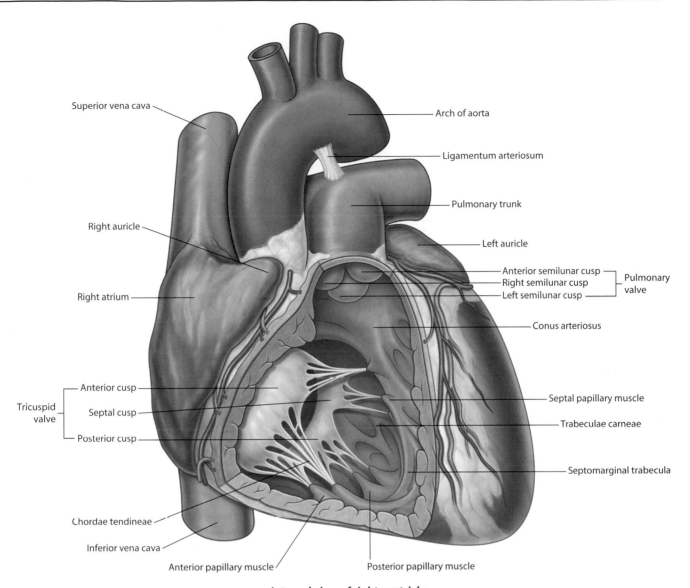

Superior vena cava

Arch of aorta

Ligamentum arteriosum

Pulmonary trunk

Right auricle

Left auricle

Anterior semilunar cusp
Right semilunar cusp
Left semilunar cusp　} Pulmonary valve

Right atrium

Conus arteriosus

Anterior cusp

Septal cusp

Posterior cusp

Tricuspid valve

Septal papillary muscle

Trabeculae carneae

Septomarginal trabecula

Chordae tendineae

Inferior vena cava

Anterior papillary muscle

Posterior papillary muscle

Internal view of right ventricle

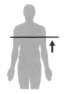

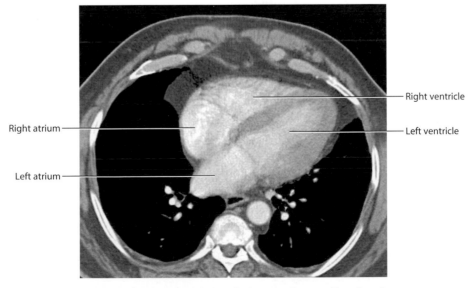

Right ventricle

Right atrium

Left ventricle

Left atrium

Positioning of right ventricle in relation to other cardiac chambers.
CT image, with contrast, in axial plane

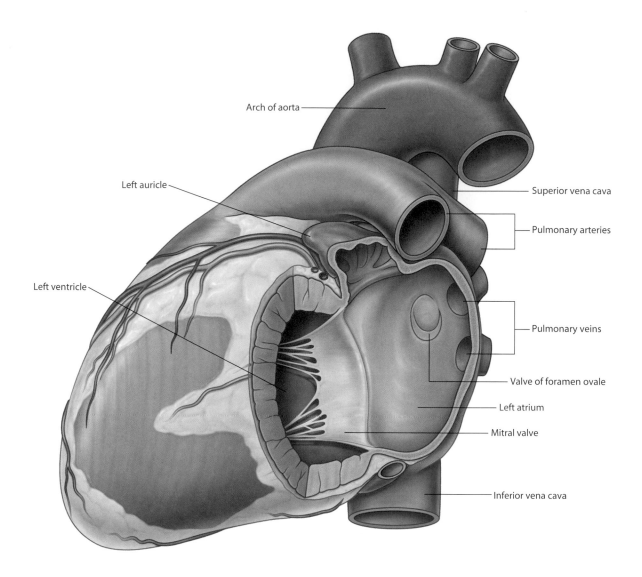

Arch of aorta

Left auricle

Left ventricle

Superior vena cava

Pulmonary arteries

Pulmonary veins

Valve of foramen ovale

Left atrium

Mitral valve

Inferior vena cava

Internal view of left atrium

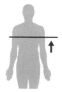

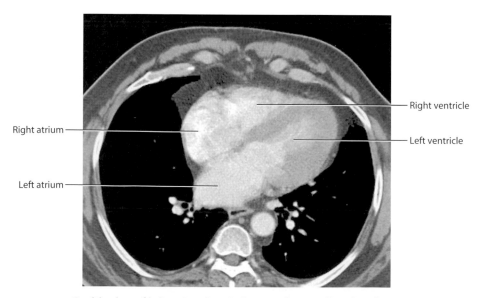

Right ventricle

Right atrium

Left ventricle

Left atrium

Positioning of left atrium in relation to other cardiac chambers.
CT image, with contrast, in axial plane

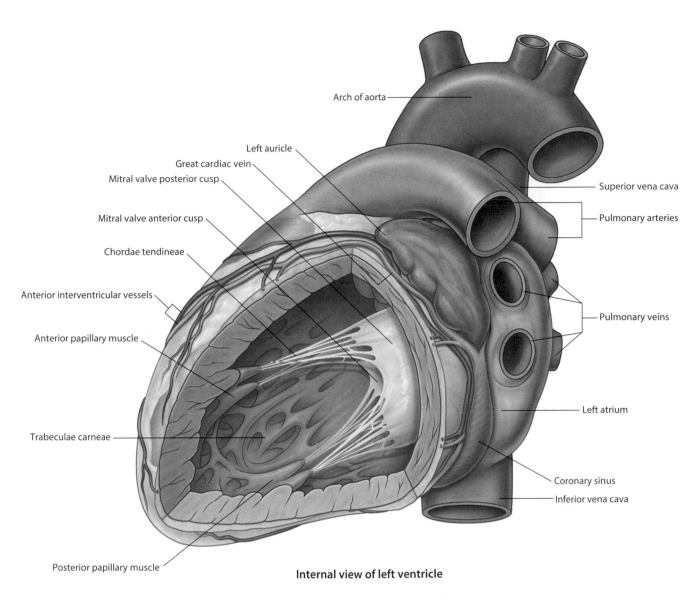

Arch of aorta

Left auricle

Great cardiac vein

Mitral valve posterior cusp

Mitral valve anterior cusp

Chordae tendineae

Anterior interventricular vessels

Anterior papillary muscle

Trabeculae carneae

Posterior papillary muscle

Superior vena cava

Pulmonary arteries

Pulmonary veins

Left atrium

Coronary sinus

Inferior vena cava

Internal view of left ventricle

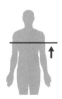

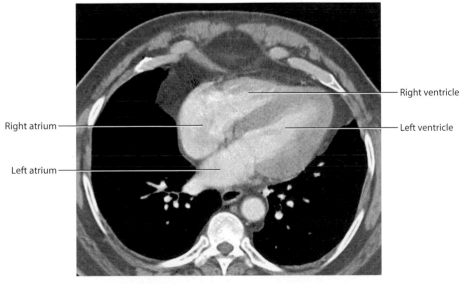

Right atrium

Left atrium

Right ventricle

Left ventricle

Positioning of left ventricle in relation to other cardiac chambers.
CT image, with contrast, in axial plane

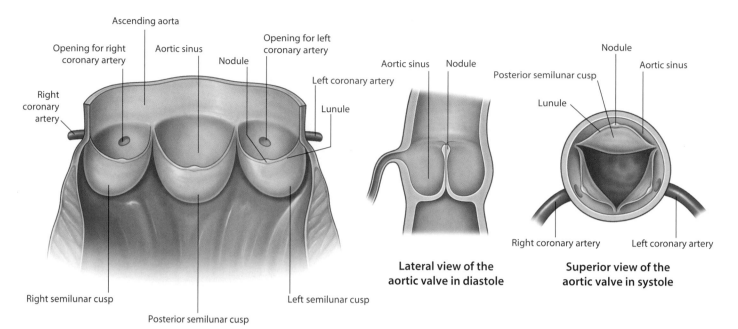

Ascending aorta

Opening for right
coronary artery

Aortic sinus

Nodule

Opening for left
coronary artery

Left coronary artery

Right
coronary
artery

Lunule

Right semilunar cusp

Posterior semilunar cusp

Left semilunar cusp

**Anterior view of the aortic valve
(resected and opened out)**

Aortic sinus

Nodule

**Lateral view of the
aortic valve in diastole**

Nodule

Posterior semilunar cusp

Aortic sinus

Lunule

Right coronary artery

Left coronary artery

**Superior view of the
aortic valve in systole**

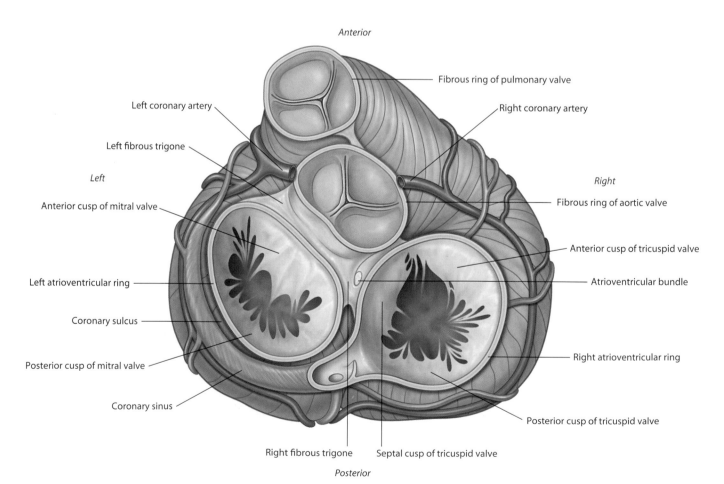

Anterior

Left coronary artery

Left fibrous trigone

Left

Anterior cusp of mitral valve

Left atrioventricular ring

Coronary sulcus

Posterior cusp of mitral valve

Coronary sinus

Fibrous ring of pulmonary valve

Right coronary artery

Right

Fibrous ring of aortic valve

Anterior cusp of tricuspid valve

Atrioventricular bundle

Right atrioventricular ring

Posterior cusp of tricuspid valve

Right fibrous trigone

Septal cusp of tricuspid valve

Posterior

**Cardiac skeleton (superior view;
atria removed)**

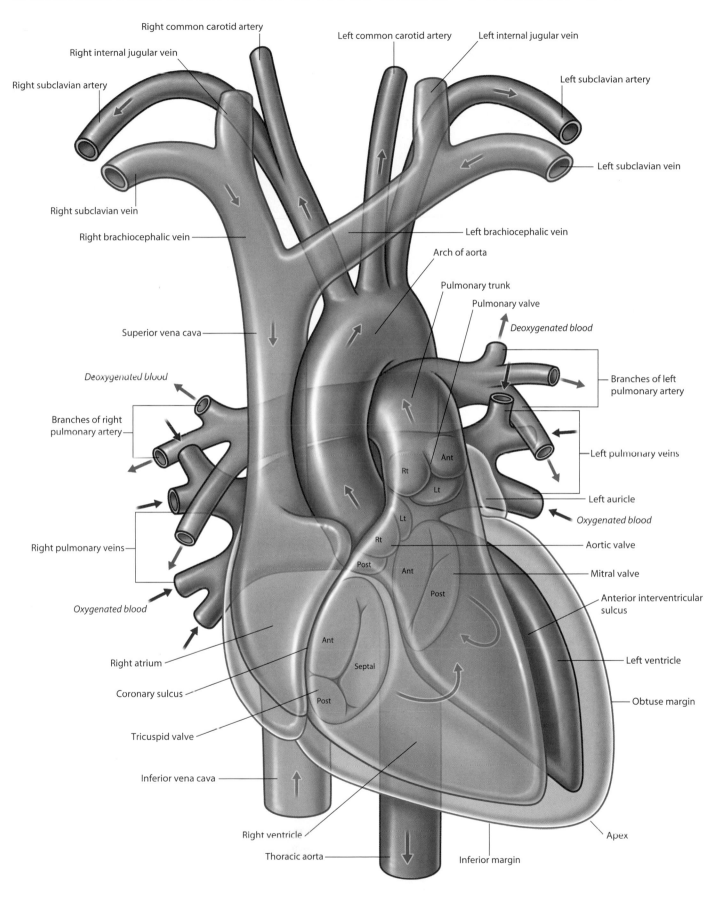

Right common carotid artery

Right internal jugular vein

Right subclavian artery

Left common carotid artery

Left internal jugular vein

Left subclavian artery

Left subclavian vein

Right subclavian vein

Right brachiocephalic vein

Left brachiocephalic vein

Arch of aorta

Pulmonary trunk

Pulmonary valve

Superior vena cava

Deoxygenated blood

Deoxygenated blood

Branches of left
pulmonary artery

Branches of right
pulmonary artery

Ant

Rt

Lt

Left pulmonary veins

Lt

Left auricle

Rt

Oxygenated blood

Right pulmonary veins

Post

Ant

Aortic valve

Post

Mitral valve

Oxygenated blood

Ant

Anterior interventricular
sulcus

Right atrium

Septal

Left ventricle

Coronary sulcus

Post

Obtuse margin

Tricuspid valve

Inferior vena cava

Right ventricle

Thoracic aorta

Inferior margin

Apex

Cardiac chambers and direction of blood flow

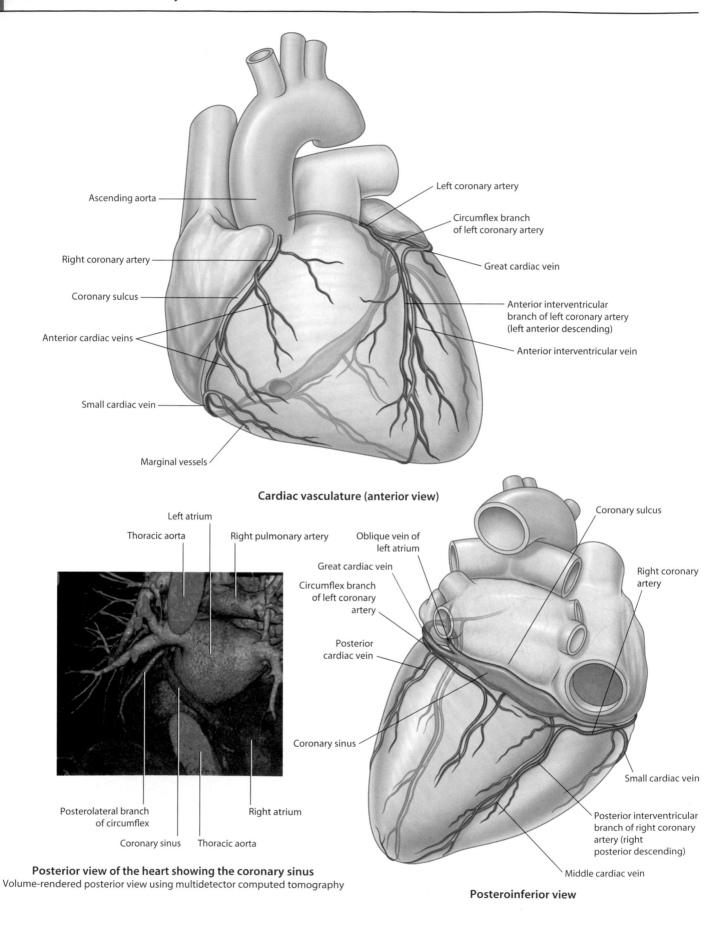

Ascending aorta

Right coronary artery

Coronary sulcus

Anterior cardiac veins

Small cardiac vein

Marginal vessels

Left coronary artery

Circumflex branch
of left coronary artery

Great cardiac vein

Anterior interventricular
branch of left coronary artery
(left anterior descending)

Anterior interventricular vein

Cardiac vasculature (anterior view)

Thoracic aorta

Left atrium

Right pulmonary artery

Posterolateral branch
of circumflex

Coronary sinus

Thoracic aorta

Right atrium

Posterior view of the heart showing the coronary sinus
Volume-rendered posterior view using multidetector computed tomography

Coronary sulcus

Oblique vein of
left atrium

Great cardiac vein

Circumflex branch
of left coronary
artery

Right coronary
artery

Posterior
cardiac vein

Coronary sinus

Small cardiac vein

Posterior interventricular
branch of right coronary
artery (right
posterior descending)

Middle cardiac vein

Posteroinferior view

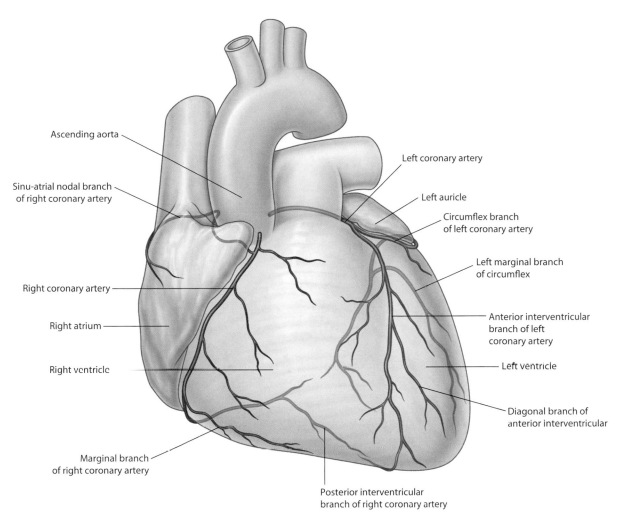

Ascending aorta

Sinu-atrial nodal branch
of right coronary artery

Right coronary artery

Right atrium

Right ventricle

Left coronary artery

Left auricle

Circumflex branch
of left coronary artery

Left marginal branch
of circumflex

Anterior interventricular
branch of left
coronary artery

Left ventricle

Diagonal branch of
anterior interventricular

Marginal branch
of right coronary artery

Posterior interventricular
branch of right coronary artery

Coronary arteries (right dominant system)

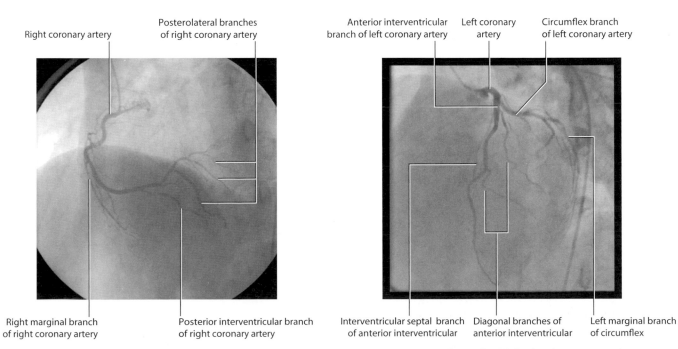

Right coronary artery

Posterolateral branches
of right coronary artery

Anterior interventricular
branch of left coronary artery

Left coronary
artery

Circumflex branch
of left coronary artery

Right marginal branch
of right coronary artery

Posterior interventricular branch
of right coronary artery

Interventricular septal branch
of anterior interventricular

Diagonal branches of
anterior interventricular

Left marginal branch
of circumflex

Coronary angiography (right dominant system).
Left anterior oblique projection, cranial angulation, of right coronary artery

Coronary angiography (right dominant system).
Left anterior oblique projection, cranial angulation, of left coronary artery

103

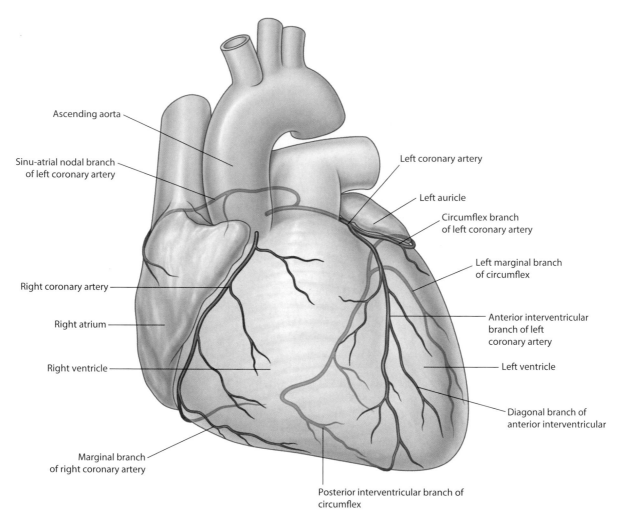

Ascending aorta

Sinu-atrial nodal branch
of left coronary artery

Right coronary artery

Right atrium

Right ventricle

Marginal branch
of right coronary artery

Left coronary artery

Left auricle

Circumflex branch
of left coronary artery

Left marginal branch
of circumflex

Anterior interventricular
branch of left
coronary artery

Left ventricle

Diagonal branch of
anterior interventricular

Posterior interventricular branch of
circumflex

Coronary arteries (left dominant system)

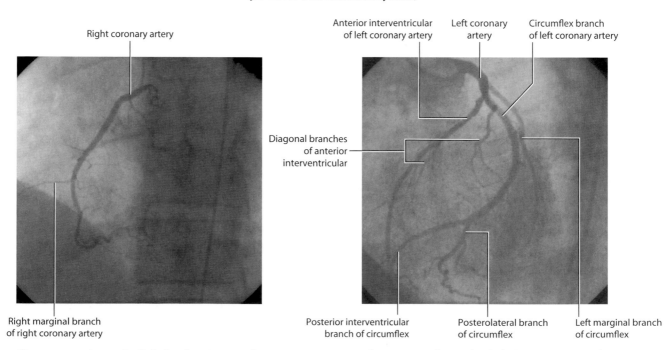

Right coronary artery

Right marginal branch
of right coronary artery

Coronary angiography (left dominant system).
Left anterior oblique projection, cranial angulation, of right coronary artery

Anterior interventricular
of left coronary artery

Left coronary
artery

Circumflex branch
of left coronary artery

Diagonal branches
of anterior
interventricular

Posterior interventricular
branch of circumflex

Posterolateral branch
of circumflex

Left marginal branch
of circumflex

Coronary angiography (left dominant system).
Left anterior oblique projection, cranial angulation, of left coronary artery

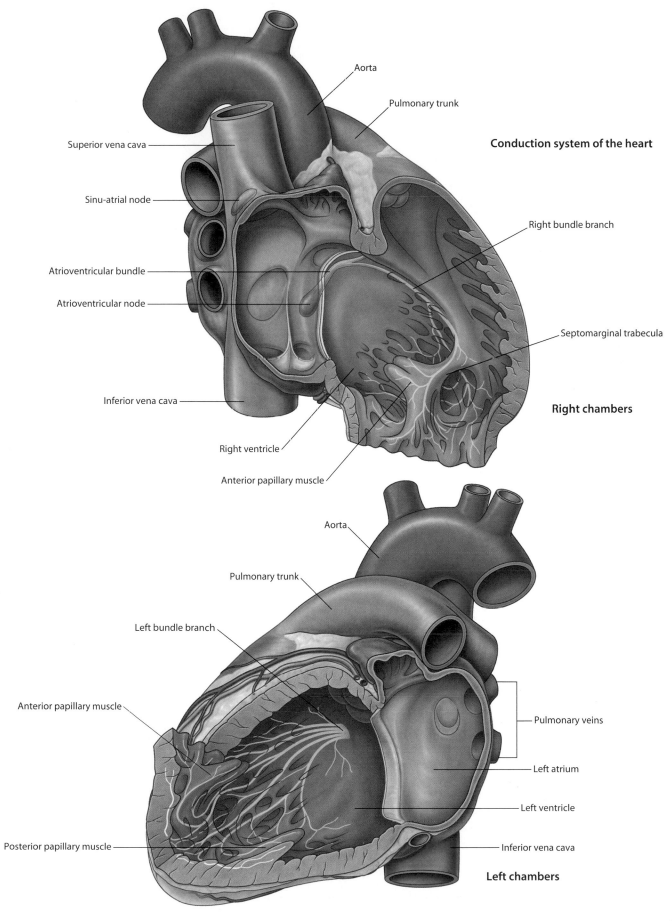

Conduction system of the heart

Aorta

Pulmonary trunk

Superior vena cava

Sinu-atrial node

Right bundle branch

Atrioventricular bundle

Atrioventricular node

Septomarginal trabecula

Inferior vena cava

Right chambers

Right ventricle

Anterior papillary muscle

Aorta

Pulmonary trunk

Left bundle branch

Anterior papillary muscle

Pulmonary veins

Left atrium

Left ventricle

Posterior papillary muscle

Inferior vena cava

Left chambers

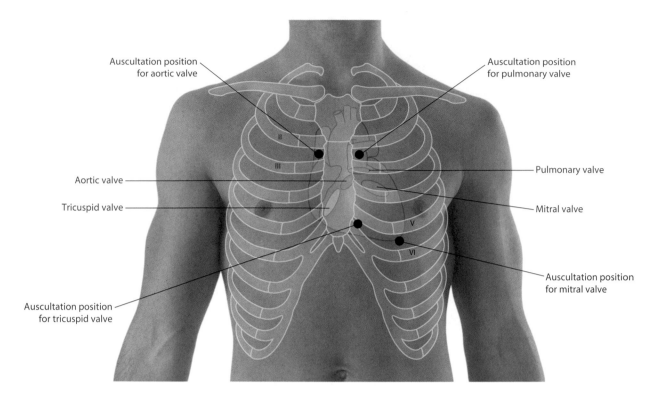

Auscultation position for aortic valve

Auscultation position for pulmonary valve

II

III

Aortic valve

Pulmonary valve

Tricuspid valve

Mitral valve

V

VI

Auscultation position for mitral valve

Auscultation position for tricuspid valve

Auscultation points

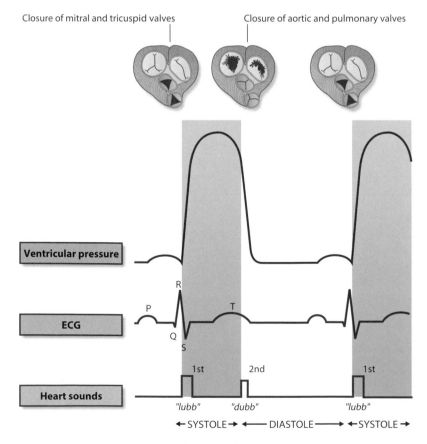

Closure of mitral and tricuspid valves

Closure of aortic and pulmonary valves

Ventricular pressure

R

P

T

ECG

Q

S

1st

2nd

1st

Heart sounds

"lubb"

"dubb"

"lubb"

← SYSTOLE → ← DIASTOLE → ← SYSTOLE →

Cardiac auscultation

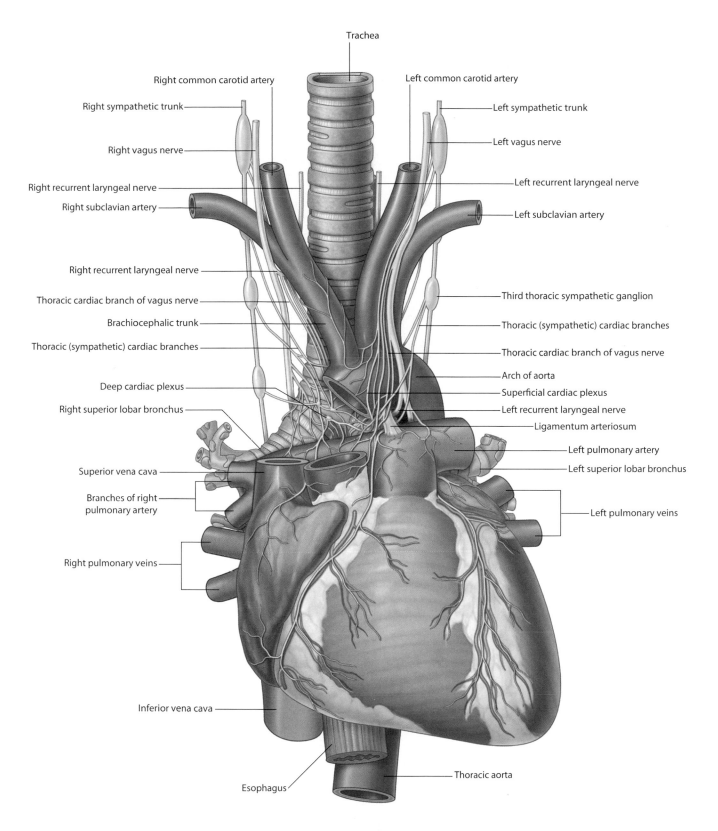

Trachea

Right common carotid artery

Right sympathetic trunk

Right vagus nerve

Right recurrent laryngeal nerve

Right subclavian artery

Right recurrent laryngeal nerve

Thoracic cardiac branch of vagus nerve

Brachiocephalic trunk

Thoracic (sympathetic) cardiac branches

Deep cardiac plexus

Right superior lobar bronchus

Superior vena cava

Branches of right
pulmonary artery

Right pulmonary veins

Inferior vena cava

Esophagus

Left common carotid artery

Left sympathetic trunk

Left vagus nerve

Left recurrent laryngeal nerve

Left subclavian artery

Third thoracic sympathetic ganglion

Thoracic (sympathetic) cardiac branches

Thoracic cardiac branch of vagus nerve

Arch of aorta

Superficial cardiac plexus

Left recurrent laryngeal nerve

Ligamentum arteriosum

Left pulmonary artery

Left superior lobar bronchus

Left pulmonary veins

Thoracic aorta

Cardiac plexus and nerves of the heart

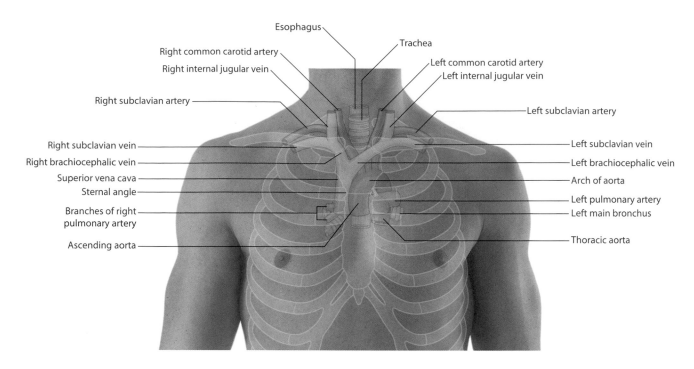

Esophagus
Trachea
Right common carotid artery
Right internal jugular vein
Left common carotid artery
Left internal jugular vein
Right subclavian artery
Left subclavian artery
Right subclavian vein
Left subclavian vein
Right brachiocephalic vein
Left brachiocephalic vein
Superior vena cava
Arch of aorta
Sternal angle
Left pulmonary artery
Branches of right
pulmonary artery
Left main bronchus
Ascending aorta
Thoracic aorta

Surface projections of structures in the superior mediastinum

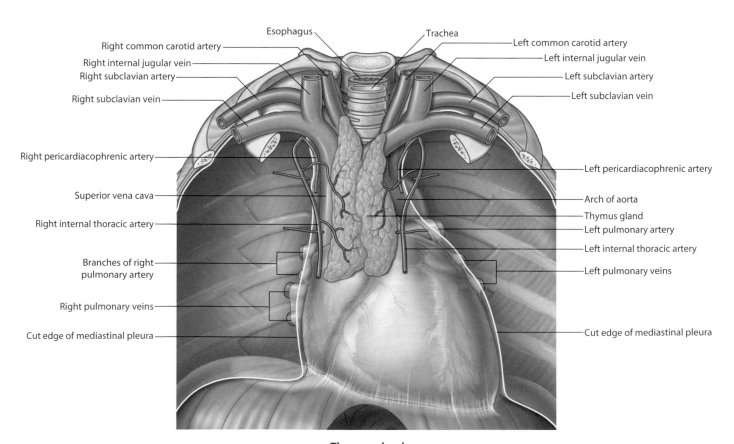

Esophagus
Trachea
Right common carotid artery
Left common carotid artery
Right internal jugular vein
Left internal jugular vein
Right subclavian artery
Left subclavian artery
Right subclavian vein
Left subclavian vein
Right pericardiacophrenic artery
Left pericardiacophrenic artery
Superior vena cava
Arch of aorta
Thymus gland
Right internal thoracic artery
Left pulmonary artery
Left internal thoracic artery
Branches of right
pulmonary artery
Left pulmonary veins
Right pulmonary veins
Cut edge of mediastinal pleura
Cut edge of mediastinal pleura

Thymus gland

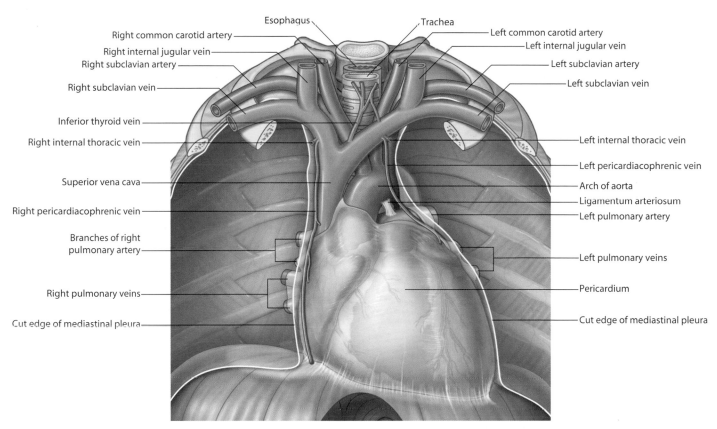

Esophagus — Trachea

Right common carotid artery — Left common carotid artery

Right internal jugular vein — Left internal jugular vein

Right subclavian artery — Left subclavian artery

Right subclavian vein — Left subclavian vein

Inferior thyroid vein — Left internal thoracic vein

Right internal thoracic vein — Left pericardiacophrenic vein

Superior vena cava — Arch of aorta

Right pericardiacophrenic vein — Ligamentum arteriosum

— Left pulmonary artery

Branches of right pulmonary artery — Left pulmonary veins

Right pulmonary veins — Pericardium

Cut edge of mediastinal pleura — Cut edge of mediastinal pleura

Veins of the superior mediastinum

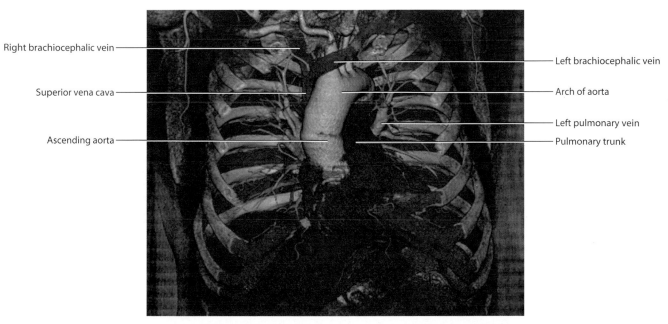

Right brachiocephalic vein — Left brachiocephalic vein

Superior vena cava — Arch of aorta

— Left pulmonary vein

Ascending aorta — Pulmonary trunk

Anterior view of the superior mediastinum showing venous and arterial channels.
Volume-rendered anterior view using multidetector computed tomography

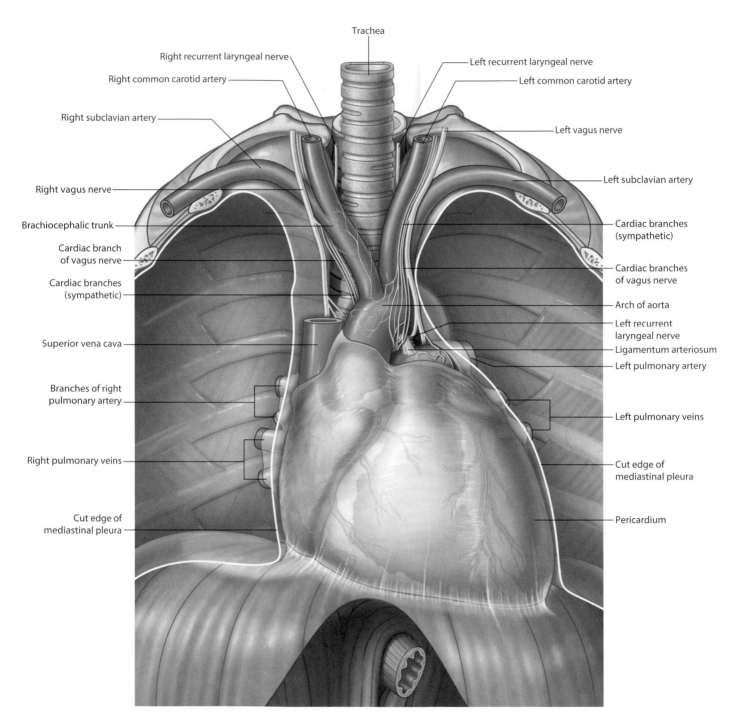

Trachea

Right recurrent laryngeal nerve

Right common carotid artery

Right subclavian artery

Right vagus nerve

Brachiocephalic trunk

Cardiac branch of vagus nerve

Cardiac branches (sympathetic)

Superior vena cava

Branches of right pulmonary artery

Right pulmonary veins

Cut edge of mediastinal pleura

Left recurrent laryngeal nerve

Left common carotid artery

Left vagus nerve

Left subclavian artery

Cardiac branches (sympathetic)

Cardiac branches of vagus nerve

Arch of aorta

Left recurrent laryngeal nerve

Ligamentum arteriosum

Left pulmonary artery

Left pulmonary veins

Cut edge of mediastinal pleura

Pericardium

Arteries and nerves of the superior mediastinum

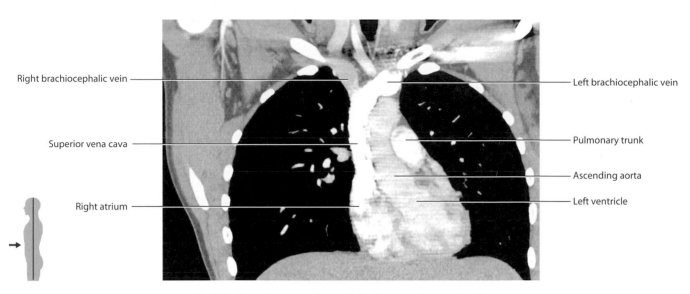

Right brachiocephalic vein

Superior vena cava

Right atrium

Left brachiocephalic vein

Pulmonary trunk

Ascending aorta

Left ventricle

Positioning of venous channels in the superior mediastinum.
CT image, with contrast, in coronal plane

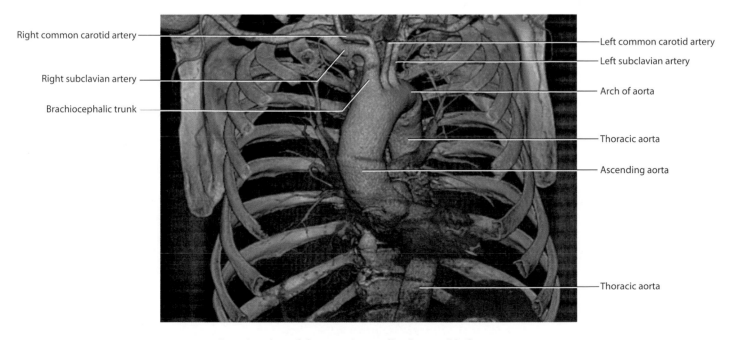

Right common carotid artery

Right subclavian artery

Brachiocephalic trunk

Left common carotid artery

Left subclavian artery

Arch of aorta

Thoracic aorta

Ascending aorta

Thoracic aorta

Anterior view of the superior mediastinum with the venous channels, pulmonary trunk, and heart removed.
Volume-rendered anterior view using multidetector computed tomography

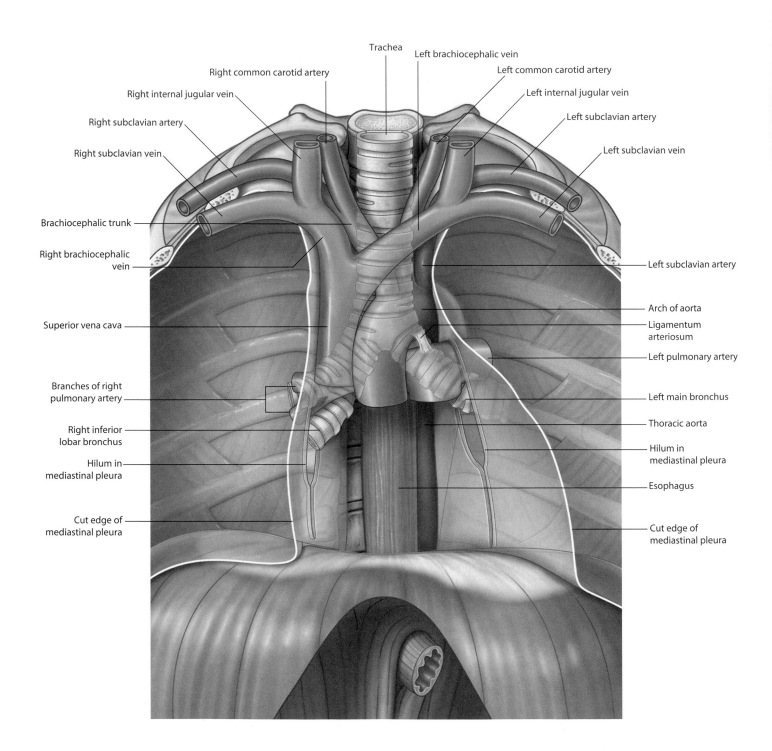

Trachea

Left brachiocephalic vein

Right common carotid artery

Left common carotid artery

Right internal jugular vein

Left internal jugular vein

Right subclavian artery

Left subclavian artery

Right subclavian vein

Left subclavian vein

Brachiocephalic trunk

Right brachiocephalic vein

Left subclavian artery

Arch of aorta

Superior vena cava

Ligamentum arteriosum

Left pulmonary artery

Branches of right pulmonary artery

Left main bronchus

Right inferior lobar bronchus

Thoracic aorta

Hilum in mediastinal pleura

Hilum in mediastinal pleura

Esophagus

Cut edge of mediastinal pleura

Cut edge of mediastinal pleura

Trachea and structures relating to it in the superior mediastinum

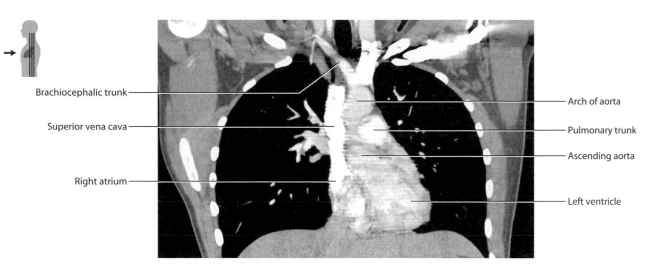

Brachiocephalic trunk

Superior vena cava

Right atrium

Arch of aorta

Pulmonary trunk

Ascending aorta

Left ventricle

Positioning of brachiocephalic trunk in relation to other structures in the superior mediastinum.
CT image, with contrast, in coronal plane

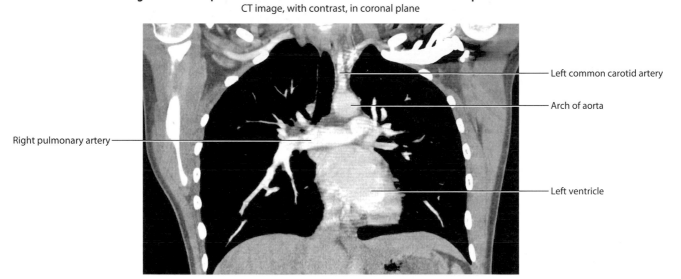

Right pulmonary artery

Left common carotid artery

Arch of aorta

Left ventricle

Positioning of left common carotid artery in relation to other structures in the superior mediastinum.
CT image, with contrast, in coronal plane

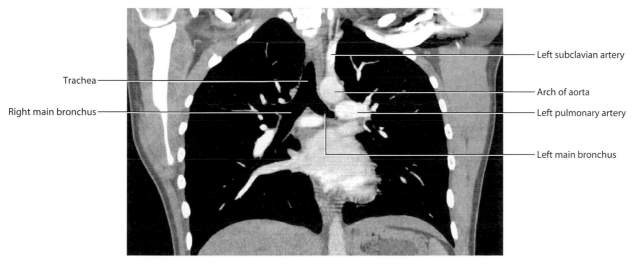

Trachea

Right main bronchus

Left subclavian artery

Arch of aorta

Left pulmonary artery

Left main bronchus

Positioning of left subclavian artery and the bifurcation of the trachea in relation to other structures in the superior mediastinum.
CT image, with contrast, in coronal plane

113

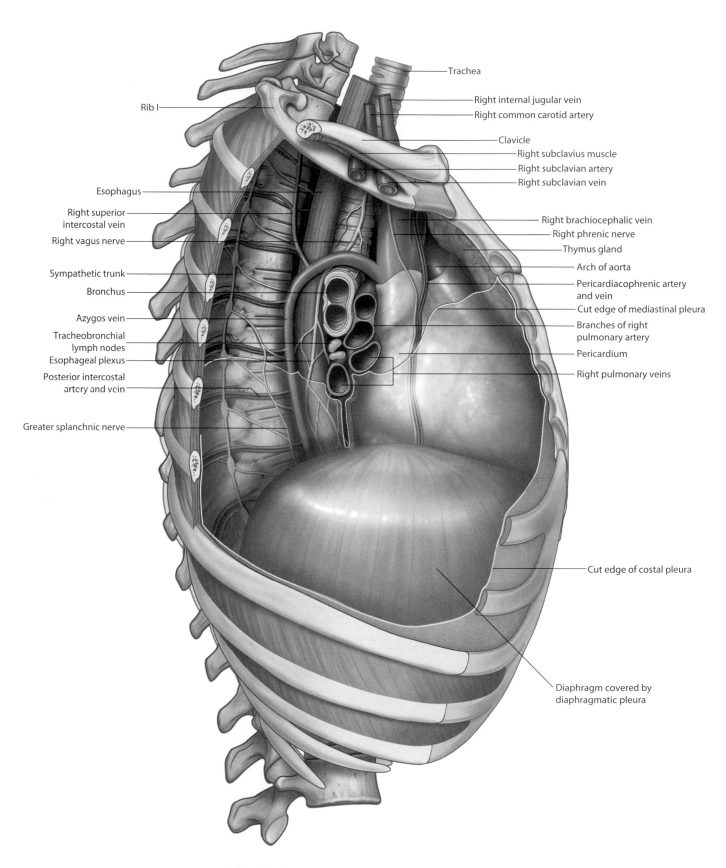

Trachea

Right internal jugular vein

Right common carotid artery

Rib I

Clavicle

Right subclavius muscle

Right subclavian artery

Right subclavian vein

Esophagus

Right superior
intercostal vein

Right brachiocephalic vein

Right phrenic nerve

Right vagus nerve

Thymus gland

Sympathetic trunk

Arch of aorta

Bronchus

Pericardiacophrenic artery
and vein

Azygos vein

Cut edge of mediastinal pleura

Tracheobronchial
lymph nodes

Branches of right
pulmonary artery

Esophageal plexus

Pericardium

Posterior intercostal
artery and vein

Right pulmonary veins

Greater splanchnic nerve

Cut edge of costal pleura

Diaphragm covered by
diaphragmatic pleura

Right side of mediastinum and right thoracic cavity

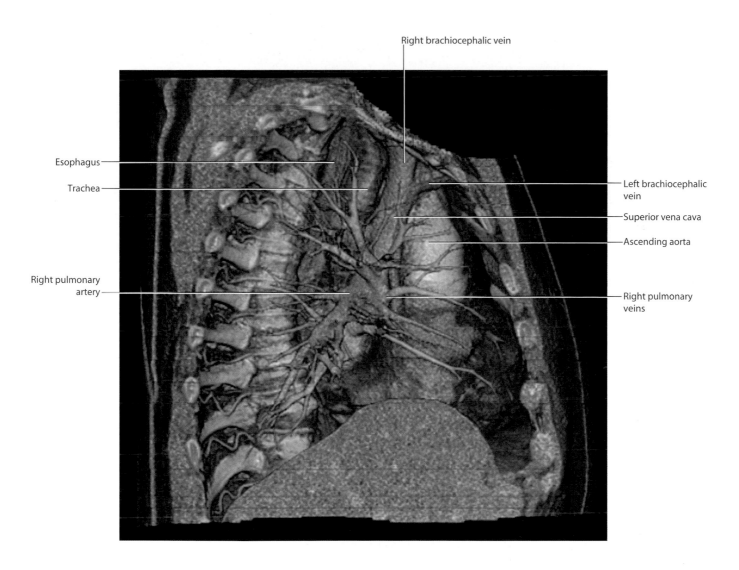

Right brachiocephalic vein

Esophagus

Trachea

Right pulmonary artery

Left brachiocephalic vein

Superior vena cava

Ascending aorta

Right pulmonary veins

View of mediastinal structures from the right side of the thorax.
Volume-rendered lateral view from the right side using multidetector computed tomography

115

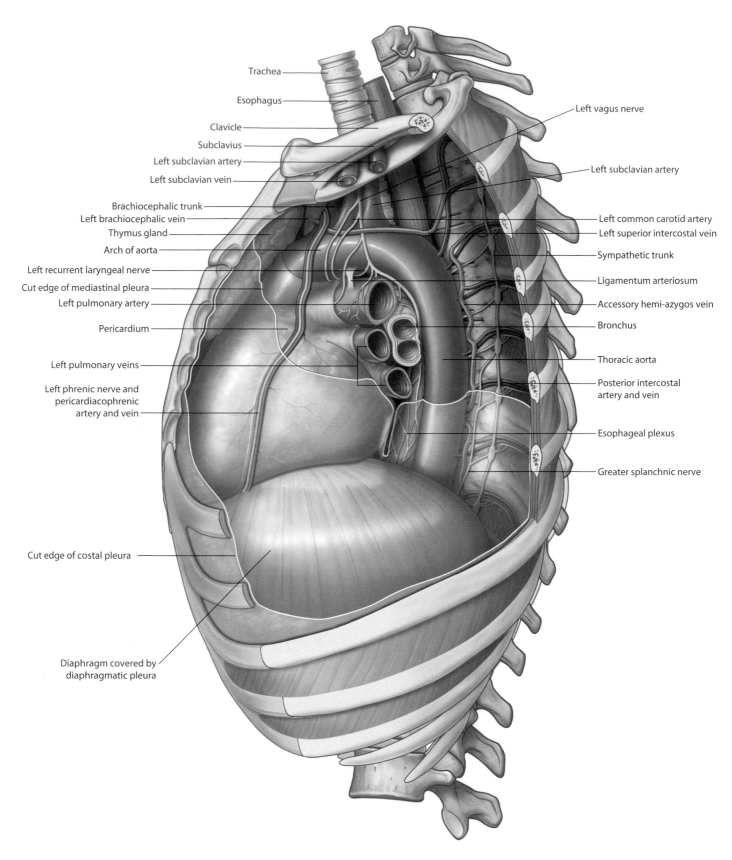

Trachea

Esophagus

Clavicle

Subclavius

Left subclavian artery

Left subclavian vein

Brachiocephalic trunk

Left brachiocephalic vein

Thymus gland

Arch of aorta

Left recurrent laryngeal nerve

Cut edge of mediastinal pleura

Left pulmonary artery

Pericardium

Left pulmonary veins

Left phrenic nerve and
pericardiacophrenic
artery and vein

Cut edge of costal pleura

Diaphragm covered by
diaphragmatic pleura

Left vagus nerve

Left subclavian artery

Left common carotid artery

Left superior intercostal vein

Sympathetic trunk

Ligamentum arteriosum

Accessory hemi-azygos vein

Bronchus

Thoracic aorta

Posterior intercostal
artery and vein

Esophageal plexus

Greater splanchnic nerve

Left side of mediastinum and left thoracic cavity

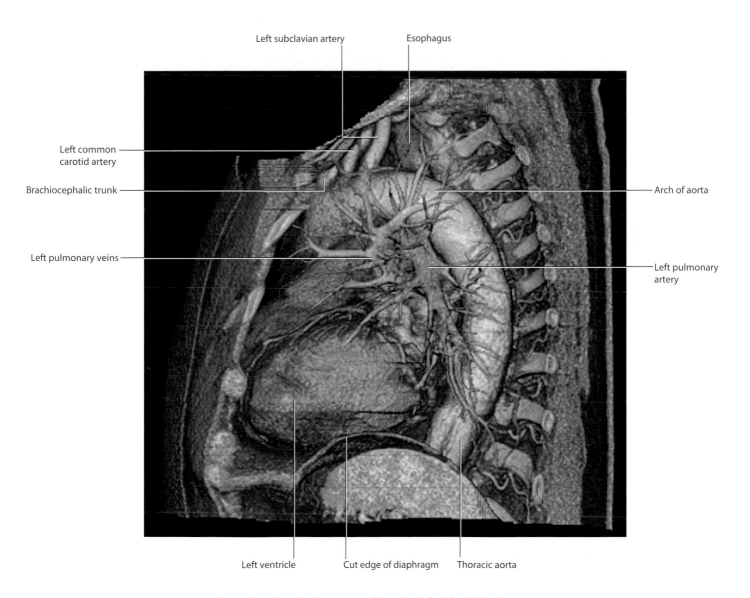

Left subclavian artery   Esophagus

Left common
carotid artery

Brachiocephalic trunk

Arch of aorta

Left pulmonary veins

Left pulmonary
artery

Left ventricle   Cut edge of diaphragm   Thoracic aorta

View of mediastinal structures from the left side of the thorax.
Volume-rendered lateral view from the left side using multidetector computed tomography

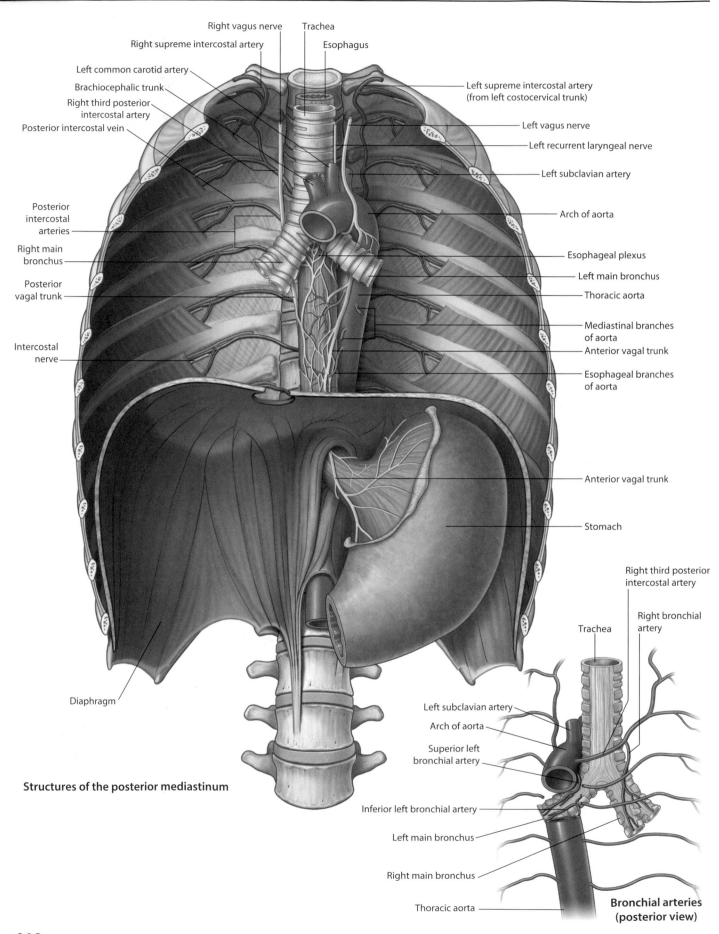

Right vagus nerve

Trachea

Esophagus

Right supreme intercostal artery

Left common carotid artery

Brachiocephalic trunk

Right third posterior intercostal artery

Posterior intercostal vein

Posterior intercostal arteries

Right main bronchus

Posterior vagal trunk

Intercostal nerve

Diaphragm

Left supreme intercostal artery (from left costocervical trunk)

Left vagus nerve

Left recurrent laryngeal nerve

Left subclavian artery

Arch of aorta

Esophageal plexus

Left main bronchus

Thoracic aorta

Mediastinal branches of aorta

Anterior vagal trunk

Esophageal branches of aorta

Anterior vagal trunk

Stomach

Structures of the posterior mediastinum

Right third posterior intercostal artery

Right bronchial artery

Trachea

Left subclavian artery

Arch of aorta

Superior left bronchial artery

Inferior left bronchial artery

Left main bronchus

Right main bronchus

Thoracic aorta

Bronchial arteries (posterior view)

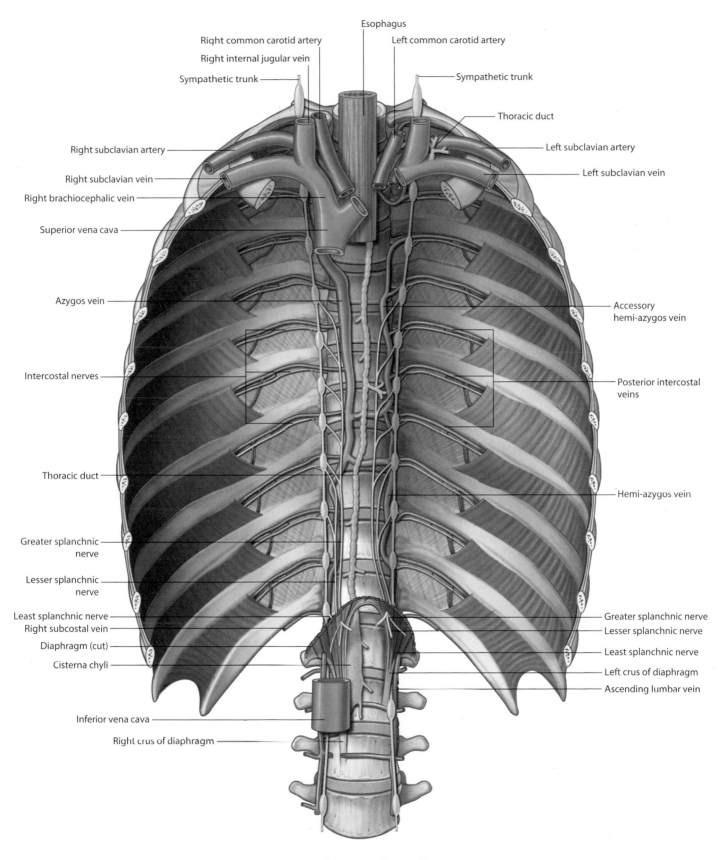

Right common carotid artery

Right internal jugular vein

Sympathetic trunk

Esophagus

Left common carotid artery

Sympathetic trunk

Thoracic duct

Right subclavian artery

Left subclavian artery

Right subclavian vein

Left subclavian vein

Right brachiocephalic vein

Superior vena cava

Azygos vein

Accessory
hemi-azygos vein

Intercostal nerves

Posterior intercostal
veins

Thoracic duct

Hemi-azygos vein

Greater splanchnic
nerve

Lesser splanchnic
nerve

Least splanchnic nerve

Greater splanchnic nerve

Right subcostal vein

Lesser splanchnic nerve

Diaphragm (cut)

Least splanchnic nerve

Cisterna chyli

Left crus of diaphragm

Ascending lumbar vein

Inferior vena cava

Right crus of diaphragm

**Structures of the posterior mediastinum
(thoracic aorta and esophagus removed)**

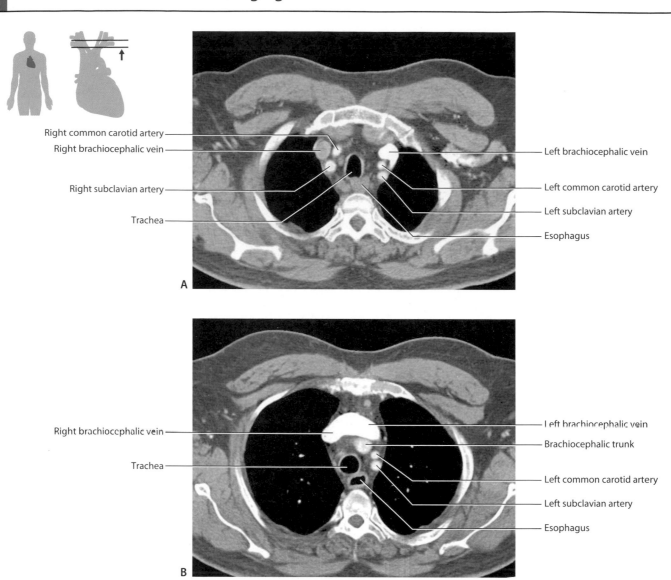

Right common carotid artery
Right brachiocephalic vein

Right subclavian artery

Trachea

Left brachiocephalic vein

Left common carotid artery

Left subclavian artery

Esophagus

A

Right brachiocephalic vein

Trachea

Left brachiocephalic vein

Brachiocephalic trunk

Left common carotid artery

Left subclavian artery

Esophagus

B

A through I – This is a series of images that pass through the thorax from superior to inferior showing the various mediastinal structures and their relationships with each other.

CT images, with contrast, in axial plane

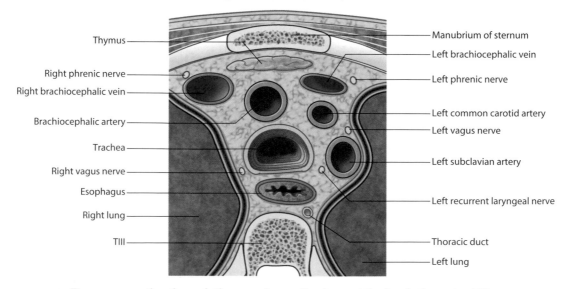

Thymus

Right phrenic nerve

Right brachiocephalic vein

Brachiocephalic artery

Trachea

Right vagus nerve

Esophagus

Right lung

TIII

Manubrium of sternum

Left brachiocephalic vein

Left phrenic nerve

Left common carotid artery

Left vagus nerve

Left subclavian artery

Left recurrent laryngeal nerve

Thoracic duct

Left lung

Transverse section through the superior mediastinum at the level of vertebra TIII

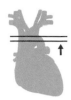

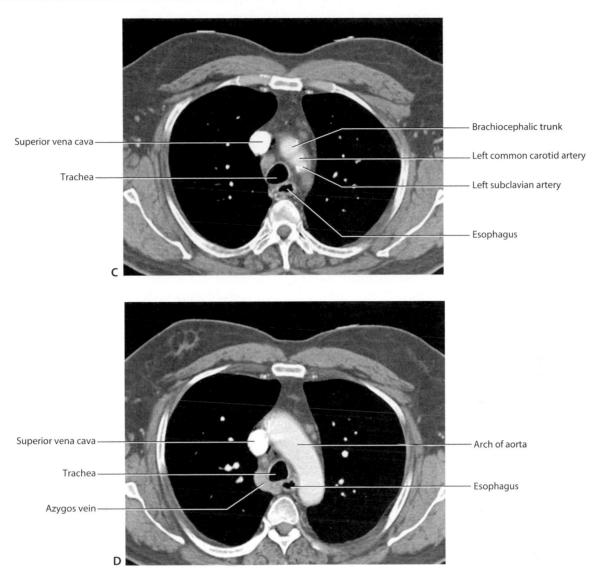

Superior vena cava — Brachiocephalic trunk

Left common carotid artery

Trachea — Left subclavian artery

Esophagus

C

Superior vena cava — Arch of aorta

Trachea — Esophagus

Azygos vein —

D

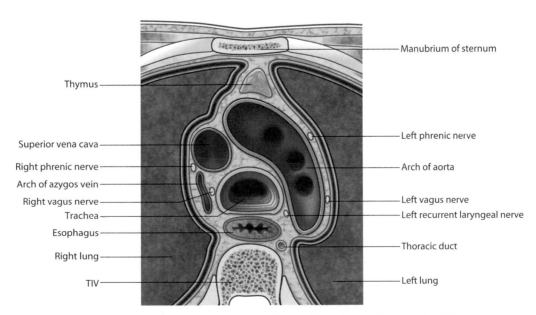

Manubrium of sternum

Thymus —

Superior vena cava — Left phrenic nerve

Right phrenic nerve — Arch of aorta

Arch of azygos vein —

Right vagus nerve — Left vagus nerve

Trachea — Left recurrent laryngeal nerve

Esophagus — Thoracic duct

Right lung —

TIV — Left lung

Transverse section through the superior mediastinum at the level of vertebra TIV

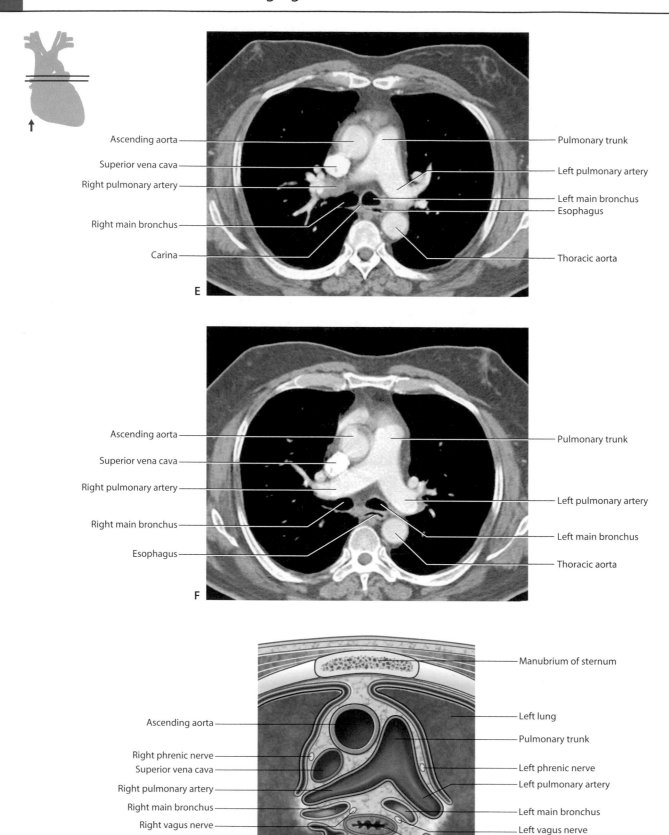

Ascending aorta — Pulmonary trunk

Superior vena cava — Left pulmonary artery

Right pulmonary artery — Left main bronchus
— Esophagus

Right main bronchus

Carina — Thoracic aorta

E

Ascending aorta — Pulmonary trunk

Superior vena cava

Right pulmonary artery — Left pulmonary artery

Right main bronchus — Left main bronchus

Esophagus — Thoracic aorta

F

Ascending aorta — Manubrium of sternum

— Left lung

— Pulmonary trunk

Right phrenic nerve — Left phrenic nerve

Superior vena cava

Right pulmonary artery — Left pulmonary artery

Right main bronchus — Left main bronchus

Right vagus nerve — Left vagus nerve

Azygos vein — Esophagus

Right lung — Thoracic duct

TV — Thoracic aorta

Transverse section through the superior mediastinum at the level of vertebra TV

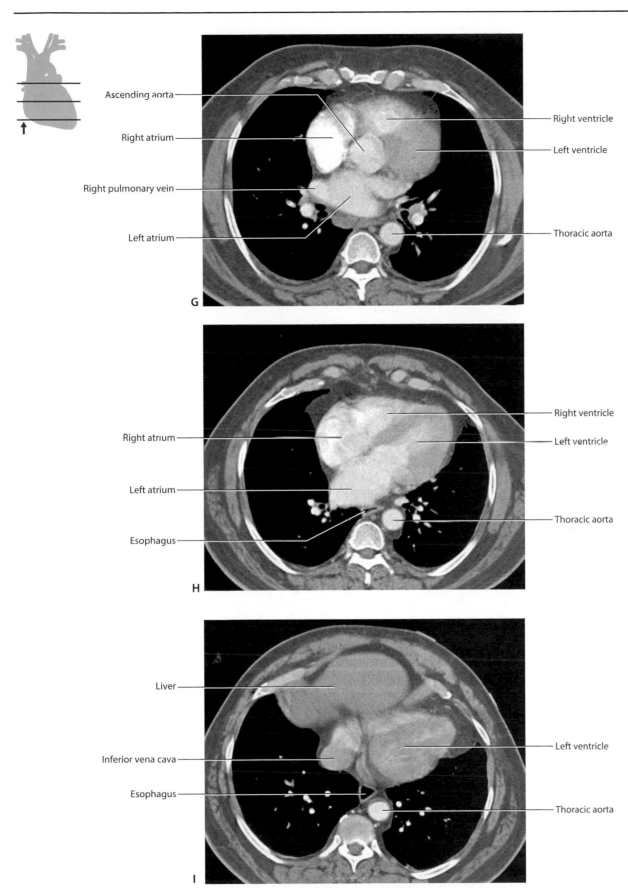

A through I – This is a series of images that pass through the thorax from superior to inferior showing the various mediastinal structures and their relationships with each other.

CT images, with contrast, in axial plane

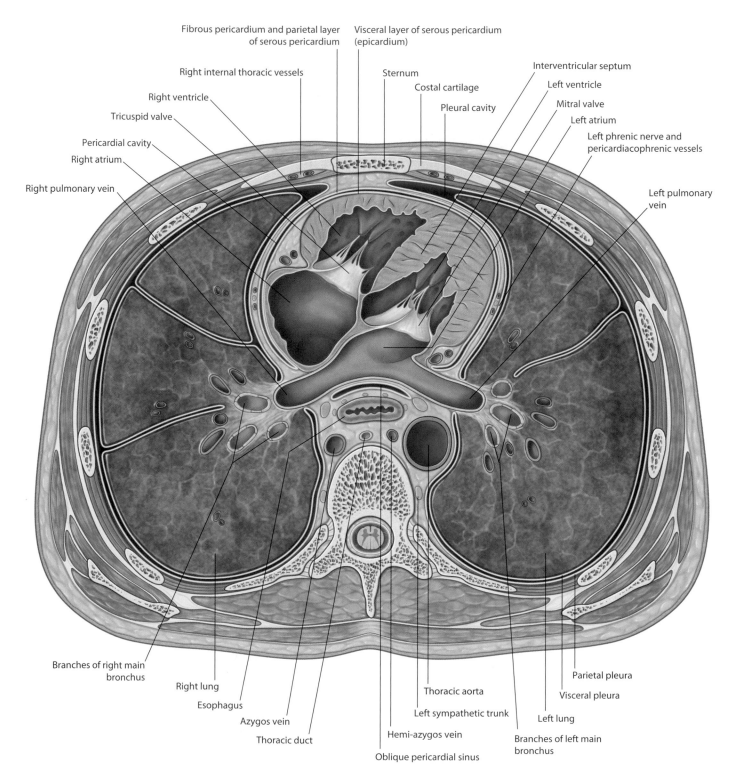

Fibrous pericardium and parietal layer of serous pericardium

Right internal thoracic vessels

Right ventricle

Tricuspid valve

Pericardial cavity

Right atrium

Right pulmonary vein

Visceral layer of serous pericardium (epicardium)

Sternum

Costal cartilage

Pleural cavity

Interventricular septum

Left ventricle

Mitral valve

Left atrium

Left phrenic nerve and pericardiacophrenic vessels

Left pulmonary vein

Branches of right main bronchus

Right lung

Esophagus

Azygos vein

Thoracic duct

Oblique pericardial sinus

Hemi-azygos vein

Left sympathetic trunk

Thoracic aorta

Left lung

Branches of left main bronchus

Visceral pleura

Parietal pleura

**Transverse section through thorax
(approximately TVII)**

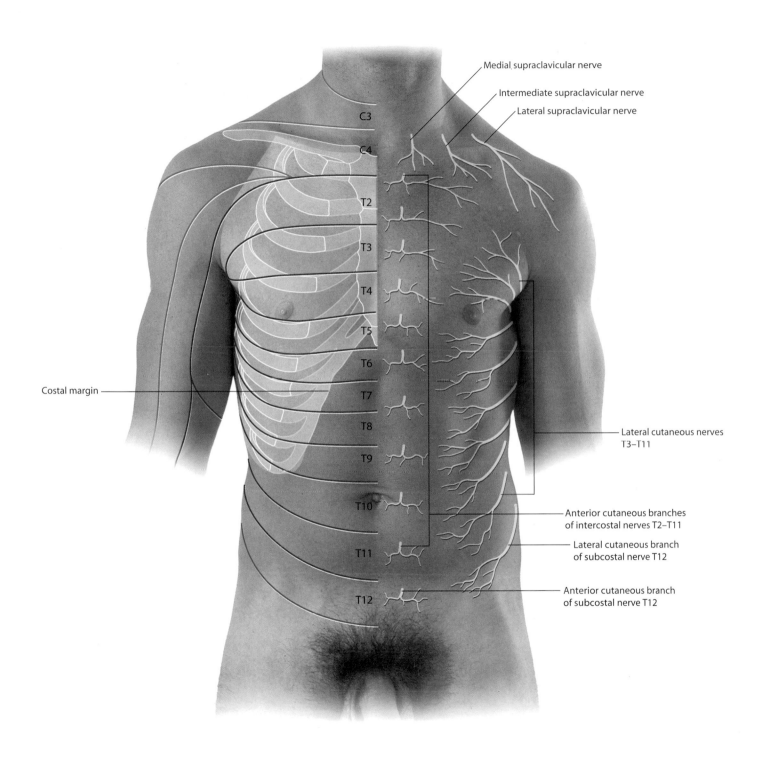

C3
C4
T2
T3
T4
T5
T6
T7
T8
T9
T10
T11
T12

Medial supraclavicular nerve

Intermediate supraclavicular nerve

Lateral supraclavicular nerve

Costal margin

Lateral cutaneous nerves
T3–T11

Anterior cutaneous branches
of intercostal nerves T2–T11

Lateral cutaneous branch
of subcostal nerve T12

Anterior cutaneous branch
of subcostal nerve T12

Dermatomes and cutaneous nerves of the thoracic region

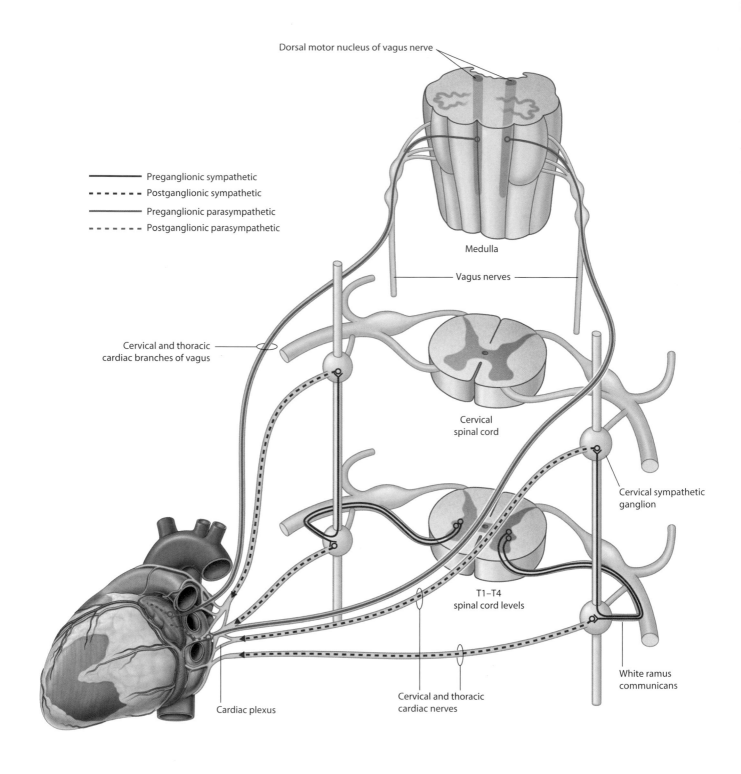

Dorsal motor nucleus of vagus nerve

Preganglionic sympathetic
Postganglionic sympathetic
Preganglionic parasympathetic
Postganglionic parasympathetic

Medulla

Vagus nerves

Cervical and thoracic
cardiac branches of vagus

Cervical
spinal cord

Cervical sympathetic
ganglion

T1–T4
spinal cord levels

White ramus
communicans

Cardiac plexus

Cervical and thoracic
cardiac nerves

**Visceral efferent (motor) innervation of the heart
(sympathetic and parasympathetic)**

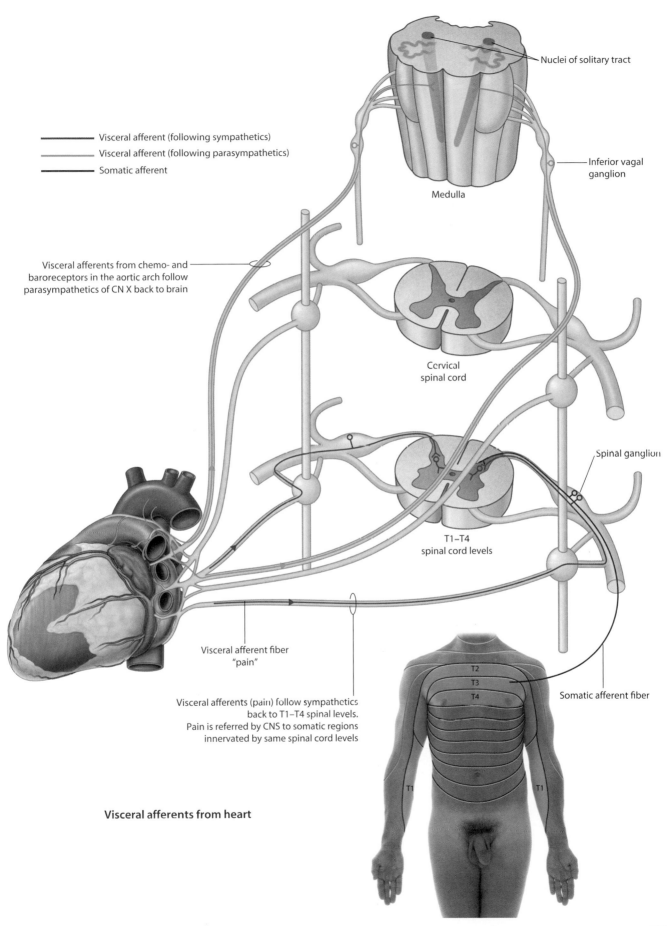

Nuclei of solitary tract

Inferior vagal ganglion

Medulla

Visceral afferent (following sympathetics)

Visceral afferent (following parasympathetics)

Somatic afferent

Visceral afferents from chemo- and baroreceptors in the aortic arch follow parasympathetics of CN X back to brain

Cervical spinal cord

Spinal ganglion

T1–T4 spinal cord levels

Visceral afferent fiber "pain"

Somatic afferent fiber

Visceral afferents (pain) follow sympathetics back to T1–T4 spinal levels. Pain is referred by CNS to somatic regions innervated by same spinal cord levels

T2

T3

T4

T1

T1

Visceral afferents from heart

Muscles of the pectoral region

Muscle		Origin	Insertion	Innervation	Function
Pectoralis major	1	Medial half of clavicle and anterior surface of sternum, first seven costal cartilages, aponeurosis of external oblique	Lateral lip of intertubercular sulcus of humerus	Medial and lateral pectoral nerves	Adduction, medial rotation, and flexion of the humerus at the shoulder joint
Subclavius	2	Rib I at junction between rib and costal cartilage	Groove on inferior surface of middle third of clavicle	Nerve to subclavius	Pulls clavicle medially to stabilize sternoclavicular joint; depresses tip of shoulder
Pectoralis minor	3	Anterior surfaces of the third, fourth, and fifth ribs, and deep fascia overlying the related intercostal spaces	Coracoid process of scapula	Medial pectoral nerves	Depresses tip of shoulder; protracts scapula

Muscles of the thoracic wall

Muscle		Origin	Insertion	Innervation	Function
External intercostal	4	Inferior margin of rib above	Superior margin of rib below	Intercostal nerves; T1–T11	Most active during inspiration; supports intercostal space; moves ribs superiorly
Internal intercostal	5	Lateral edge of costal groove of rib above	Superior margin of rib below deep to the attachment of the related external intercostal	Intercostal nerves; T1–T11	Most active during expiration; supports intercostal space; moves ribs inferiorly
Innermost intercostal	6	Medial edge of costal groove of rib above	Internal aspect of superior margin of rib below	Intercostal nerves; T1–T11	Acts with internal intercostal muscles
Subcostales	7	Internal surface (near angle) of lower ribs	Internal surface of second or third rib below	Related intercostal nerves	May depress ribs
Transversus thoracis	8	Inferior margins and internal surfaces of costal cartilages of second to sixth ribs	Inferior aspect of deep surface of body of sternum, xiphoid process, and costal cartilages ribs IV–VII	Related intercostal nerves	Depresses costal cartilages

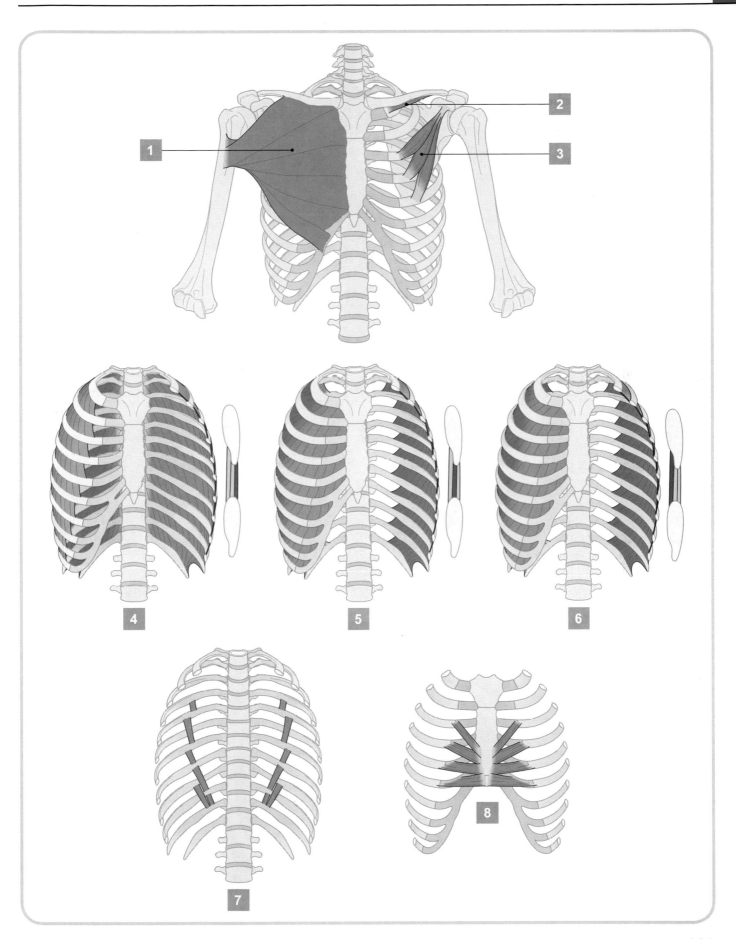

Branches of the thoracic aorta

Branches		Origin and course
Pericardial branches	1	A few small vessels to the posterior surface of the pericardial sac
Bronchial branches	2	Vary in number, size, and origin—usually, two left bronchial arteries from the thoracic aorta and one right bronchial artery from the third posterior intercostal artery or the superior left bronchial artery
Esophageal branches	3	Four or five vessels from the anterior aspect of the thoracic aorta, which form a continuous anastomotic chain—anastomotic connections include esophageal branches of the inferior thyroid artery superiorly, and esophageal branches of the left inferior phrenic and the left gastric arteries inferiorly
Mediastinal branches	4	Several small branches supplying lymph nodes, vessels, nerves, and areolar tissue in the posterior mediastinum
Posterior intercostal arteries	5	Usually nine pairs of vessels branching from the posterior surface of the thoracic aorta—usually supply lower nine intercostal spaces (first two spaces are supplied by the supreme intercostal artery—a branch of the costocervical trunk)
Superior phrenic arteries	6	Small vessels from the lower part of the thoracic aorta supplying the posterior part of the superior surface of the diaphragm—they anastomose with the musculophrenic and pericardiacophrenic arteries
Subcostal artery	7	The lowest pair of branches from the thoracic aorta located inferior to rib XII

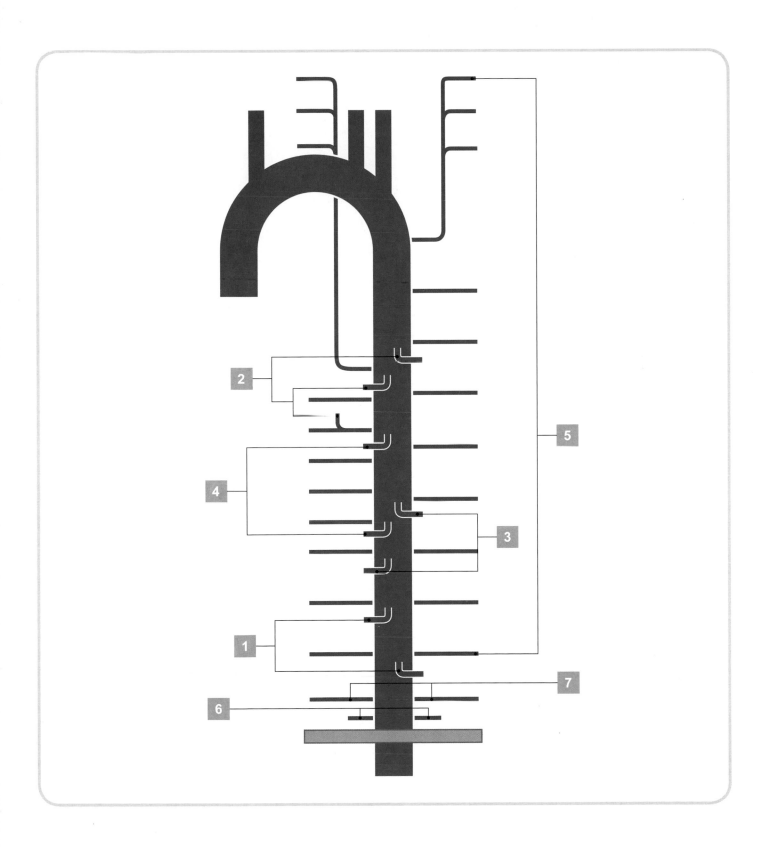

4

ABDOMEN

CONTENTS

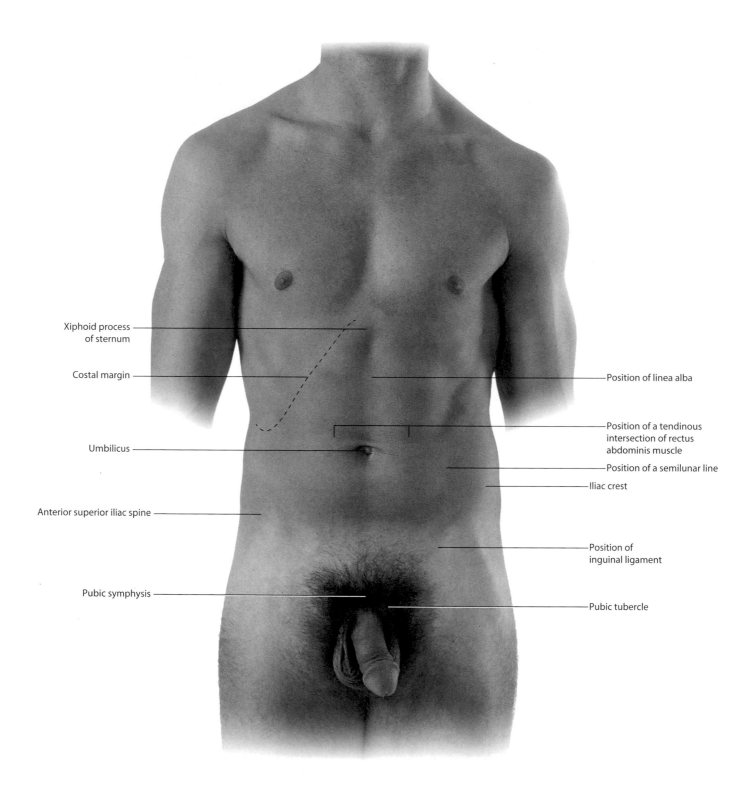

Xiphoid process
of sternum

Costal margin

Umbilicus

Anterior superior iliac spine

Pubic symphysis

Position of linea alba

Position of a tendinous
intersection of rectus
abdominis muscle

Position of a semilunar line

Iliac crest

Position of
inguinal ligament

Pubic tubercle

Anterior abdominal wall surface anatomy

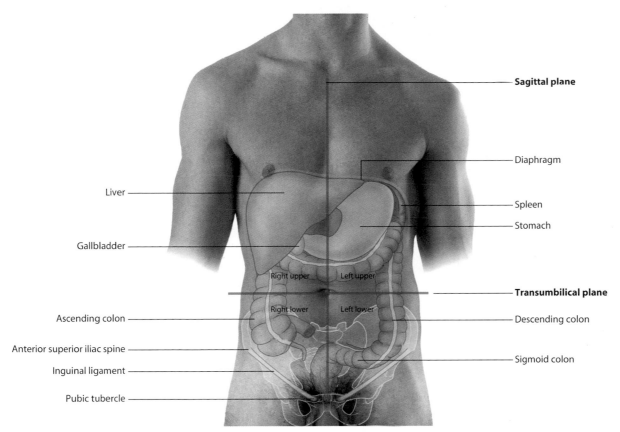

Sagittal plane

Diaphragm

Spleen

Stomach

Liver

Gallbladder

Right upper | Left upper

Transumbilical plane

Right lower | Left lower

Ascending colon

Descending colon

Anterior superior iliac spine

Inguinal ligament

Sigmoid colon

Pubic tubercle

Abdominal quadrants and the positions of major viscera

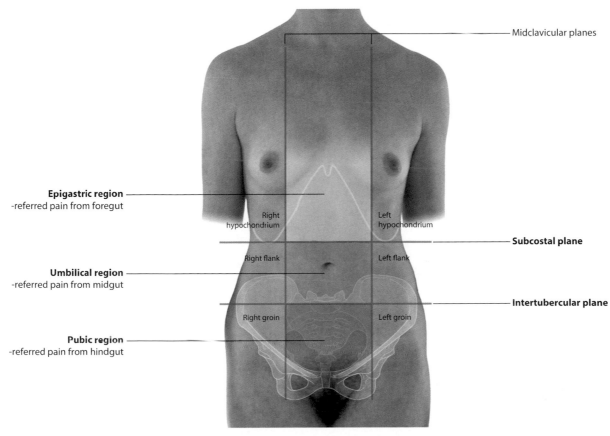

Midclavicular planes

Epigastric region
-referred pain from foregut

Right hypochondrium | Left hypochondrium

Subcostal plane

Right flank | Left flank

Umbilical region
-referred pain from midgut

Intertubercular plane

Right groin | Left groin

Pubic region
-referred pain from hindgut

The nine regions of the abdomen

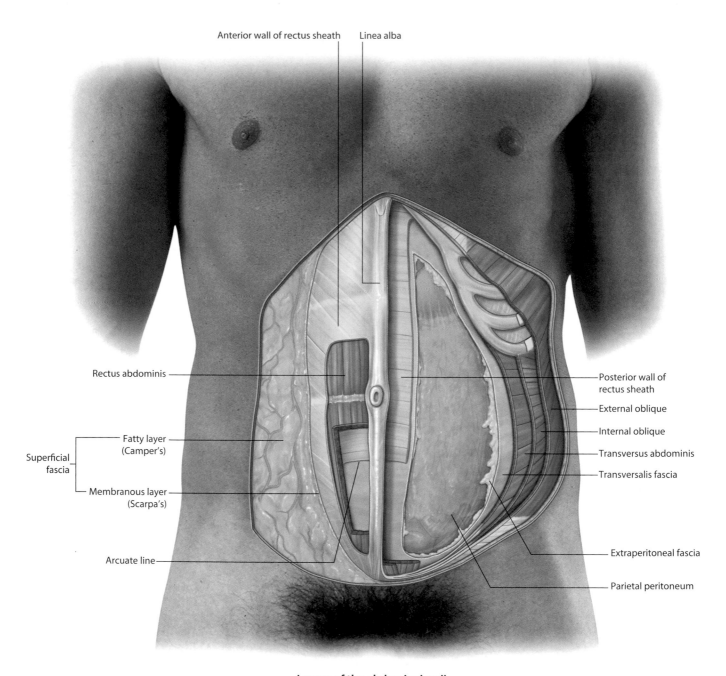

Anterior wall of rectus sheath
Linea alba

Rectus abdominis

Superficial fascia
Fatty layer (Camper's)
Membranous layer (Scarpa's)

Arcuate line

Posterior wall of rectus sheath
External oblique
Internal oblique
Transversus abdominis
Transversalis fascia

Extraperitoneal fascia
Parietal peritoneum

Layers of the abdominal wall

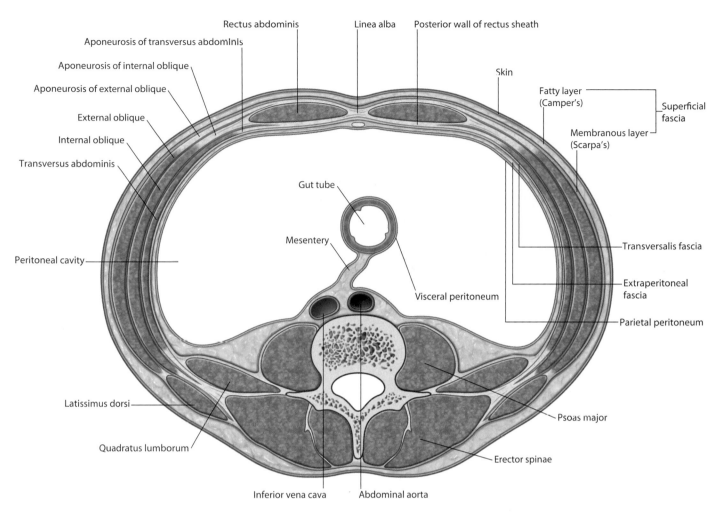

Transverse section showing the layers of the abdominal wall (above umbilicus)

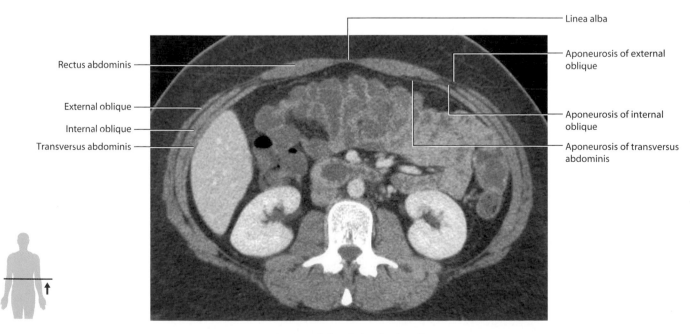

Layers of the abdominal wall.
CT image, with contrast, in axial plane

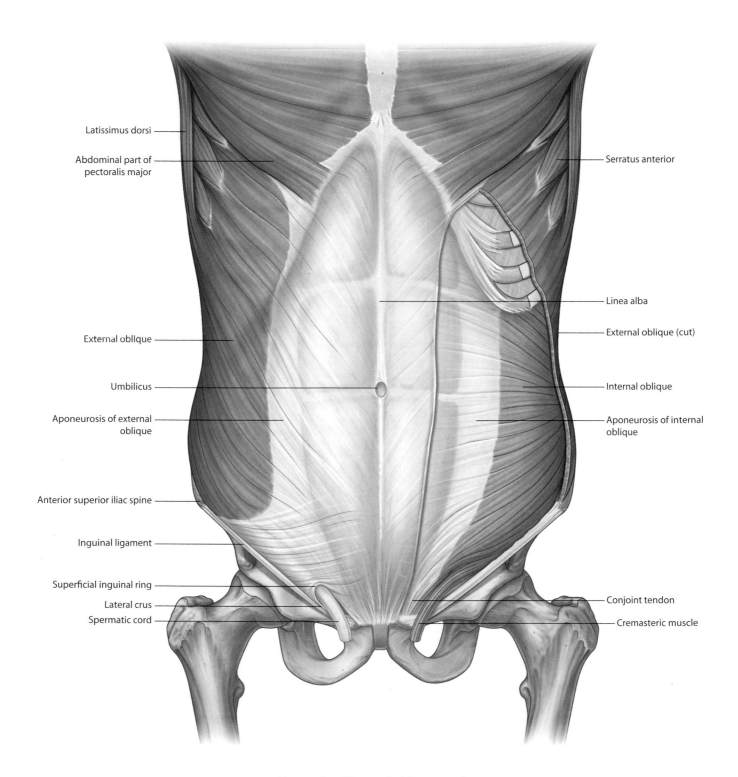

Latissimus dorsi

Abdominal part of pectoralis major

Serratus anterior

Linea alba

External oblique

External oblique (cut)

Umbilicus

Internal oblique

Aponeurosis of external oblique

Aponeurosis of internal oblique

Anterior superior iliac spine

Inguinal ligament

Superficial inguinal ring

Lateral crus

Conjoint tendon

Spermatic cord

Cremasteric muscle

External and internal oblique muscles

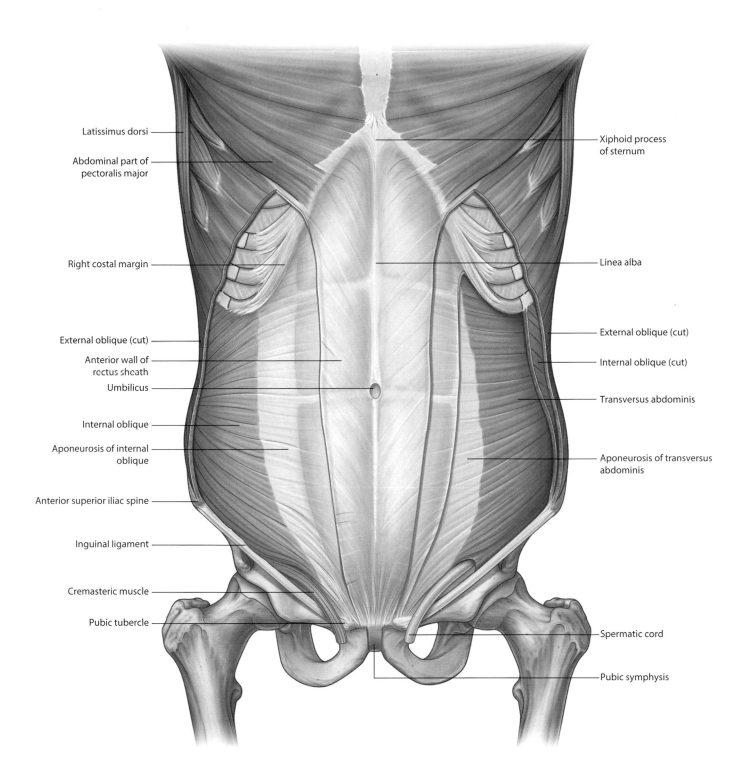

Latissimus dorsi

Abdominal part of pectoralis major

Right costal margin

External oblique (cut)

Anterior wall of rectus sheath

Umbilicus

Internal oblique

Aponeurosis of internal oblique

Anterior superior iliac spine

Inguinal ligament

Cremasteric muscle

Pubic tubercle

Xiphoid process of sternum

Linea alba

External oblique (cut)

Internal oblique (cut)

Transversus abdominis

Aponeurosis of transversus abdominis

Spermatic cord

Pubic symphysis

Internal oblique and transversus abdominis muscles

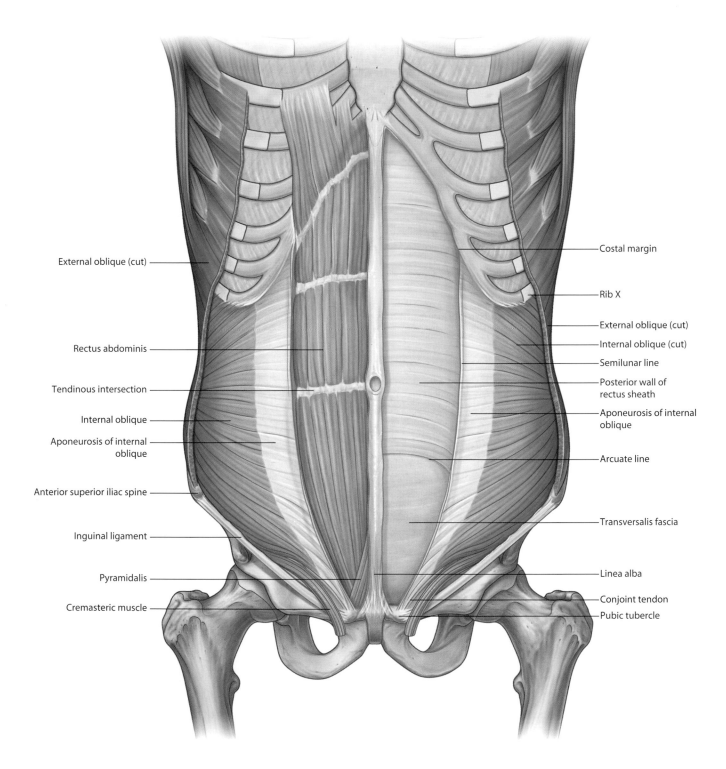

External oblique (cut)

Rectus abdominis

Tendinous intersection

Internal oblique

Aponeurosis of internal oblique

Anterior superior iliac spine

Inguinal ligament

Pyramidalis

Cremasteric muscle

Costal margin

Rib X

External oblique (cut)

Internal oblique (cut)

Semilunar line

Posterior wall of rectus sheath

Aponeurosis of internal oblique

Arcuate line

Transversalis fascia

Linea alba

Conjoint tendon

Pubic tubercle

Rectus abdominis and pyramidalis muscles

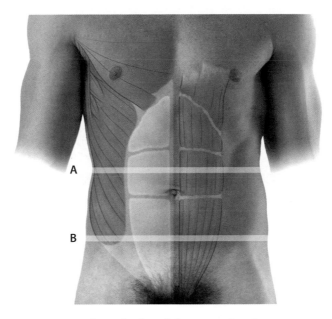

Organization of the rectus sheath.
A. Transverse section through the upper three quarters of the rectus sheath
B. Transverse section through the lower one quarter of the rectus sheath

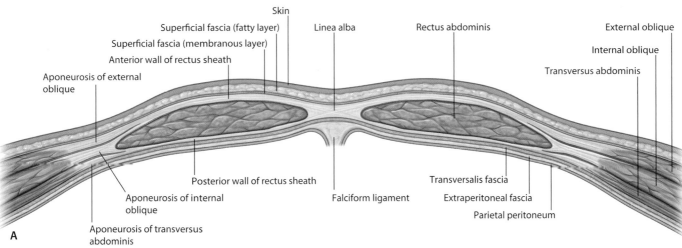

Skin

Superficial fascia (fatty layer)

Superficial fascia (membranous layer)

Anterior wall of rectus sheath

Aponeurosis of external oblique

Linea alba

Rectus abdominis

External oblique

Internal oblique

Transversus abdominis

Posterior wall of rectus sheath

Aponeurosis of internal oblique

Aponeurosis of transversus abdominis

Falciform ligament

Transversalis fascia

Extraperitoneal fascia

Parietal peritoneum

A

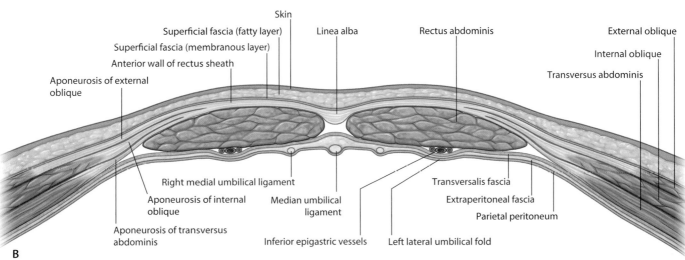

Skin

Superficial fascia (fatty layer)

Superficial fascia (membranous layer)

Anterior wall of rectus sheath

Aponeurosis of external oblique

Linea alba

Rectus abdominis

External oblique

Internal oblique

Transversus abdominis

Right medial umbilical ligament

Aponeurosis of internal oblique

Aponeurosis of transversus abdominis

Median umbilical ligament

Inferior epigastric vessels

Left lateral umbilical fold

Transversalis fascia

Extraperitoneal fascia

Parietal peritoneum

B

141

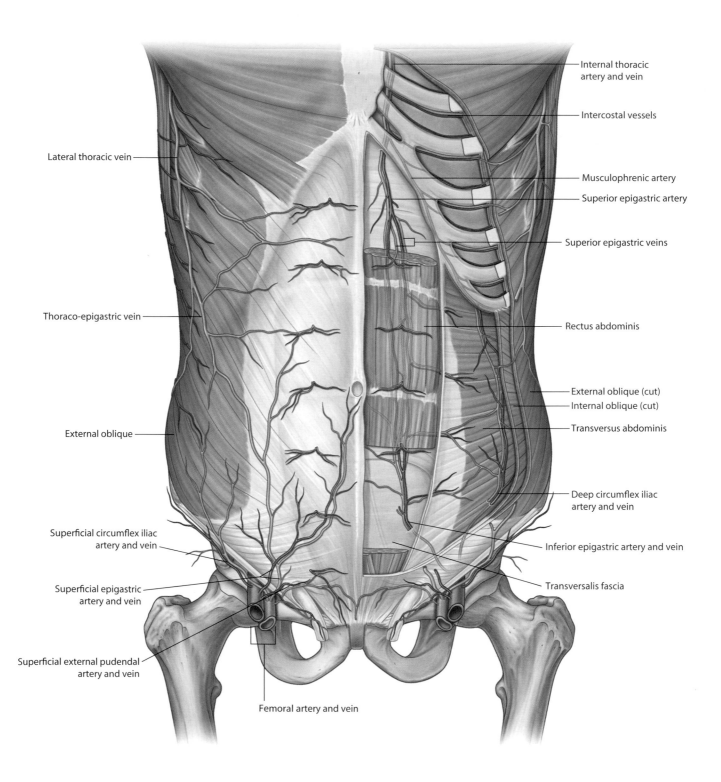

Lateral thoracic vein

Thoraco-epigastric vein

External oblique

Superficial circumflex iliac
artery and vein

Superficial epigastric
artery and vein

Superficial external pudendal
artery and vein

Femoral artery and vein

Internal thoracic
artery and vein

Intercostal vessels

Musculophrenic artery

Superior epigastric artery

Superior epigastric veins

Rectus abdominis

External oblique (cut)
Internal oblique (cut)
Transversus abdominis

Deep circumflex iliac
artery and vein

Inferior epigastric artery and vein

Transversalis fascia

Vasculature of the anterior abdominal wall

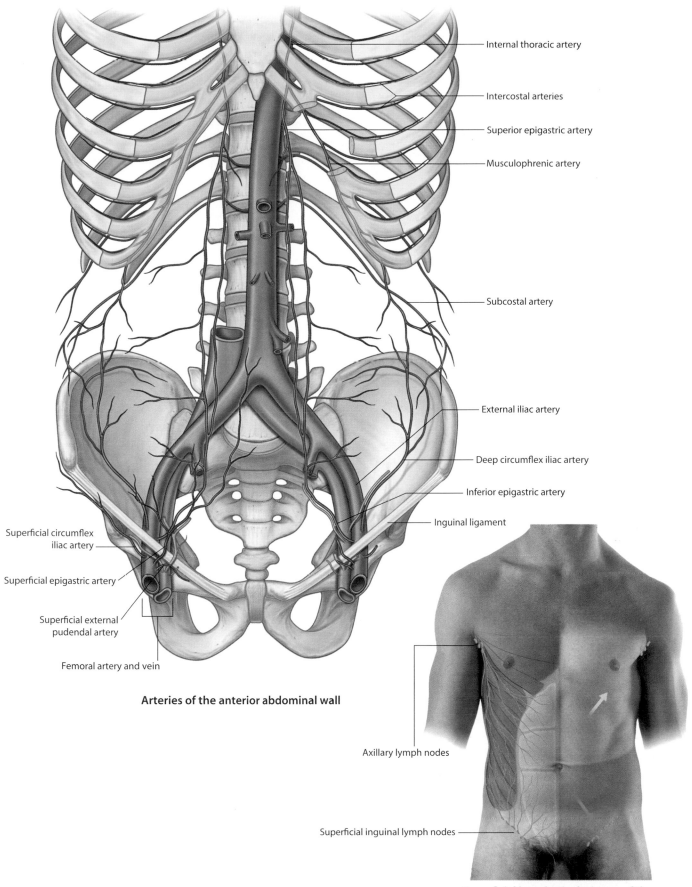

Internal thoracic artery

Intercostal arteries

Superior epigastric artery

Musculophrenic artery

Subcostal artery

External iliac artery

Deep circumflex iliac artery

Inferior epigastric artery

Inguinal ligament

Superficial circumflex iliac artery

Superficial epigastric artery

Superficial external pudendal artery

Femoral artery and vein

Arteries of the anterior abdominal wall

Axillary lymph nodes

Superficial inguinal lymph nodes

Superficial lymphatic drainage of the anterolateral abdominal wall

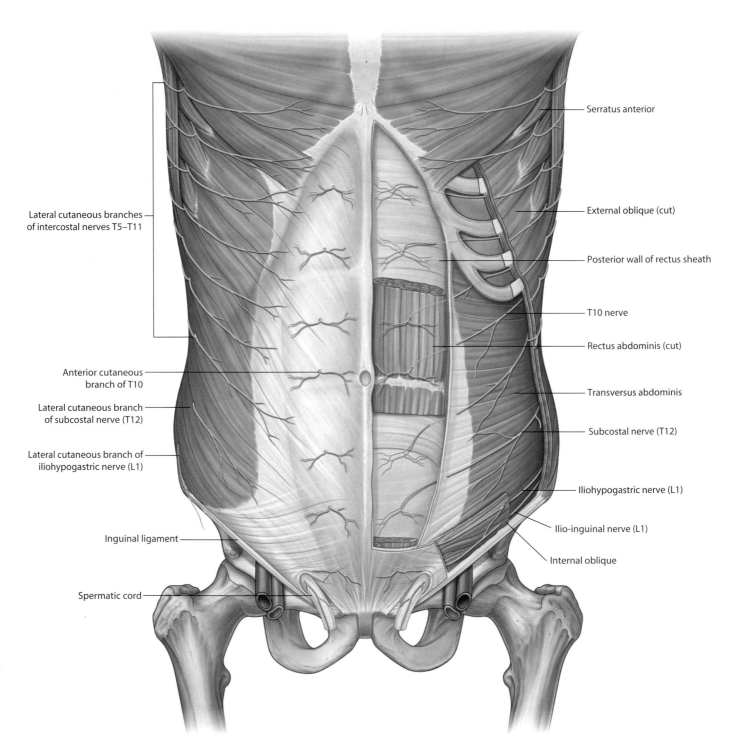

Serratus anterior

External oblique (cut)

Posterior wall of rectus sheath

T10 nerve

Rectus abdominis (cut)

Transversus abdominis

Subcostal nerve (T12)

Iliohypogastric nerve (L1)

Ilio-inguinal nerve (L1)

Internal oblique

Lateral cutaneous branches of intercostal nerves T5–T11

Anterior cutaneous branch of T10

Lateral cutaneous branch of subcostal nerve (T12)

Lateral cutaneous branch of iliohypogastric nerve (L1)

Inguinal ligament

Spermatic cord

Nerves of the anterolateral abdominal wall

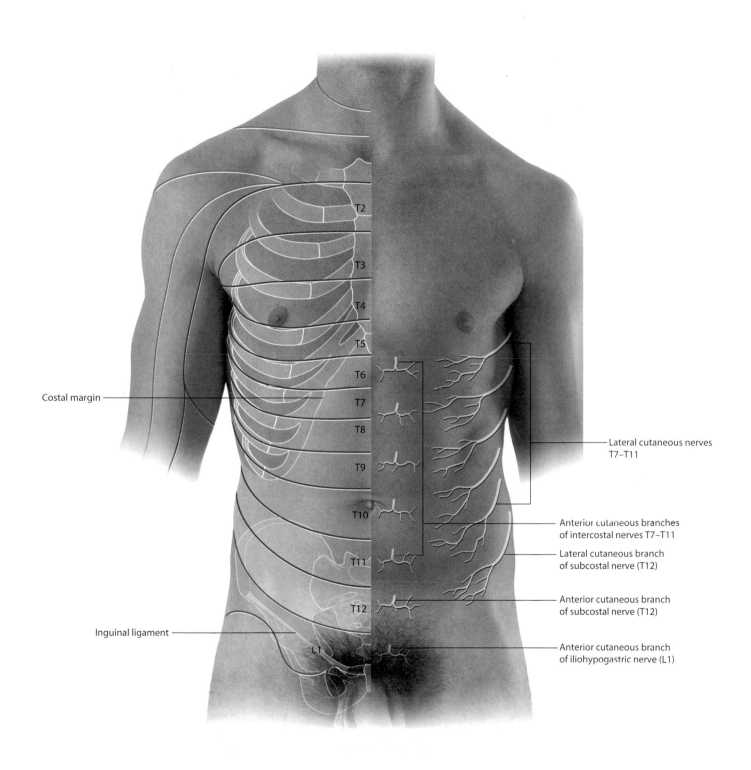

Costal margin

Inguinal ligament

Lateral cutaneous nerves T7–T11

Anterior cutaneous branches of intercostal nerves T7–T11

Lateral cutaneous branch of subcostal nerve (T12)

Anterior cutaneous branch of subcostal nerve (T12)

Anterior cutaneous branch of iliohypogastric nerve (L1)

T2
T3
T4
T5
T6
T7
T8
T9
T10
T11
T12
L1

Dermatomes and cutaneous nerves of the anterolateral abdominal wall

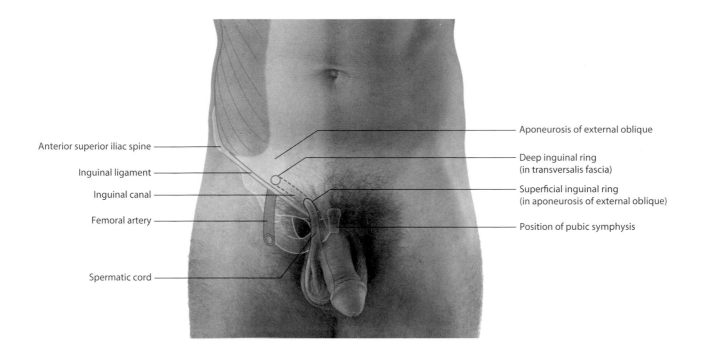

Anterior superior iliac spine

Inguinal ligament

Inguinal canal

Femoral artery

Spermatic cord

Aponeurosis of external oblique

Deep inguinal ring
(in transversalis fascia)

Superficial inguinal ring
(in aponeurosis of external oblique)

Position of pubic symphysis

Inguinal region in a man

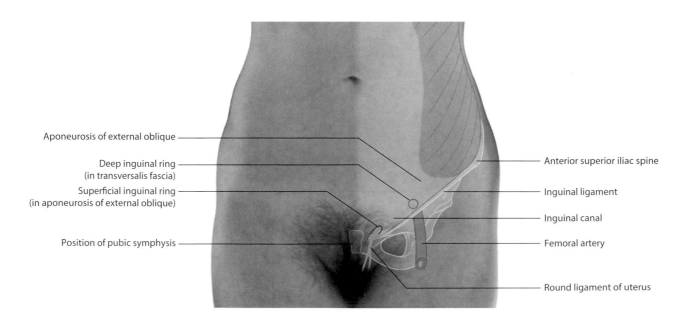

Aponeurosis of external oblique

Deep inguinal ring
(in transversalis fascia)

Superficial inguinal ring
(in aponeurosis of external oblique)

Position of pubic symphysis

Anterior superior iliac spine

Inguinal ligament

Inguinal canal

Femoral artery

Round ligament of uterus

Inguinal region in a woman

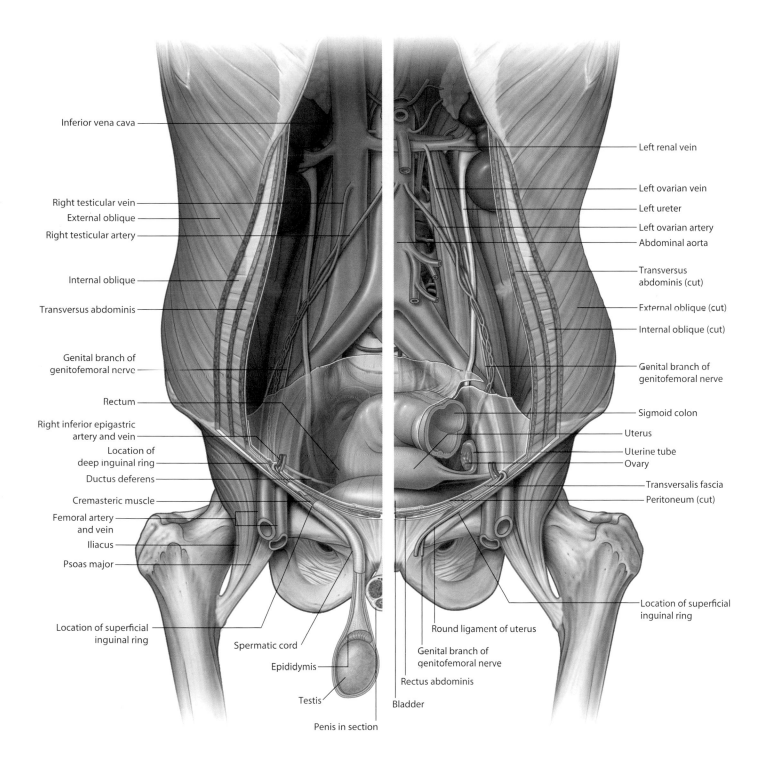

Inferior vena cava

Right testicular vein
External oblique
Right testicular artery

Internal oblique

Transversus abdominis

Genital branch of
genitofemoral nerve

Rectum

Right inferior epigastric
artery and vein

Location of
deep inguinal ring

Ductus deferens

Cremasteric muscle

Femoral artery
and vein

Iliacus

Psoas major

Location of superficial
inguinal ring

Spermatic cord

Epididymis

Testis

Penis in section

Left renal vein

Left ovarian vein

Left ureter

Left ovarian artery

Abdominal aorta

Transversus
abdominis (cut)

External oblique (cut)

Internal oblique (cut)

Genital branch of
genitofemoral nerve

Sigmoid colon

Uterus

Uterine tube

Ovary

Transversalis fascia

Peritoneum (cut)

Location of superficial
inguinal ring

Round ligament of uterus

Genital branch of
genitofemoral nerve

Rectus abdominis

Bladder

Inguinal region in men

Inguinal region in women

147

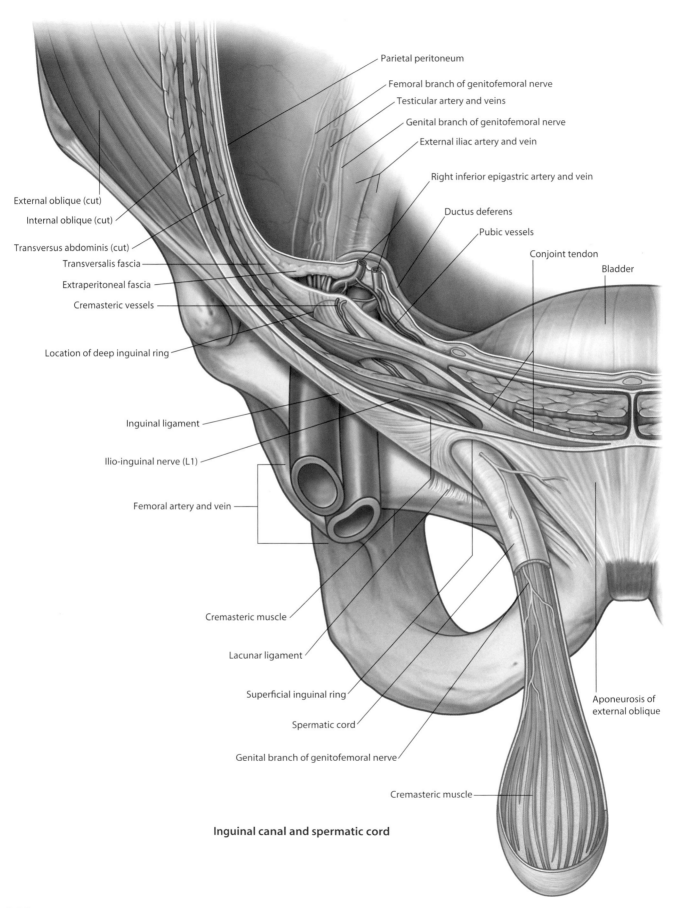

Parietal peritoneum

Femoral branch of genitofemoral nerve

Testicular artery and veins

Genital branch of genitofemoral nerve

External iliac artery and vein

Right inferior epigastric artery and vein

Ductus deferens

Pubic vessels

Conjoint tendon

Bladder

External oblique (cut)

Internal oblique (cut)

Transversus abdominis (cut)

Transversalis fascia

Extraperitoneal fascia

Cremasteric vessels

Location of deep inguinal ring

Inguinal ligament

Ilio-inguinal nerve (L1)

Femoral artery and vein

Aponeurosis of external oblique

Cremasteric muscle

Lacunar ligament

Superficial inguinal ring

Spermatic cord

Genital branch of genitofemoral nerve

Cremasteric muscle

Inguinal canal and spermatic cord

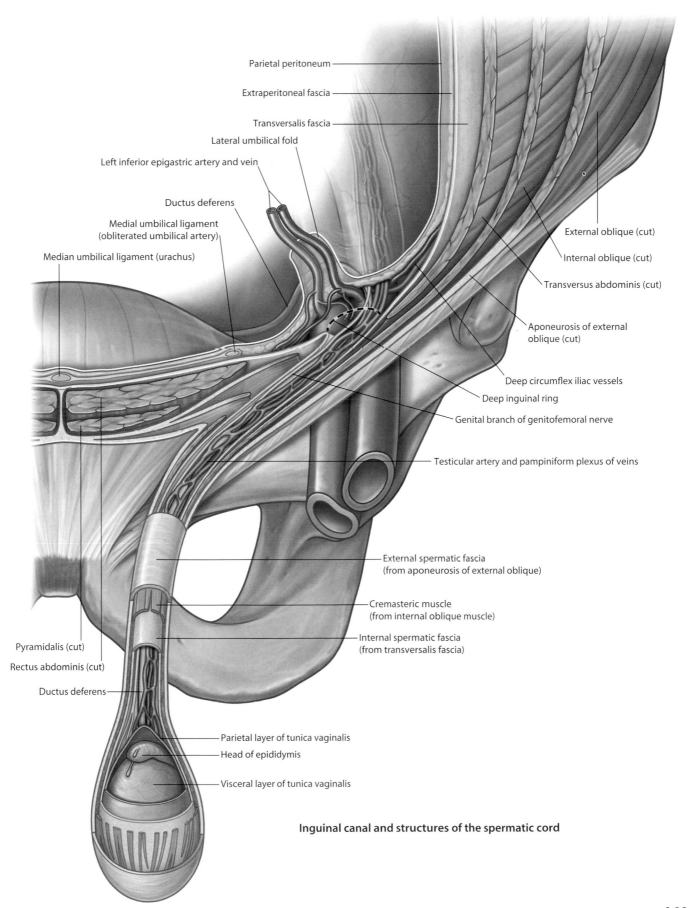

Parietal peritoneum

Extraperitoneal fascia

Transversalis fascia

Lateral umbilical fold

Left inferior epigastric artery and vein

Ductus deferens

Medial umbilical ligament
(obliterated umbilical artery)

Median umbilical ligament (urachus)

External oblique (cut)

Internal oblique (cut)

Transversus abdominis (cut)

Aponeurosis of external
oblique (cut)

Deep circumflex iliac vessels

Deep inguinal ring

Genital branch of genitofemoral nerve

Testicular artery and pampiniform plexus of veins

External spermatic fascia
(from aponeurosis of external oblique)

Cremasteric muscle
(from internal oblique muscle)

Internal spermatic fascia
(from transversalis fascia)

Pyramidalis (cut)

Rectus abdominis (cut)

Ductus deferens

Parietal layer of tunica vaginalis

Head of epididymis

Visceral layer of tunica vaginalis

Inguinal canal and structures of the spermatic cord

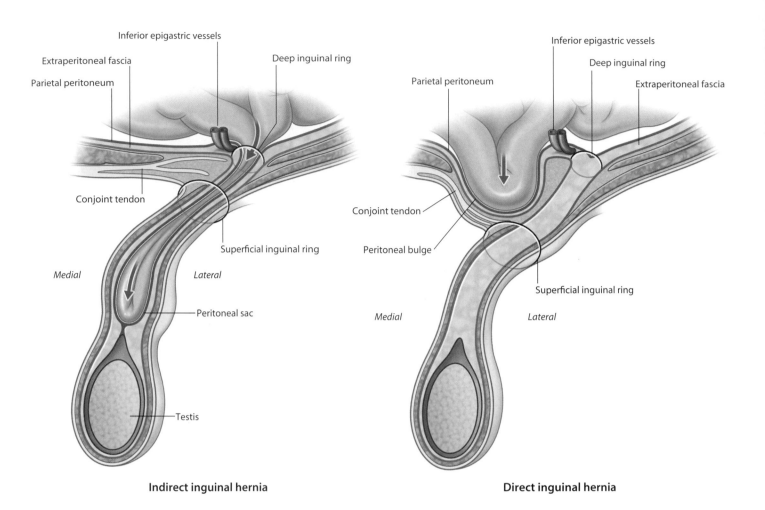

Inferior epigastric vessels

Extraperitoneal fascia

Parietal peritoneum

Deep inguinal ring

Conjoint tendon

Superficial inguinal ring

Medial

Lateral

Peritoneal sac

Testis

Indirect inguinal hernia

Parietal peritoneum

Inferior epigastric vessels

Deep inguinal ring

Extraperitoneal fascia

Conjoint tendon

Peritoneal bulge

Superficial inguinal ring

Medial

Lateral

Direct inguinal hernia

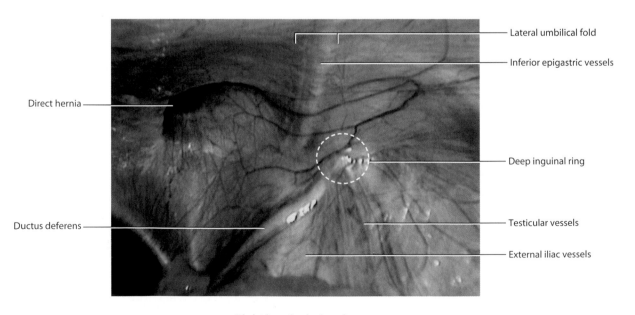

Lateral umbilical fold

Inferior epigastric vessels

Direct hernia

Deep inguinal ring

Ductus deferens

Testicular vessels

External iliac vessels

Right inguinal triangle.
Laparoscopic view showing the parietal peritoneum still covering the area
(inside the peritoneal cavity looking anteroinferior)

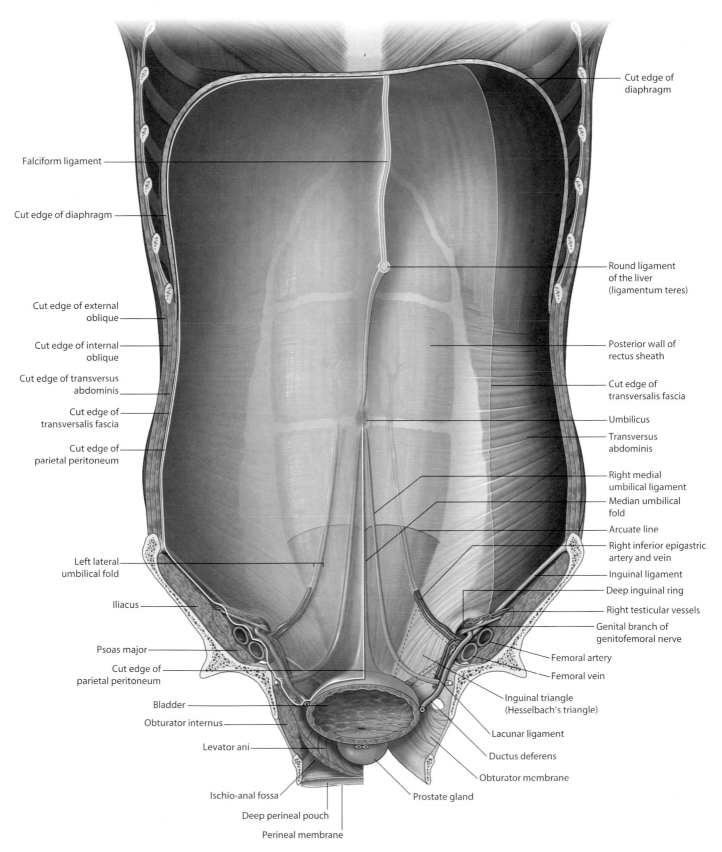

Internal view of anterior abdominal wall in men

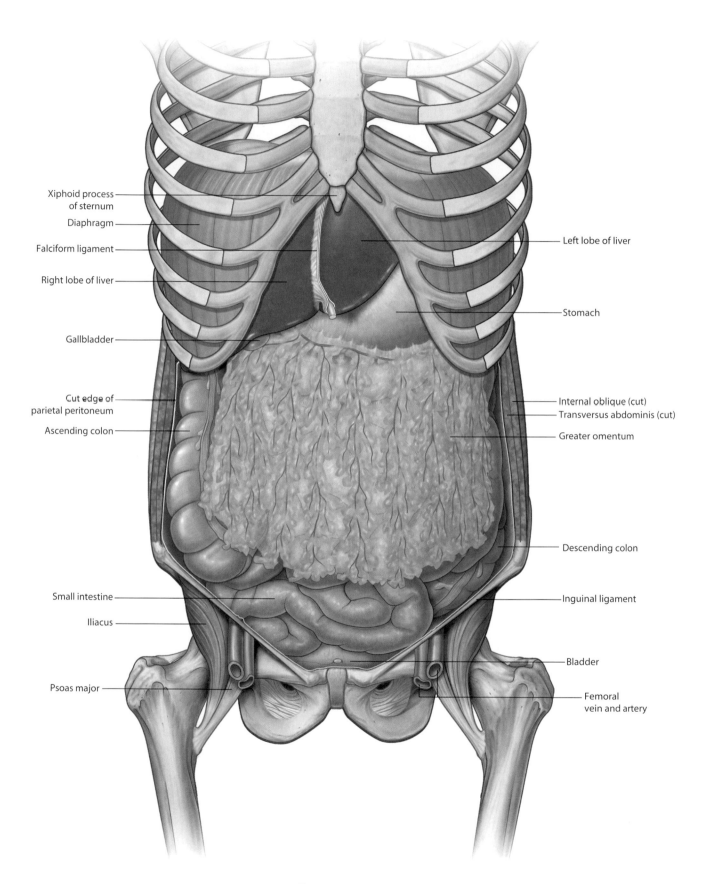

Xiphoid process
of sternum

Diaphragm

Falciform ligament

Right lobe of liver

Gallbladder

Cut edge of
parietal peritoneum

Ascending colon

Small intestine

Iliacus

Psoas major

Left lobe of liver

Stomach

Internal oblique (cut)

Transversus abdominis (cut)

Greater omentum

Descending colon

Inguinal ligament

Bladder

Femoral
vein and artery

Greater omentum

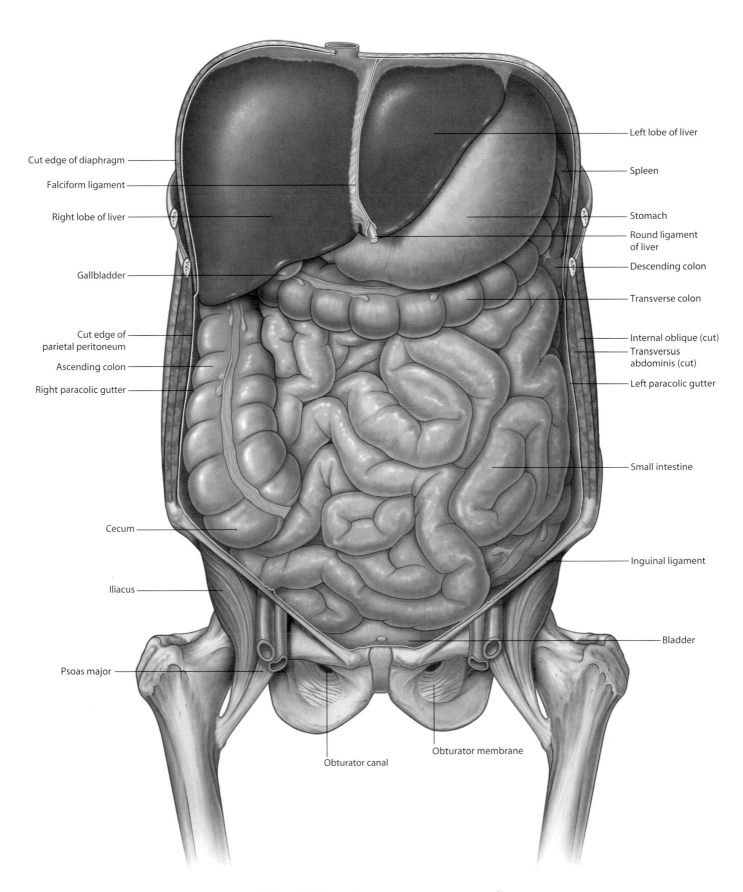

Cut edge of diaphragm

Falciform ligament

Right lobe of liver

Gallbladder

Cut edge of
parietal peritoneum

Ascending colon

Right paracolic gutter

Cecum

Iliacus

Psoas major

Left lobe of liver

Spleen

Stomach

Round ligament
of liver

Descending colon

Transverse colon

Internal oblique (cut)

Transversus
abdominis (cut)

Left paracolic gutter

Small intestine

Inguinal ligament

Bladder

Obturator membrane

Obturator canal

Abdominal viscera (greater omentum removed)

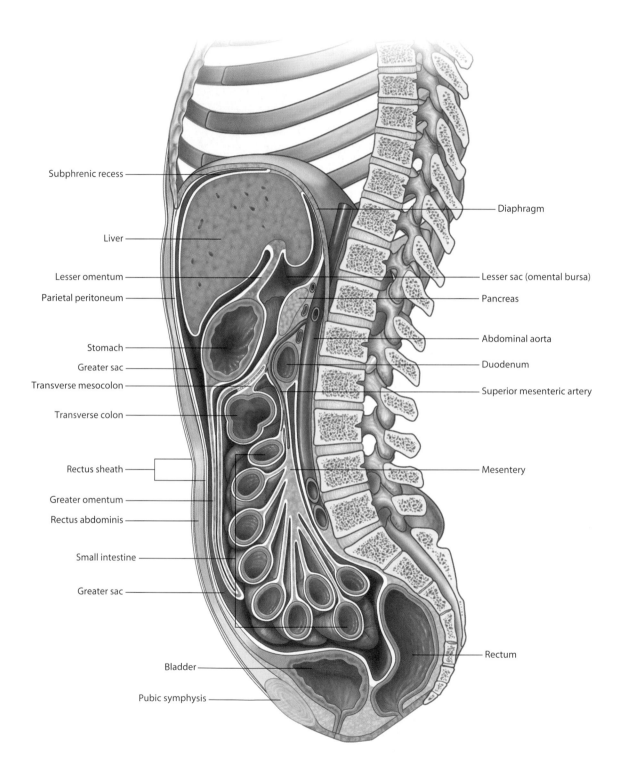

Subphrenic recess

Liver

Lesser omentum

Parietal peritoneum

Stomach

Greater sac

Transverse mesocolon

Transverse colon

Rectus sheath

Greater omentum

Rectus abdominis

Small intestine

Greater sac

Bladder

Pubic symphysis

Diaphragm

Lesser sac (omental bursa)

Pancreas

Abdominal aorta

Duodenum

Superior mesenteric artery

Mesentery

Rectum

Greater and lesser sacs of the peritoneal cavity

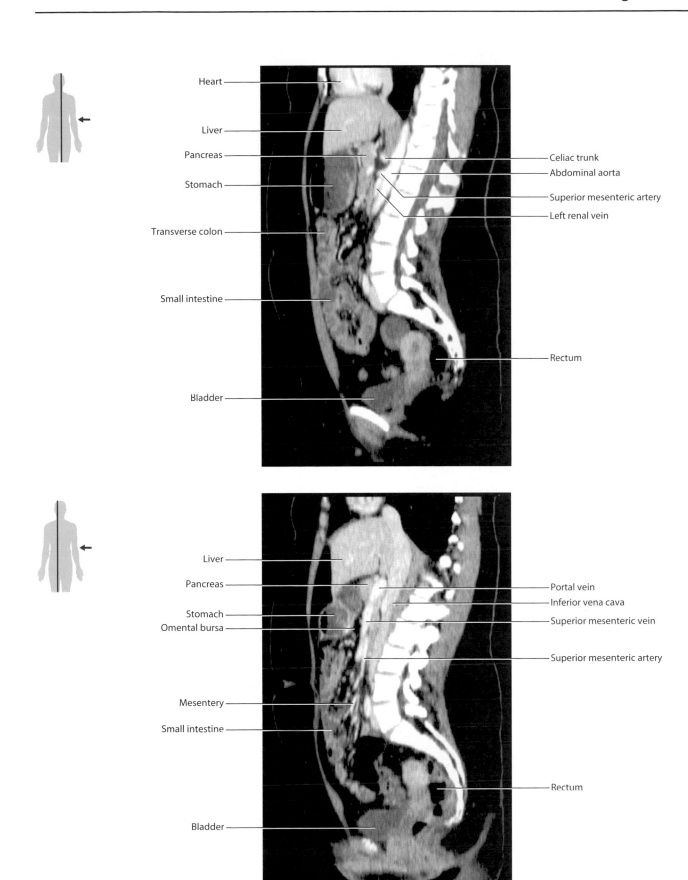

Heart

Liver

Pancreas

Stomach

Transverse colon

Small intestine

Bladder

Celiac trunk

Abdominal aorta

Superior mesenteric artery

Left renal vein

Rectum

Liver

Pancreas

Stomach

Omental bursa

Mesentery

Small intestine

Bladder

Portal vein

Inferior vena cava

Superior mesenteric vein

Superior mesenteric artery

Rectum

Arrangement of abdominal contents in peritoneal cavity.
CT images, with contrast, in sagittal plane

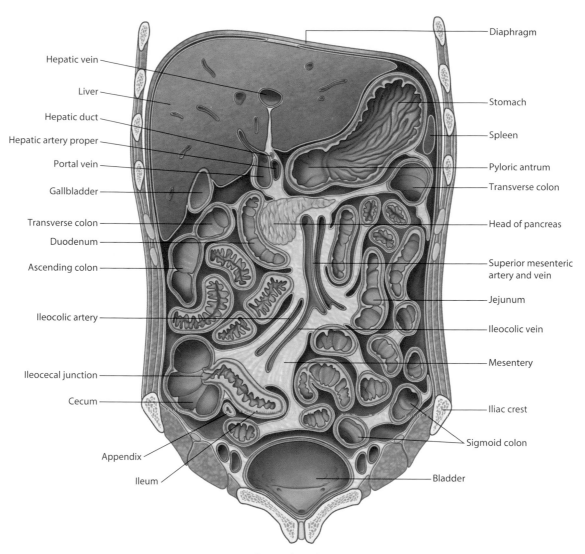

Hepatic vein

Liver

Hepatic duct

Hepatic artery proper

Portal vein

Gallbladder

Transverse colon

Duodenum

Ascending colon

Ileocolic artery

Ileocecal junction

Cecum

Appendix

Ileum

Diaphragm

Stomach

Spleen

Pyloric antrum

Transverse colon

Head of pancreas

Superior mesenteric artery and vein

Jejunum

Ileocolic vein

Mesentery

Iliac crest

Sigmoid colon

Bladder

Coronal section

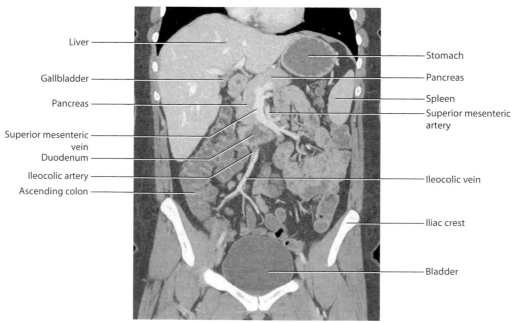

Liver

Gallbladder

Pancreas

Superior mesenteric vein

Duodenum

Ileocolic artery

Ascending colon

Stomach

Pancreas

Spleen

Superior mesenteric artery

Ileocolic vein

Iliac crest

Bladder

Coronal section.
CT image, with contrast, in coronal plane

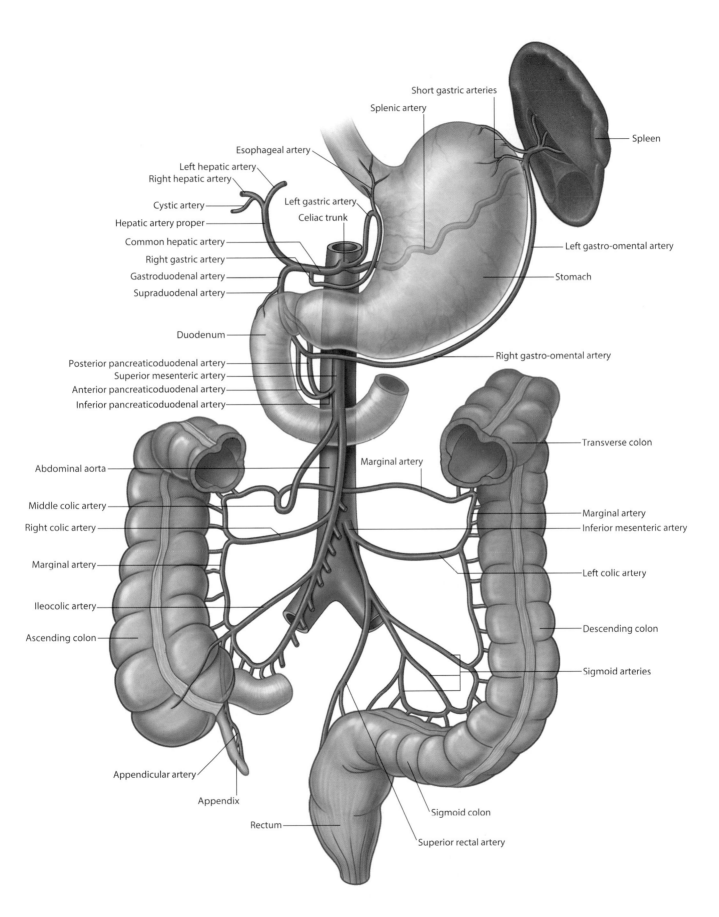

Short gastric arteries

Splenic artery

Spleen

Esophageal artery

Left hepatic artery

Right hepatic artery

Cystic artery

Left gastric artery

Hepatic artery proper

Celiac trunk

Common hepatic artery

Right gastric artery

Gastroduodenal artery

Supraduodenal artery

Left gastro-omental artery

Stomach

Duodenum

Right gastro-omental artery

Posterior pancreaticoduodenal artery

Superior mesenteric artery

Anterior pancreaticoduodenal artery

Inferior pancreaticoduodenal artery

Transverse colon

Abdominal aorta

Marginal artery

Middle colic artery

Marginal artery

Right colic artery

Inferior mesenteric artery

Marginal artery

Left colic artery

Ileocolic artery

Descending colon

Ascending colon

Sigmoid arteries

Appendicular artery

Appendix

Sigmoid colon

Rectum

Superior rectal artery

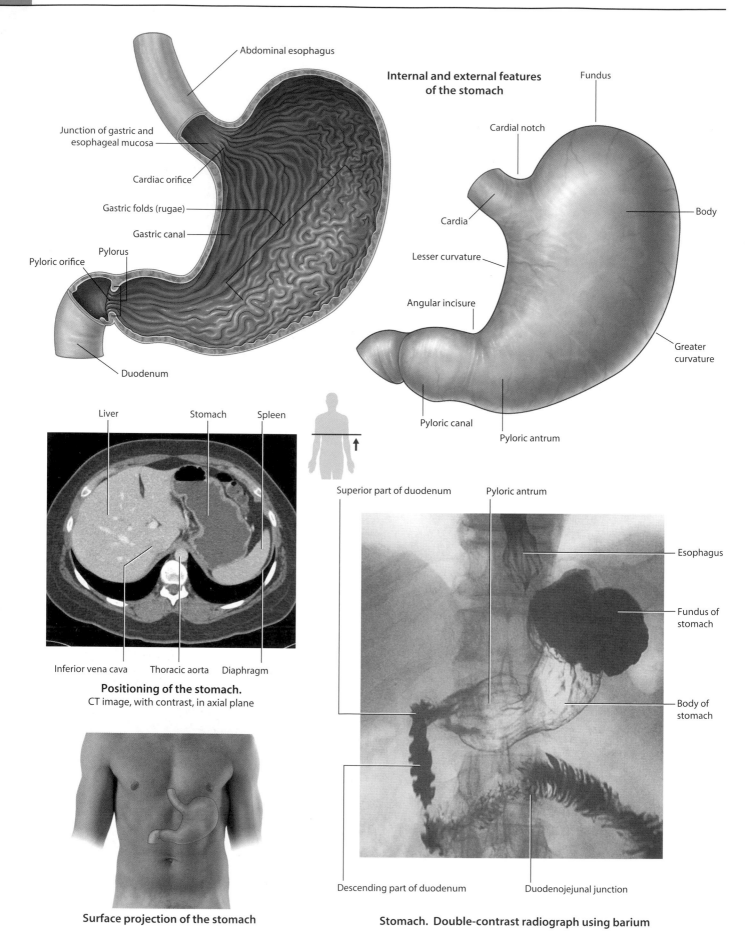

Abdominal esophagus

Junction of gastric and esophageal mucosa

Cardiac orifice

Gastric folds (rugae)

Gastric canal

Pyloric orifice

Pylorus

Duodenum

Internal and external features of the stomach

Fundus

Cardial notch

Cardia

Lesser curvature

Angular incisure

Pyloric canal

Pyloric antrum

Body

Greater curvature

Liver

Stomach

Spleen

Inferior vena cava

Thoracic aorta

Diaphragm

Positioning of the stomach.
CT image, with contrast, in axial plane

Surface projection of the stomach

Superior part of duodenum

Pyloric antrum

Esophagus

Fundus of stomach

Body of stomach

Descending part of duodenum

Duodenojejunal junction

Stomach. Double-contrast radiograph using barium

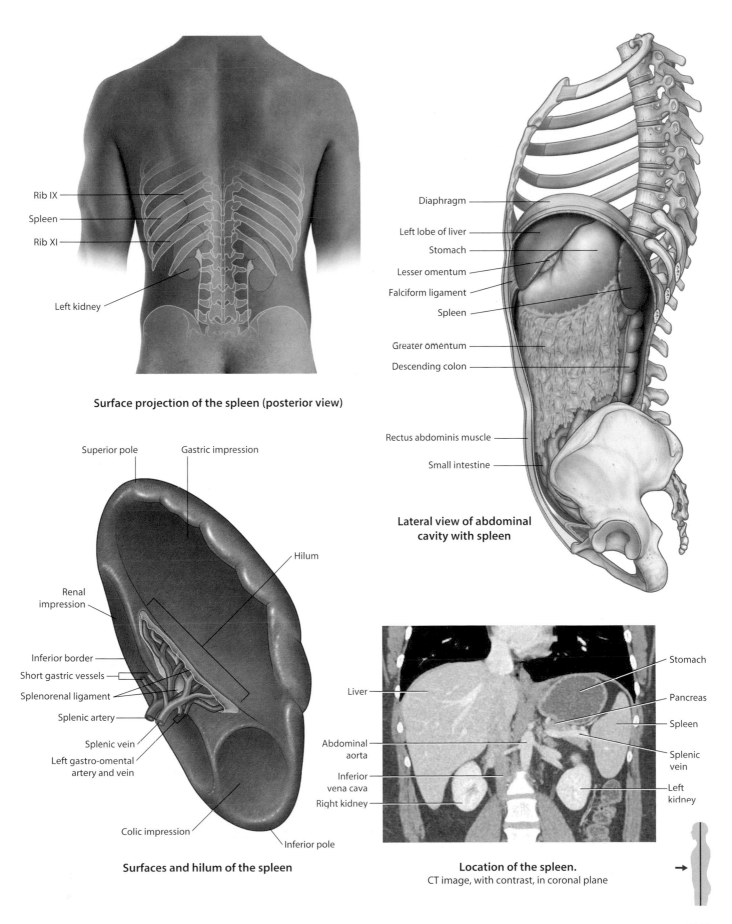

Surface projection of the spleen (posterior view)

- Rib IX
- Spleen
- Rib XI
- Left kidney

Lateral view of abdominal cavity with spleen

- Diaphragm
- Left lobe of liver
- Stomach
- Lesser omentum
- Falciform ligament
- Spleen
- Greater omentum
- Descending colon
- Rectus abdominis muscle
- Small intestine

Surfaces and hilum of the spleen

- Superior pole
- Gastric impression
- Hilum
- Renal impression
- Inferior border
- Short gastric vessels
- Splenorenal ligament
- Splenic artery
- Splenic vein
- Left gastro-omental artery and vein
- Colic impression
- Inferior pole

Location of the spleen.
CT image, with contrast, in coronal plane

- Liver
- Abdominal aorta
- Inferior vena cava
- Right kidney
- Stomach
- Pancreas
- Spleen
- Splenic vein
- Left kidney

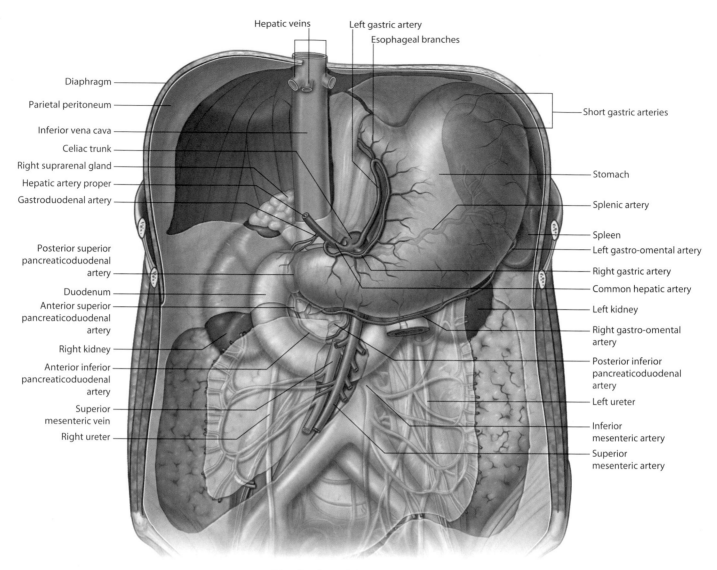

Hepatic veins
Left gastric artery
Esophageal branches
Diaphragm
Parietal peritoneum
Inferior vena cava
Celiac trunk
Right suprarenal gland
Hepatic artery proper
Gastroduodenal artery
Short gastric arteries
Stomach
Splenic artery
Spleen
Left gastro-omental artery
Right gastric artery
Common hepatic artery
Posterior superior pancreaticoduodenal artery
Duodenum
Anterior superior pancreaticoduodenal artery
Right kidney
Anterior inferior pancreaticoduodenal artery
Superior mesenteric vein
Right ureter
Left kidney
Right gastro-omental artery
Posterior inferior pancreaticoduodenal artery
Left ureter
Inferior mesenteric artery
Superior mesenteric artery

Distribution of the celiac trunk

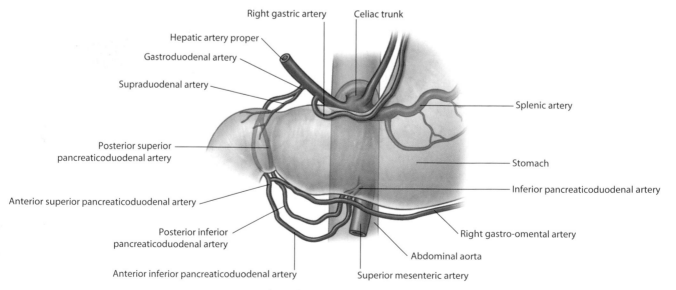

Right gastric artery
Celiac trunk
Hepatic artery proper
Gastroduodenal artery
Supraduodenal artery
Splenic artery
Posterior superior pancreaticoduodenal artery
Stomach
Inferior pancreaticoduodenal artery
Anterior superior pancreaticoduodenal artery
Posterior inferior pancreaticoduodenal artery
Right gastro-omental artery
Anterior inferior pancreaticoduodenal artery
Abdominal aorta
Superior mesenteric artery

Branches of the gastroduodenal artery

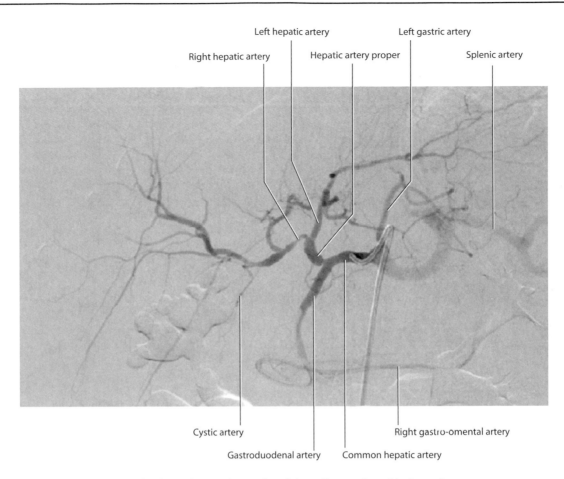

Right hepatic artery

Left hepatic artery

Hepatic artery proper

Left gastric artery

Splenic artery

Cystic artery

Gastroduodenal artery

Common hepatic artery

Right gastro-omental artery

Digital subtraction angiography of the celiac trunk and its branches

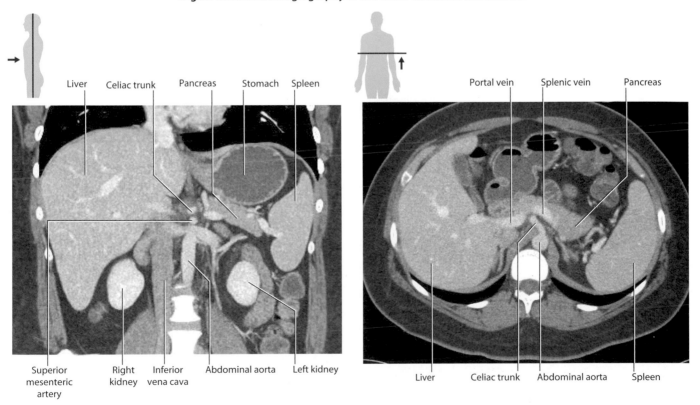

Liver   Celiac trunk   Pancreas   Stomach   Spleen

Portal vein   Splenic vein   Pancreas

Superior mesenteric artery

Right kidney

Inferior vena cava

Abdominal aorta

Left kidney

Liver   Celiac trunk   Abdominal aorta   Spleen

Positioning of the celiac trunk in relation to other structures.
CT image, with contrast, in coronal plane

Branching of the celiac trunk from the abdominal aorta.
CT image, with contrast, in axial plane

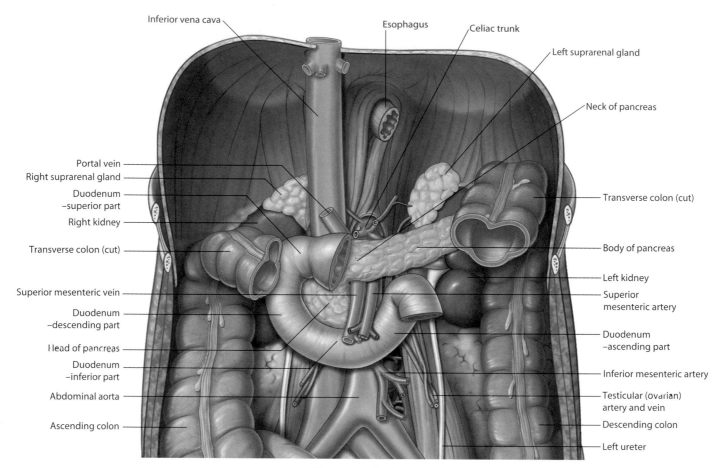

Inferior vena cava

Esophagus

Celiac trunk

Left suprarenal gland

Neck of pancreas

Portal vein

Right suprarenal gland

Duodenum –superior part

Right kidney

Transverse colon (cut)

Superior mesenteric vein

Duodenum –descending part

Head of pancreas

Duodenum –inferior part

Abdominal aorta

Ascending colon

Transverse colon (cut)

Body of pancreas

Left kidney

Superior mesenteric artery

Duodenum –ascending part

Inferior mesenteric artery

Testicular (ovarian) artery and vein

Descending colon

Left ureter

Duodenum in situ

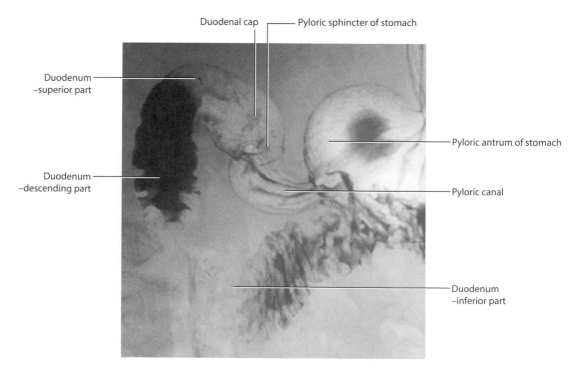

Duodenal cap

Pyloric sphincter of stomach

Duodenum –superior part

Duodenum –descending part

Pyloric antrum of stomach

Pyloric canal

Duodenum –inferior part

Double-contrast radiograph showing the duodenal cap

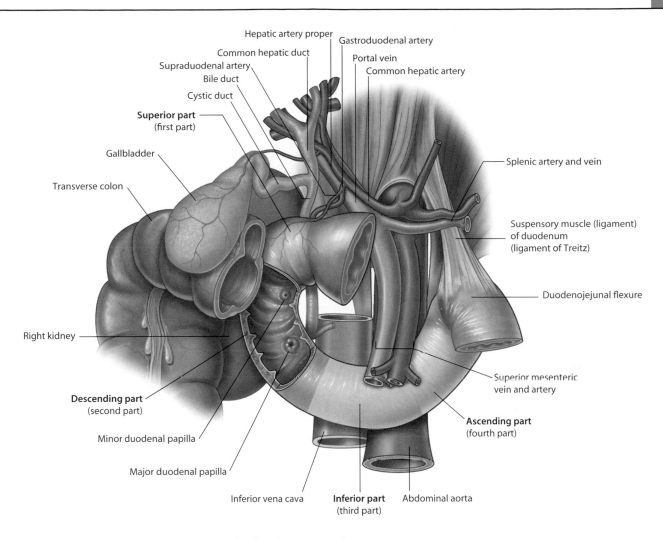

Hepatic artery proper
Common hepatic duct
Gastroduodenal artery
Portal vein
Supraduodenal artery
Common hepatic artery
Bile duct
Cystic duct
Superior part (first part)
Gallbladder
Splenic artery and vein
Transverse colon
Suspensory muscle (ligament) of duodenum (ligament of Treitz)
Duodenojejunal flexure
Right kidney
Superior mesenteric vein and artery
Descending part (second part)
Ascending part (fourth part)
Minor duodenal papilla
Major duodenal papilla
Inferior vena cava
Inferior part (third part)
Abdominal aorta

Parts of the duodenum and related structures

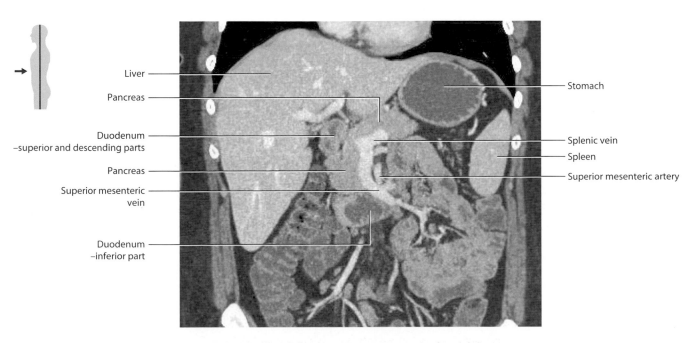

Liver
Stomach
Pancreas
Duodenum –superior and descending parts
Splenic vein
Spleen
Pancreas
Superior mesenteric artery
Superior mesenteric vein
Duodenum –inferior part

Relationship of duodenum to structures in the vicinity.
CT image, with contrast, in coronal plane

163

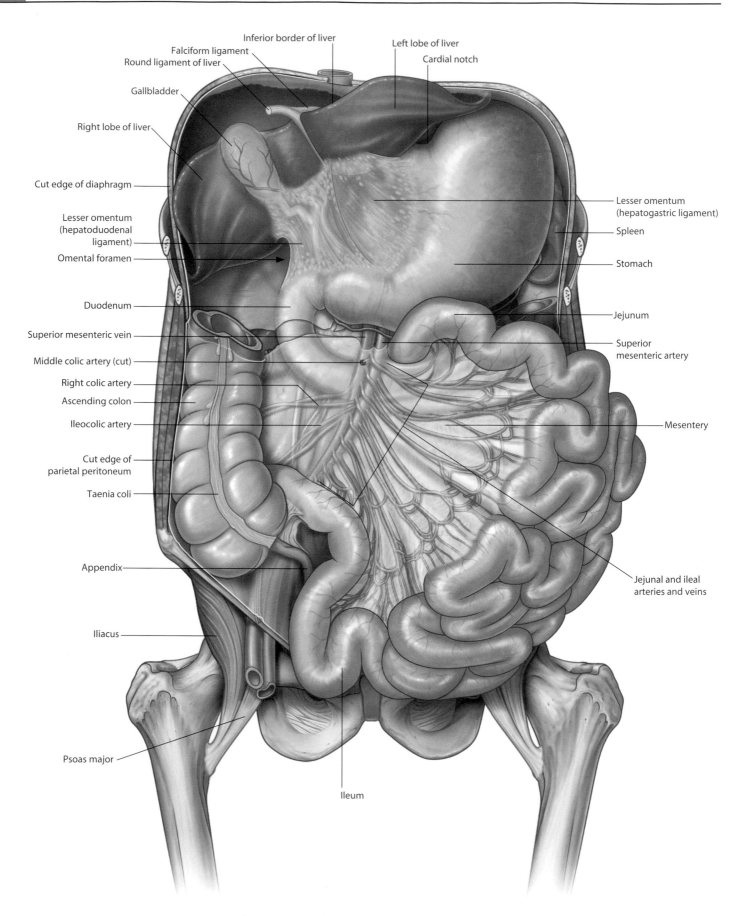

Inferior border of liver

Falciform ligament

Round ligament of liver

Gallbladder

Right lobe of liver

Cut edge of diaphragm

Lesser omentum (hepatoduodenal ligament)

Omental foramen

Duodenum

Superior mesenteric vein

Middle colic artery (cut)

Right colic artery

Ascending colon

Ileocolic artery

Cut edge of parietal peritoneum

Taenia coli

Appendix

Iliacus

Psoas major

Left lobe of liver

Cardial notch

Lesser omentum (hepatogastric ligament)

Spleen

Stomach

Jejunum

Superior mesenteric artery

Mesentery

Jejunal and ileal arteries and veins

Ileum

Small intestine displaced to show superior mesenteric vessels

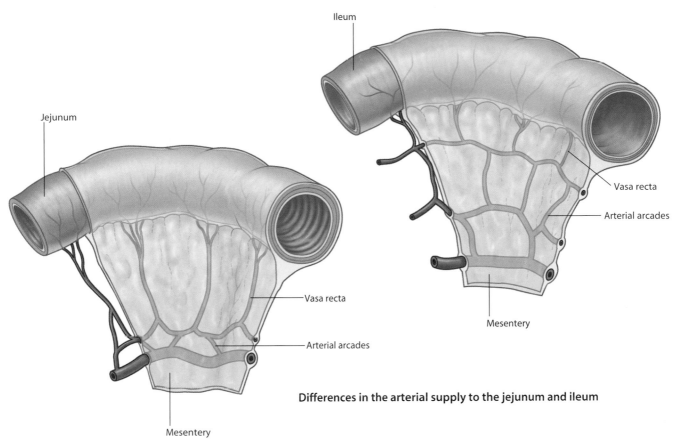

Jejunum

Ileum

Vasa recta

Vasa recta

Arterial arcades

Mesentery

Arterial arcades

Mesentery

Differences in the arterial supply to the jejunum and ileum

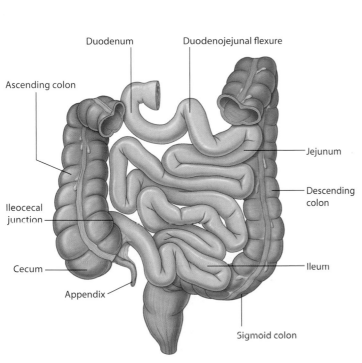

Duodenum

Duodenojejunal flexure

Ascending colon

Jejunum

Ileocecal junction

Descending colon

Cecum

Ileum

Appendix

Sigmoid colon

Jejunum and ileum

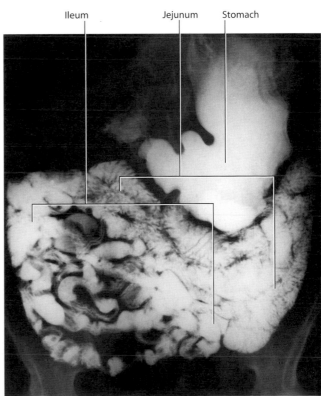

Ileum

Jejunum

Stomach

Radiograph using barium, showing jejunum and ileum

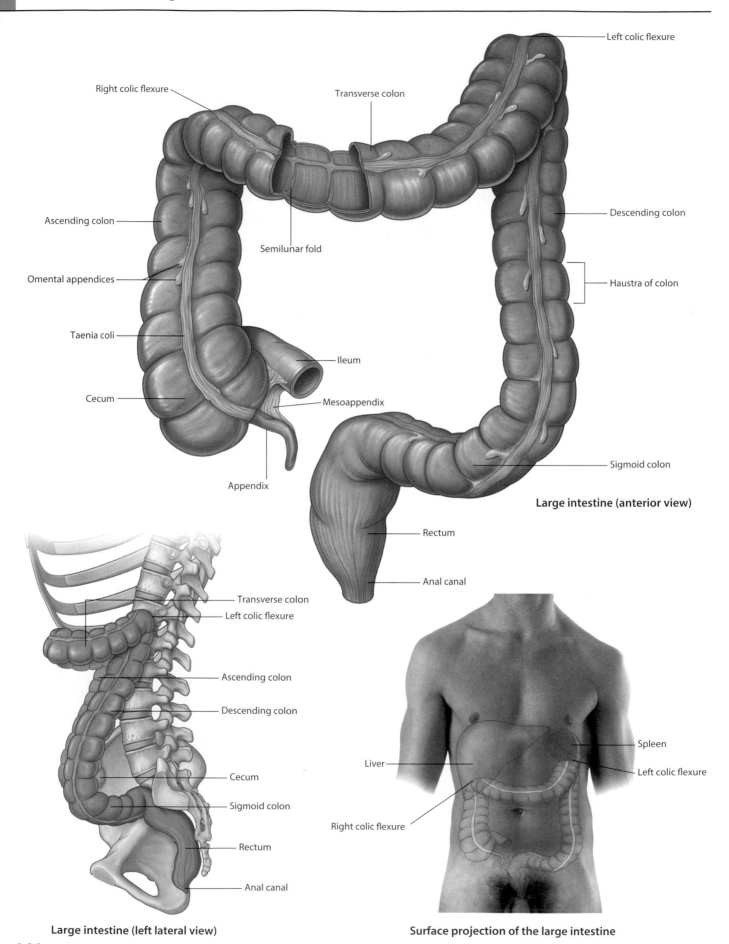

Right colic flexure

Transverse colon

Left colic flexure

Ascending colon

Descending colon

Semilunar fold

Haustra of colon

Omental appendices

Taenia coli

Ileum

Cecum

Mesoappendix

Sigmoid colon

Appendix

Large intestine (anterior view)

Rectum

Anal canal

Transverse colon

Left colic flexure

Ascending colon

Descending colon

Spleen

Cecum

Left colic flexure

Sigmoid colon

Liver

Rectum

Right colic flexure

Anal canal

Large intestine (left lateral view)

Surface projection of the large intestine

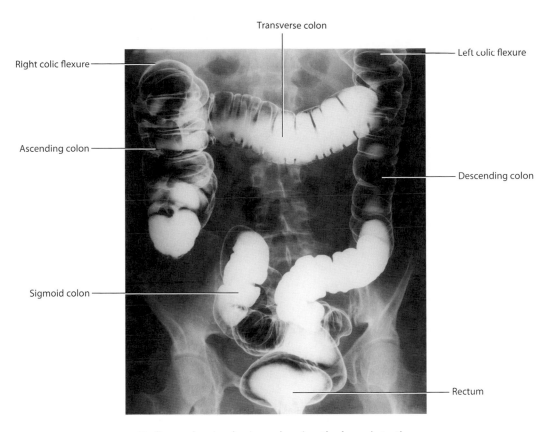

Radiograph using barium, showing the large intestine

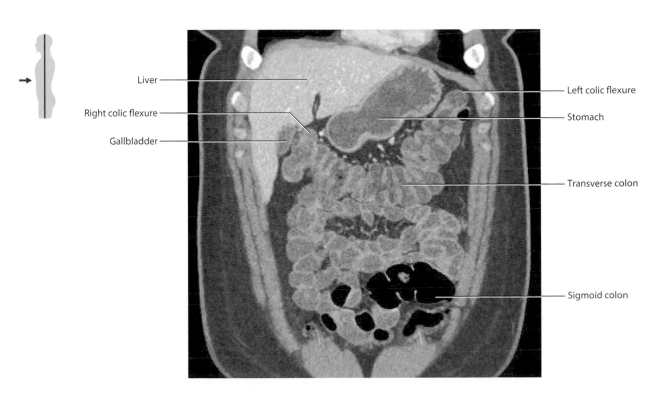

Transverse colon showing right and left colic flexures.
CT image, with contrast, in coronal plane

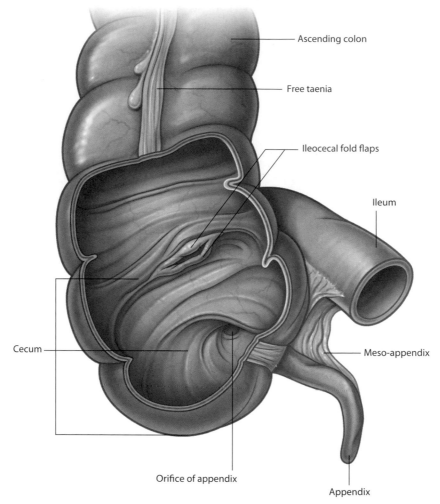

Ascending colon

Free taenia

Ileocecal fold flaps

Ileum

Cecum

Meso-appendix

Orifice of appendix

Appendix

Ileocecal junction

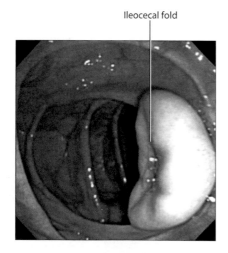

Ileocecal fold

Colonoscopy showing ileocecal fold

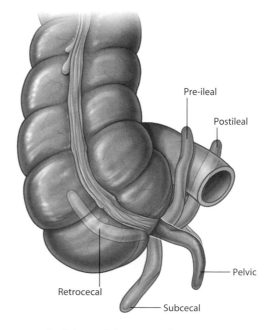

Pre-ileal

Postileal

Pelvic

Retrocecal

Subcecal

Positions of the appendix

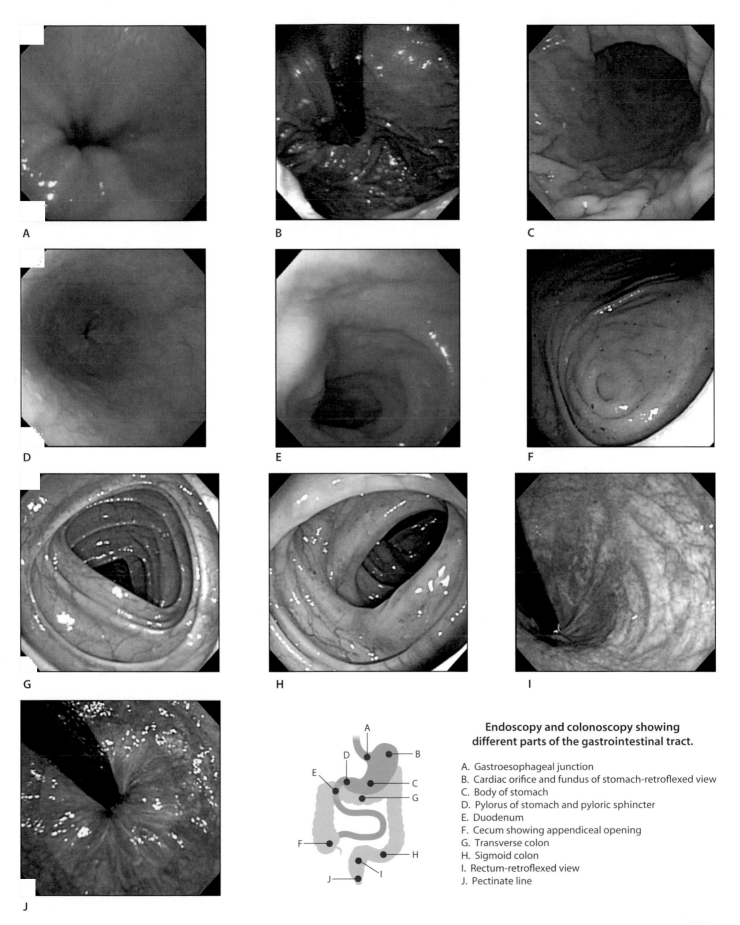

Endoscopy and colonoscopy showing different parts of the gastrointestinal tract.

A. Gastroesophageal junction
B. Cardiac orifice and fundus of stomach-retroflexed view
C. Body of stomach
D. Pylorus of stomach and pyloric sphincter
E. Duodenum
F. Cecum showing appendiceal opening
G. Transverse colon
H. Sigmoid colon
I. Rectum-retroflexed view
J. Pectinate line

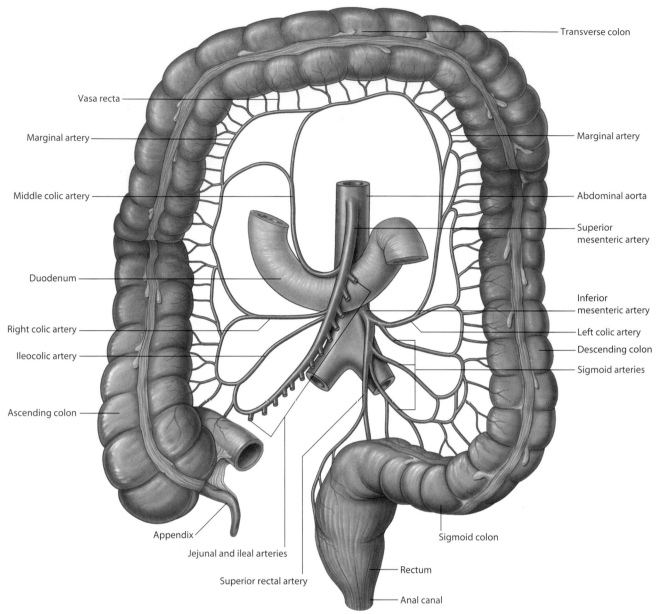

Transverse colon

Vasa recta

Marginal artery

Middle colic artery

Duodenum

Right colic artery

Ileocolic artery

Ascending colon

Marginal artery

Abdominal aorta

Superior mesenteric artery

Inferior mesenteric artery

Left colic artery

Descending colon

Sigmoid arteries

Appendix

Jejunal and ileal arteries

Superior rectal artery

Sigmoid colon

Rectum

Anal canal

Superior and inferior mesenteric arteries

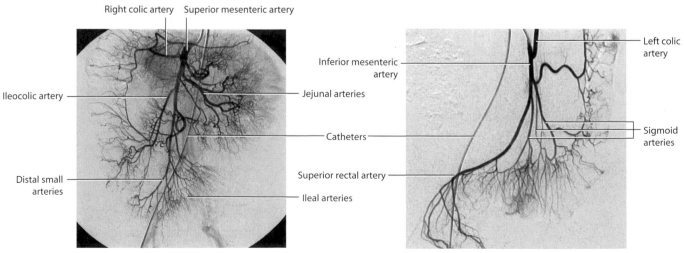

Right colic artery

Superior mesenteric artery

Ileocolic artery

Distal small arteries

Inferior mesenteric artery

Jejunal arteries

Catheters

Superior rectal artery

Ileal arteries

Left colic artery

Sigmoid arteries

Digital subtraction angiography of the superior mesenteric artery and its branches

Digital subtraction angiography of the inferior mesenteric artery and its branches

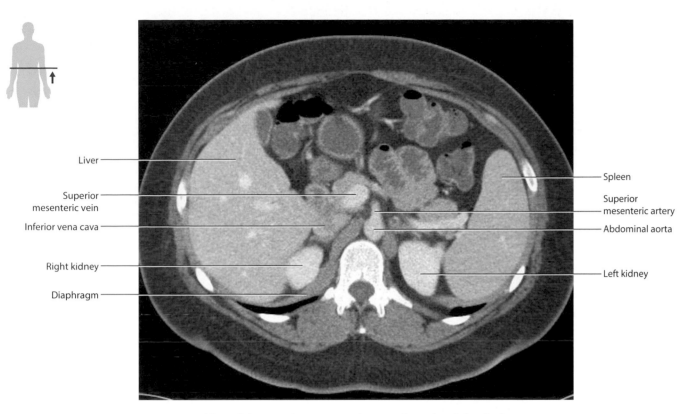

Liver

Superior mesenteric vein

Inferior vena cava

Right kidney

Diaphragm

Spleen

Superior mesenteric artery

Abdominal aorta

Left kidney

Branching of the superior mesenteric artery from the abdominal aorta.
CT image, with contrast, in axial plane

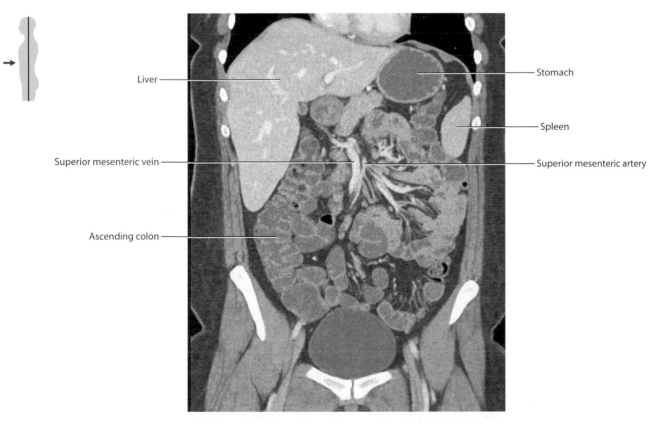

Liver

Superior mesenteric vein

Ascending colon

Stomach

Spleen

Superior mesenteric artery

Positioning of the superior mesenteric artery in relation to other structures.
CT image, with contrast, in coronal plane

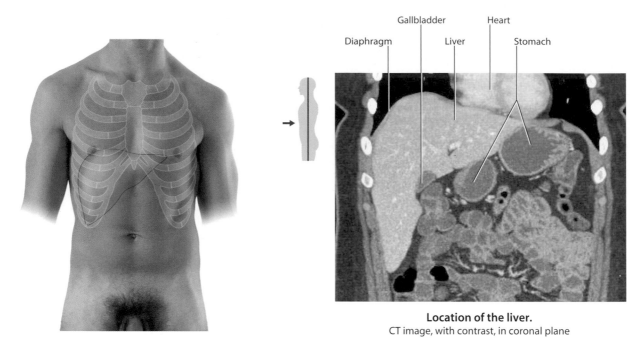

Surface projection of the liver (anterior view)

Location of the liver.
CT image, with contrast, in coronal plane

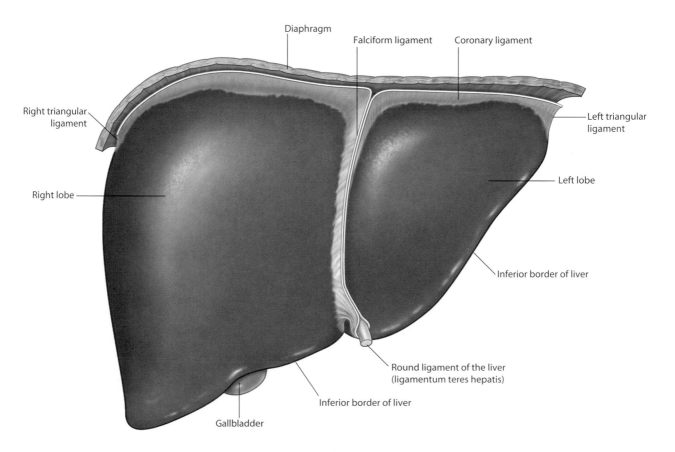

Anterior surface of liver

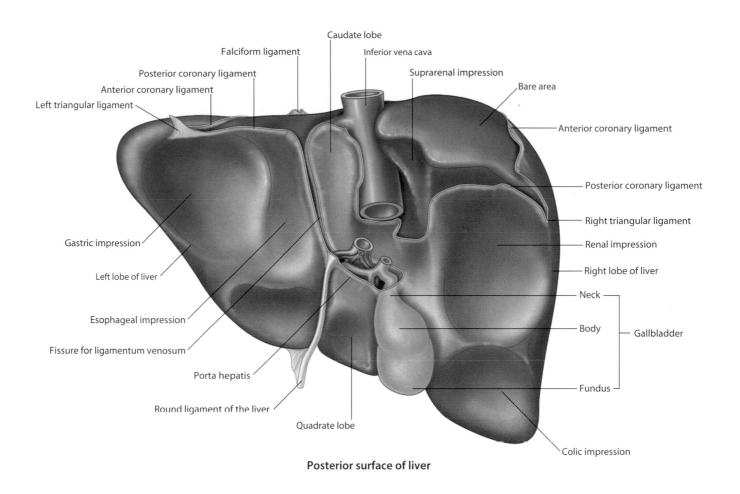

Posterior surface of liver

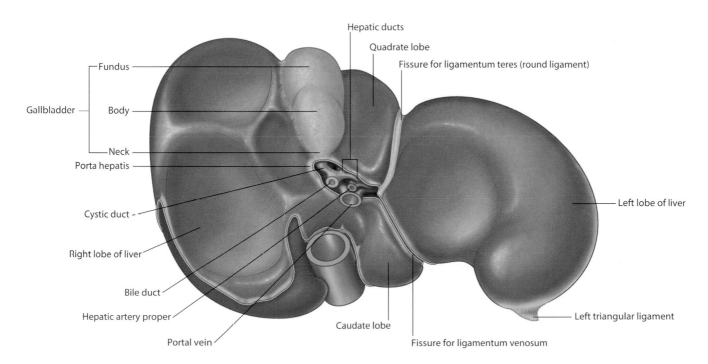

Visceral surface of liver

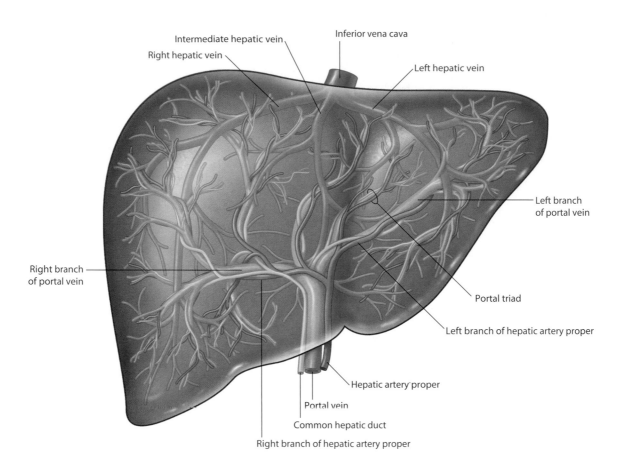

Intermediate hepatic vein

Right hepatic vein

Inferior vena cava

Left hepatic vein

Left branch of portal vein

Right branch of portal vein

Portal triad

Left branch of hepatic artery proper

Hepatic artery proper

Portal vein

Common hepatic duct

Right branch of hepatic artery proper

Anterior surface of liver with hepatic veins, portal vein, and associated vessels

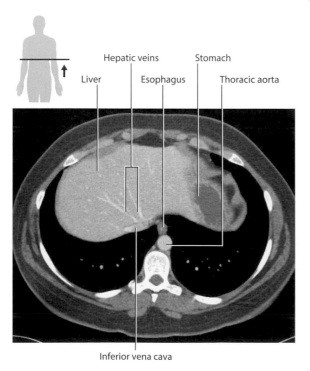

Liver

Hepatic veins

Esophagus

Stomach

Thoracic aorta

Inferior vena cava

**Hepatic veins entering the inferior vena cava
in the substance of the liver.**
CT image, with contrast, in axial plane

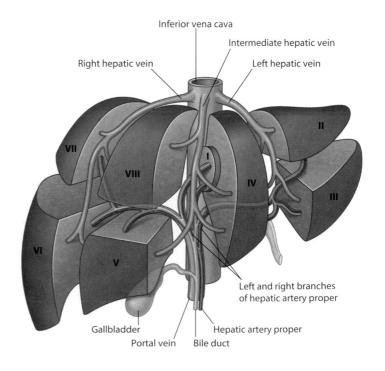

Inferior vena cava

Intermediate hepatic vein

Right hepatic vein

Left hepatic vein

II

VII

I

VIII

IV

III

VI

V

Left and right branches
of hepatic artery proper

Gallbladder

Portal vein

Bile duct

Hepatic artery proper

Arrangement of the hepatic venous segments

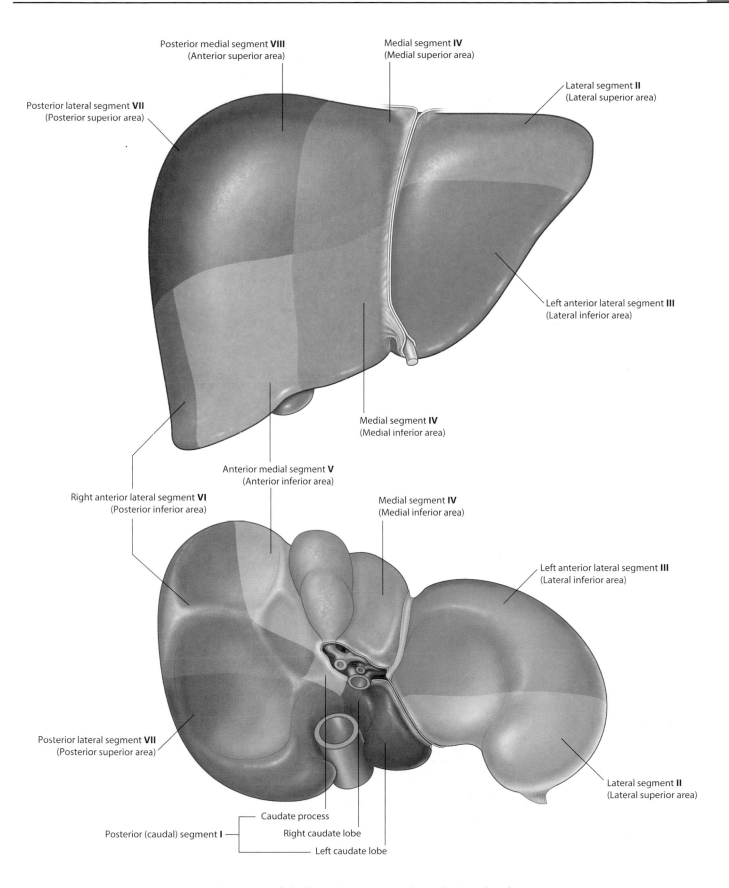

Posterior medial segment **VIII**
(Anterior superior area)

Medial segment **IV**
(Medial superior area)

Lateral segment **II**
(Lateral superior area)

Posterior lateral segment **VII**
(Posterior superior area)

Left anterior lateral segment **III**
(Lateral inferior area)

Medial segment **IV**
(Medial inferior area)

Anterior medial segment **V**
(Anterior inferior area)

Medial segment **IV**
(Medial inferior area)

Right anterior lateral segment **VI**
(Posterior inferior area)

Left anterior lateral segment **III**
(Lateral inferior area)

Posterior lateral segment **VII**
(Posterior superior area)

Lateral segment **II**
(Lateral superior area)

Caudate process

Posterior (caudal) segment **I**

Right caudate lobe

Left caudate lobe

Segments of the liver shown on anterior and visceral surfaces

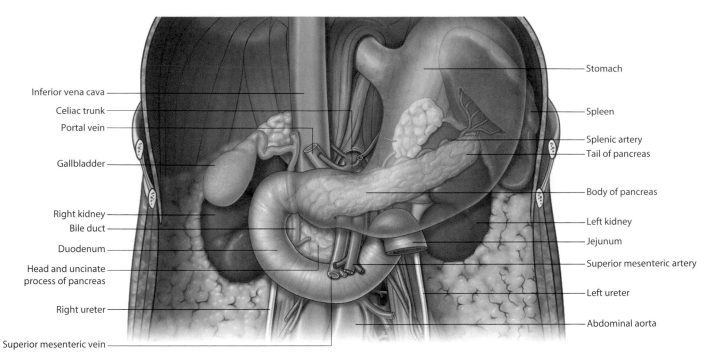

Inferior vena cava

Celiac trunk

Portal vein

Gallbladder

Right kidney

Bile duct

Duodenum

Head and uncinate process of pancreas

Right ureter

Superior mesenteric vein

Stomach

Spleen

Splenic artery

Tail of pancreas

Body of pancreas

Left kidney

Jejunum

Superior mesenteric artery

Left ureter

Abdominal aorta

Pancreas with related structures

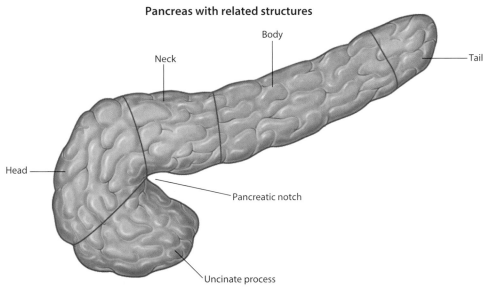

Neck

Body

Tail

Head

Pancreatic notch

Uncinate process

Anterior surface of the pancreas

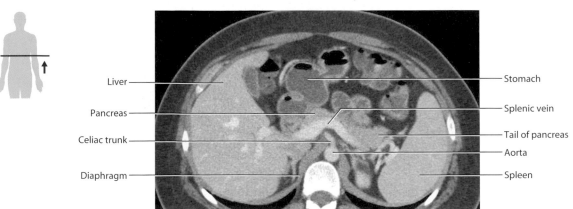

Liver

Pancreas

Celiac trunk

Diaphragm

Stomach

Splenic vein

Tail of pancreas

Aorta

Spleen

Pancreas.
CT image, with contrast, in axial plane

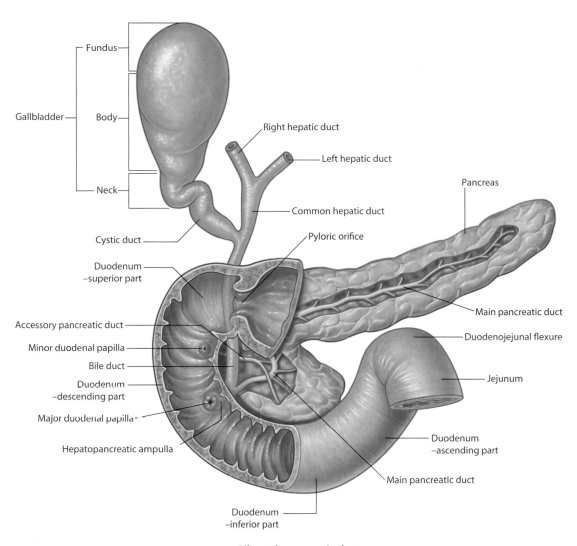

Fundus

Gallbladder

Body

Neck

Right hepatic duct

Left hepatic duct

Common hepatic duct

Cystic duct

Pyloric orifice

Pancreas

Duodenum
–superior part

Accessory pancreatic duct

Minor duodenal papilla

Bile duct

Duodenum
–descending part

Major duodenal papilla

Hepatopancreatic ampulla

Main pancreatic duct

Duodenojejunal flexure

Jejunum

Duodenum
–ascending part

Main pancreatic duct

Duodenum
–inferior part

Bile and pancreatic ducts

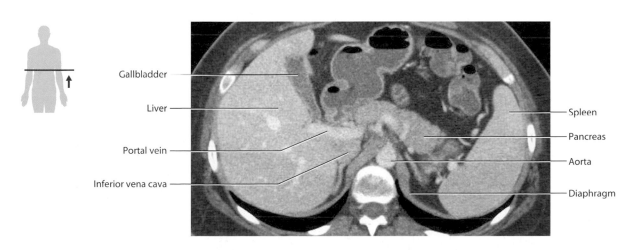

Gallbladder

Liver

Portal vein

Inferior vena cava

Spleen

Pancreas

Aorta

Diaphragm

Positioning of the gallbladder in relation to other structures.
CT image, with contrast, in axial plane

177

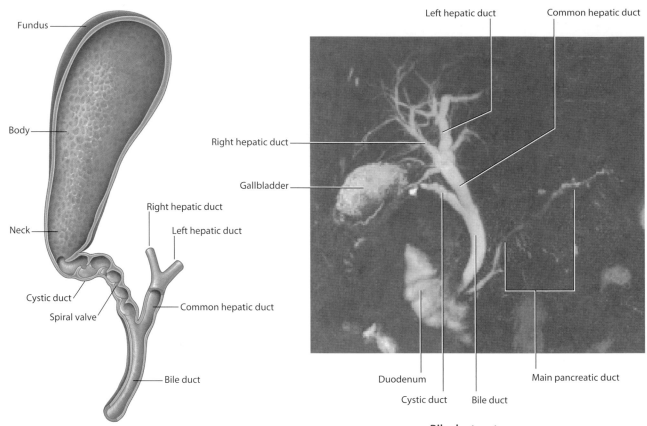

Section through gallbladder and bile ducts

Fundus
Body
Neck
Cystic duct
Spiral valve
Right hepatic duct
Left hepatic duct
Common hepatic duct
Bile duct

Left hepatic duct
Common hepatic duct
Right hepatic duct
Gallbladder
Duodenum
Cystic duct
Bile duct
Main pancreatic duct

Bile duct system.
Magnetic resonance cholecystopancreatogram

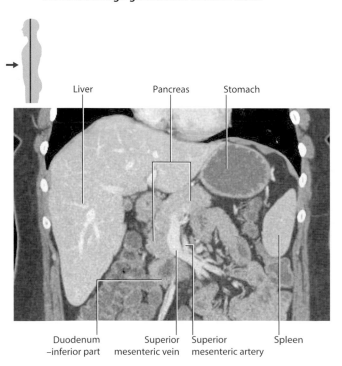

Liver
Pancreas
Stomach
Duodenum
–inferior part
Superior
mesenteric vein
Superior
mesenteric artery
Spleen

Positioning of the pancreas in relation to other structures.
CT image, with contrast, in coronal plane

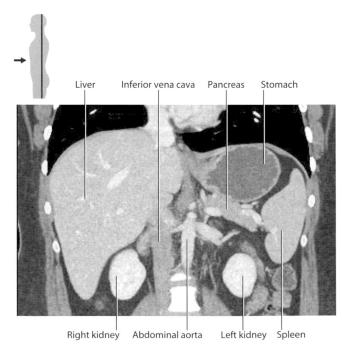

Liver
Inferior vena cava
Pancreas
Stomach
Right kidney
Abdominal aorta
Left kidney
Spleen

Relationship of pancreas to the stomach and spleen.
CT image, with contrast, in coronal plane

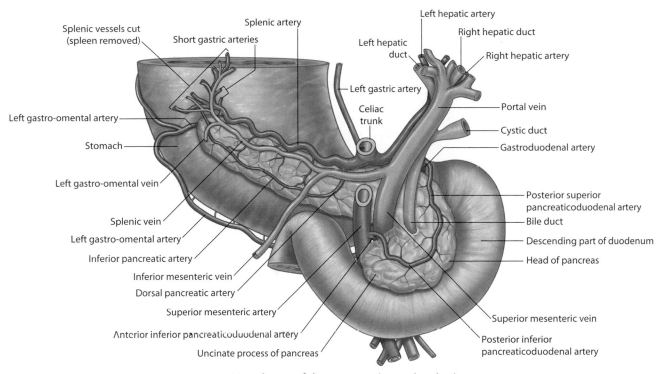

Splenic vessels cut (spleen removed)
Short gastric arteries
Splenic artery
Left hepatic artery
Right hepatic duct
Left hepatic duct
Right hepatic artery
Left gastric artery
Celiac trunk
Portal vein
Cystic duct
Gastroduodenal artery
Left gastro-omental artery
Stomach
Left gastro-omental vein
Splenic vein
Left gastro-omental artery
Inferior pancreatic artery
Inferior mesenteric vein
Dorsal pancreatic artery
Superior mesenteric artery
Anterior inferior pancreaticoduodenal artery
Uncinate process of pancreas
Posterior superior pancreaticoduodenal artery
Bile duct
Descending part of duodenum
Head of pancreas
Superior mesenteric vein
Posterior inferior pancreaticoduodenal artery

Vasculature of the pancreas (posterior view)

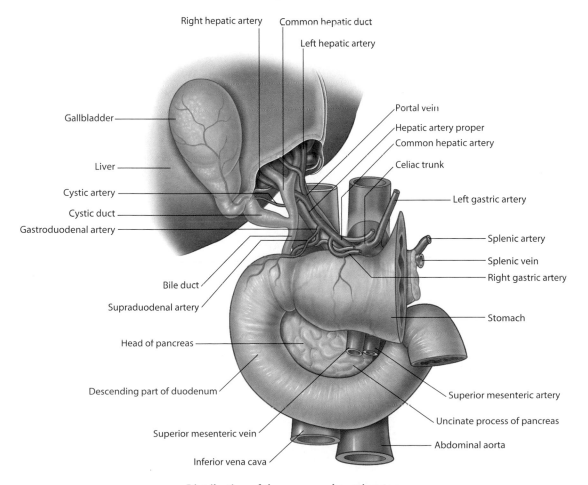

Right hepatic artery
Common hepatic duct
Left hepatic artery
Gallbladder
Liver
Cystic artery
Cystic duct
Gastroduodenal artery
Bile duct
Supraduodenal artery
Head of pancreas
Descending part of duodenum
Superior mesenteric vein
Inferior vena cava
Portal vein
Hepatic artery proper
Common hepatic artery
Celiac trunk
Left gastric artery
Splenic artery
Splenic vein
Right gastric artery
Stomach
Superior mesenteric artery
Uncinate process of pancreas
Abdominal aorta

Distribution of the common hepatic artery

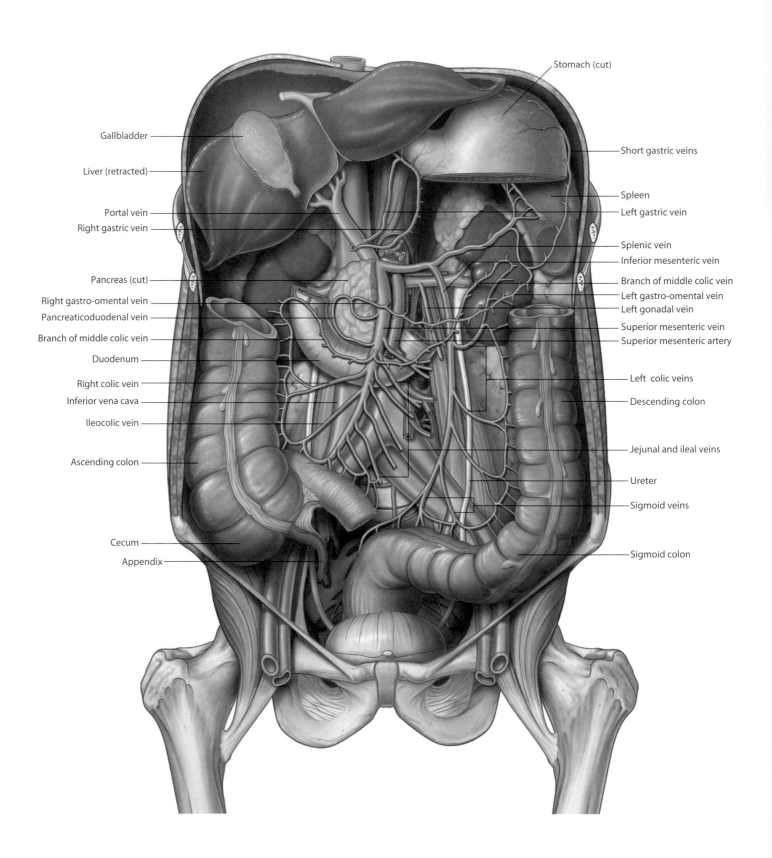

Gallbladder

Liver (retracted)

Portal vein

Right gastric vein

Pancreas (cut)

Right gastro-omental vein

Pancreaticoduodenal vein

Branch of middle colic vein

Duodenum

Right colic vein

Inferior vena cava

Ileocolic vein

Ascending colon

Cecum

Appendix

Stomach (cut)

Short gastric veins

Spleen

Left gastric vein

Splenic vein

Inferior mesenteric vein

Branch of middle colic vein

Left gastro-omental vein

Left gonadal vein

Superior mesenteric vein

Superior mesenteric artery

Left colic veins

Descending colon

Jejunal and ileal veins

Ureter

Sigmoid veins

Sigmoid colon

Venous drainage of the abdominal portion of the gastrointestinal tract in situ

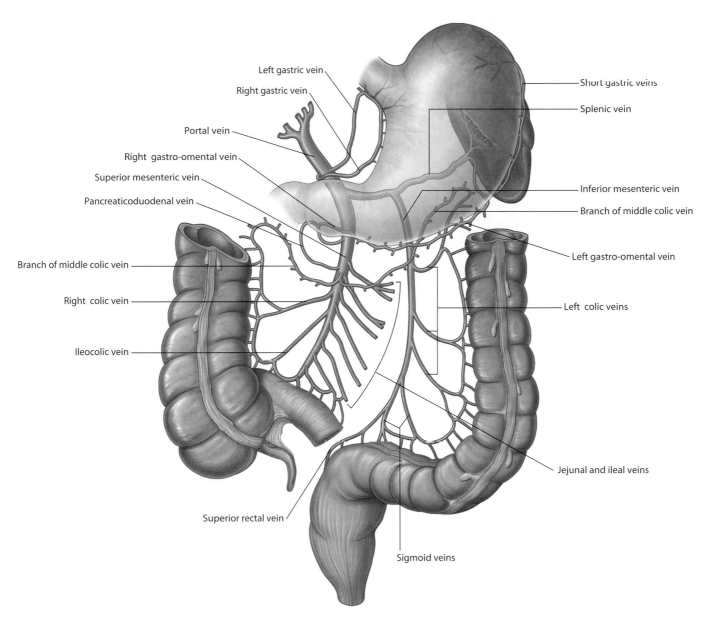

Venous drainage of the abdominal portion of the gastrointestinal tract

Labels (clockwise from top): Left gastric vein, Right gastric vein, Portal vein, Right gastro-omental vein, Superior mesenteric vein, Pancreaticoduodenal vein, Branch of middle colic vein, Right colic vein, Ileocolic vein, Superior rectal vein, Sigmoid veins, Jejunal and ileal veins, Left colic veins, Left gastro-omental vein, Branch of middle colic vein, Inferior mesenteric vein, Splenic vein, Short gastric veins

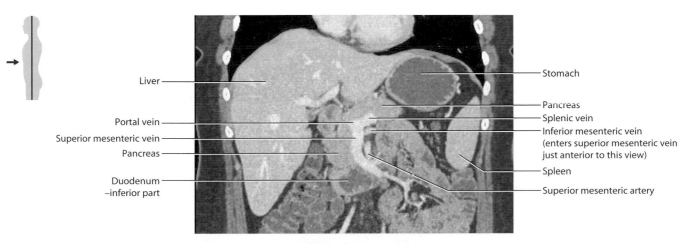

Labels: Liver, Portal vein, Superior mesenteric vein, Pancreas, Duodenum –inferior part, Stomach, Pancreas, Splenic vein, Inferior mesenteric vein (enters superior mesenteric vein just anterior to this view), Spleen, Superior mesenteric artery

Formation of the portal vein.
CT image, with contrast, in coronal plane

181

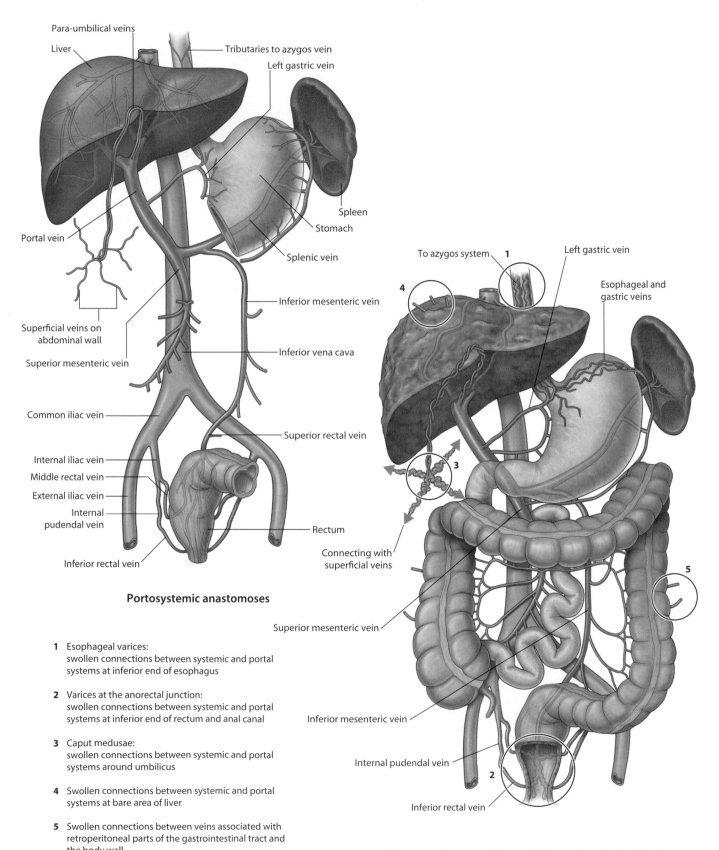

Para-umbilical veins

Liver

Tributaries to azygos vein

Left gastric vein

Portal vein

Spleen

Stomach

Splenic vein

Inferior mesenteric vein

Superficial veins on abdominal wall

Superior mesenteric vein

Inferior vena cava

Common iliac vein

Superior rectal vein

Internal iliac vein

Middle rectal vein

External iliac vein

Internal pudendal vein

Rectum

Inferior rectal vein

To azygos system

1

Left gastric vein

4

Esophageal and gastric veins

3

5

Connecting with superficial veins

Superior mesenteric vein

Inferior mesenteric vein

Internal pudendal vein

2

Inferior rectal vein

Portosystemic anastomoses

1 Esophageal varices:
   swollen connections between systemic and portal
   systems at inferior end of esophagus

2 Varices at the anorectal junction:
   swollen connections between systemic and portal
   systems at inferior end of rectum and anal canal

3 Caput medusae:
   swollen connections between systemic and portal
   systems around umbilicus

4 Swollen connections between systemic and portal
   systems at bare area of liver

5 Swollen connections between veins associated with
   retroperitoneal parts of the gastrointestinal tract and
   the body wall

Venous enlargement in portal hypertension (varices)

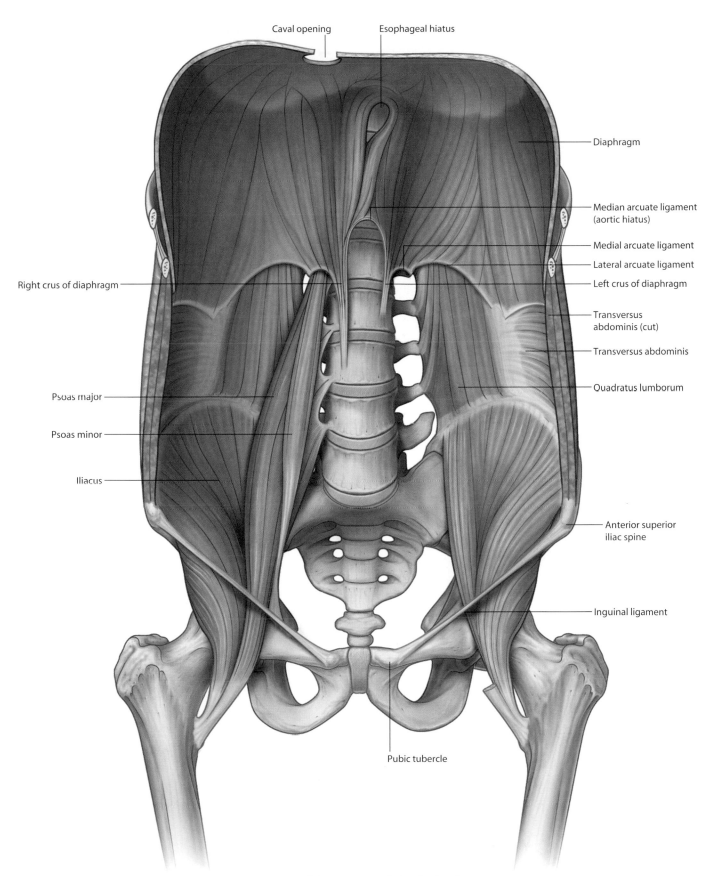

Caval opening

Esophageal hiatus

Diaphragm

Median arcuate ligament
(aortic hiatus)

Medial arcuate ligament

Lateral arcuate ligament

Right crus of diaphragm

Left crus of diaphragm

Transversus
abdominis (cut)

Transversus abdominis

Quadratus lumborum

Psoas major

Psoas minor

Iliacus

Anterior superior
iliac spine

Inguinal ligament

Pubic tubercle

Muscles of the posterior abdominal wall

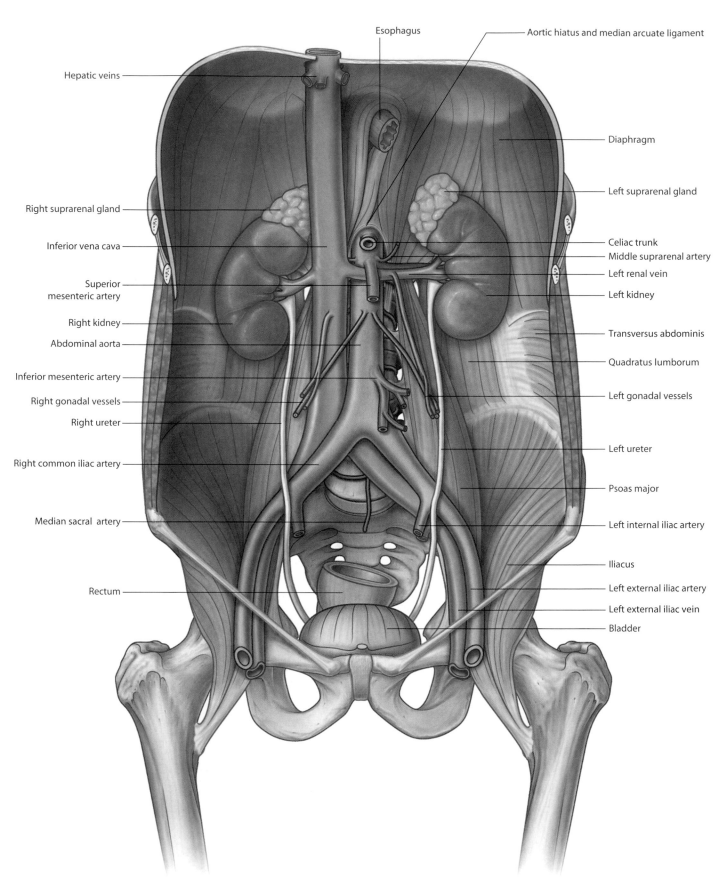

Esophagus

Aortic hiatus and median arcuate ligament

Hepatic veins

Diaphragm

Right suprarenal gland

Left suprarenal gland

Inferior vena cava

Celiac trunk

Middle suprarenal artery

Left renal vein

Superior mesenteric artery

Left kidney

Right kidney

Transversus abdominis

Abdominal aorta

Quadratus lumborum

Inferior mesenteric artery

Left gonadal vessels

Right gonadal vessels

Right ureter

Left ureter

Right common iliac artery

Psoas major

Median sacral artery

Left internal iliac artery

Iliacus

Left external iliac artery

Left external iliac vein

Rectum

Bladder

Vessels and their relationship to the posterior abdominal wall

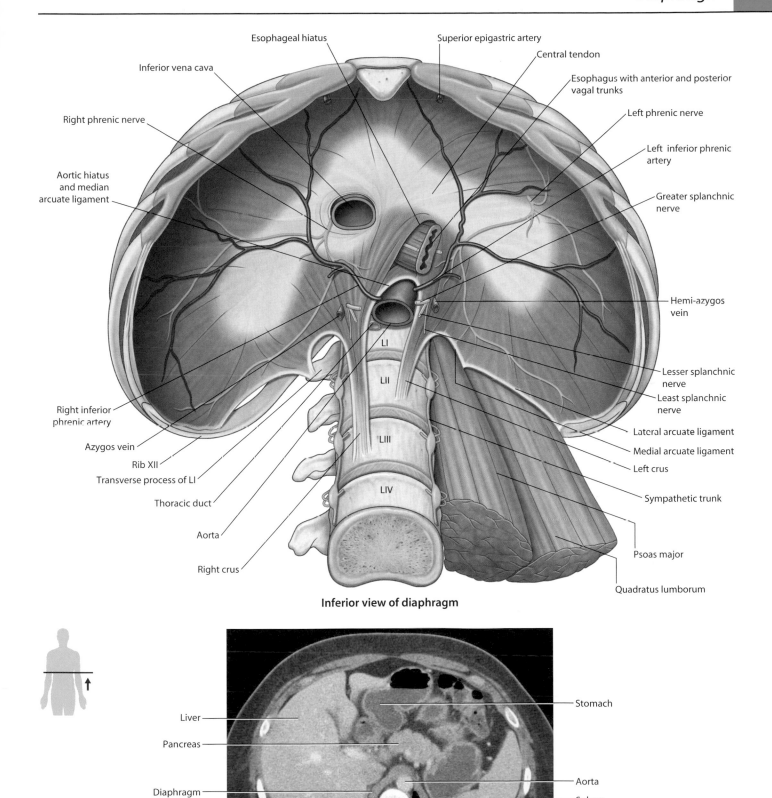

Esophageal hiatus

Inferior vena cava

Right phrenic nerve

Aortic hiatus and median arcuate ligament

Right inferior phrenic artery

Azygos vein

Rib XII

Transverse process of LI

Thoracic duct

Aorta

Right crus

Superior epigastric artery

Central tendon

Esophagus with anterior and posterior vagal trunks

Left phrenic nerve

Left inferior phrenic artery

Greater splanchnic nerve

Hemi-azygos vein

Lesser splanchnic nerve

Least splanchnic nerve

Lateral arcuate ligament

Medial arcuate ligament

Left crus

Sympathetic trunk

Psoas major

Quadratus lumborum

LI

LII

LIII

LIV

Inferior view of diaphragm

Liver

Pancreas

Diaphragm

Stomach

Aorta

Spleen

Pleural cavity

Positioning of the diaphragm in relation to other structures.
CT image, with contrast, in axial plane

185

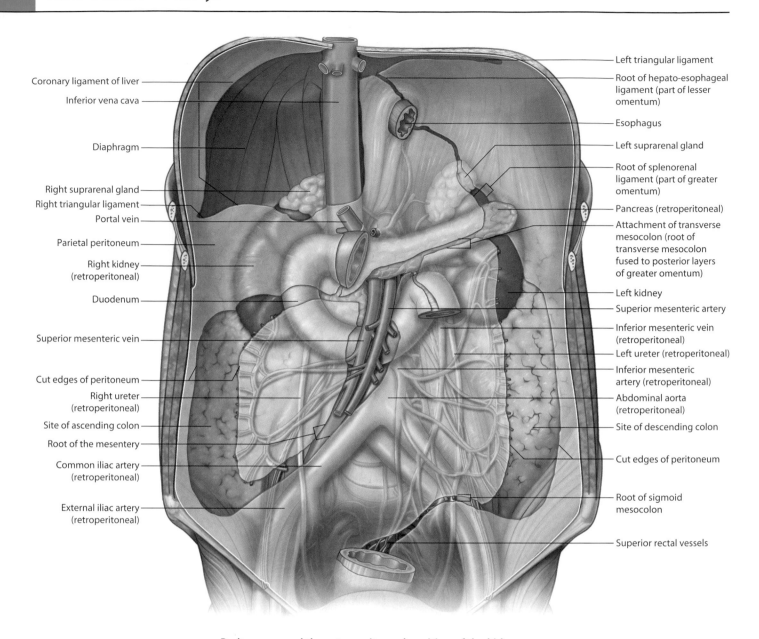

Coronary ligament of liver

Inferior vena cava

Diaphragm

Right suprarenal gland

Right triangular ligament

Portal vein

Parietal peritoneum

Right kidney (retroperitoneal)

Duodenum

Superior mesenteric vein

Cut edges of peritoneum

Right ureter (retroperitoneal)

Site of ascending colon

Root of the mesentery

Common iliac artery (retroperitoneal)

External iliac artery (retroperitoneal)

Left triangular ligament

Root of hepato-esophageal ligament (part of lesser omentum)

Esophagus

Left suprarenal gland

Root of splenorenal ligament (part of greater omentum)

Pancreas (retroperitoneal)

Attachment of transverse mesocolon (root of transverse mesocolon fused to posterior layers of greater omentum)

Left kidney

Superior mesenteric artery

Inferior mesenteric vein (retroperitoneal)

Left ureter (retroperitoneal)

Inferior mesenteric artery (retroperitoneal)

Abdominal aorta (retroperitoneal)

Site of descending colon

Cut edges of peritoneum

Root of sigmoid mesocolon

Superior rectal vessels

Peritoneum and the retroperitoneal position of the kidneys

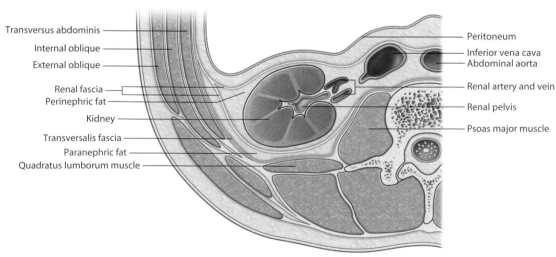

Transversus abdominis

Internal oblique

External oblique

Renal fascia

Perinephric fat

Kidney

Transversalis fascia

Paranephric fat

Quadratus lumborum muscle

Peritoneum

Inferior vena cava

Abdominal aorta

Renal artery and vein

Renal pelvis

Psoas major muscle

Organization of fat and fascia surrounding the kidneys

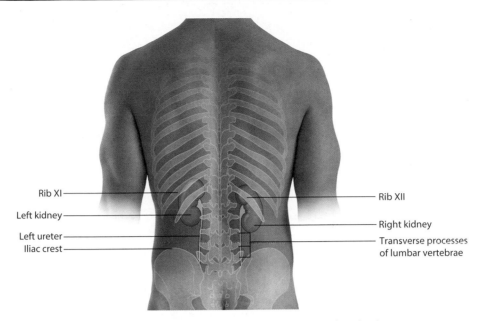

Surface projection of the kidneys and ureters (posterior view)

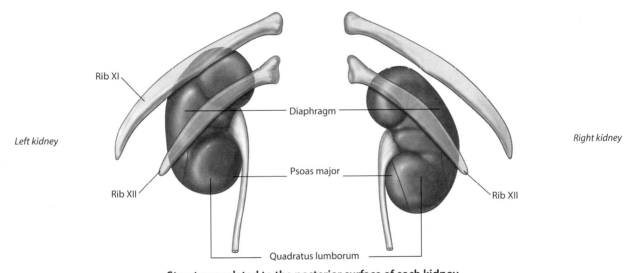

Structures related to the posterior surface of each kidney

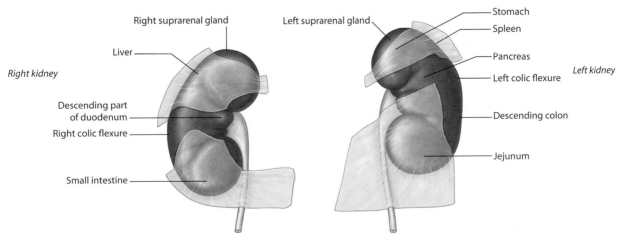

Structures related to the anterior surface of each kidney

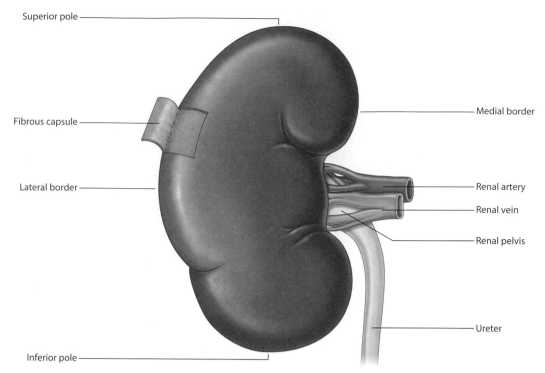

Superior pole

Fibrous capsule

Lateral border

Medial border

Renal artery

Renal vein

Renal pelvis

Ureter

Inferior pole

Anterior surface of right kidney

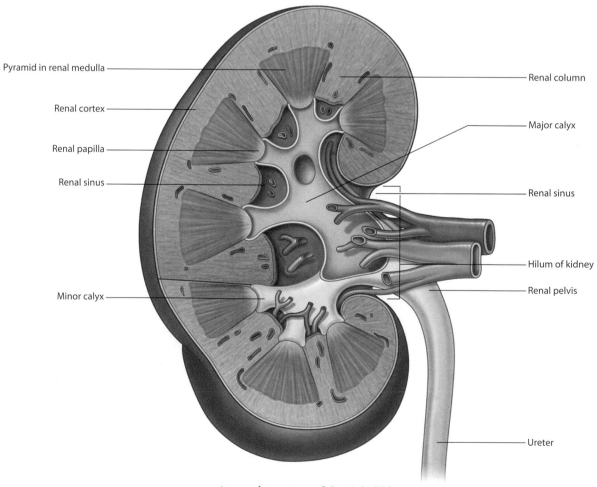

Pyramid in renal medulla

Renal cortex

Renal papilla

Renal sinus

Minor calyx

Renal column

Major calyx

Renal sinus

Hilum of kidney

Renal pelvis

Ureter

Internal structure of the right kidney

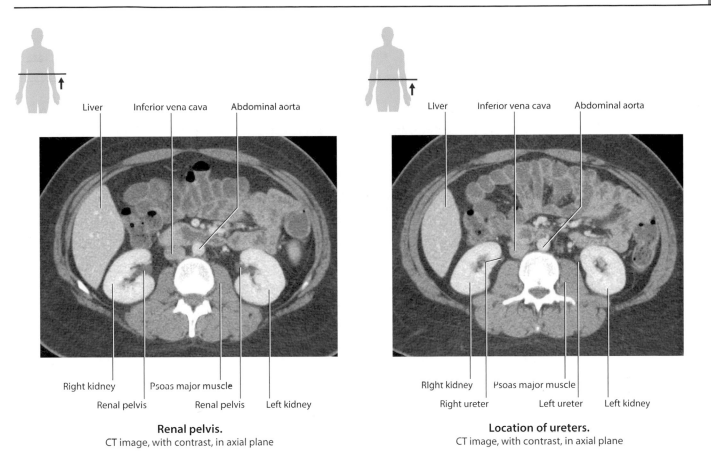

Liver   Inferior vena cava   Abdominal aorta

Right kidney   Psoas major muscle
Renal pelvis   Renal pelvis   Left kidney

Renal pelvis.
CT image, with contrast, in axial plane

Liver   Inferior vena cava   Abdominal aorta

Right kidney   Psoas major muscle
Right ureter   Left ureter   Left kidney

Location of ureters.
CT image, with contrast, in axial plane

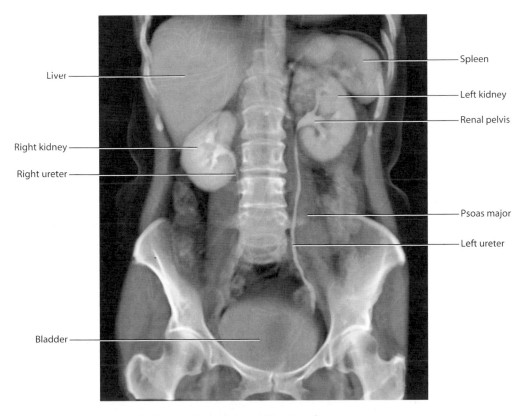

Liver

Spleen

Left kidney

Renal pelvis

Right kidney

Right ureter

Psoas major

Left ureter

Bladder

Pathway of ureter in relation to other structures.
Coronal view of 3-D urogram using multidetector computed tomography

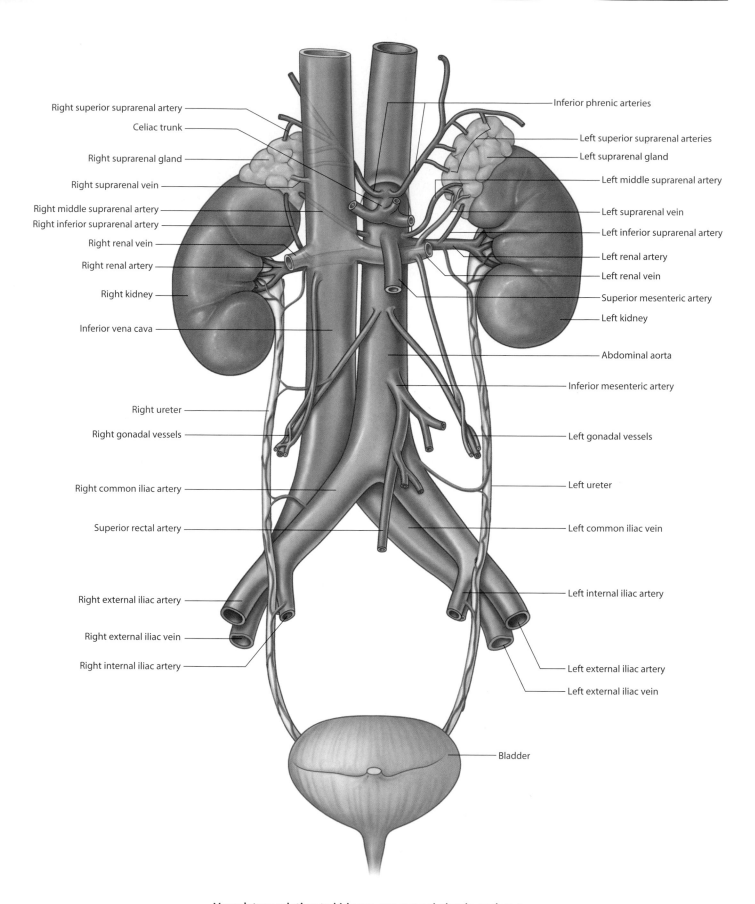

Right superior suprarenal artery

Celiac trunk

Right suprarenal gland

Right suprarenal vein

Right middle suprarenal artery

Right inferior suprarenal artery

Right renal vein

Right renal artery

Right kidney

Inferior vena cava

Right ureter

Right gonadal vessels

Right common iliac artery

Superior rectal artery

Right external iliac artery

Right external iliac vein

Right internal iliac artery

Inferior phrenic arteries

Left superior suprarenal arteries

Left suprarenal gland

Left middle suprarenal artery

Left suprarenal vein

Left inferior suprarenal artery

Left renal artery

Left renal vein

Superior mesenteric artery

Left kidney

Abdominal aorta

Inferior mesenteric artery

Left gonadal vessels

Left ureter

Left common iliac vein

Left internal iliac artery

Left external iliac artery

Left external iliac vein

Bladder

Vasculature relating to kidneys, suprarenal glands, and ureters

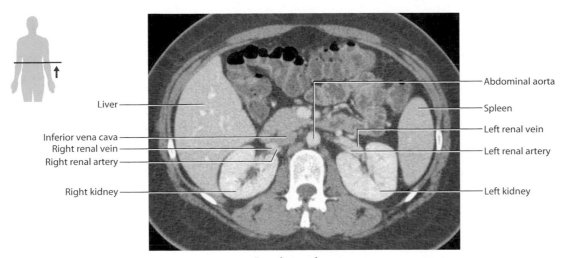

Liver

Inferior vena cava
Right renal vein
Right renal artery

Right kidney

Abdominal aorta

Spleen

Left renal vein

Left renal artery

Left kidney

Renal vasculature.
CT image, with contrast, in axial plane

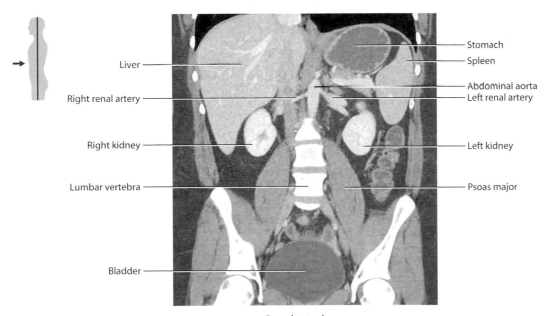

Liver

Right renal artery

Right kidney

Lumbar vertebra

Bladder

Stomach

Spleen

Abdominal aorta
Left renal artery

Left kidney

Psoas major

Renal arteries.
CT image, with contrast, in coronal plane

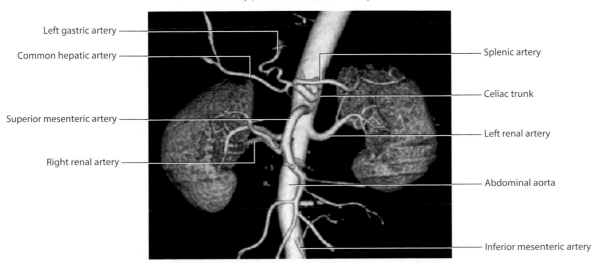

Left gastric artery

Common hepatic artery

Superior mesenteric artery

Right renal artery

Splenic artery

Celiac trunk

Left renal artery

Abdominal aorta

Inferior mesenteric artery

Renal arteries.
Volume-rendered anterior view using multidetector computer tomography

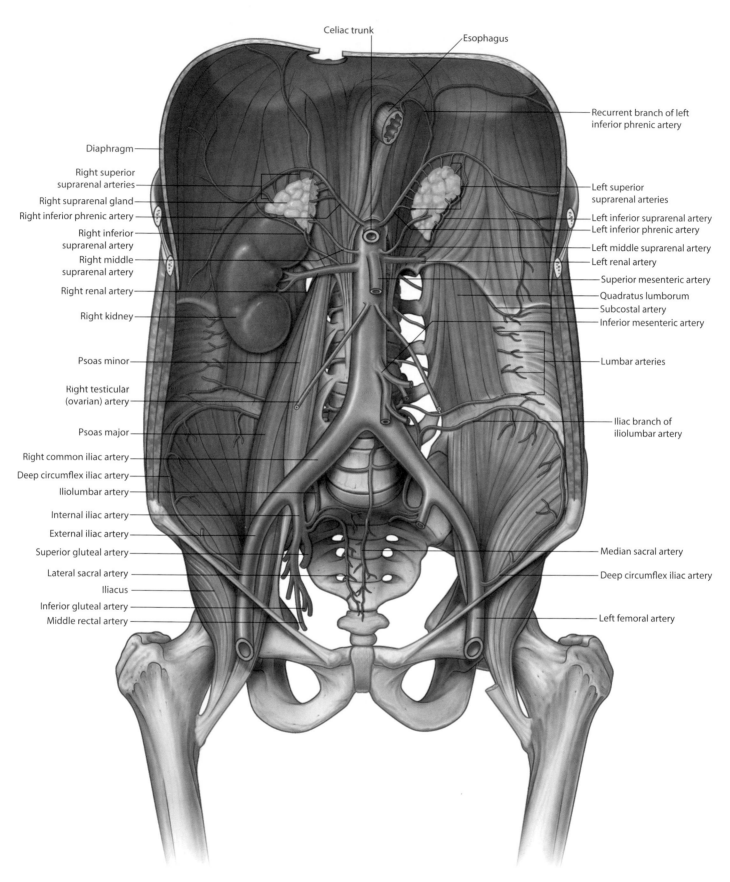

Celiac trunk

Esophagus

Recurrent branch of left inferior phrenic artery

Diaphragm

Right superior suprarenal arteries

Right suprarenal gland

Right inferior phrenic artery

Right inferior suprarenal artery

Right middle suprarenal artery

Right renal artery

Right kidney

Psoas minor

Right testicular (ovarian) artery

Psoas major

Right common iliac artery

Deep circumflex iliac artery

Iliolumbar artery

Internal iliac artery

External iliac artery

Superior gluteal artery

Lateral sacral artery

Iliacus

Inferior gluteal artery

Middle rectal artery

Left superior suprarenal arteries

Left inferior suprarenal artery

Left inferior phrenic artery

Left middle suprarenal artery

Left renal artery

Superior mesenteric artery

Quadratus lumborum

Subcostal artery

Inferior mesenteric artery

Lumbar arteries

Iliac branch of iliolumbar artery

Median sacral artery

Deep circumflex iliac artery

Left femoral artery

Abdominal aorta and branches

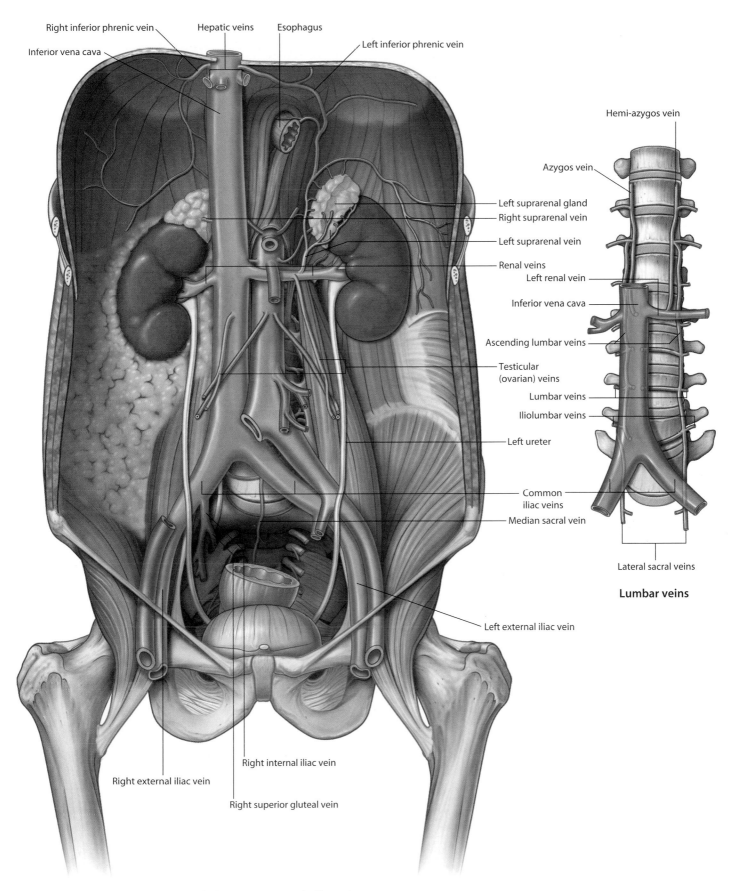

Right inferior phrenic vein

Inferior vena cava

Hepatic veins

Esophagus

Left inferior phrenic vein

Hemi-azygos vein

Azygos vein

Left suprarenal gland

Right suprarenal vein

Left suprarenal vein

Renal veins

Left renal vein

Inferior vena cava

Ascending lumbar veins

Testicular (ovarian) veins

Lumbar veins

Iliolumbar veins

Left ureter

Common iliac veins

Median sacral vein

Lateral sacral veins

Lumbar veins

Left external iliac vein

Right external iliac vein

Right internal iliac vein

Right superior gluteal vein

Inferior vena cava and tributaries

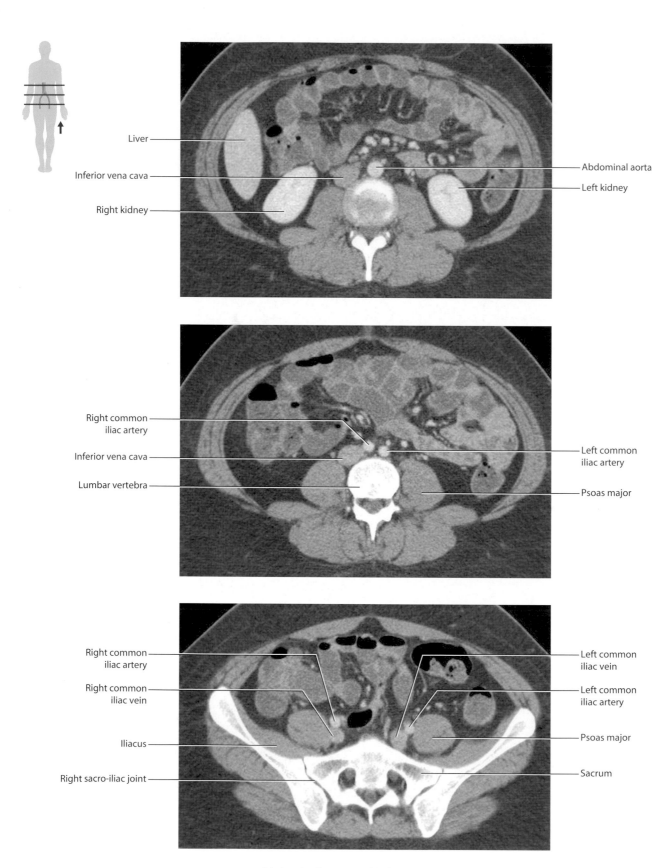

Abdominal aorta and inferior vena cava.
CT images, with contrast, in axial plane

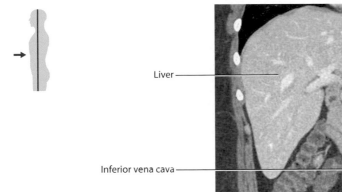

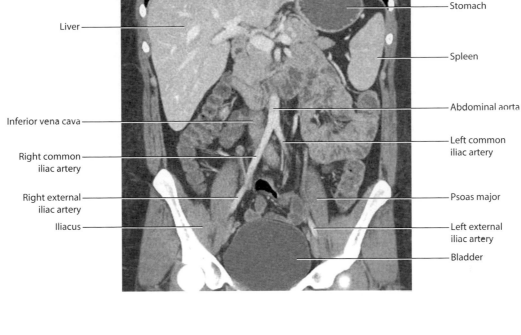

Liver —

Inferior vena cava —

Right common — iliac artery

Right external — iliac artery

Iliacus —

— Stomach

— Spleen

— Abdominal aorta

— Left common iliac artery

— Psoas major

— Left external iliac artery

— Bladder

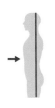

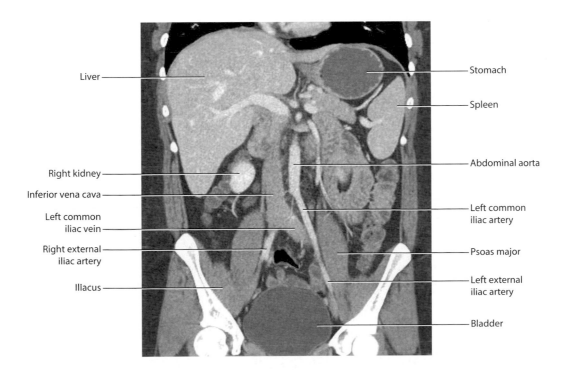

Liver —

Right kidney —

Inferior vena cava —

Left common — iliac vein

Right external — iliac artery

Illacus —

— Stomach

— Spleen

— Abdominal aorta

— Left common iliac artery

— Psoas major

— Left external iliac artery

— Bladder

Positioning of the abdominal aorta and inferior vena cava in relation to other structures.
CT images, with contrast, in coronal plane

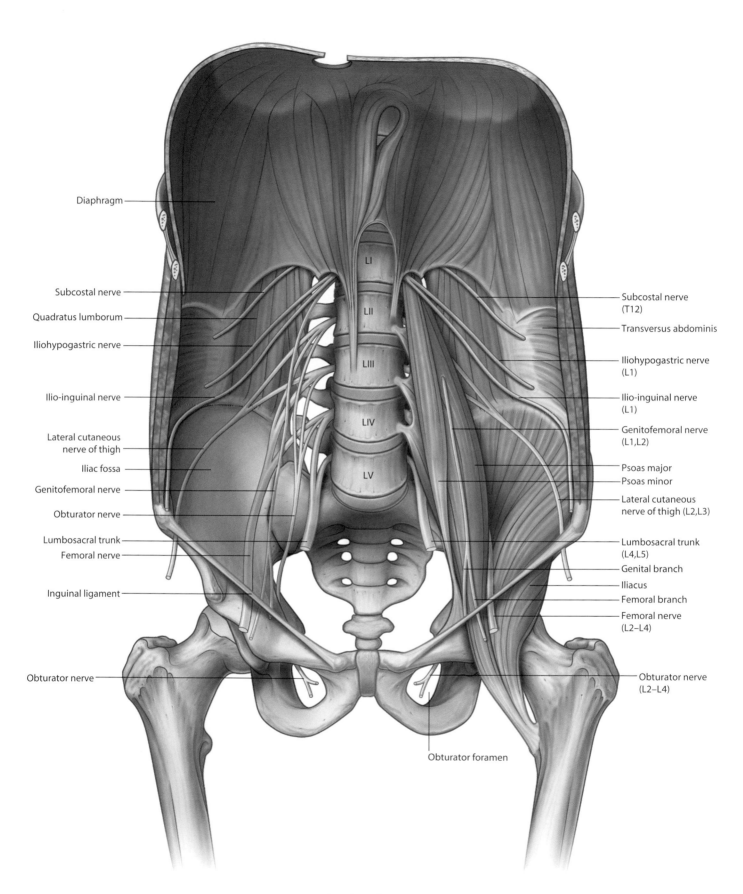

Diaphragm

Subcostal nerve

Quadratus lumborum

Iliohypogastric nerve

Ilio-inguinal nerve

Lateral cutaneous
nerve of thigh

Iliac fossa

Genitofemoral nerve

Obturator nerve

Lumbosacral trunk

Femoral nerve

Inguinal ligament

Obturator nerve

LI

LII

LIII

LIV

LV

Subcostal nerve
(T12)

Transversus abdominis

Iliohypogastric nerve
(L1)

Ilio-inguinal nerve
(L1)

Genitofemoral nerve
(L1,L2)

Psoas major

Psoas minor

Lateral cutaneous
nerve of thigh (L2,L3)

Lumbosacral trunk
(L4,L5)

Genital branch

Iliacus

Femoral branch

Femoral nerve
(L2–L4)

Obturator nerve
(L2–L4)

Obturator foramen

Lumbar plexus

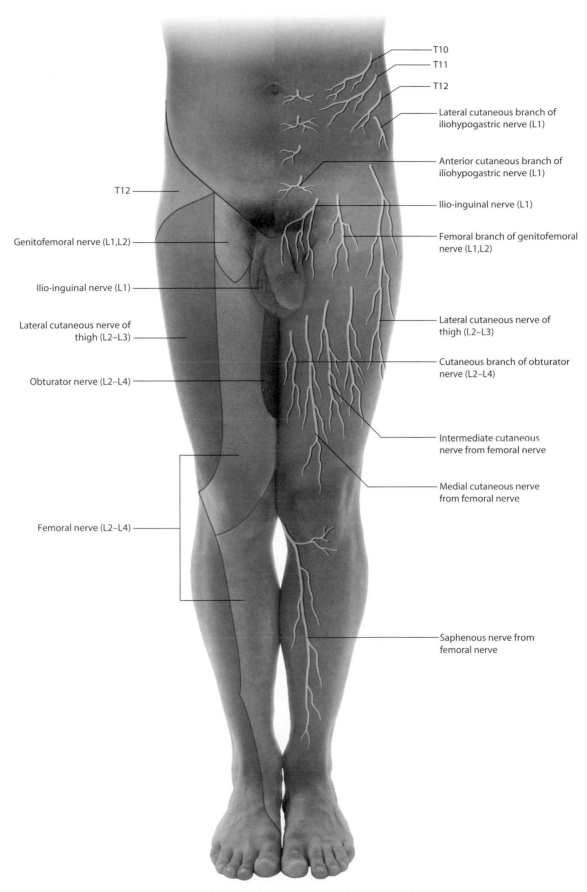

T10
T11
T12
Lateral cutaneous branch of iliohypogastric nerve (L1)
Anterior cutaneous branch of iliohypogastric nerve (L1)
Ilio-inguinal nerve (L1)
Femoral branch of genitofemoral nerve (L1,L2)
Lateral cutaneous nerve of thigh (L2–L3)
Cutaneous branch of obturator nerve (L2–L4)
Intermediate cutaneous nerve from femoral nerve
Medial cutaneous nerve from femoral nerve
Saphenous nerve from femoral nerve

T12
Genitofemoral nerve (L1,L2)
Ilio-inguinal nerve (L1)
Lateral cutaneous nerve of thigh (L2–L3)
Obturator nerve (L2–L4)
Femoral nerve (L2–L4)

Cutaneous distribution of the nerves from the lumbar plexus

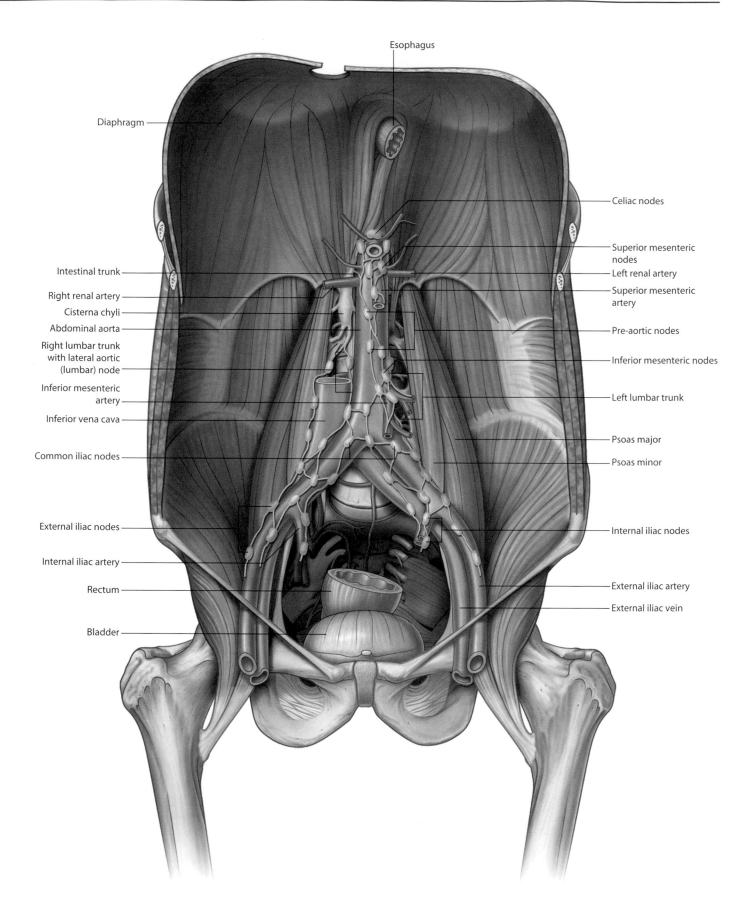

Esophagus

Diaphragm

Celiac nodes

Superior mesenteric nodes

Intestinal trunk

Left renal artery

Right renal artery

Superior mesenteric artery

Cisterna chyli

Abdominal aorta

Pre-aortic nodes

Right lumbar trunk with lateral aortic (lumbar) node

Inferior mesenteric nodes

Inferior mesenteric artery

Left lumbar trunk

Inferior vena cava

Psoas major

Common iliac nodes

Psoas minor

External iliac nodes

Internal iliac nodes

Internal iliac artery

Rectum

External iliac artery

External iliac vein

Bladder

Abdominal lymphatics

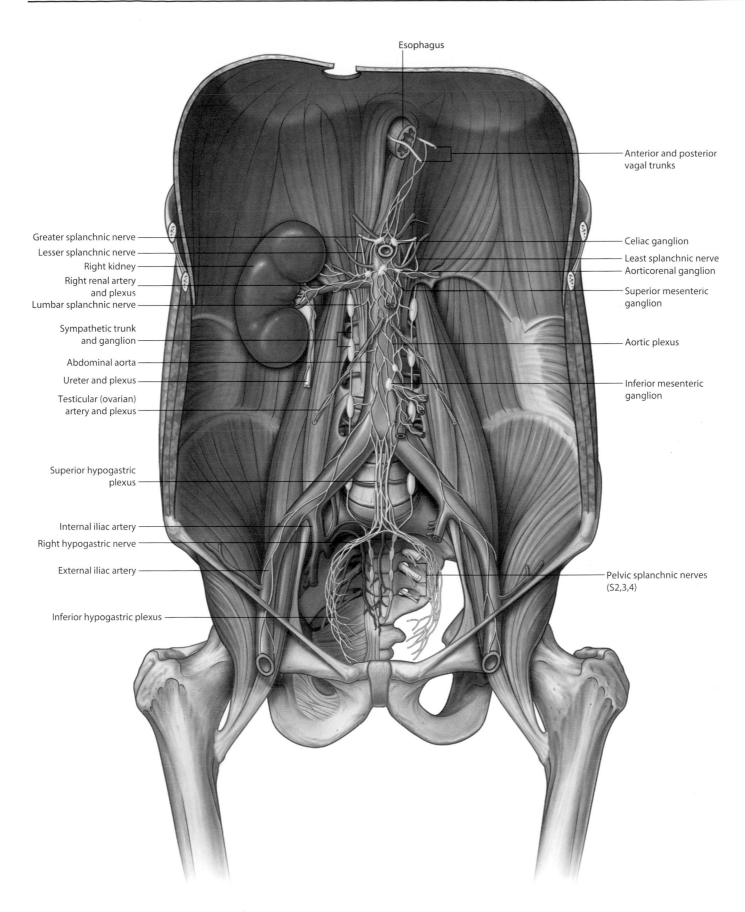

Esophagus

Anterior and posterior vagal trunks

Greater splanchnic nerve

Lesser splanchnic nerve

Right kidney

Right renal artery and plexus

Lumbar splanchnic nerve

Sympathetic trunk and ganglion

Abdominal aorta

Ureter and plexus

Testicular (ovarian) artery and plexus

Superior hypogastric plexus

Internal iliac artery

Right hypogastric nerve

External iliac artery

Inferior hypogastric plexus

Celiac ganglion

Least splanchnic nerve

Aorticorenal ganglion

Superior mesenteric ganglion

Aortic plexus

Inferior mesenteric ganglion

Pelvic splanchnic nerves (S2,3,4)

Prevertebral plexuses and ganglia with sympathetic trunks

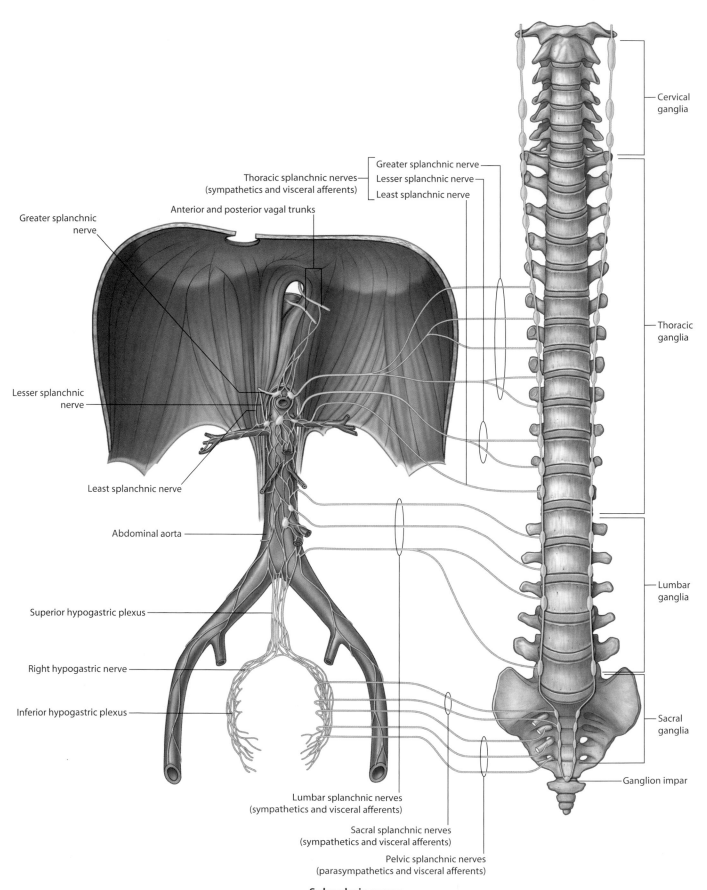

Greater splanchnic nerve

Thoracic splanchnic nerves (sympathetics and visceral afferents)

Anterior and posterior vagal trunks

Greater splanchnic nerve

Lesser splanchnic nerve

Least splanchnic nerve

Cervical ganglia

Thoracic ganglia

Lesser splanchnic nerve

Least splanchnic nerve

Abdominal aorta

Superior hypogastric plexus

Right hypogastric nerve

Inferior hypogastric plexus

Lumbar ganglia

Sacral ganglia

Ganglion impar

Lumbar splanchnic nerves (sympathetics and visceral afferents)

Sacral splanchnic nerves (sympathetics and visceral afferents)

Pelvic splanchnic nerves (parasympathetics and visceral afferents)

Splanchnic nerves

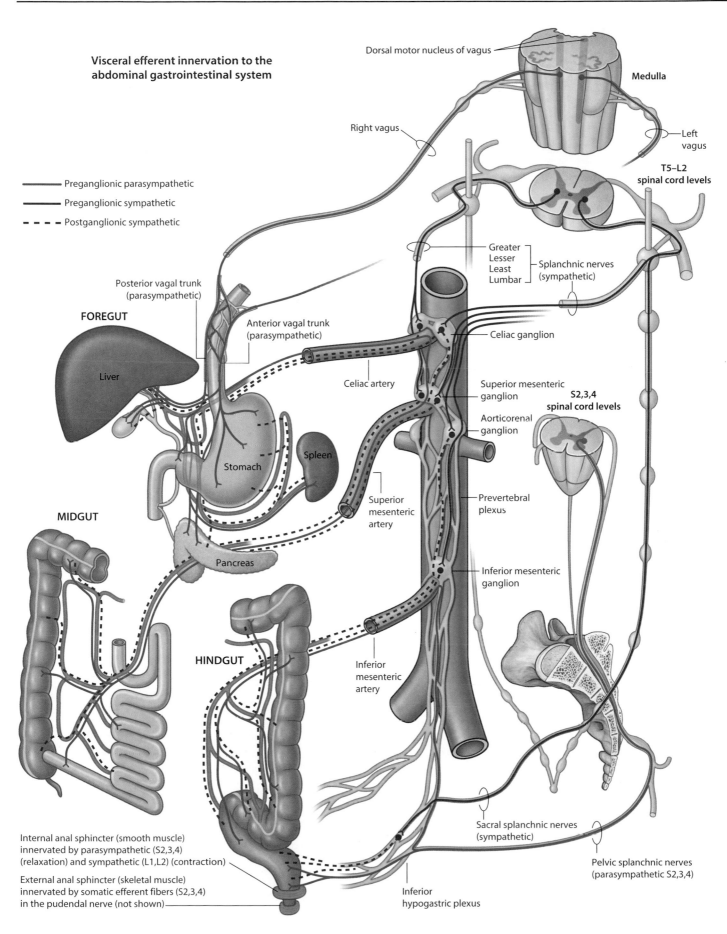

Visceral efferent innervation to the
abdominal gastrointestinal system

Dorsal motor nucleus of vagus

Medulla

Right vagus

Left vagus

T5–L2
spinal cord levels

Preganglionic parasympathetic
Preganglionic sympathetic
Postganglionic sympathetic

Greater
Lesser
Least
Lumbar — Splanchnic nerves
(sympathetic)

Posterior vagal trunk
(parasympathetic)

FOREGUT

Anterior vagal trunk
(parasympathetic)

Celiac ganglion

Celiac artery

Liver

Superior mesenteric
ganglion

S2,3,4
spinal cord levels

Aorticorenal
ganglion

Spleen

Stomach

Prevertebral
plexus

Superior
mesenteric
artery

MIDGUT

Pancreas

Inferior mesenteric
ganglion

HINDGUT

Inferior
mesenteric
artery

Sacral splanchnic nerves
(sympathetic)

Internal anal sphincter (smooth muscle)
innervated by parasympathetic (S2,3,4)
(relaxation) and sympathetic (L1,L2) (contraction)

External anal sphincter (skeletal muscle)
innervated by somatic efferent fibers (S2,3,4)
in the pudendal nerve (not shown)

Inferior
hypogastric plexus

Pelvic splanchnic nerves
(parasympathetic S2,3,4)

201

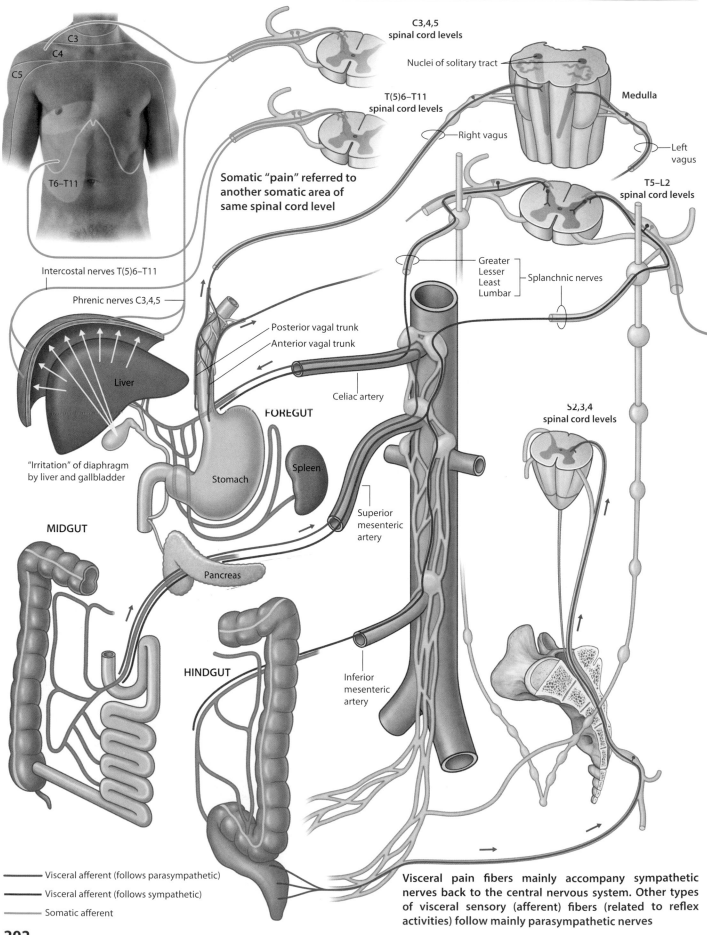

C3,4,5
spinal cord levels

Nuclei of solitary tract

Medulla

T(5)6–T11
spinal cord levels

Right vagus

Left vagus

T5–L2
spinal cord levels

C3

C4

C5

T6–T11

Somatic "pain" referred to
another somatic area of
same spinal cord level

Intercostal nerves T(5)6–T11

Phrenic nerves C3,4,5

Greater
Lesser
Least
Lumbar

Splanchnic nerves

Posterior vagal trunk

Anterior vagal trunk

Celiac artery

FOREGUT

Liver

"Irritation" of diaphragm
by liver and gallbladder

Stomach

Spleen

S2,3,4
spinal cord levels

MIDGUT

Pancreas

Superior
mesenteric
artery

HINDGUT

Inferior
mesenteric
artery

Visceral afferent (follows parasympathetic)

Visceral afferent (follows sympathetic)

Somatic afferent

**Visceral pain fibers mainly accompany sympathetic
nerves back to the central nervous system. Other types
of visceral sensory (afferent) fibers (related to reflex
activities) follow mainly parasympathetic nerves**

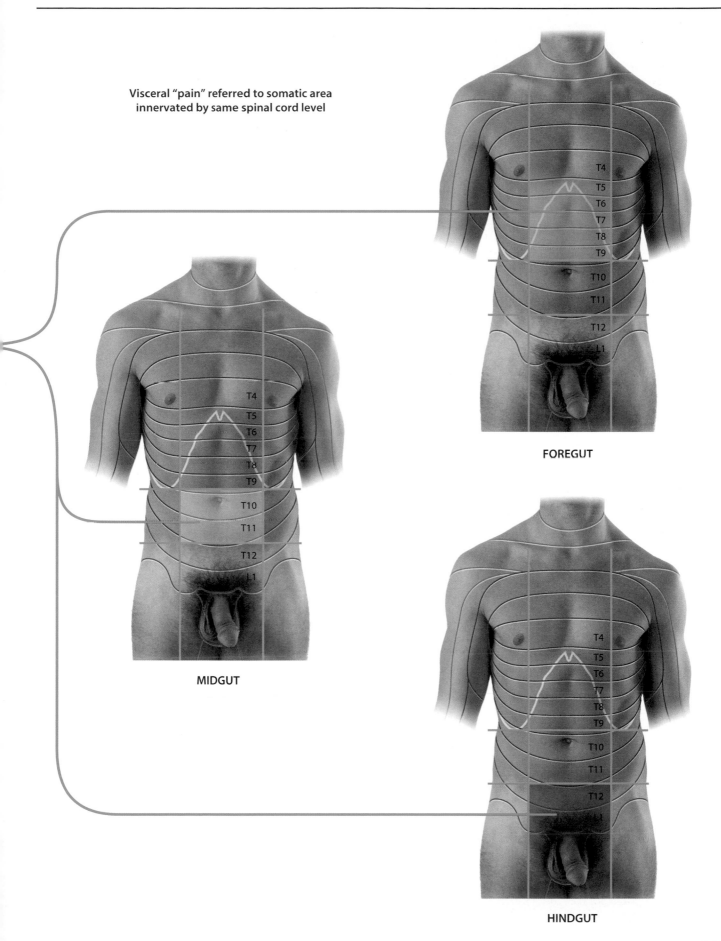

Visceral "pain" referred to somatic area
innervated by same spinal cord level

FOREGUT

MIDGUT

HINDGUT

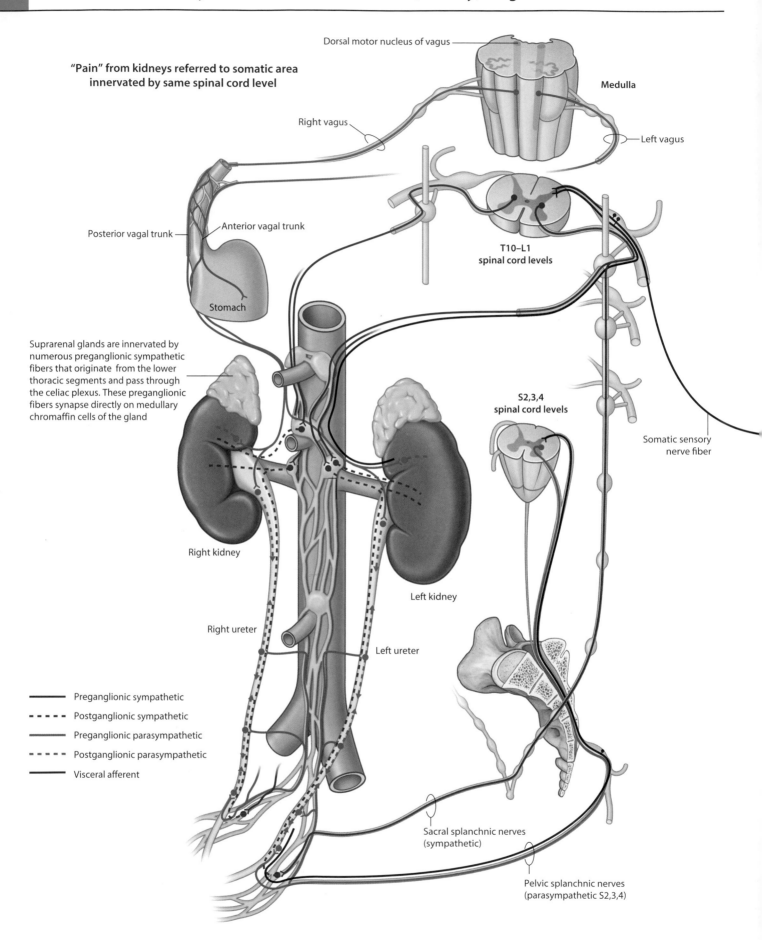

"Pain" from kidneys referred to somatic area
innervated by same spinal cord level

Dorsal motor nucleus of vagus

Medulla

Right vagus

Left vagus

Posterior vagal trunk

Anterior vagal trunk

T10–L1
spinal cord levels

Stomach

Suprarenal glands are innervated by
numerous preganglionic sympathetic
fibers that originate from the lower
thoracic segments and pass through
the celiac plexus. These preganglionic
fibers synapse directly on medullary
chromaffin cells of the gland

S2,3,4
spinal cord levels

Somatic sensory
nerve fiber

Right kidney

Left kidney

Right ureter

Left ureter

———— Preganglionic sympathetic

- - - - Postganglionic sympathetic

———— Preganglionic parasympathetic

- - - - Postganglionic parasympathetic

———— Visceral afferent

Sacral splanchnic nerves
(sympathetic)

Pelvic splanchnic nerves
(parasympathetic S2,3,4)

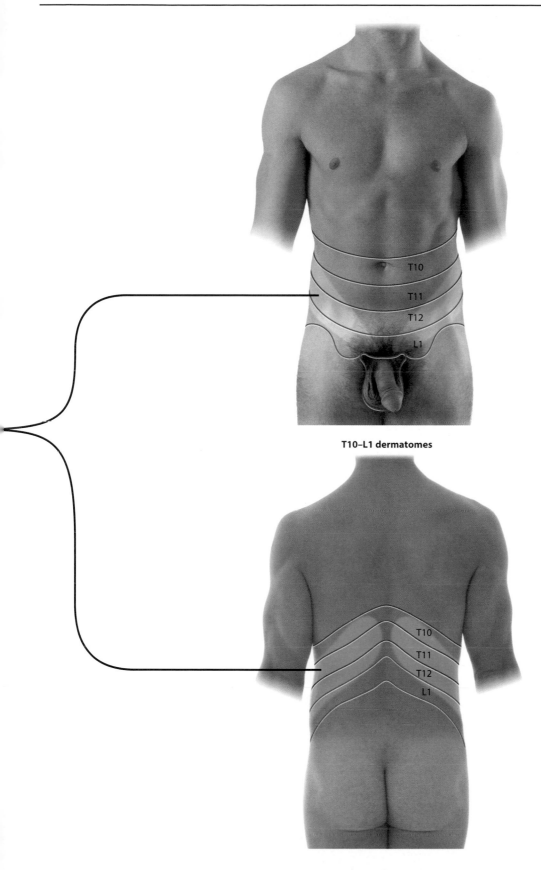

T10–L1 dermatomes

Pain fibers mainly follow sympathetic nerves to the central nervous system (CNS). This pain is 'referred' by the CNS to the somatic area innervated by the same spinal levels. Other types of visceral afferent (sensory) fibers (related to reflex activities) follow mainly parasympathetic nerves

Abdominal wall muscles

Muscle		Origin	Insertion	Innervation	Function
External oblique	1	Muscular slips from the outer surfaces of the lower eight ribs (ribs V to XII)	Lateral lip of iliac crest; aponeurosis ending in midline raphe (linea alba)	Anterior rami of lower six thoracic spinal nerves (T7 to T12)	Compress abdominal contents; both muscles flex trunk; each muscle bends trunk to same side, turning anterior part of abdomen to opposite side
Internal oblique	2	Thoracolumbar fascia; iliac crest between origins of external and transversus; lateral two thirds of inguinal ligament	Inferior border of the lower three or four ribs; aponeurosis ending in linea alba; pubic crest and pectineal line	Anterior rami of lower six thoracic spinal nerves (T7 to T12) and L1	Compress abdominal contents; both muscles flex trunk; each muscle bends trunk and turns anterior part of abdomen to same side
Transversus abdominis	3	Thoracolumbar fascia; medial lip of iliac crest; lateral one third of inguinal ligament; costal cartilages lower six ribs (ribs VII to XII)	Aponeurosis ending in linea alba; pubic crest and pectineal line	Anterior rami of lower six thoracic spinal nerves (T7 to T12) and L1	Compress abdominal contents
Rectus abdominis	4	Pubic crest, pubic tubercle, and pubic symphysis	Costal cartilages of ribs V to VII; xiphoid process	Anterior rami of lower seven thoracic spinal nerves (T7 to T12)	Compress abdominal contents; flex vertebral column; tense abdominal wall
Pyramidalis	5	Front of pubis and pubic symphysis	Into linea alba	Anterior ramus of T12	Tenses the linea alba

Posterior abdominal wall muscles

Muscle		Origin	Insertion	Innervation	Function
Psoas major	6	Lateral surface of bodies of TXII and LI to LV vertebrae, transverse processes of the lumbar vertebrae, and the intervertebral discs between TXII and LI to LV vertebrae	Lesser trochanter of the femur	Anterior rami of L1 to L3	Flexion of thigh at hip joint
Psoas minor	7	Lateral surface of bodies of TXII and LI vertebrae and intervening intervertebral disc	Pectineal line of the pelvic brim and iliopubic eminence	Anterior rami of L1	Weak flexion of lumbar vertebral column
Quadratus lumborum	8	Transverse process of LV vertebra, iliolumbar ligament, and iliac crest	Transverse processes of LI to LIV vertebrae and inferior border of rib XII	Anterior rami of T12 and L1 to L4	Depress and stabilize rib XII and some lateral bending of trunk
Iliacus	9	Upper two thirds of iliac fossa, anterior sacro-iliac and iliolumbar ligaments, and upper lateral surface of sacrum	Lesser trochanter of femur	Femoral nerve (L2 to L4)	Flexion of thigh at hip joint

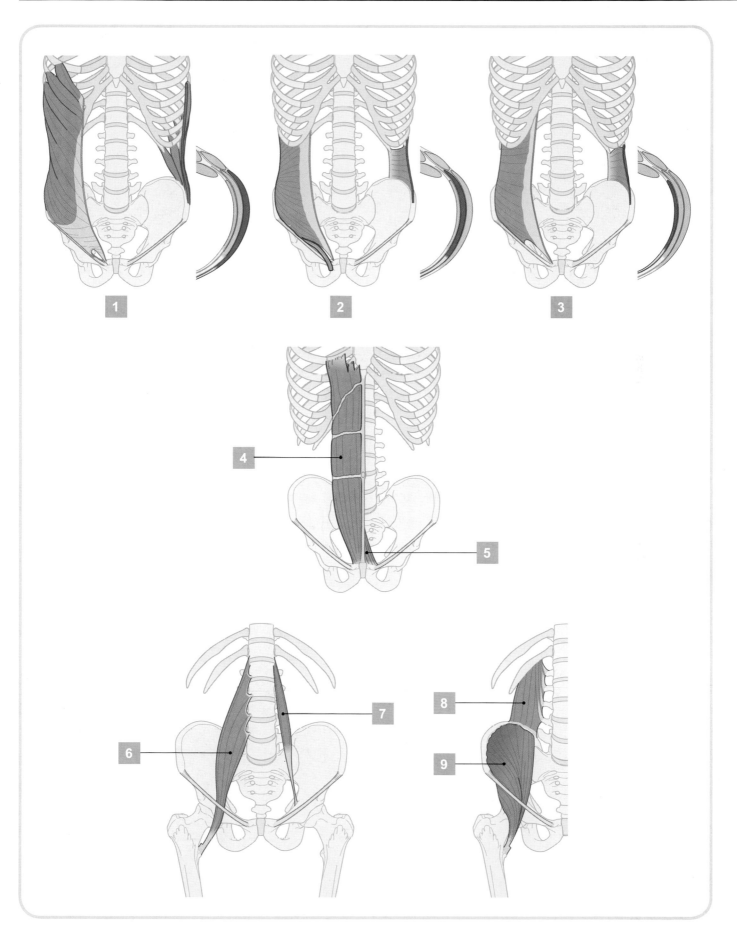

Branches of the abdominal aorta

Artery		Branch	Origin	Parts supplied
Celiac trunk	1	Anterior	Immediately inferior to the aortic hiatus of the diaphragm	Abdominal foregut
Superior mesenteric artery	2	Anterior	Immediately inferior to the celiac trunk	Abdominal midgut
Inferior mesenteric artery	3	Anterior	Inferior to the renal arteries	Abdominal hindgut
Middle suprarenal arteries	4	Lateral	Immediately superior to the renal arteries	Suprarenal glands
Renal arteries	5	Lateral	Immediately inferior to the superior mesenteric artery	Kidneys
Testicular or ovarian arteries	6	Paired anterior	Inferior to the renal arteries	Testes in male and ovaries in female
Inferior phrenic arteries	7	Lateral	Immediately inferior to the aortic hiatus	Diaphragm
Lumbar arteries	8	Posterior	Usually four pairs	Posterior abdominal wall and spinal cord
Median sacral artery	9	Posterior	Just superior to the aortic bifurcation, passes inferiorly across lumbar vertebrae, sacrum, and coccyx	
Common iliac arteries	10	Terminal	Bifurcation usually occurs at the level of LIV vertebra	

Branches of the lumbar plexus

Branch		Origin	Spinal segments	Function: motor	Function: sensory
Iliohypogastric	1	Anterior ramus L1	L1	Internal oblique and transversus abdominis	Posterolateral gluteal skin and skin in pubic region
Ilio-inguinal	2	Anterior ramus L1	L1	Internal oblique and transversus abdominis	Skin in the upper medial thigh, and either the skin over the root of the penis and anterior scrotum or the mons pubis and labium majus
Genitofemoral	3	Anterior rami L1 and L2	L1, L2	Genital branch—male cremasteric muscle	Genital branch—skin of anterior scrotum or skin of mons pubis and labium majus; femoral branch—skin of upper anterior thigh
Lateral cutaneous nerve of thigh	4	Anterior rami L2 and L3	L2, L3		Skin on anterior and lateral thigh to the knee
Obturator	5	Anterior rami L2 to L4	L2 to L4	Obturator externus, pectineus, and muscles in medial compartment of thigh	Skin on medial aspect of the thigh
Femoral	6	Anterior rami L2 to L4	L2 to L4	Iliacus, pectineus, and muscles in anterior compartment of thigh	Skin on anterior thigh and medial surface of leg

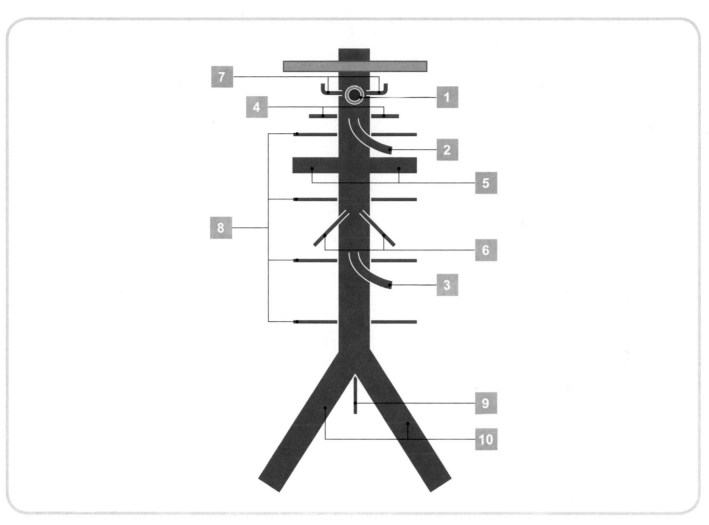

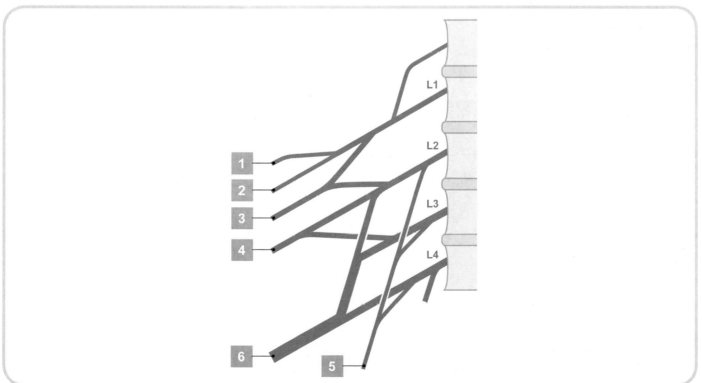

CONTENTS

PELVIS AND PERINEUM

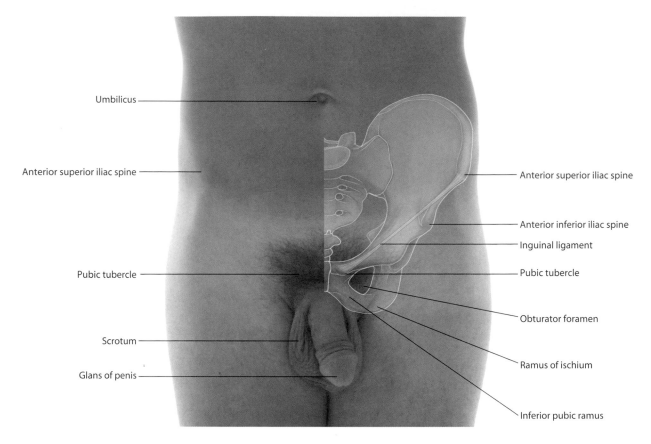

Umbilicus

Anterior superior iliac spine

Anterior superior iliac spine

Anterior inferior iliac spine

Inguinal ligament

Pubic tubercle

Pubic tubercle

Obturator foramen

Scrotum

Ramus of ischium

Glans of penis

Inferior pubic ramus

Surface anatomy with bones (anterior view)

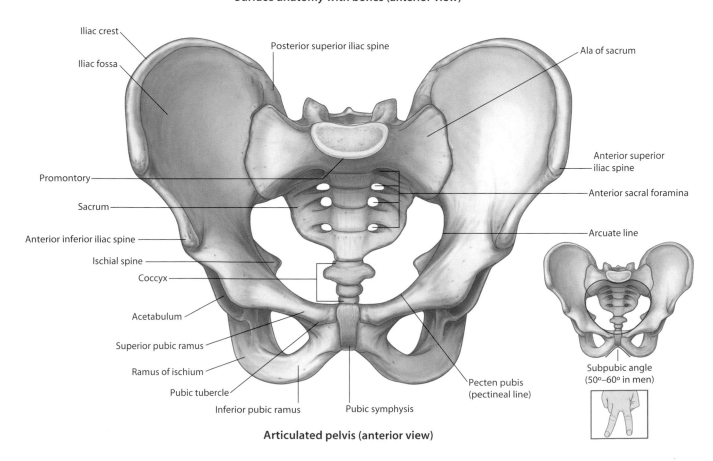

Iliac crest

Posterior superior iliac spine

Ala of sacrum

Iliac fossa

Promontory

Anterior superior iliac spine

Sacrum

Anterior sacral foramina

Anterior inferior iliac spine

Arcuate line

Ischial spine

Coccyx

Acetabulum

Superior pubic ramus

Ramus of ischium

Pubic tubercle

Pecten pubis (pectineal line)

Inferior pubic ramus

Pubic symphysis

Subpubic angle (50°–60° in men)

Articulated pelvis (anterior view)

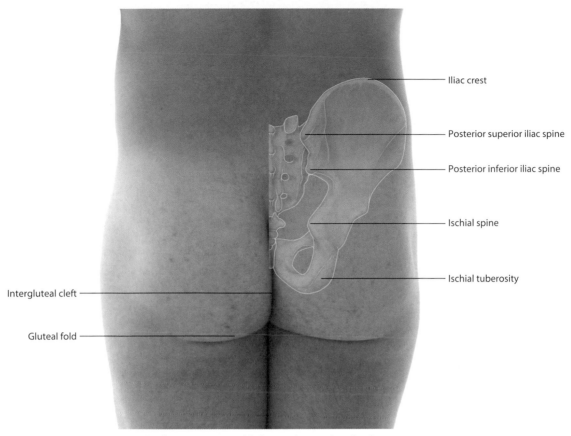

Surface anatomy with bones (posterior view)

Iliac crest

Posterior superior iliac spine

Posterior inferior iliac spine

Ischial spine

Ischial tuberosity

Intergluteal cleft

Gluteal fold

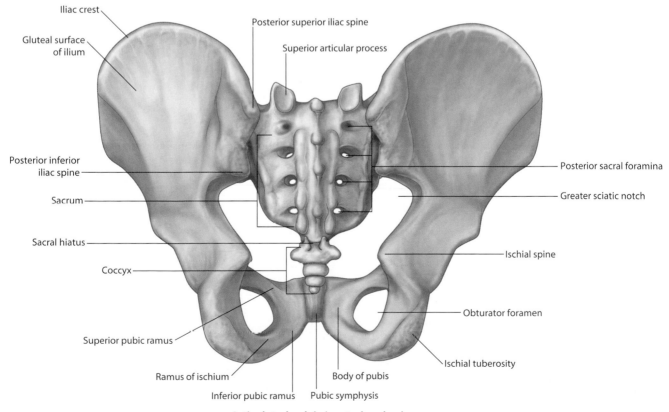

Articulated pelvis (posterior view)

Iliac crest

Gluteal surface of ilium

Posterior superior iliac spine

Superior articular process

Posterior inferior iliac spine

Sacrum

Sacral hiatus

Coccyx

Superior pubic ramus

Ramus of ischium

Inferior pubic ramus

Body of pubis

Pubic symphysis

Posterior sacral foramina

Greater sciatic notch

Ischial spine

Obturator foramen

Ischial tuberosity

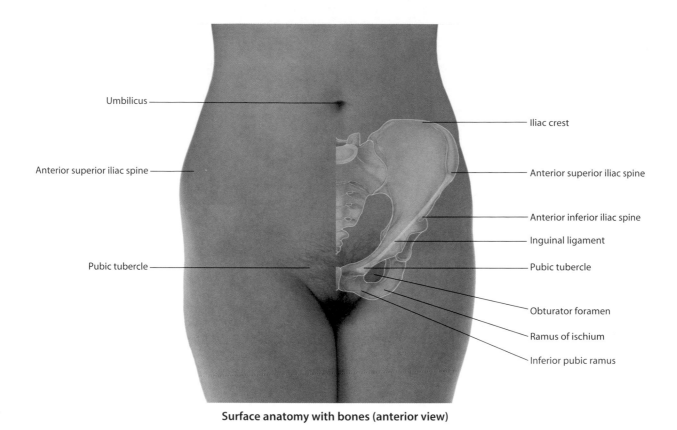

Umbilicus

Iliac crest

Anterior superior iliac spine

Anterior superior iliac spine

Anterior inferior iliac spine

Inguinal ligament

Pubic tubercle

Pubic tubercle

Obturator foramen

Ramus of ischium

Inferior pubic ramus

Surface anatomy with bones (anterior view)

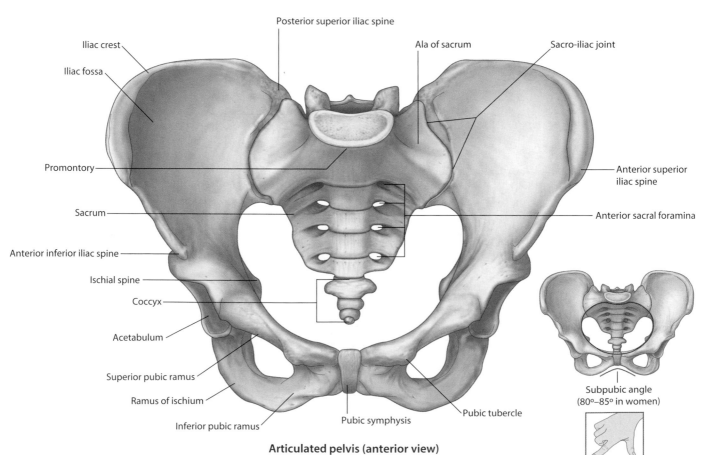

Posterior superior iliac spine

Ala of sacrum

Sacro-iliac joint

Iliac crest

Iliac fossa

Anterior superior iliac spine

Promontory

Sacrum

Anterior sacral foramina

Anterior inferior iliac spine

Ischial spine

Coccyx

Acetabulum

Superior pubic ramus

Ramus of ischium

Inferior pubic ramus

Pubic symphysis

Pubic tubercle

Subpubic angle (80º–85º in women)

Articulated pelvis (anterior view)

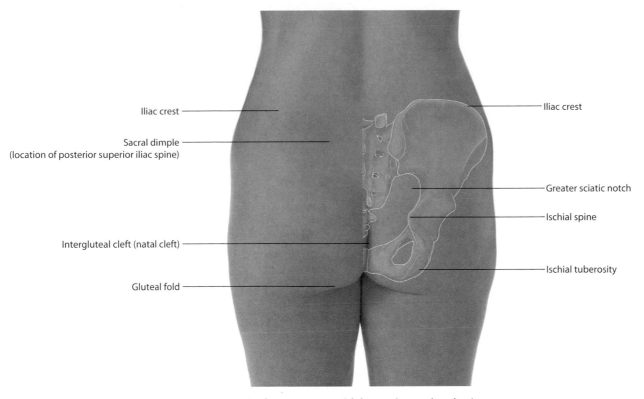

Iliac crest

Sacral dimple
(location of posterior superior iliac spine)

Intergluteal cleft (natal cleft)

Gluteal fold

Iliac crest

Greater sciatic notch

Ischial spine

Ischial tuberosity

Surface anatomy with bones (posterior view)

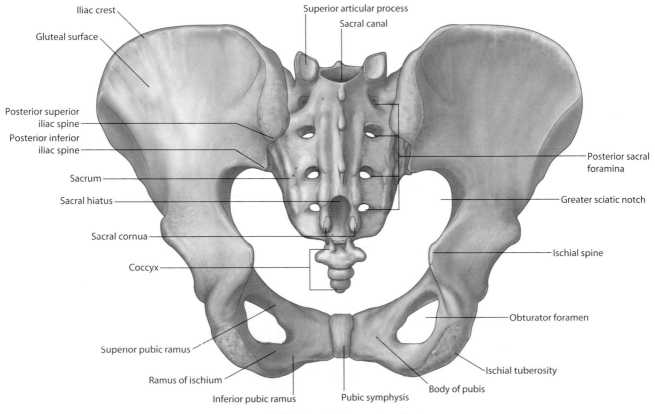

Iliac crest

Gluteal surface

Posterior superior
iliac spine

Posterior inferior
iliac spine

Sacrum

Sacral hiatus

Sacral cornua

Coccyx

Superior pubic ramus

Ramus of ischium

Inferior pubic ramus

Superior articular process

Sacral canal

Posterior sacral
foramina

Greater sciatic notch

Ischial spine

Obturator foramen

Ischial tuberosity

Pubic symphysis

Body of pubis

Articulated pelvis (posterior view)

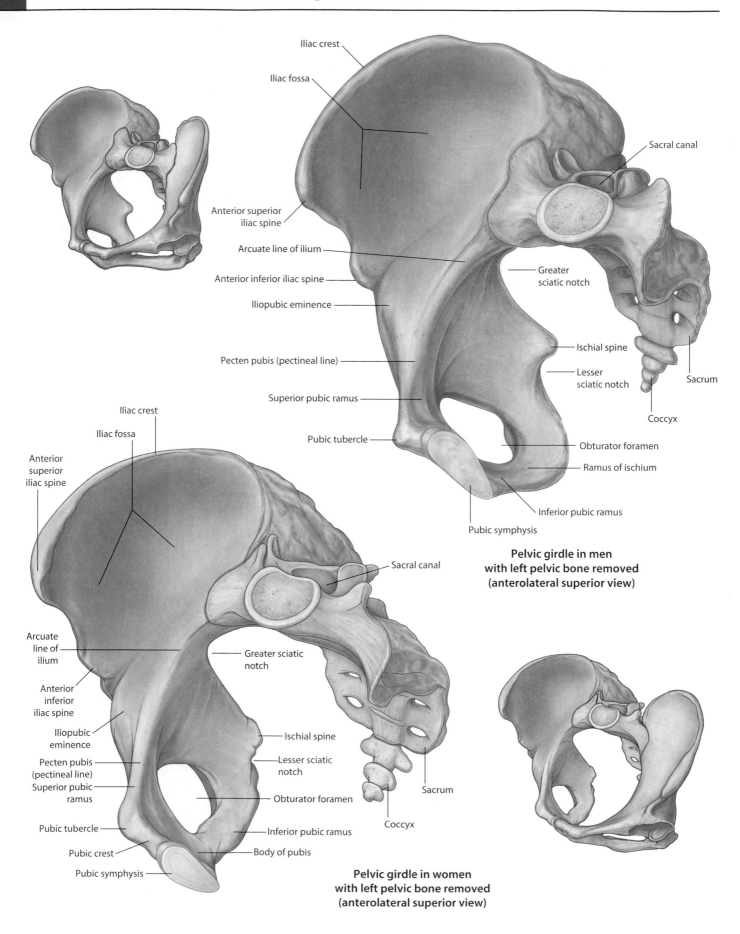

Iliac crest

Iliac fossa

Sacral canal

Anterior superior
iliac spine

Arcuate line of ilium

Greater
sciatic notch

Anterior inferior iliac spine

Iliopubic eminence

Pecten pubis (pectineal line)

Ischial spine

Superior pubic ramus

Lesser
sciatic notch

Sacrum

Pubic tubercle

Coccyx

Obturator foramen

Ramus of ischium

Inferior pubic ramus

Pubic symphysis

**Pelvic girdle in men
with left pelvic bone removed
(anterolateral superior view)**

Iliac crest

Iliac fossa

Anterior
superior
iliac spine

Sacral canal

Arcuate
line of
ilium

Greater sciatic
notch

Anterior
inferior
iliac spine

Iliopubic
eminence

Ischial spine

Pecten pubis
(pectineal line)

Lesser sciatic
notch

Superior pubic
ramus

Obturator foramen

Sacrum

Pubic tubercle

Inferior pubic ramus

Coccyx

Pubic crest

Body of pubis

Pubic symphysis

**Pelvic girdle in women
with left pelvic bone removed
(anterolateral superior view)**

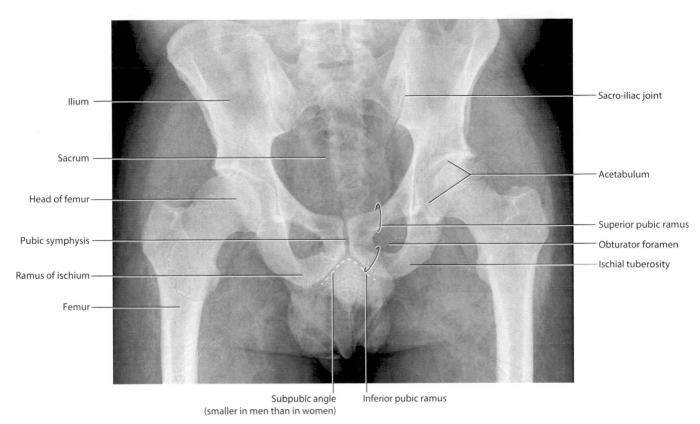

Ilium

Sacrum

Head of femur

Pubic symphysis

Ramus of ischium

Femur

Sacro-iliac joint

Acetabulum

Superior pubic ramus

Obturator foramen

Ischial tuberosity

Subpubic angle
(smaller in men than in women)

Inferior pubic ramus

Male bony pelvis.
Radiograph, AP view

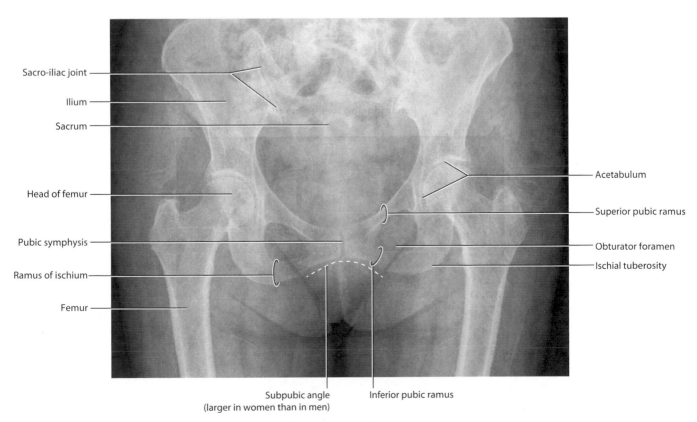

Sacro-iliac joint

Ilium

Sacrum

Head of femur

Pubic symphysis

Ramus of ischium

Femur

Acetabulum

Superior pubic ramus

Obturator foramen

Ischial tuberosity

Subpubic angle
(larger in women than in men)

Inferior pubic ramus

Female bony pelvis.
Radiograph, AP view

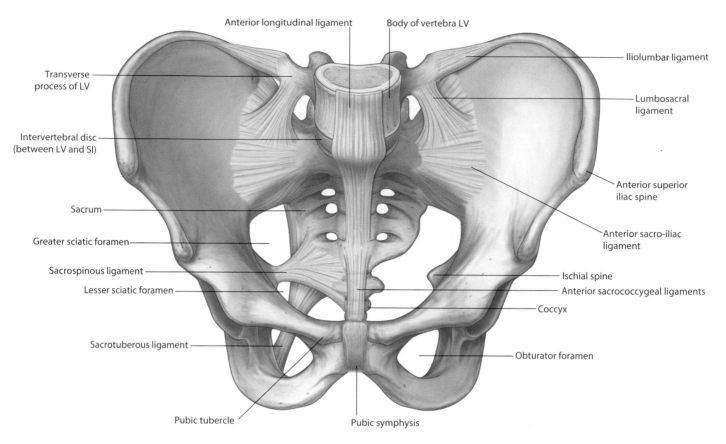

Lumbosacral joints and associated ligaments (anterior view)

Anterior longitudinal ligament

Body of vertebra LV

Iliolumbar ligament

Transverse process of LV

Lumbosacral ligament

Intervertebral disc (between LV and SI)

Anterior superior iliac spine

Sacrum

Anterior sacro-iliac ligament

Greater sciatic foramen

Sacrospinous ligament

Ischial spine

Lesser sciatic foramen

Anterior sacrococcygeal ligaments

Coccyx

Sacrotuberous ligament

Obturator foramen

Pubic tubercle

Pubic symphysis

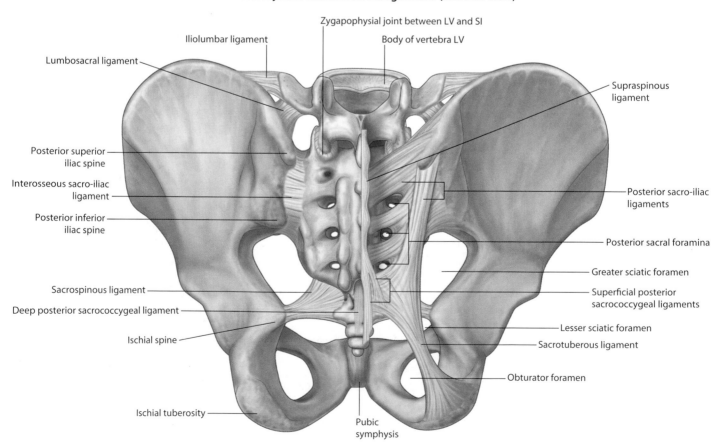

Lumbosacral joints and associated ligaments (posterior view)

Iliolumbar ligament

Zygapophysial joint between LV and SI

Body of vertebra LV

Lumbosacral ligament

Supraspinous ligament

Posterior superior iliac spine

Posterior sacro-iliac ligaments

Interosseous sacro-iliac ligament

Posterior inferior iliac spine

Posterior sacral foramina

Greater sciatic foramen

Sacrospinous ligament

Superficial posterior sacrococcygeal ligaments

Deep posterior sacrococcygeal ligament

Lesser sciatic foramen

Ischial spine

Sacrotuberous ligament

Obturator foramen

Ischial tuberosity

Pubic symphysis

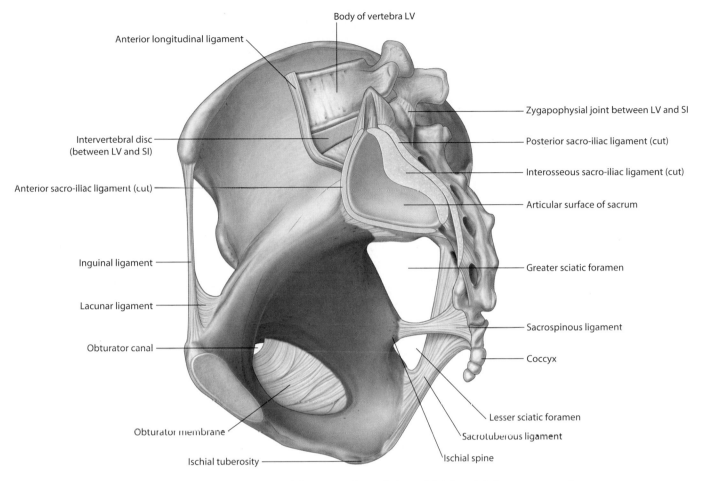

Body of vertebra LV

Anterior longitudinal ligament

Zygapophysial joint between LV and SI

Intervertebral disc (between LV and SI)

Posterior sacro-iliac ligament (cut)

Interosseous sacro-iliac ligament (cut)

Anterior sacro-iliac ligament (cut)

Articular surface of sacrum

Inguinal ligament

Greater sciatic foramen

Lacunar ligament

Sacrospinous ligament

Obturator canal

Coccyx

Lesser sciatic foramen

Obturator membrane

Sacrotuberous ligament

Ischial tuberosity

Ischial spine

Sacro-iliac joints and associated ligaments (lateral view with left pelvic bone removed)

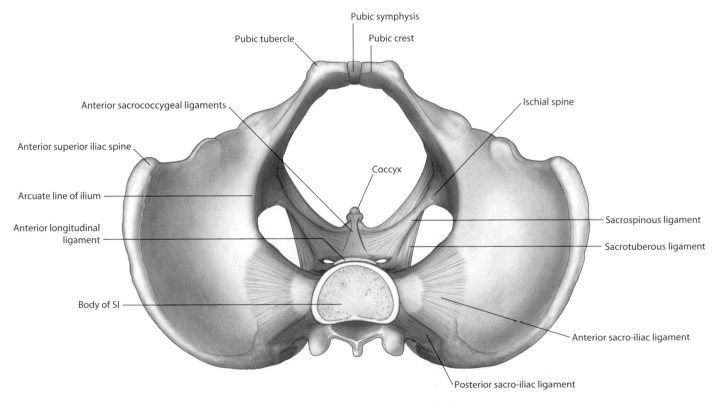

Pubic symphysis

Pubic tubercle

Pubic crest

Anterior sacrococcygeal ligaments

Ischial spine

Anterior superior iliac spine

Coccyx

Arcuate line of ilium

Anterior longitudinal ligament

Sacrospinous ligament

Sacrotuberous ligament

Body of SI

Anterior sacro-iliac ligament

Posterior sacro-iliac ligament

Sacro-iliac joints (anterosuperior view)

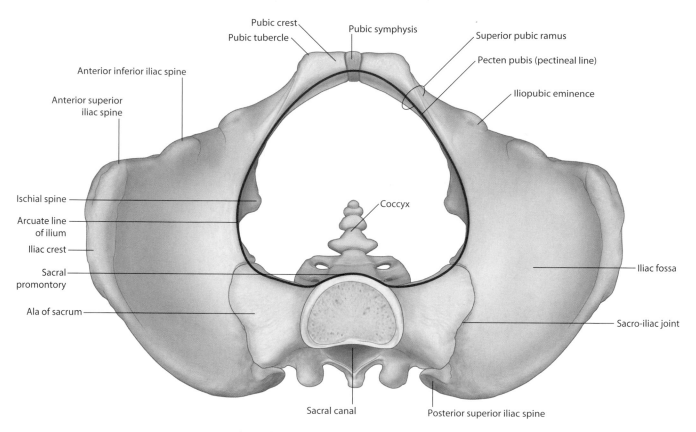

Pubic crest
Pubic tubercle
Pubic symphysis
Superior pubic ramus
Pecten pubis (pectineal line)
Iliopubic eminence

Anterior inferior iliac spine
Anterior superior iliac spine

Ischial spine
Arcuate line of ilium
Iliac crest
Sacral promontory
Ala of sacrum

Coccyx

Iliac fossa

Sacro-iliac joint

Sacral canal
Posterior superior iliac spine

Pelvic inlet (shown in red; anterosuperior view)

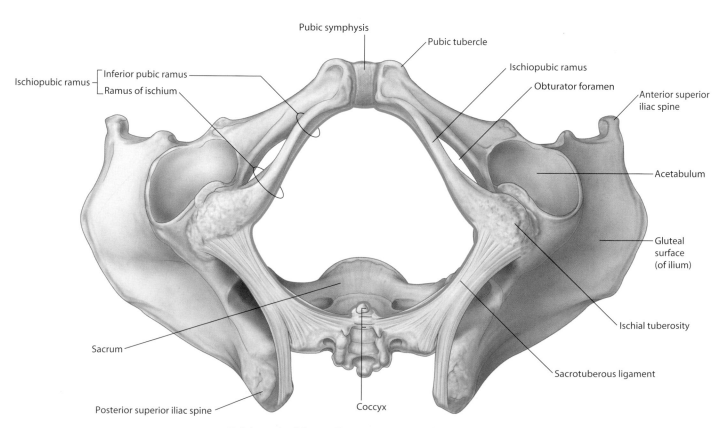

Pubic symphysis
Pubic tubercle
Ischiopubic ramus
Obturator foramen
Anterior superior iliac spine

Ischiopubic ramus
 Inferior pubic ramus
 Ramus of ischium

Acetabulum

Gluteal surface (of ilium)

Sacrum

Ischial tuberosity

Posterior superior iliac spine
Coccyx
Sacrotuberous ligament

Pelvic outlet (shown in green; anteroinferior view)

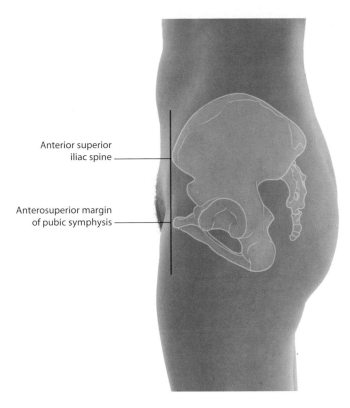

Anterior superior
iliac spine

Anterosuperior margin
of pubic symphysis

Pelvic orientation in anatomical position (lateral view)

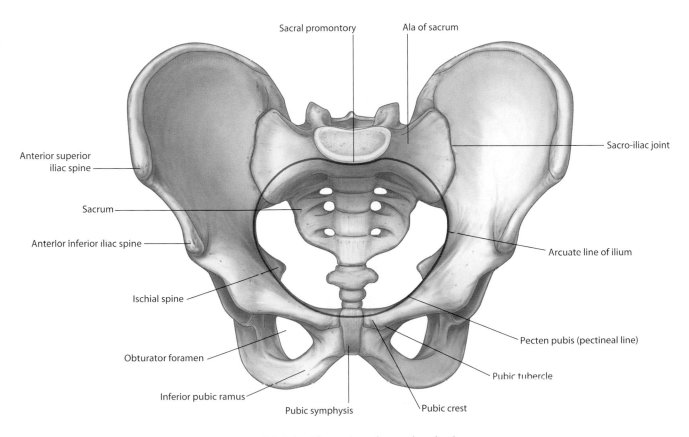

Sacral promontory

Ala of sacrum

Sacro-iliac joint

Anterior superior
iliac spine

Sacrum

Anterior inferior iliac spine

Ischial spine

Obturator foramen

Inferior pubic ramus

Pubic symphysis

Pubic crest

Pubic tubercle

Pecten pubis (pectineal line)

Arcuate line of ilium

Pelvic inlet (shown in red; anterior view)

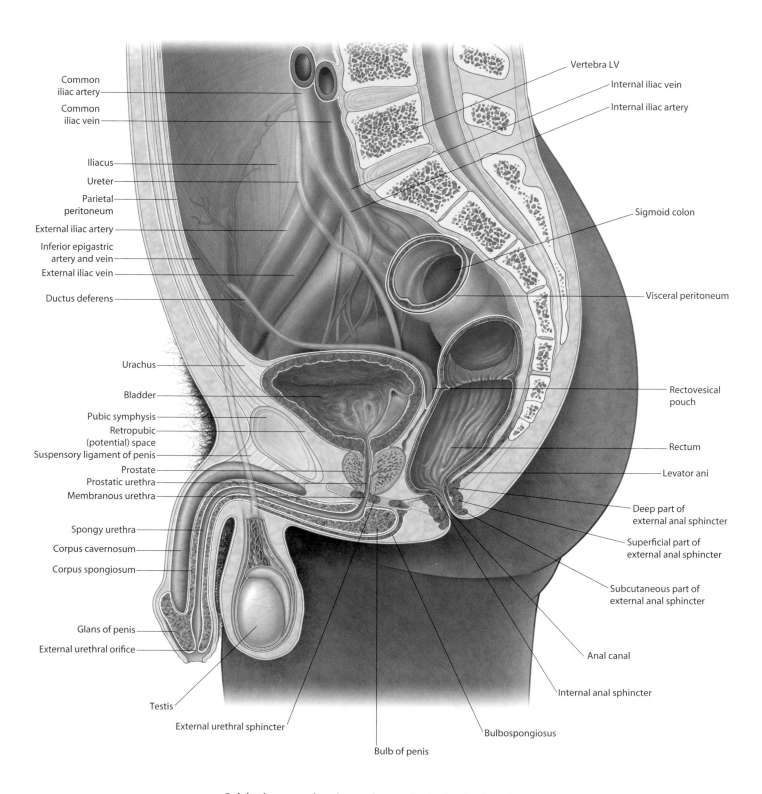

Common iliac artery

Common iliac vein

Iliacus

Ureter

Parietal peritoneum

External iliac artery

Inferior epigastric artery and vein

External iliac vein

Ductus deferens

Urachus

Bladder

Pubic symphysis

Retropubic (potential) space

Suspensory ligament of penis

Prostate

Prostatic urethra

Membranous urethra

Spongy urethra

Corpus cavernosum

Corpus spongiosum

Glans of penis

External urethral orifice

Testis

External urethral sphincter

Bulb of penis

Vertebra LV

Internal iliac vein

Internal iliac artery

Sigmoid colon

Visceral peritoneum

Rectovesical pouch

Rectum

Levator ani

Deep part of external anal sphincter

Superficial part of external anal sphincter

Subcutaneous part of external anal sphincter

Anal canal

Internal anal sphincter

Bulbospongiosus

Pelvic viscera and perineum in men *in situ* (sagittal section)

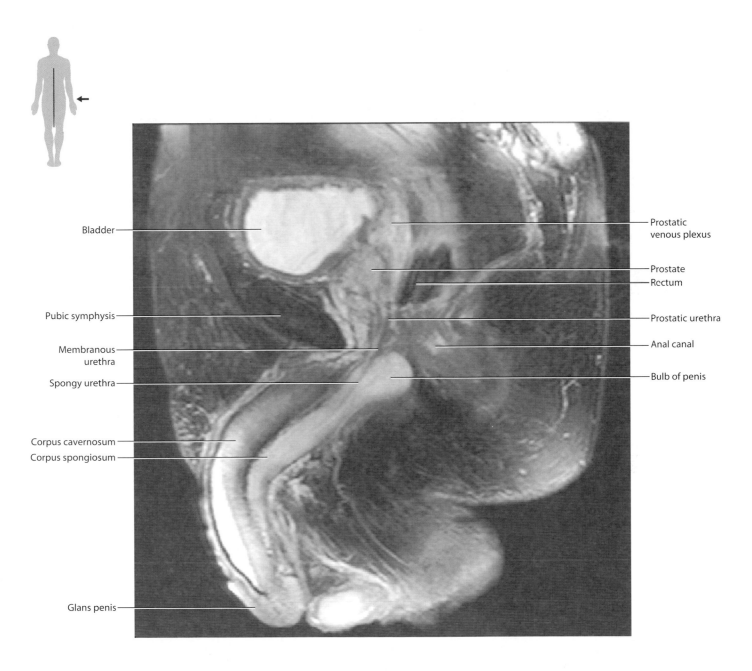

Bladder

Pubic symphysis

Membranous urethra

Spongy urethra

Corpus cavernosum

Corpus spongiosum

Glans penis

Prostatic venous plexus

Prostate

Rectum

Prostatic urethra

Anal canal

Bulb of penis

Pelvic viscera in men.
Fat-saturated T2-weighted MR image in sagittal plane

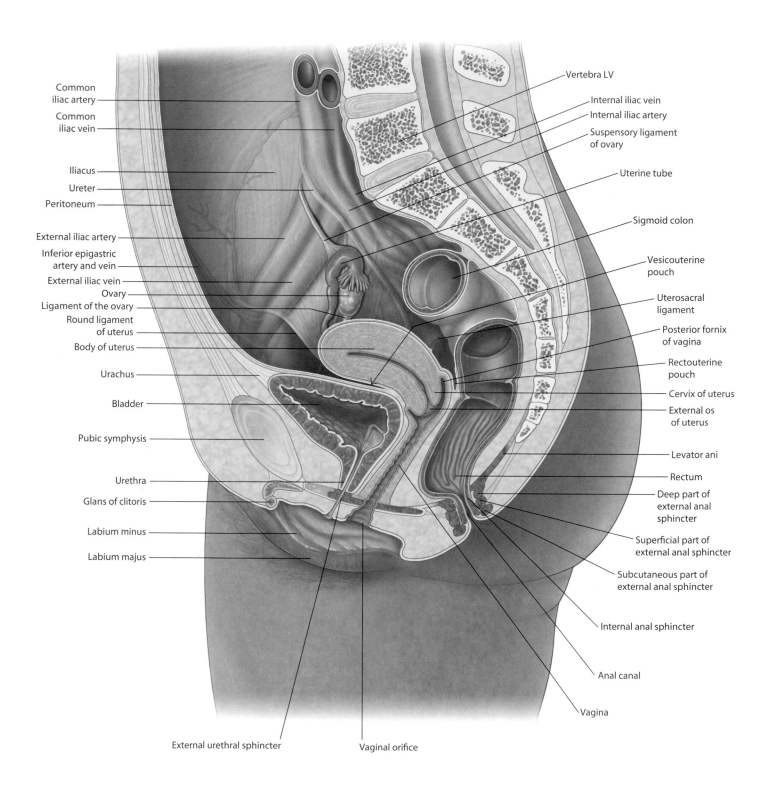

Common iliac artery
Common iliac vein
Iliacus
Ureter
Peritoneum
External iliac artery
Inferior epigastric artery and vein
External iliac vein
Ovary
Ligament of the ovary
Round ligament of uterus
Body of uterus
Urachus
Bladder
Pubic symphysis
Urethra
Glans of clitoris
Labium minus
Labium majus

Vertebra LV
Internal iliac vein
Internal iliac artery
Suspensory ligament of ovary
Uterine tube
Sigmoid colon
Vesicouterine pouch
Uterosacral ligament
Posterior fornix of vagina
Rectouterine pouch
Cervix of uterus
External os of uterus
Levator ani
Rectum
Deep part of external anal sphincter
Superficial part of external anal sphincter
Subcutaneous part of external anal sphincter
Internal anal sphincter
Anal canal
Vagina

External urethral sphincter
Vaginal orifice

Pelvic viscera and perineum in women *in situ* **(sagittal section)**

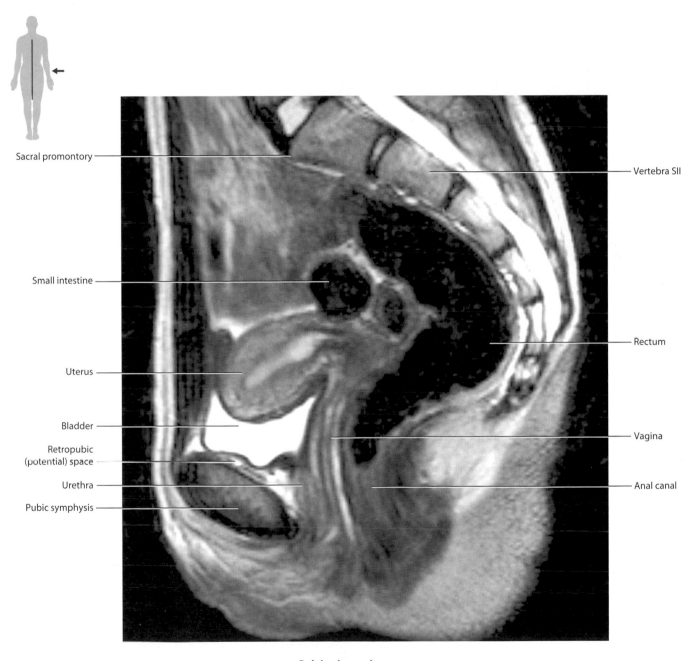

Sacral promontory

Small intestine

Uterus

Bladder

Retropubic
(potential) space

Urethra

Pubic symphysis

Vertebra SII

Rectum

Vagina

Anal canal

Pelvic viscera in women.
T2-weighted MR image in sagittal plane

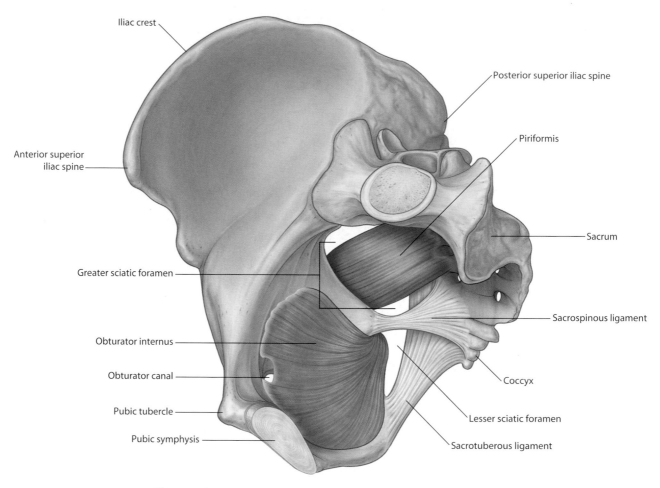

Iliac crest

Posterior superior iliac spine

Piriformis

Anterior superior
iliac spine

Sacrum

Greater sciatic foramen

Sacrospinous ligament

Obturator internus

Obturator canal

Coccyx

Pubic tubercle

Lesser sciatic foramen

Pubic symphysis

Sacrotuberous ligament

Obturator internus and piriformis muscles (oblique medial view)

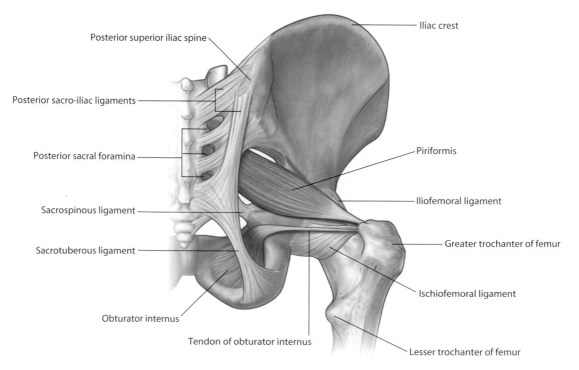

Iliac crest

Posterior superior iliac spine

Posterior sacro-iliac ligaments

Piriformis

Posterior sacral foramina

Iliofemoral ligament

Sacrospinous ligament

Sacrotuberous ligament

Greater trochanter of femur

Ischiofemoral ligament

Obturator internus

Lesser trochanter of femur

Tendon of obturator internus

Obturator internus and piriformis muscles (posterior view)

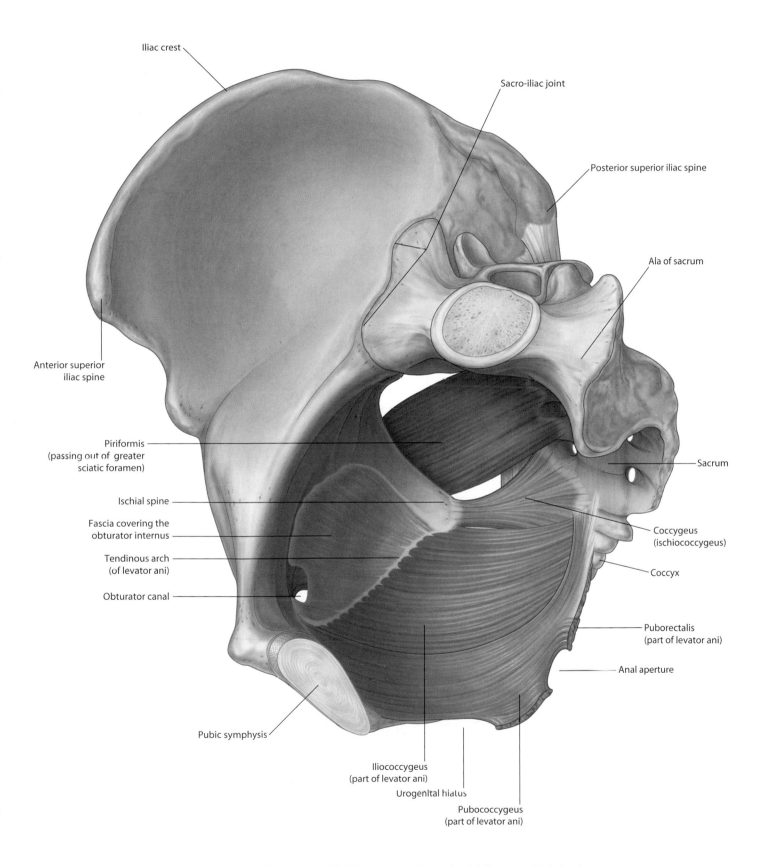

Iliac crest

Sacro-iliac joint

Posterior superior iliac spine

Ala of sacrum

Anterior superior
iliac spine

Piriformis
(passing out of greater
sciatic foramen)

Ischial spine

Fascia covering the
obturator internus

Tendinous arch
(of levator ani)

Obturator canal

Sacrum

Coccygeus
(ischiococcygeus)

Coccyx

Puborectalis
(part of levator ani)

Anal aperture

Pubic symphysis

Iliococcygeus
(part of levator ani)

Urogenital hiatus

Pubococcygeus
(part of levator ani)

Levator ani and coccygeus (ischiococcygeus) muscles (oblique sagittal view)

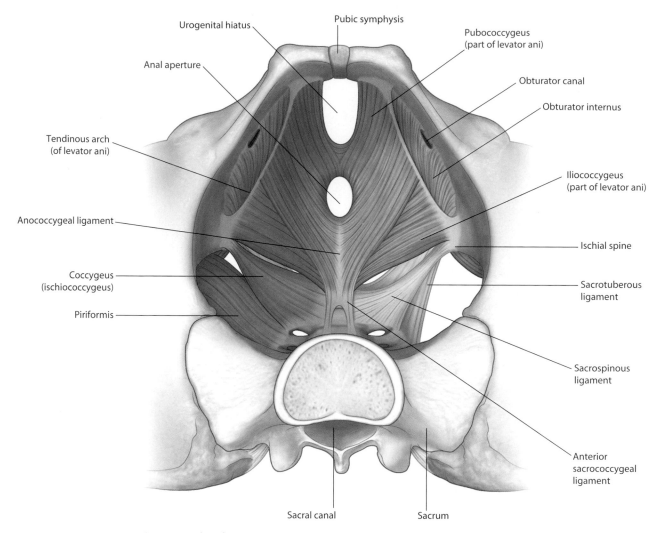

Urogenital hiatus

Pubic symphysis

Pubococcygeus
(part of levator ani)

Anal aperture

Obturator canal

Obturator internus

Tendinous arch
(of levator ani)

Iliococcygeus
(part of levator ani)

Anococcygeal ligament

Ischial spine

Coccygeus
(ischiococcygeus)

Sacrotuberous
ligament

Piriformis

Sacrospinous
ligament

Anterior
sacrococcygeal
ligament

Sacral canal

Sacrum

Levator ani and coccygeus (ischiococcygeus) muscles (anterosuperior view)

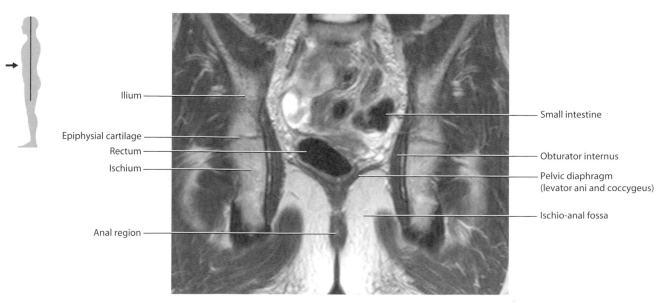

Ilium

Small intestine

Epiphysial cartilage

Rectum

Obturator internus

Ischium

Pelvic diaphragm
(levator ani and coccygeus)

Ischio-anal fossa

Anal region

**Pelvic diaphragm in relation to other structures in
the pelvic cavity and perineum.**
T2-weighted MR image in coronal plane

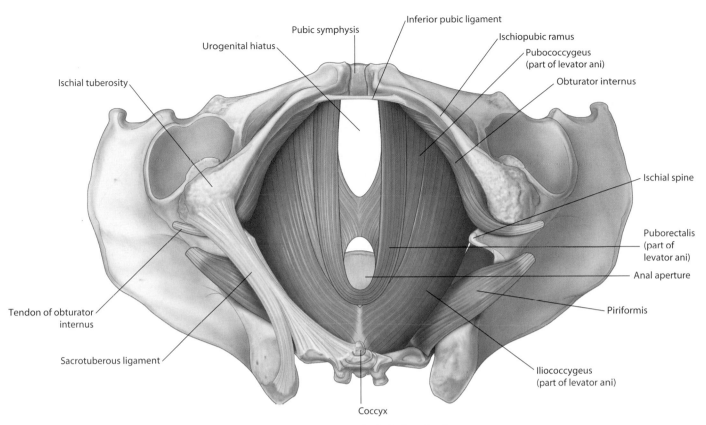

Levator ani muscle (inferior view)

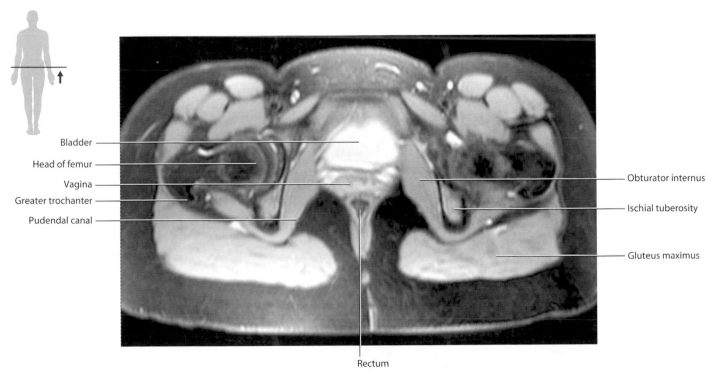

Obturator internus muscle and its relationship to other pelvic structures.
Fat-saturated T2-weighted MR image in axial plane

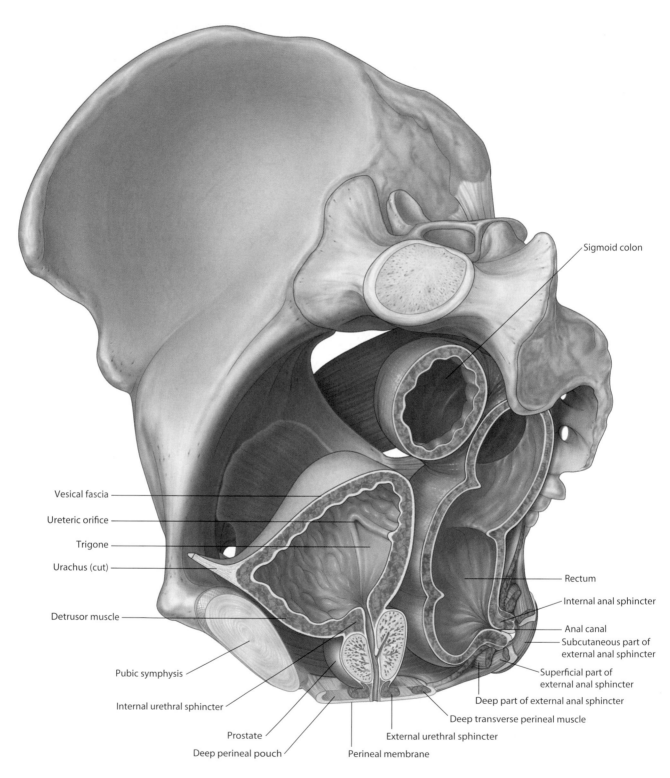

Bladder, prostate, and rectum within pelvic cavity in men (oblique sagittal view)

Sigmoid colon

Vesical fascia

Ureteric orifice

Trigone

Urachus (cut)

Detrusor muscle

Pubic symphysis

Internal urethral sphincter

Prostate

Deep perineal pouch

Perineal membrane

External urethral sphincter

Deep transverse perineal muscle

Deep part of external anal sphincter

Superficial part of
external anal sphincter

Subcutaneous part of
external anal sphincter

Anal canal

Internal anal sphincter

Rectum

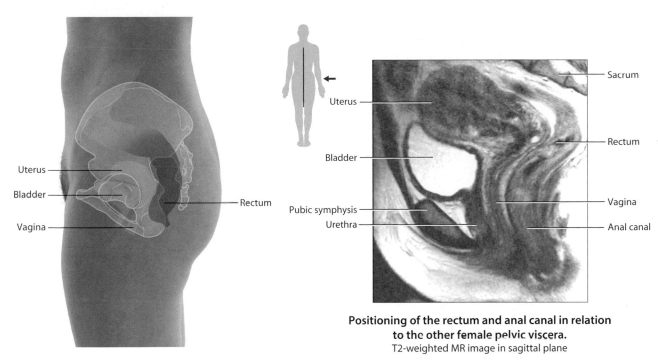

Surface projection of the rectum in women

Positioning of the rectum and anal canal in relation to the other female pelvic viscera.
T2-weighted MR image in sagittal plane

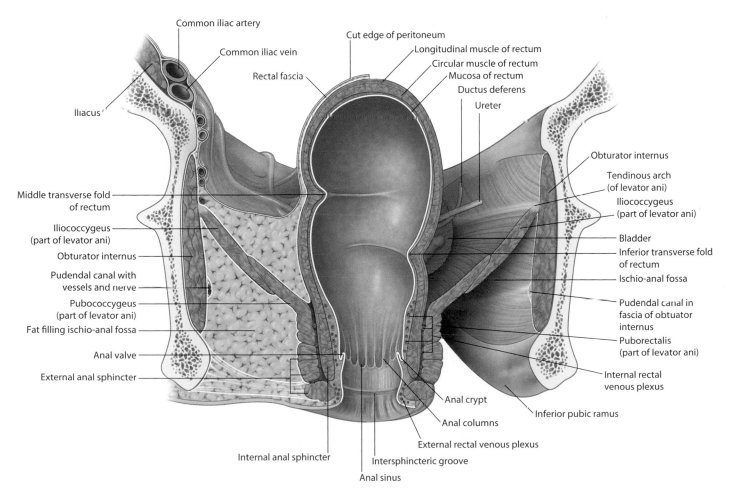

Coronal section through rectum and anal canal (posterior view)

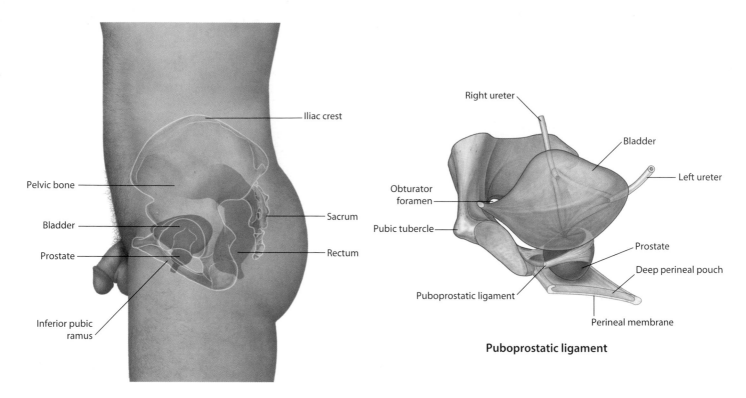

Surface projection of the bladder in men (lateral view)

Iliac crest

Pelvic bone

Bladder

Prostate

Inferior pubic ramus

Sacrum

Rectum

Puboprostatic ligament

Right ureter

Bladder

Left ureter

Obturator foramen

Pubic tubercle

Prostate

Deep perineal pouch

Puboprostatic ligament

Perineal membrane

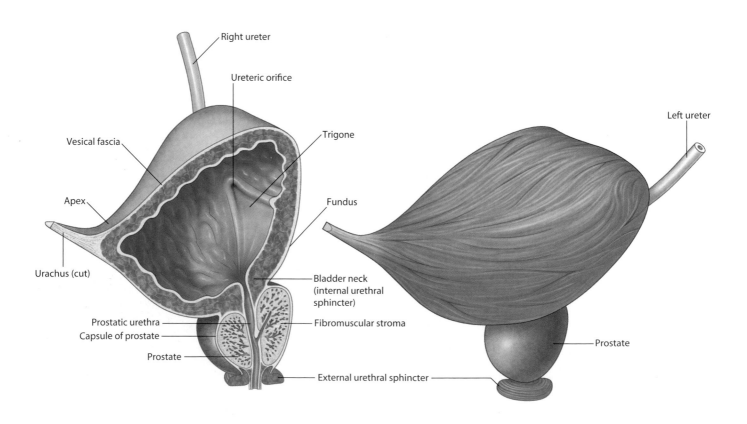

Right ureter

Ureteric orifice

Vesical fascia

Trigone

Apex

Fundus

Urachus (cut)

Bladder neck (internal urethral sphincter)

Prostatic urethra

Fibromuscular stroma

Capsule of prostate

Prostate

External urethral sphincter

Left ureter

Prostate

Urinary bladder in men

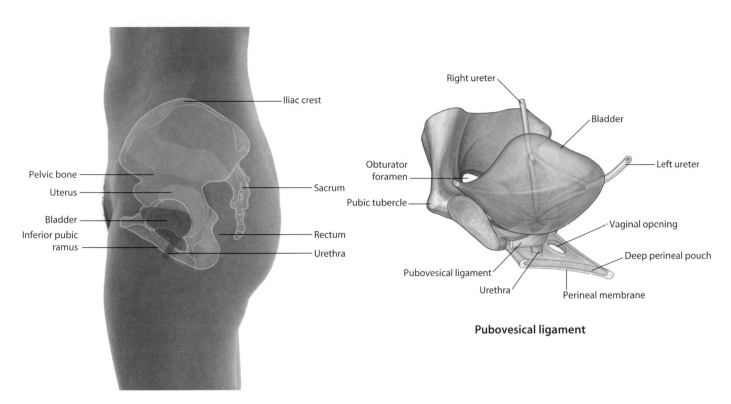

Surface projection of the bladder in women (lateral view)

Pubovesical ligament

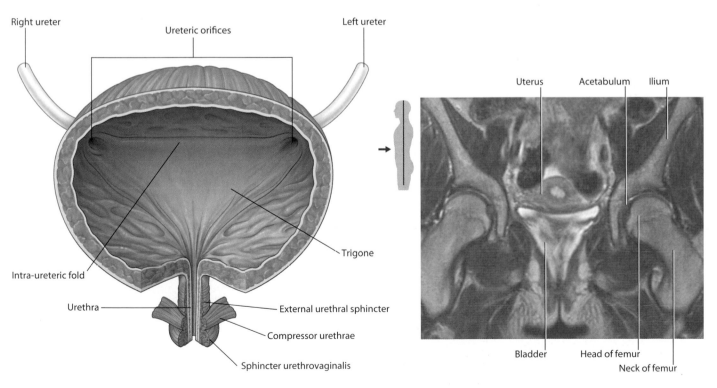

Urinary bladder and urethral sphincter muscles in women (anterior view of posterior wall)

Appearance and positioning of the bladder in relation to other structures in the female pelvic cavity.
T2-weighted MR image in coronal plane

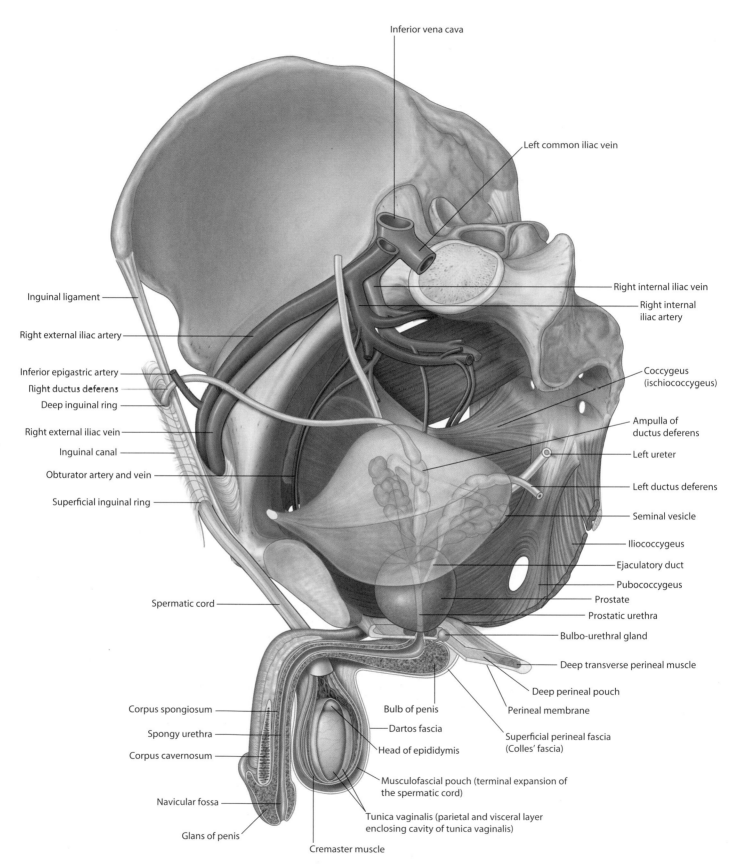

Inferior vena cava

Left common iliac vein

Right internal iliac vein

Right internal iliac artery

Inguinal ligament

Right external iliac artery

Inferior epigastric artery

Right ductus deferens

Deep inguinal ring

Right external iliac vein

Inguinal canal

Obturator artery and vein

Superficial inguinal ring

Coccygeus (ischiococcygeus)

Ampulla of ductus deferens

Left ureter

Left ductus deferens

Seminal vesicle

Iliococcygeus

Ejaculatory duct

Pubococcygeus

Prostate

Prostatic urethra

Bulbo-urethral gland

Deep transverse perineal muscle

Deep perineal pouch

Perineal membrane

Superficial perineal fascia (Colles' fascia)

Spermatic cord

Corpus spongiosum

Spongy urethra

Corpus cavernosum

Navicular fossa

Glans of penis

Bulb of penis

Dartos fascia

Head of epididymis

Musculofascial pouch (terminal expansion of the spermatic cord)

Tunica vaginalis (parietal and visceral layer enclosing cavity of tunica vaginalis)

Cremaster muscle

Reproductive system in men (oblique sagittal view)

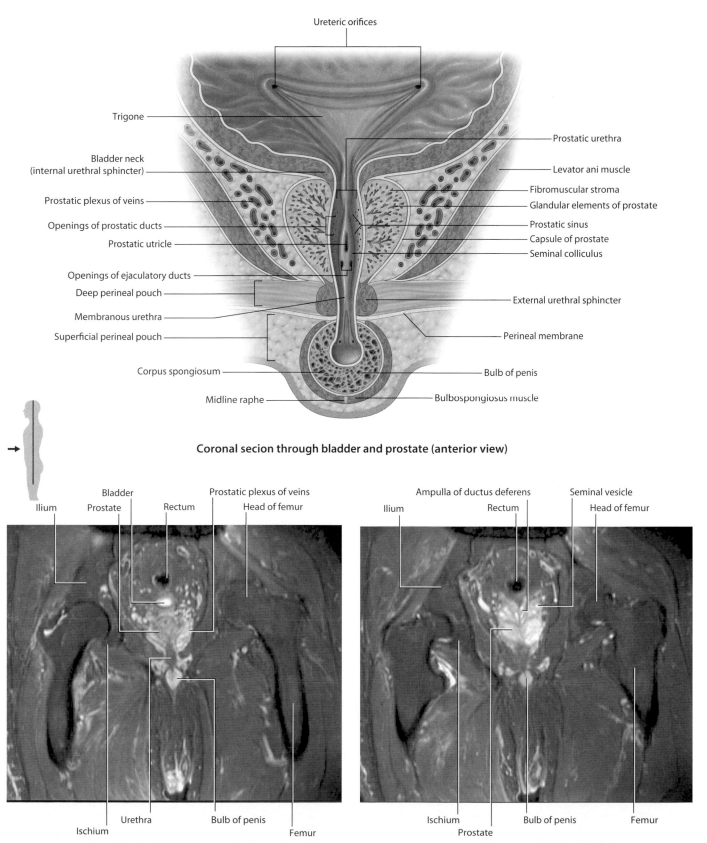

Ureteric orifices

Trigone

Bladder neck
(internal urethral sphincter)

Prostatic plexus of veins

Openings of prostatic ducts

Prostatic utricle

Openings of ejaculatory ducts

Deep perineal pouch

Membranous urethra

Superficial perineal pouch

Corpus spongiosum

Midline raphe

Prostatic urethra

Levator ani muscle

Fibromuscular stroma

Glandular elements of prostate

Prostatic sinus

Capsule of prostate

Seminal colliculus

External urethral sphincter

Perineal membrane

Bulb of penis

Bulbospongiosus muscle

Coronal secion through bladder and prostate (anterior view)

Ilium   Prostate   Bladder   Rectum   Prostatic plexus of veins   Head of femur

Ischium   Urethra   Bulb of penis   Femur

**Appearance and positioning of bladder and prostate in relation to
other structures in the male pelvis and perineum.**
Fat-saturated T2-weighted MR image in coronal plane

Ilium   Ampulla of ductus deferens   Rectum   Seminal vesicle   Head of femur

Ischium   Prostate   Bulb of penis   Femur

**Appearance and positioning of ductus deferens
and seminal vesicles in relation to other structures
in the male pelvis and perineum.**
Fat-saturated T2-weighted MR image in coronal plane

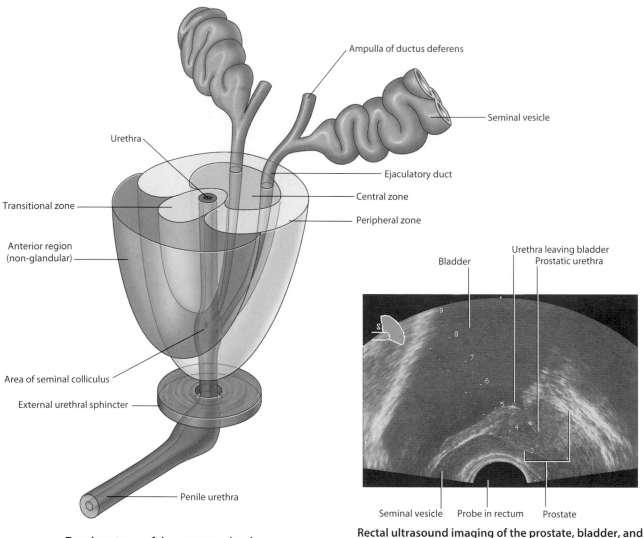

Urethra

Transitional zone

Anterior region
(non-glandular)

Area of seminal colliculus

External urethral sphincter

Ampulla of ductus deferens

Seminal vesicle

Ejaculatory duct

Central zone

Peripheral zone

Penile urethra

Zonal anatomy of the prostate gland.
Most carcinomas originate in the peripheral zone.
Benign prostatic hypertrophy (BPH)
affects mainly the transitional zone

Bladder

Urethra leaving bladder
Prostatic urethra

Seminal vesicle   Probe in rectum   Prostate

Rectal ultrasound imaging of the prostate, bladder, and
seminal vesicle. Sagittal view also showing the urethra

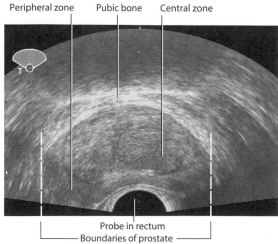

Peripheral zone   Pubic bone   Central zone

Probe in rectum
Boundaries of prostate

Rectal ultrasound imaging of the prostate.
Axial view showing the central and peripheral zones

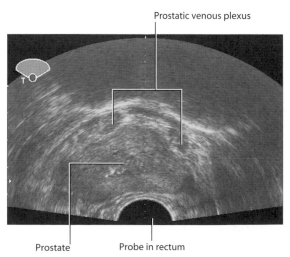

Prostatic venous plexus

Prostate   Probe in rectum

Rectal ultrasound imaging of the prostate.
Axial view showing the surrounding plexus of veins

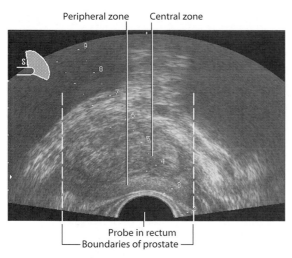

**Rectal ultrasound imaging of the prostate.
Sagittal view showing the central and peripheral zones**

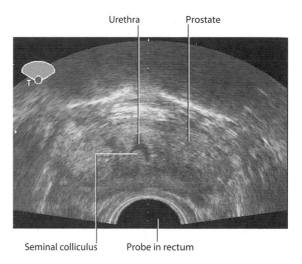

**Rectal ultrasound imaging of the prostate.
Axial view showing the urethra and seminal colliculus**

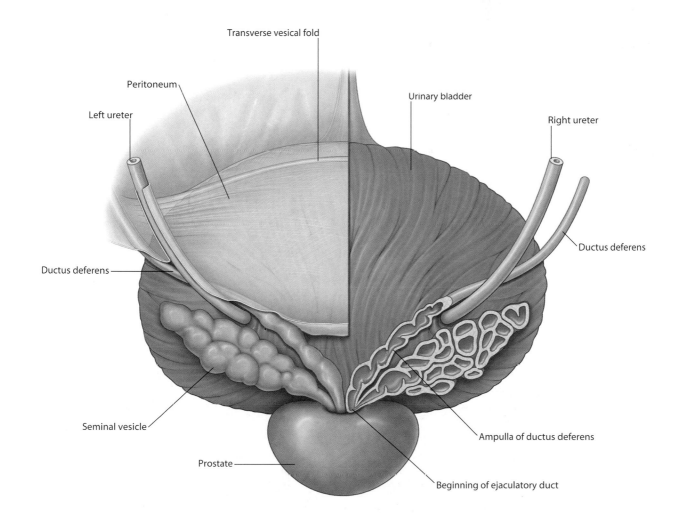

Bladder and prostate (posterior view)

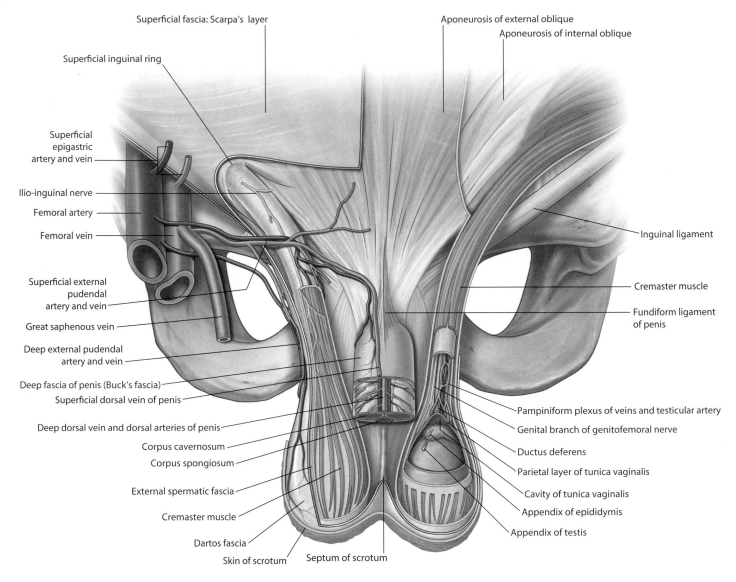

Superficial fascia: Scarpa's layer

Superficial inguinal ring

Superficial epigastric artery and vein

Ilio-inguinal nerve

Femoral artery

Femoral vein

Superficial external pudendal artery and vein

Great saphenous vein

Deep external pudendal artery and vein

Deep fascia of penis (Buck's fascia)

Superficial dorsal vein of penis

Deep dorsal vein and dorsal arteries of penis

Corpus cavernosum

Corpus spongiosum

External spermatic fascia

Cremaster muscle

Dartos fascia

Skin of scrotum

Septum of scrotum

Aponeurosis of external oblique

Aponeurosis of internal oblique

Inguinal ligament

Cremaster muscle

Fundiform ligament of penis

Pampiniform plexus of veins and testicular artery

Genital branch of genitofemoral nerve

Ductus deferens

Parietal layer of tunica vaginalis

Cavity of tunica vaginalis

Appendix of epididymis

Appendix of testis

Contents of the scrotum (anterior view)

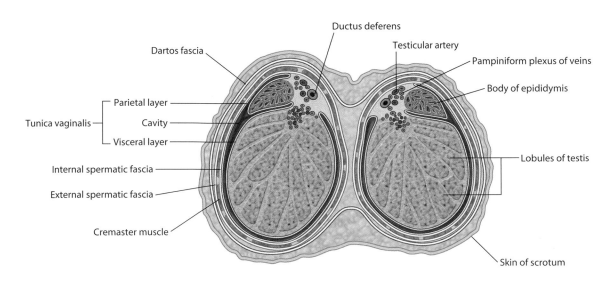

Dartos fascia

Ductus deferens

Testicular artery

Pampiniform plexus of veins

Body of epididymis

Tunica vaginalis
- Parietal layer
- Cavity
- Visceral layer

Internal spermatic fascia

External spermatic fascia

Cremaster muscle

Lobules of testis

Skin of scrotum

Transverse section through the scrotum and testes

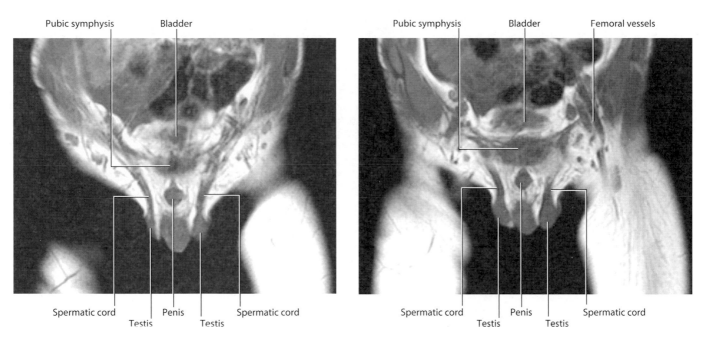

Spermatic cord appearance and positioning in a young male.
T1-weighted MR images in coronal plane

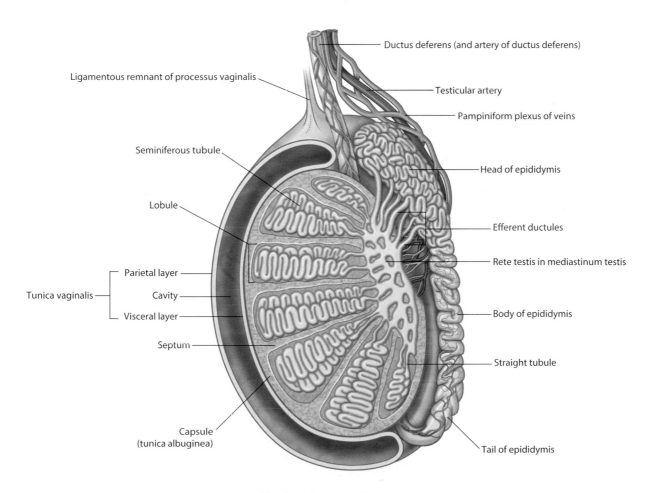

Testis and surrounding structures

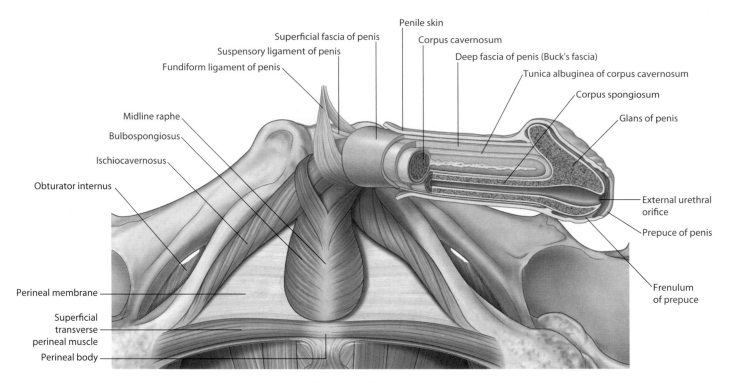

Superficial fascia of penis

Suspensory ligament of penis

Fundiform ligament of penis

Penile skin

Corpus cavernosum

Deep fascia of penis (Buck's fascia)

Tunica albuginea of corpus cavernosum

Corpus spongiosum

Glans of penis

Midline raphe

Bulbospongiosus

Ischiocavernosus

Obturator internus

External urethral orifice

Prepuce of penis

Perineal membrane

Frenulum of prepuce

Superficial transverse perineal muscle

Perineal body

Structure of the penis

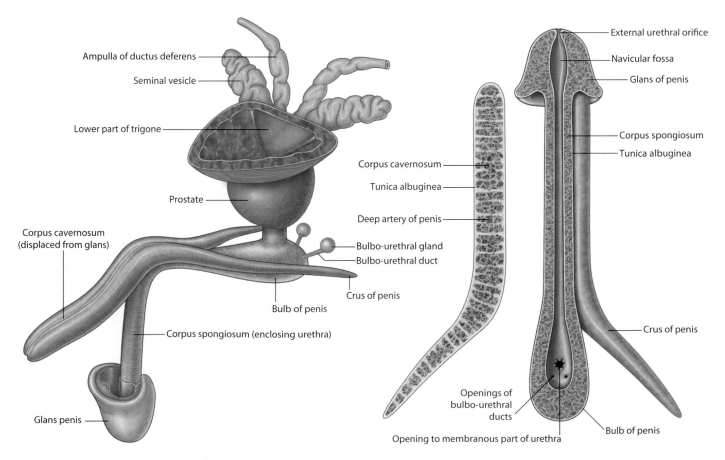

Ampulla of ductus deferens

Seminal vesicle

Lower part of trigone

Prostate

Corpus cavernosum (displaced from glans)

Bulbo-urethral gland

Bulbo-urethral duct

Crus of penis

Bulb of penis

Corpus spongiosum (enclosing urethra)

Glans penis

External urethral orifice

Navicular fossa

Glans of penis

Corpus spongiosum

Tunica albuginea

Corpus cavernosum

Tunica albuginea

Deep artery of penis

Crus of penis

Openings of bulbo-urethral ducts

Opening to membranous part of urethra

Bulb of penis

Structure of the penis

Roof of spongy urethra (inferior view)

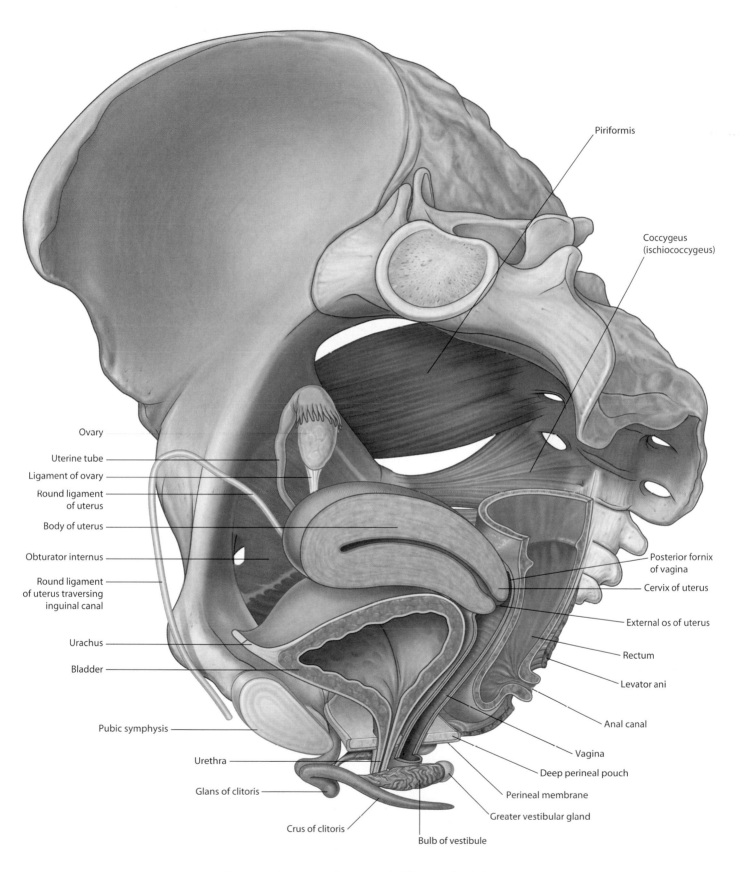

Piriformis

Coccygeus (ischiococcygeus)

Ovary

Uterine tube

Ligament of ovary

Round ligament of uterus

Body of uterus

Obturator internus

Round ligament of uterus traversing inguinal canal

Urachus

Bladder

Pubic symphysis

Urethra

Glans of clitoris

Crus of clitoris

Bulb of vestibule

Posterior fornix of vagina

Cervix of uterus

External os of uterus

Rectum

Levator ani

Anal canal

Vagina

Deep perineal pouch

Perineal membrane

Greater vestibular gland

Reproductive system in women (oblique sagittal view)

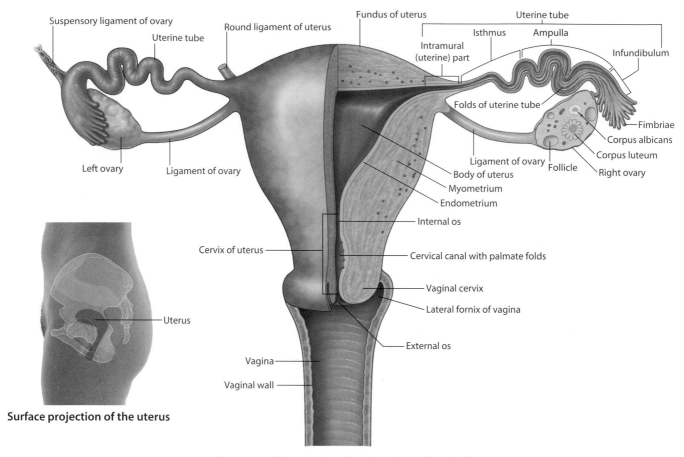

Suspensory ligament of ovary

Uterine tube

Round ligament of uterus

Fundus of uterus

Uterine tube

Isthmus

Ampulla

Intramural (uterine) part

Infundibulum

Folds of uterine tube

Fimbriae

Corpus albicans

Corpus luteum

Left ovary

Ligament of ovary

Ligament of ovary

Follicle

Right ovary

Body of uterus

Myometrium

Endometrium

Internal os

Cervix of uterus

Cervical canal with palmate folds

Vaginal cervix

Lateral fornix of vagina

External os

Uterus

Vagina

Vaginal wall

Surface projection of the uterus

Structure of the uterus and ovaries (posterior view)

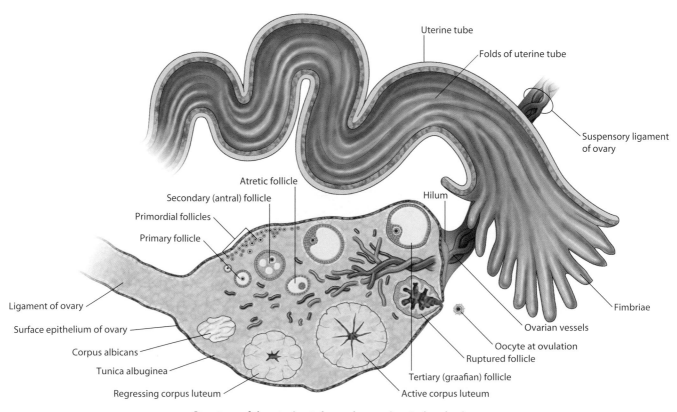

Uterine tube

Folds of uterine tube

Suspensory ligament of ovary

Atretic follicle

Hilum

Secondary (antral) follicle

Primordial follicles

Primary follicle

Ligament of ovary

Surface epithelium of ovary

Corpus albicans

Tunica albuginea

Regressing corpus luteum

Fimbriae

Ovarian vessels

Oocyte at ovulation

Ruptured follicle

Tertiary (graafian) follicle

Active corpus luteum

Structure of the uterine tube and ovary (posterior view)

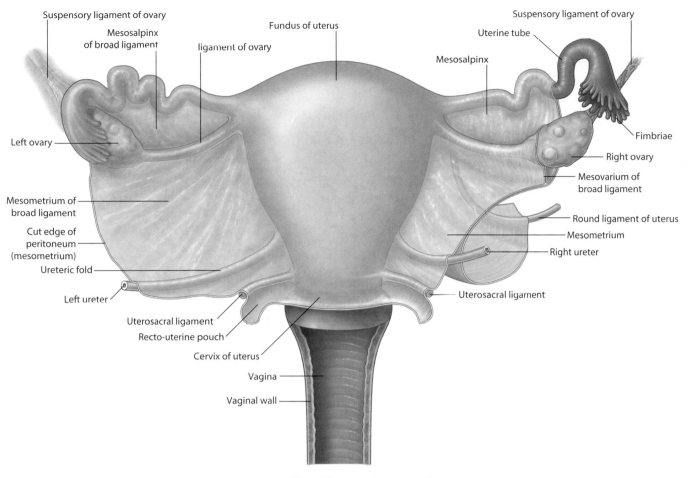

Suspensory ligament of ovary

Mesosalpinx of broad ligament

ligament of ovary

Fundus of uterus

Suspensory ligament of ovary

Uterine tube

Mesosalpinx

Fimbriae

Left ovary

Right ovary

Mesovarium of broad ligament

Mesometrium of broad ligament

Round ligament of uterus

Mesometrium

Cut edge of peritoneum (mesometrium)

Right ureter

Ureteric fold

Uterosacral ligament

Left ureter

Uterosacral ligament

Recto-uterine pouch

Cervix of uterus

Vagina

Vaginal wall

Uterus and broad ligament (posterior view)

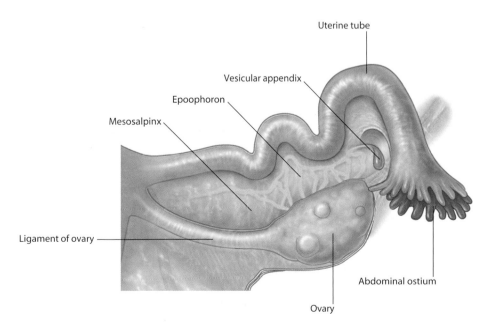

Uterine tube

Vesicular appendix

Epoophoron

Mesosalpinx

Ligament of ovary

Abdominal ostium

Ovary

Uterine tube and ovary (posterior view)

A

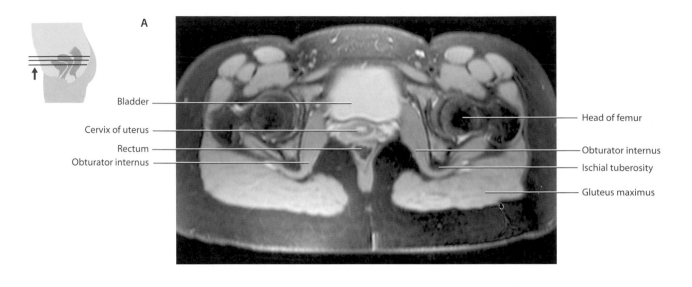

Bladder

Cervix of uterus

Rectum

Obturator internus

Head of femur

Obturator internus

Ischial tuberosity

Gluteus maximus

B

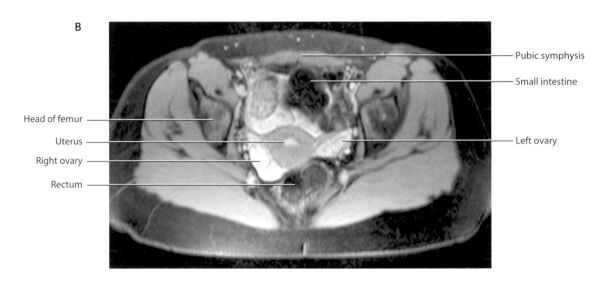

Head of femur

Uterus

Right ovary

Rectum

Pubic symphysis

Small intestine

Left ovary

C

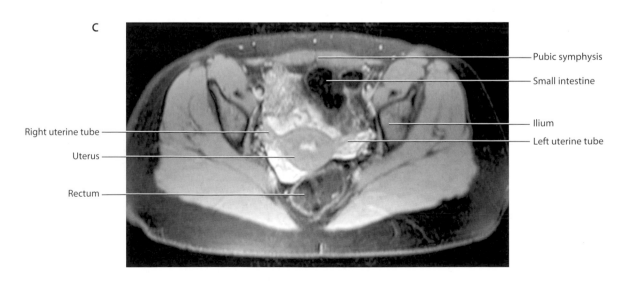

Right uterine tube

Uterus

Rectum

Pubic symphysis

Small intestine

Ilium

Left uterine tube

**Appearance of cervix of uterus, uterus, ovaries, and uterine tubes
in relation to other pelvic structures.**
Fat-saturated T2-weighted MR images in axial plane

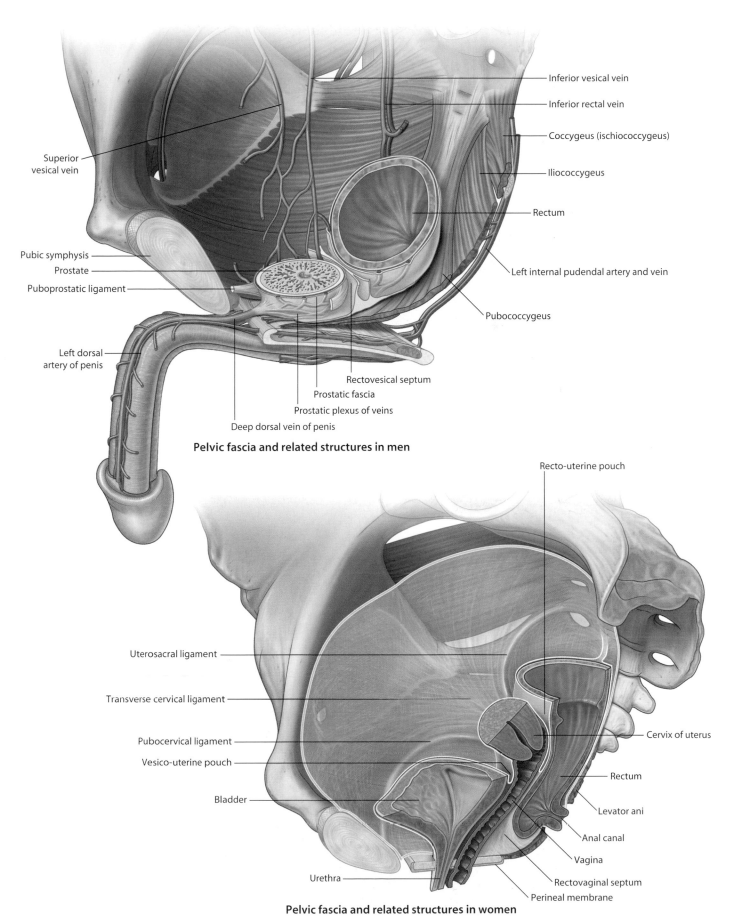

Inferior vesical vein

Inferior rectal vein

Coccygeus (ischiococcygeus)

Iliococcygeus

Rectum

Left internal pudendal artery and vein

Pubococcygeus

Superior vesical vein

Pubic symphysis

Prostate

Puboprostatic ligament

Left dorsal artery of penis

Rectovesical septum

Prostatic fascia

Prostatic plexus of veins

Deep dorsal vein of penis

Pelvic fascia and related structures in men

Recto-uterine pouch

Uterosacral ligament

Transverse cervical ligament

Pubocervical ligament

Vesico-uterine pouch

Bladder

Cervix of uterus

Rectum

Levator ani

Anal canal

Vagina

Urethra

Rectovaginal septum

Perineal membrane

Pelvic fascia and related structures in women

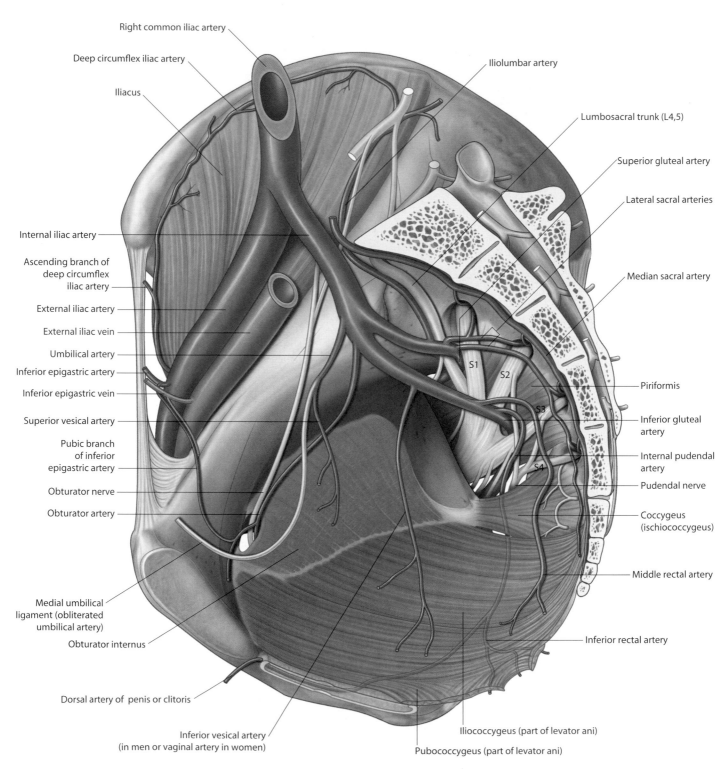

**Arterial supply to the pelvis
(right side sagittal view)**

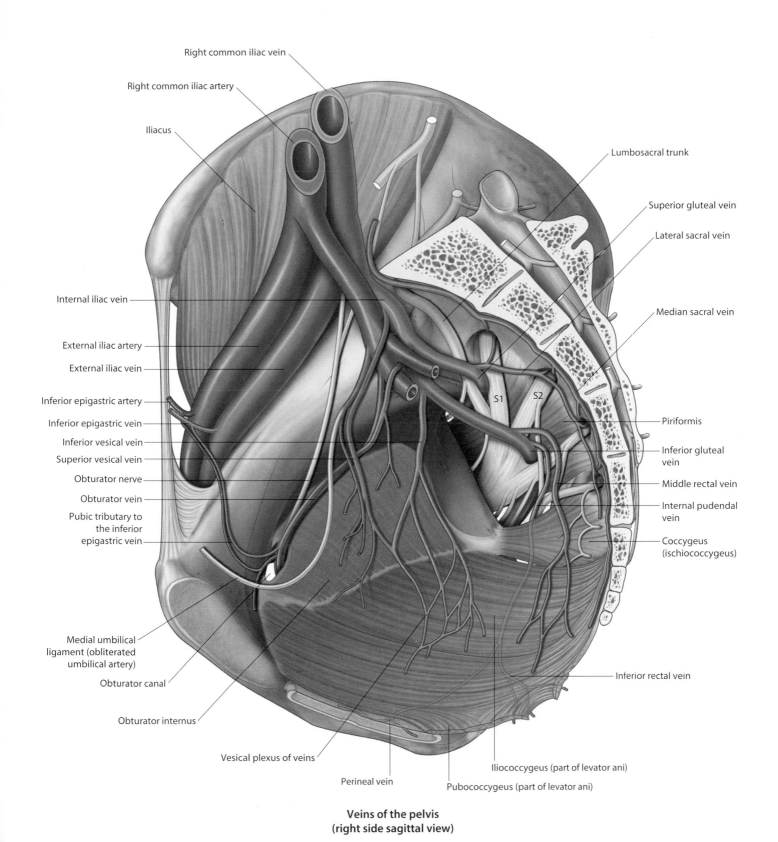

Right common iliac vein

Right common iliac artery

Iliacus

Internal iliac vein

External iliac artery

External iliac vein

Inferior epigastric artery

Inferior epigastric vein

Inferior vesical vein

Superior vesical vein

Obturator nerve

Obturator vein

Pubic tributary to the inferior epigastric vein

Medial umbilical ligament (obliterated umbilical artery)

Obturator canal

Obturator internus

Vesical plexus of veins

Perineal vein

Lumbosacral trunk

Superior gluteal vein

Lateral sacral vein

Median sacral vein

S1　S2

Piriformis

Inferior gluteal vein

Middle rectal vein

Internal pudendal vein

Coccygeus (ischiococcygeus)

Inferior rectal vein

Iliococcygeus (part of levator ani)

Pubococcygeus (part of levator ani)

**Veins of the pelvis
(right side sagittal view)**

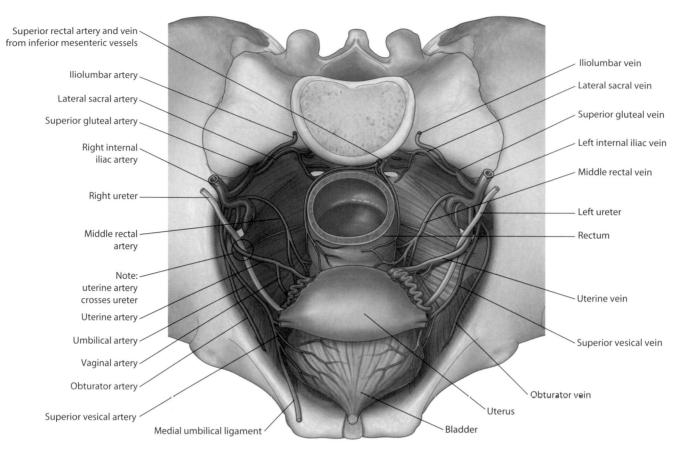

Superior rectal artery and vein from inferior mesenteric vessels

Iliolumbar artery

Lateral sacral artery

Superior gluteal artery

Right internal iliac artery

Right ureter

Middle rectal artery

Note: uterine artery crosses ureter

Uterine artery

Umbilical artery

Vaginal artery

Obturator artery

Superior vesical artery

Medial umbilical ligament

Iliolumbar vein

Lateral sacral vein

Superior gluteal vein

Left internal iliac vein

Middle rectal vein

Left ureter

Rectum

Uterine vein

Superior vesical vein

Obturator vein

Uterus

Bladder

Vasculature of the pelvic viscera in women (superior view)

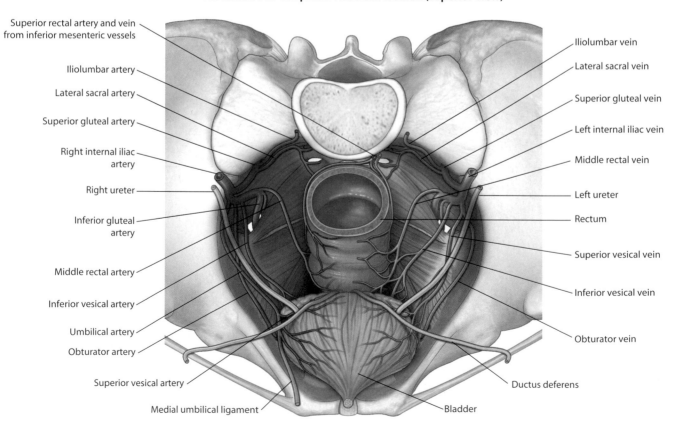

Superior rectal artery and vein from inferior mesenteric vessels

Iliolumbar artery

Lateral sacral artery

Superior gluteal artery

Right internal iliac artery

Right ureter

Inferior gluteal artery

Middle rectal artery

Inferior vesical artery

Umbilical artery

Obturator artery

Superior vesical artery

Medial umbilical ligament

Iliolumbar vein

Lateral sacral vein

Superior gluteal vein

Left internal iliac vein

Middle rectal vein

Left ureter

Rectum

Superior vesical vein

Inferior vesical vein

Obturator vein

Ductus deferens

Bladder

Vasculature of the pelvic viscera in men (superior view)

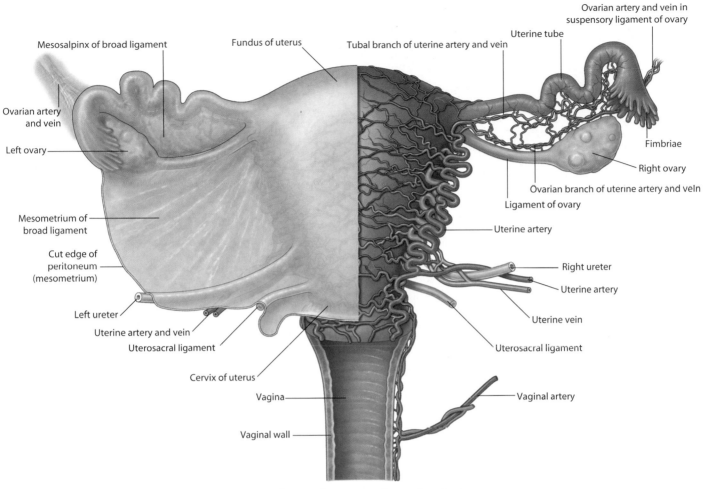

Vascular supply to uterus (posterior view)

Labels (clockwise from top left):
- Mesosalpinx of broad ligament
- Fundus of uterus
- Tubal branch of uterine artery and vein
- Uterine tube
- Ovarian artery and vein in suspensory ligament of ovary
- Fimbriae
- Right ovary
- Ovarian branch of uterine artery and vein
- Ligament of ovary
- Uterine artery
- Right ureter
- Uterine artery
- Uterine vein
- Uterosacral ligament
- Vaginal artery
- Vaginal wall
- Vagina
- Cervix of uterus
- Uterosacral ligament
- Uterine artery and vein
- Left ureter
- Cut edge of peritoneum (mesometrium)
- Mesometrium of broad ligament
- Left ovary
- Ovarian artery and vein

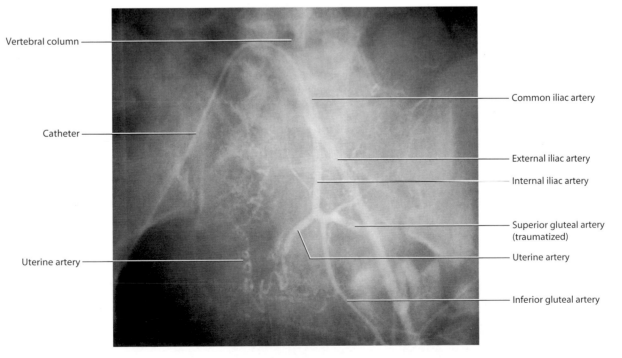

Vascular supply to uterus.
Angiogram

Labels:
- Vertebral column
- Common iliac artery
- External iliac artery
- Internal iliac artery
- Catheter
- Superior gluteal artery (traumatized)
- Uterine artery
- Uterine artery
- Inferior gluteal artery

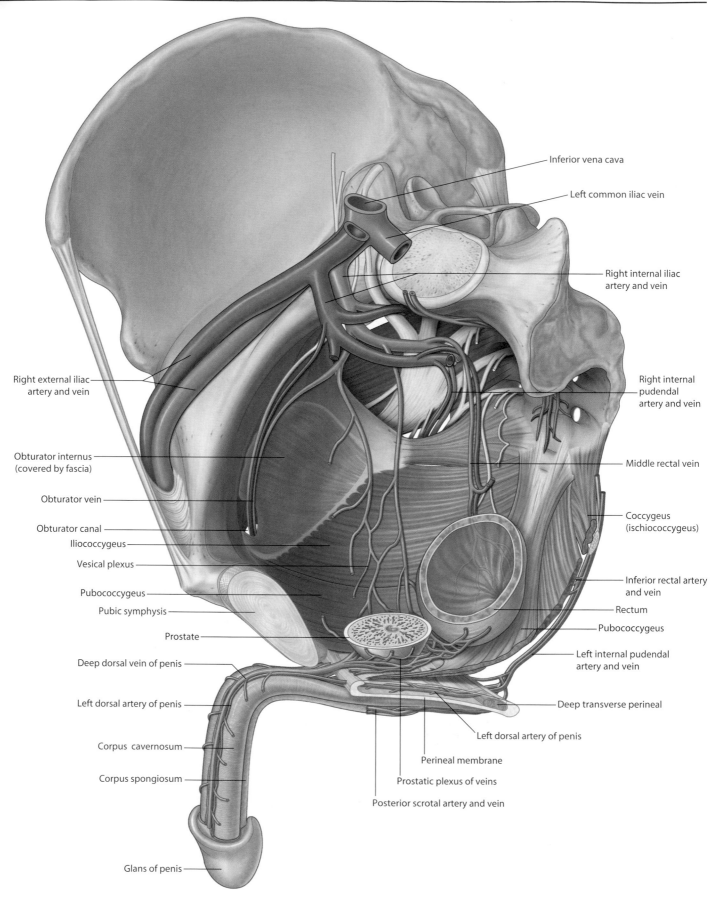

Inferior vena cava

Left common iliac vein

Right internal iliac artery and vein

Right external iliac artery and vein

Right internal pudendal artery and vein

Obturator internus (covered by fascia)

Middle rectal vein

Obturator vein

Obturator canal

Iliococcygeus

Vesical plexus

Coccygeus (ischiococcygeus)

Inferior rectal artery and vein

Pubococcygeus

Rectum

Pubic symphysis

Pubococcygeus

Prostate

Left internal pudendal artery and vein

Deep dorsal vein of penis

Left dorsal artery of penis

Deep transverse perineal

Left dorsal artery of penis

Corpus cavernosum

Perineal membrane

Corpus spongiosum

Prostatic plexus of veins

Posterior scrotal artery and vein

Glans of penis

Venous drainage of pelvic viscera in men
(oblique sagittal view)

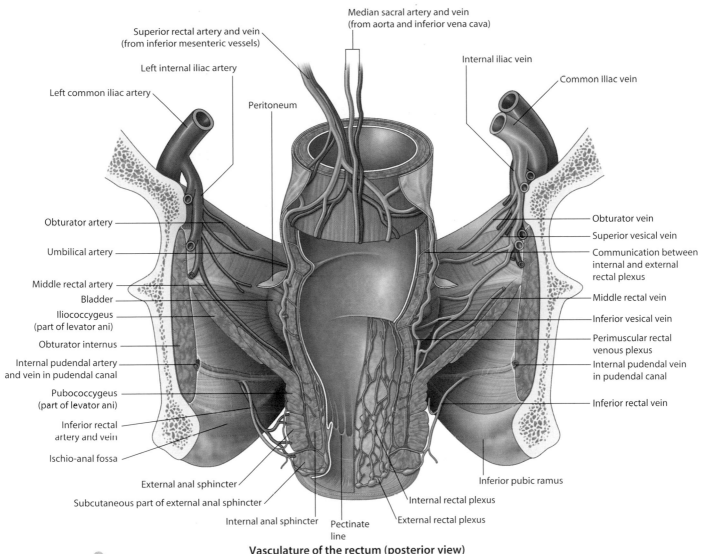

Median sacral artery and vein
(from aorta and inferior vena cava)

Superior rectal artery and vein
(from inferior mesenteric vessels)

Internal iliac vein

Left internal iliac artery

Common Iliac vein

Left common iliac artery

Peritoneum

Obturator artery

Obturator vein

Umbilical artery

Superior vesical vein

Communication between
internal and external
rectal plexus

Middle rectal artery

Bladder

Middle rectal vein

Iliococcygeus
(part of levator ani)

Inferior vesical vein

Obturator internus

Perimuscular rectal
venous plexus

Internal pudendal artery
and vein in pudendal canal

Internal pudendal vein
in pudendal canal

Pubococcygeus
(part of levator ani)

Inferior rectal vein

Inferior rectal
artery and vein

Ischio-anal fossa

External anal sphincter

Subcutaneous part of external anal sphincter

Inferior pubic ramus

Internal rectal plexus

Internal anal sphincter

Pectinate
line

External rectal plexus

Vasculature of the rectum (posterior view)

Pubic symphysis

Urethra

Femur

Vagina

Obturator internus

Pudendal canal

Ischial tuberosity

Anal region

Gluteus maximus

Inferior rectal branch to anal region

Inferior rectal neurovascular bundle crossing the ischio-anal fossa.
T2-weighted MR image in axial plane

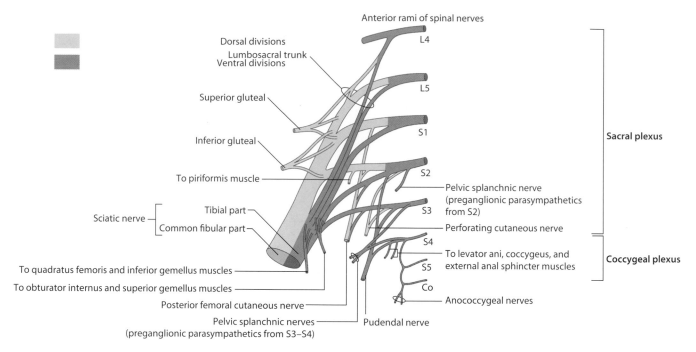

Anterior rami of spinal nerves

Dorsal divisions
Lumbosacral trunk
Ventral divisions

Superior gluteal

Inferior gluteal

To piriformis muscle

Sciatic nerve
- Tibial part
- Common fibular part

L4
L5
S1
S2
S3
S4
S5
Co

Pelvic splanchnic nerve (preganglionic parasympathetics from S2)

Perforating cutaneous nerve

To levator ani, coccygeus, and external anal sphincter muscles

Anococcygeal nerves

Sacral plexus

Coccygeal plexus

To quadratus femoris and inferior gemellus muscles
To obturator internus and superior gemellus muscles
Posterior femoral cutaneous nerve
Pelvic splanchnic nerves (preganglionic parasympathetics from S3–S4)
Pudendal nerve

Components and branches of the sacral and coccygeal nerve plexuses

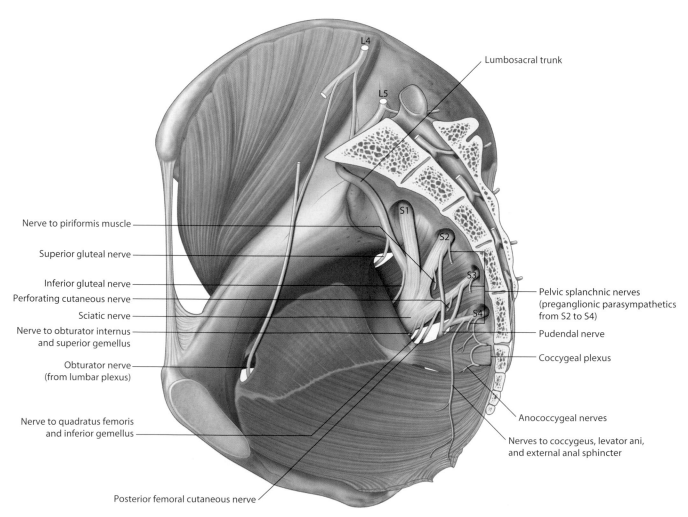

L4
L5
S1
S2
S3
S4

Lumbosacral trunk

Nerve to piriformis muscle
Superior gluteal nerve
Inferior gluteal nerve
Perforating cutaneous nerve
Sciatic nerve
Nerve to obturator internus and superior gemellus
Obturator nerve (from lumbar plexus)

Nerve to quadratus femoris and inferior gemellus

Posterior femoral cutaneous nerve

Pelvic splanchnic nerves (preganglionic parasympathetics from S2 to S4)
Pudendal nerve
Coccygeal plexus
Anococcygeal nerves
Nerves to coccygeus, levator ani, and external anal sphincter

Sacral and coccygeal nerve plexuses within the pelvic cavity (sagittal view)

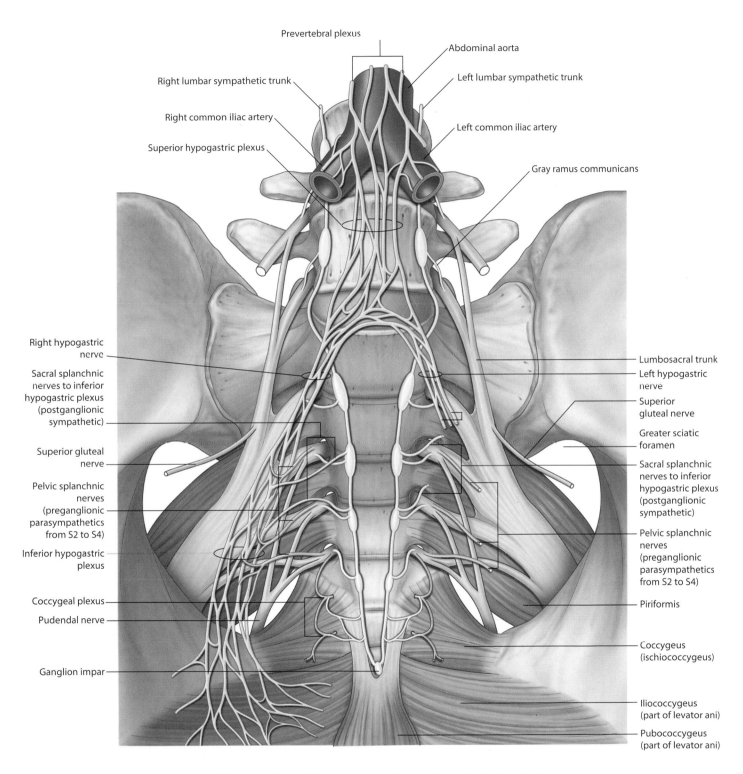

Prevertebral plexus

Abdominal aorta

Right lumbar sympathetic trunk

Left lumbar sympathetic trunk

Right common iliac artery

Left common iliac artery

Superior hypogastric plexus

Gray ramus communicans

Right hypogastric nerve

Lumbosacral trunk

Sacral splanchnic nerves to inferior hypogastric plexus (postganglionic sympathetic)

Left hypogastric nerve

Superior gluteal nerve

Greater sciatic foramen

Superior gluteal nerve

Sacral splanchnic nerves to inferior hypogastric plexus (postganglionic sympathetic)

Pelvic splanchnic nerves (preganglionic parasympathetics from S2 to S4)

Pelvic splanchnic nerves (preganglionic parasympathetics from S2 to S4)

Inferior hypogastric plexus

Piriformis

Coccygeal plexus

Pudendal nerve

Coccygeus (ischiococcygeus)

Ganglion impar

Iliococcygeus (part of levator ani)

Pubococcygeus (part of levator ani)

Pelvic extensions of the prevertebral nerve plexus (anterior view)

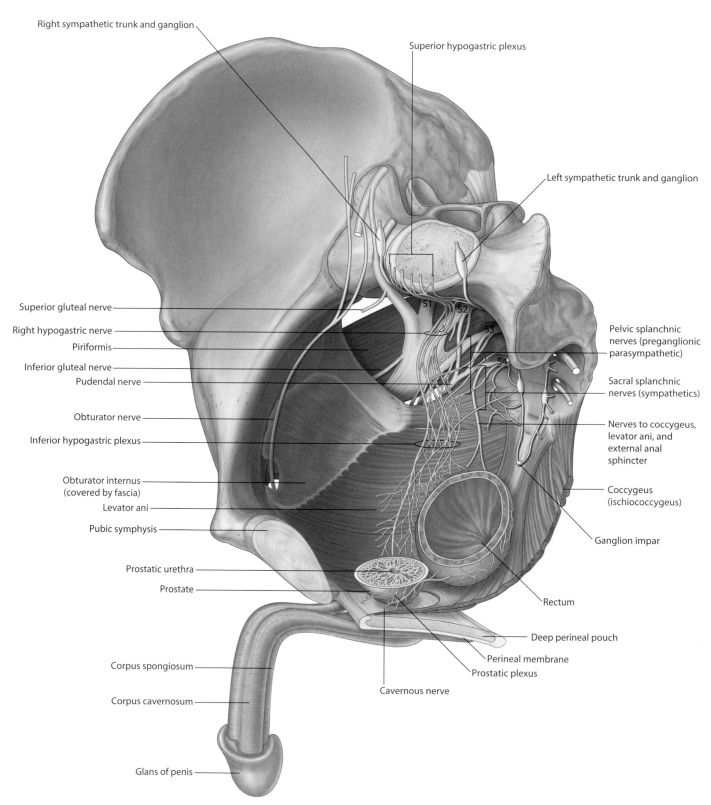

Right sympathetic trunk and ganglion

Superior hypogastric plexus

Left sympathetic trunk and ganglion

S1

S2

S3

S4

Superior gluteal nerve

Right hypogastric nerve

Piriformis

Inferior gluteal nerve

Pudendal nerve

Obturator nerve

Inferior hypogastric plexus

Obturator internus
(covered by fascia)

Levator ani

Pubic symphysis

Prostatic urethra

Prostate

Corpus spongiosum

Corpus cavernosum

Glans of penis

Pelvic splanchnic
nerves (preganglionic
parasympathetic)

Sacral splanchnic
nerves (sympathetics)

Nerves to coccygeus,
levator ani, and
external anal
sphincter

Coccygeus
(ischiococcygeus)

Ganglion impar

Rectum

Deep perineal pouch

Perineal membrane

Prostatic plexus

Cavernous nerve

Hypogastric nerve plexuses
(oblique sagittal view)

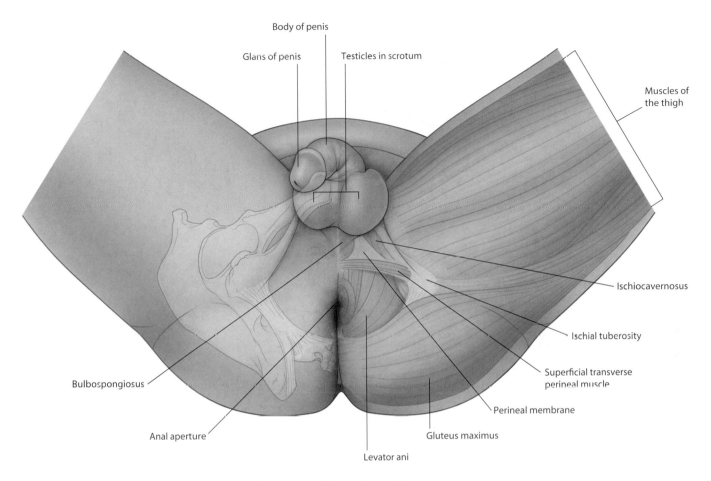

Body of penis

Glans of penis

Testicles in scrotum

Muscles of the thigh

Ischiocavernosus

Ischial tuberosity

Superficial transverse perineal muscle

Perineal membrane

Gluteus maximus

Levator ani

Anal aperture

Bulbospongiosus

Structures of the perineum in men

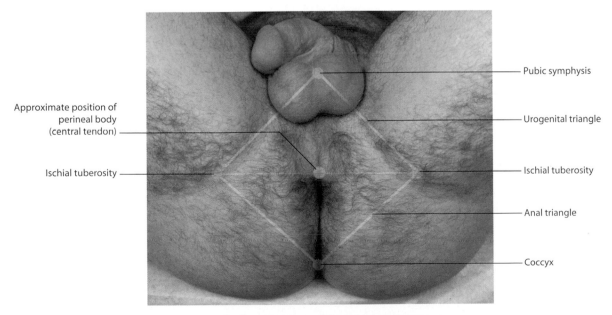

Pubic symphysis

Urogenital triangle

Approximate position of perineal body (central tendon)

Ischial tuberosity

Ischial tuberosity

Anal triangle

Coccyx

Surface anatomy of the perineum in men

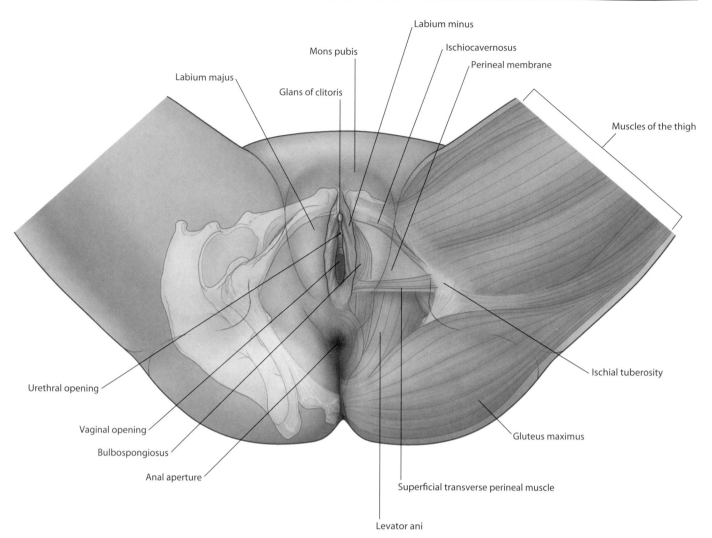

Labium minus

Mons pubis

Ischiocavernosus

Perineal membrane

Labium majus

Glans of clitoris

Muscles of the thigh

Urethral opening

Vaginal opening

Bulbospongiosus

Anal aperture

Ischial tuberosity

Gluteus maximus

Superficial transverse perineal muscle

Levator ani

Structures of the perineum in women

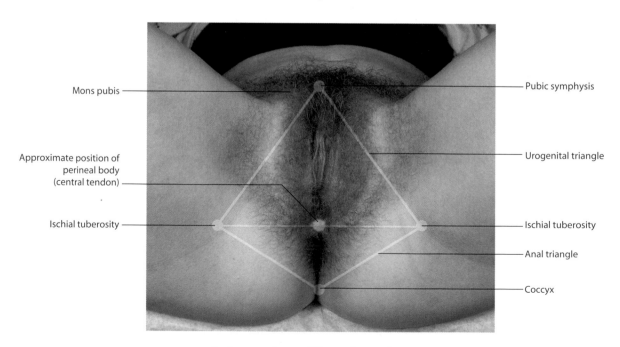

Mons pubis

Pubic symphysis

Approximate position of perineal body (central tendon)

Urogenital triangle

Ischial tuberosity

Ischial tuberosity

Anal triangle

Coccyx

Surface anatomy of the perineum in women

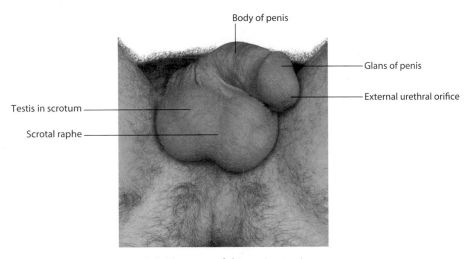

Body of penis

Glans of penis

External urethral orifice

Testis in scrotum

Scrotal raphe

Superficial features of the perineum in men

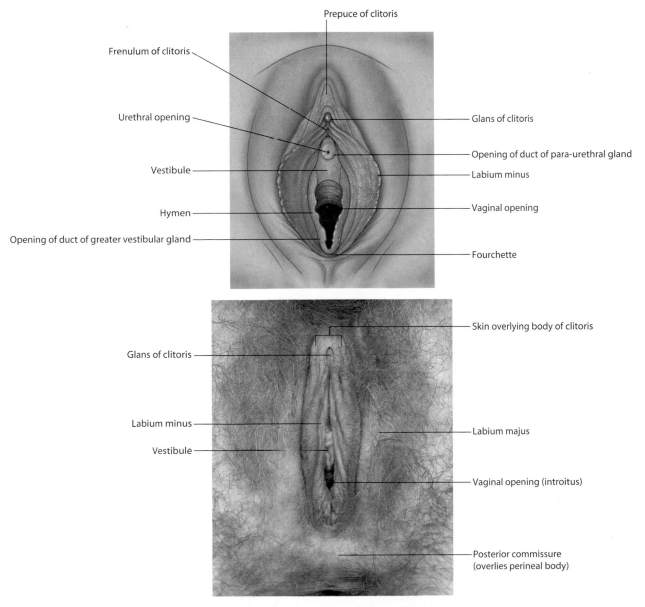

Prepuce of clitoris

Frenulum of clitoris

Urethral opening

Glans of clitoris

Opening of duct of para-urethral gland

Vestibule

Labium minus

Hymen

Vaginal opening

Opening of duct of greater vestibular gland

Fourchette

Skin overlying body of clitoris

Glans of clitoris

Labium minus

Labium majus

Vestibule

Vaginal opening (introitus)

Posterior commissure
(overlies perineal body)

Superficial features of the perineum in women

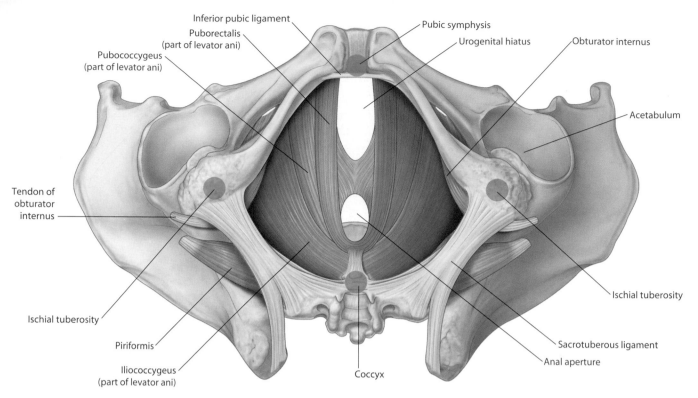

Inferior pubic ligament

Puborectalis
(part of levator ani)

Pubococcygeus
(part of levator ani)

Pubic symphysis

Urogenital hiatus

Obturator internus

Acetabulum

Tendon of
obturator
internus

Ischial tuberosity

Ischial tuberosity

Piriformis

Iliococcygeus
(part of levator ani)

Coccyx

Sacrotuberous ligament

Anal aperture

Borders and ceiling of the perineum in men

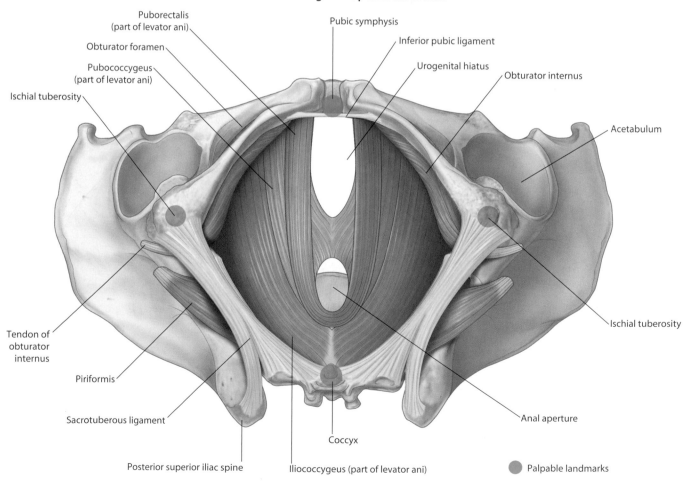

Puborectalis
(part of levator ani)

Obturator foramen

Pubococcygeus
(part of levator ani)

Ischial tuberosity

Pubic symphysis

Inferior pubic ligament

Urogenital hiatus

Obturator internus

Acetabulum

Tendon of
obturator
internus

Piriformis

Sacrotuberous ligament

Ischial tuberosity

Anal aperture

Posterior superior iliac spine

Iliococcygeus (part of levator ani)

Coccyx

● Palpable landmarks

Borders and ceiling of the perineum in women

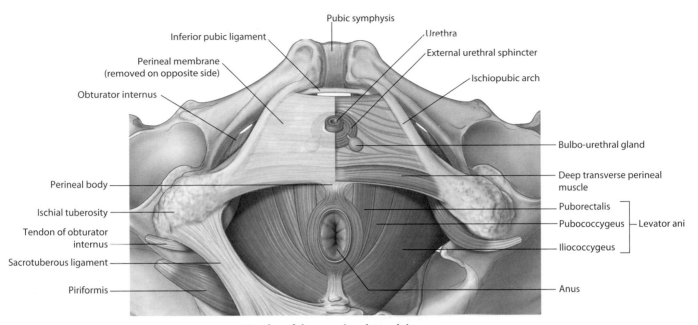

Pubic symphysis
Inferior pubic ligament
Urethra
External urethral sphincter
Perineal membrane
(removed on opposite side)
Ischiopubic arch
Obturator internus
Bulbo-urethral gland
Perineal body
Deep transverse perineal muscle
Ischial tuberosity
Puborectalis
Tendon of obturator internus
Pubococcygeus — Levator ani
Sacrotuberous ligament
Iliococcygeus
Piriformis
Anus

Muscles of deep perineal pouch in men
(perineal membrane removed on left side to expose deep perineal pouch)

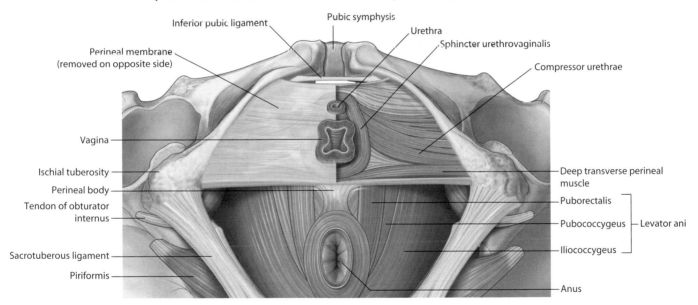

Inferior pubic ligament
Pubic symphysis
Urethra
Sphincter urethrovaginalis
Perineal membrane
(removed on opposite side)
Compressor urethrae
Vagina
Ischial tuberosity
Deep transverse perineal muscle
Perineal body
Puborectalis
Tendon of obturator internus
Pubococcygeus — Levator ani
Sacrotuberous ligament
Iliococcygeus
Piriformis
Anus

Muscles of deep perineal pouch in women
(perineal membrane removed on left side to expose deep perineal pouch)

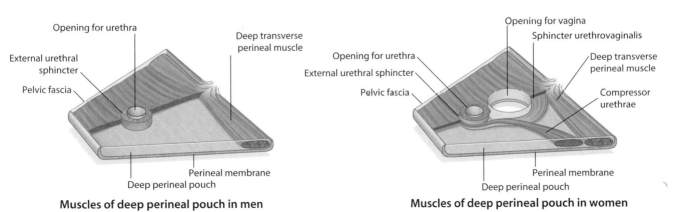

Opening for urethra
Deep transverse perineal muscle
External urethral sphincter
Pelvic fascia
Perineal membrane
Deep perineal pouch

Muscles of deep perineal pouch in men

Opening for vagina
Sphincter urethrovaginalis
Opening for urethra
Deep transverse perineal muscle
External urethral sphincter
Compressor urethrae
Pelvic fascia
Perineal membrane
Deep perineal pouch

Muscles of deep perineal pouch in women

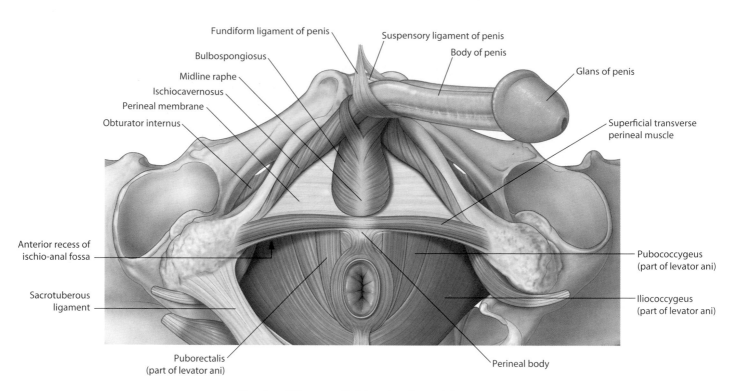

Fundiform ligament of penis
Suspensory ligament of penis
Body of penis
Glans of penis
Bulbospongiosus
Midline raphe
Ischiocavernosus
Perineal membrane
Obturator internus
Superficial transverse perineal muscle
Anterior recess of ischio-anal fossa
Sacrotuberous ligament
Pubococcygeus (part of levator ani)
Iliococcygeus (part of levator ani)
Puborectalis (part of levator ani)
Perineal body

Muscles of the superficial perineal pouch in men

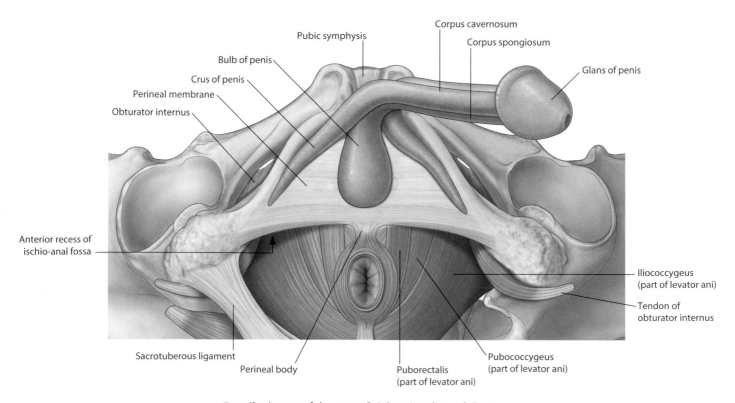

Pubic symphysis
Corpus cavernosum
Corpus spongiosum
Bulb of penis
Crus of penis
Perineal membrane
Obturator internus
Glans of penis
Anterior recess of ischio-anal fossa
Iliococcygeus (part of levator ani)
Tendon of obturator internus
Sacrotuberous ligament
Perineal body
Puborectalis (part of levator ani)
Pubococcygeus (part of levator ani)

Erectile tissues of the superficial perineal pouch in men

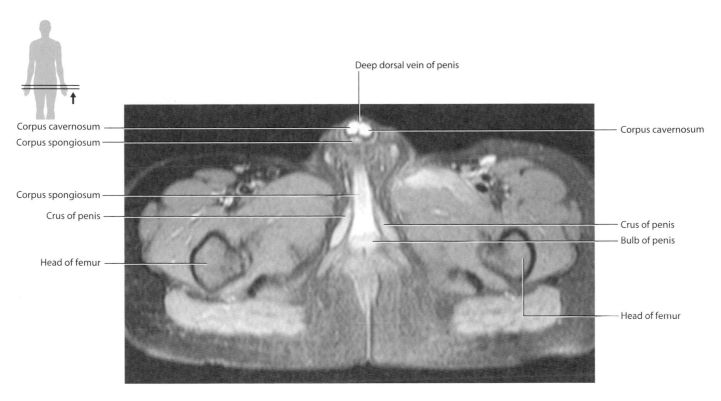

Deep dorsal vein of penis

Corpus cavernosum

Corpus spongiosum

Corpus spongiosum

Crus of penis

Head of femur

Corpus cavernosum

Crus of penis

Bulb of penis

Head of femur

Erectile tissues in relation to other structures in the male perineum.
Fat-saturated T2-weighted MR image in axial plane

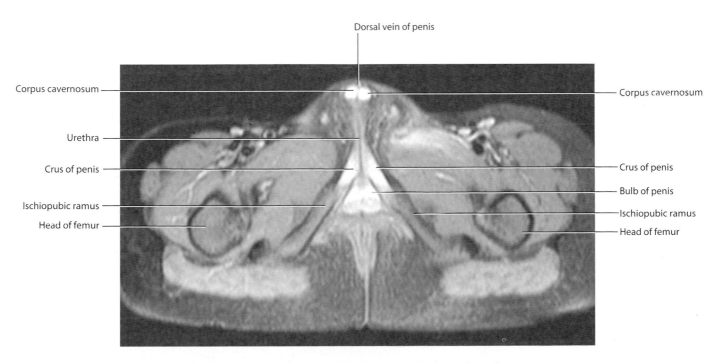

Dorsal vein of penis

Corpus cavernosum

Urethra

Crus of penis

Ischiopubic ramus

Head of femur

Corpus cavernosum

Crus of penis

Bulb of penis

Ischiopubic ramus

Head of femur

Erectile tissues in relation to other structures in the male perineum.
Fat-saturated T2-weighted MR image in axial plane

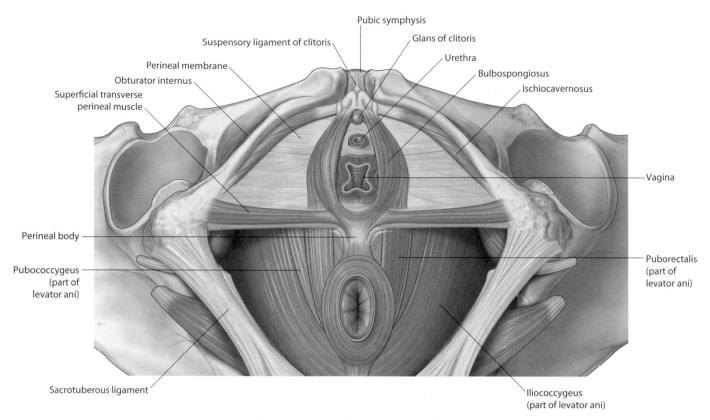

Pubic symphysis

Suspensory ligament of clitoris

Glans of clitoris

Perineal membrane

Urethra

Obturator internus

Bulbospongiosus

Superficial transverse perineal muscle

Ischiocavernosus

Vagina

Perineal body

Puborectalis (part of levator ani)

Pubococcygeus (part of levator ani)

Sacrotuberous ligament

Iliococcygeus (part of levator ani)

Muscles of the superficial perineal pouch in women

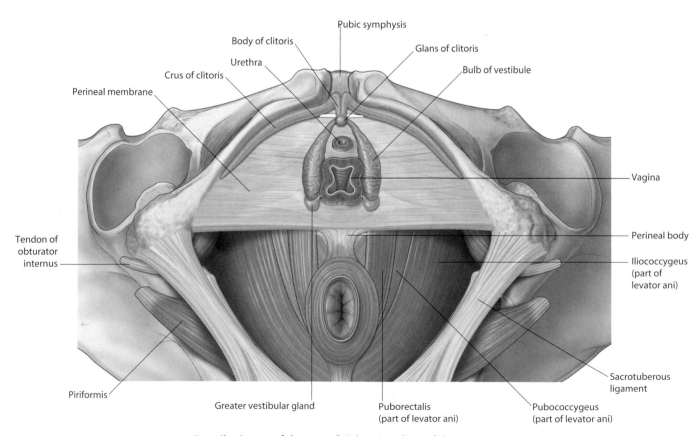

Pubic symphysis

Body of clitoris

Glans of clitoris

Urethra

Crus of clitoris

Bulb of vestibule

Perineal membrane

Vagina

Tendon of obturator internus

Perineal body

Iliococcygeus (part of levator ani)

Sacrotuberous ligament

Piriformis

Greater vestibular gland

Puborectalis (part of levator ani)

Pubococcygeus (part of levator ani)

Erectile tissues of the superficial perineal pouch in women

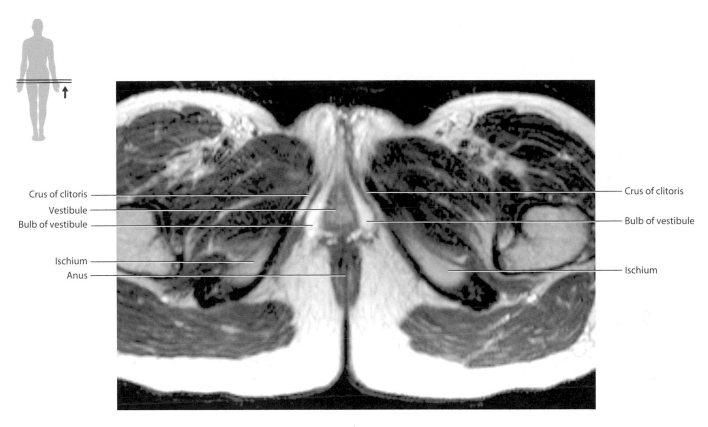

Crus of clitoris

Vestibule

Bulb of vestibule

Ischium

Anus

Crus of clitoris

Bulb of vestibule

Ischium

Erectile tissues in relation to other structures in the female perineum.
T2-weighted MR image in axial plane

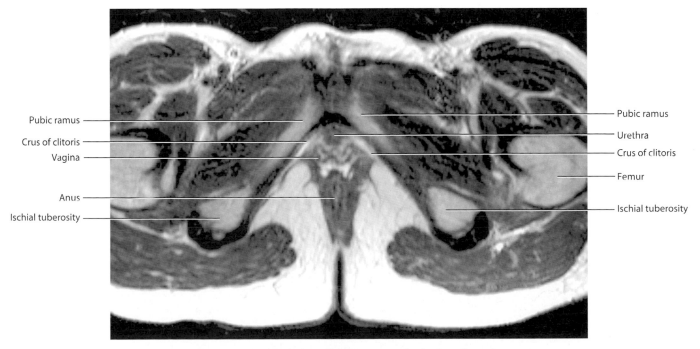

Pubic ramus

Crus of clitoris

Vagina

Anus

Ischial tuberosity

Pubic ramus

Urethra

Crus of clitoris

Femur

Ischial tuberosity

Erectile tissues in relation to other structures in the female perineum.
T2-weighted MR image in axial plane

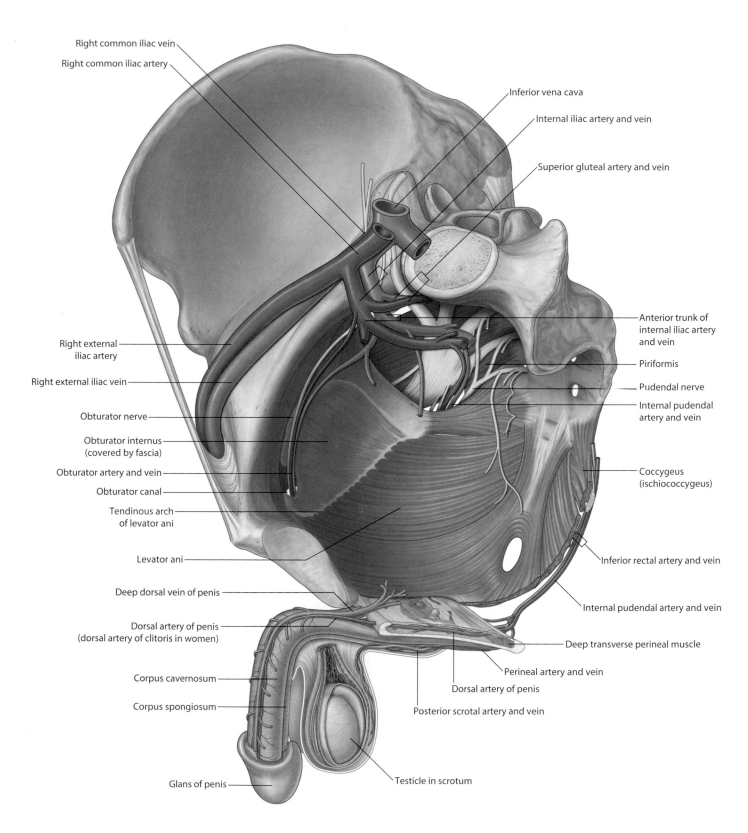

Right common iliac vein

Right common iliac artery

Inferior vena cava

Internal iliac artery and vein

Superior gluteal artery and vein

Right external iliac artery

Right external iliac vein

Obturator nerve

Obturator internus (covered by fascia)

Obturator artery and vein

Obturator canal

Tendinous arch of levator ani

Levator ani

Deep dorsal vein of penis

Dorsal artery of penis (dorsal artery of clitoris in women)

Corpus cavernosum

Corpus spongiosum

Glans of penis

Anterior trunk of internal iliac artery and vein

Piriformis

Pudendal nerve

Internal pudendal artery and vein

Coccygeus (ischiococcygeus)

Inferior rectal artery and vein

Internal pudendal artery and vein

Deep transverse perineal muscle

Perineal artery and vein

Dorsal artery of penis

Posterior scrotal artery and vein

Testicle in scrotum

Course of internal pudendal artery and vein in men (oblique sagittal view)

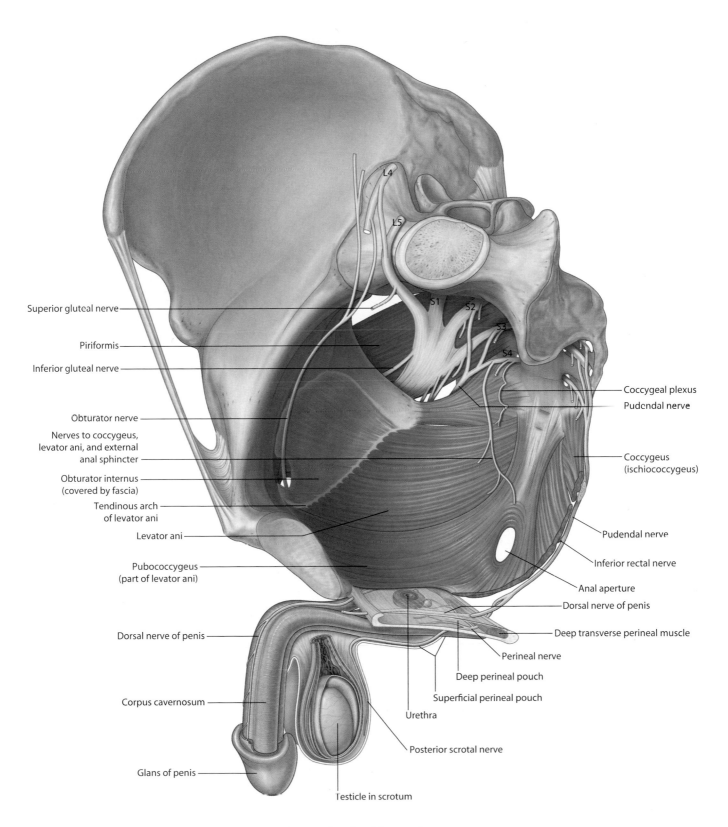

Superior gluteal nerve

Piriformis

Inferior gluteal nerve

Obturator nerve

Nerves to coccygeus,
levator ani, and external
anal sphincter

Obturator internus
(covered by fascia)

Tendinous arch
of levator ani

Levator ani

Pubococcygeus
(part of levator ani)

Dorsal nerve of penis

Corpus cavernosum

Glans of penis

L4

L5

S1

S2

S3

S4

Coccygeal plexus

Pudendal nerve

Coccygeus
(ischiococcygeus)

Pudendal nerve

Inferior rectal nerve

Anal aperture

Dorsal nerve of penis

Deep transverse perineal muscle

Perineal nerve

Deep perineal pouch

Superficial perineal pouch

Urethra

Posterior scrotal nerve

Testicle in scrotum

**Course of pudendal nerve in men
(oblique sagittal view)**

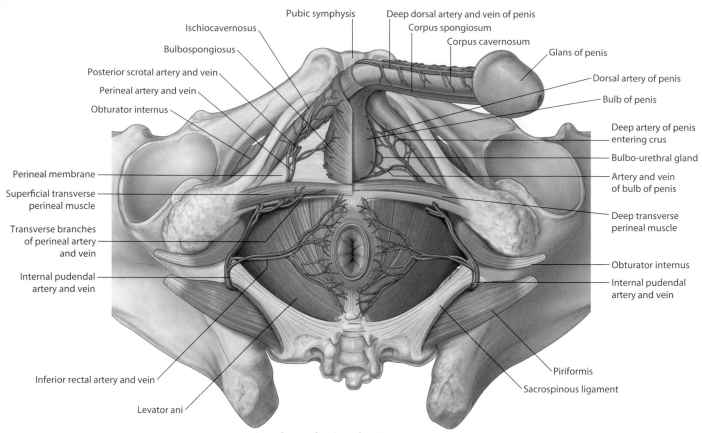

Arteries and veins of perineum in men
(perineal membrane removed on left side to expose deep perineal pouch; inferior view)

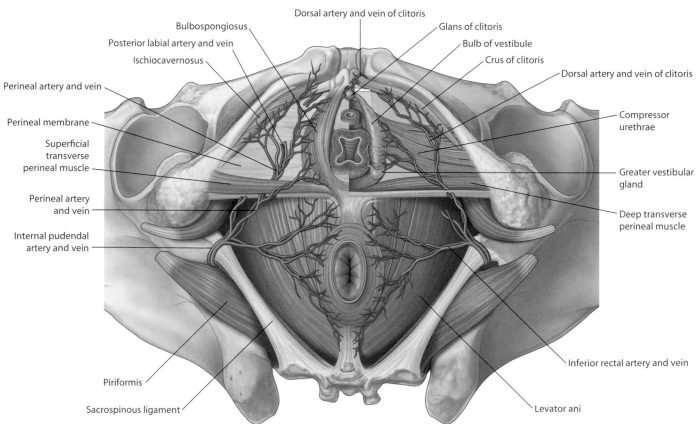

Arteries and veins of perineum in women
(perineal membrane removed on left side to expose deep perineal pouch; inferior view)

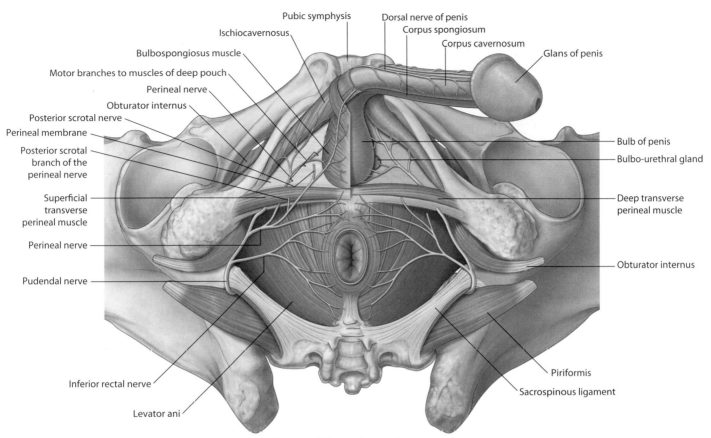

Pubic symphysis
Ischiocavernosus
Bulbospongiosus muscle
Motor branches to muscles of deep pouch
Perineal nerve
Obturator internus
Posterior scrotal nerve
Perineal membrane
Posterior scrotal branch of the perineal nerve
Superficial transverse perineal muscle
Perineal nerve
Pudendal nerve
Inferior rectal nerve
Levator ani

Dorsal nerve of penis
Corpus spongiosum
Corpus cavernosum
Glans of penis
Bulb of penis
Bulbo-urethral gland
Deep transverse perineal muscle
Obturator internus
Piriformis
Sacrospinous ligament

Nerves of the perineum in men
(perineal membrane removed on left side to expose deep perineal pouch; inferior view)

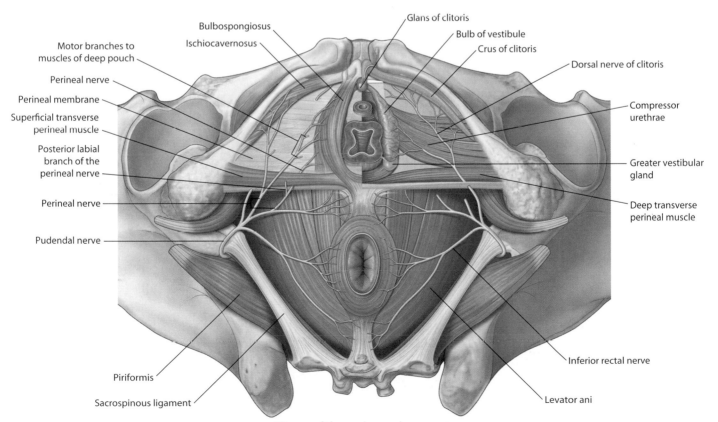

Motor branches to muscles of deep pouch
Perineal nerve
Perineal membrane
Superficial transverse perineal muscle
Posterior labial branch of the perineal nerve
Perineal nerve
Pudendal nerve
Piriformis
Sacrospinous ligament

Bulbospongiosus
Ischiocavernosus
Glans of clitoris
Bulb of vestibule
Crus of clitoris
Dorsal nerve of clitoris
Compressor urethrae
Greater vestibular gland
Deep transverse perineal muscle
Inferior rectal nerve
Levator ani

Nerves of the perineum in women
(perineal membrane removed on left side to expose deep perineal pouch; inferior view)

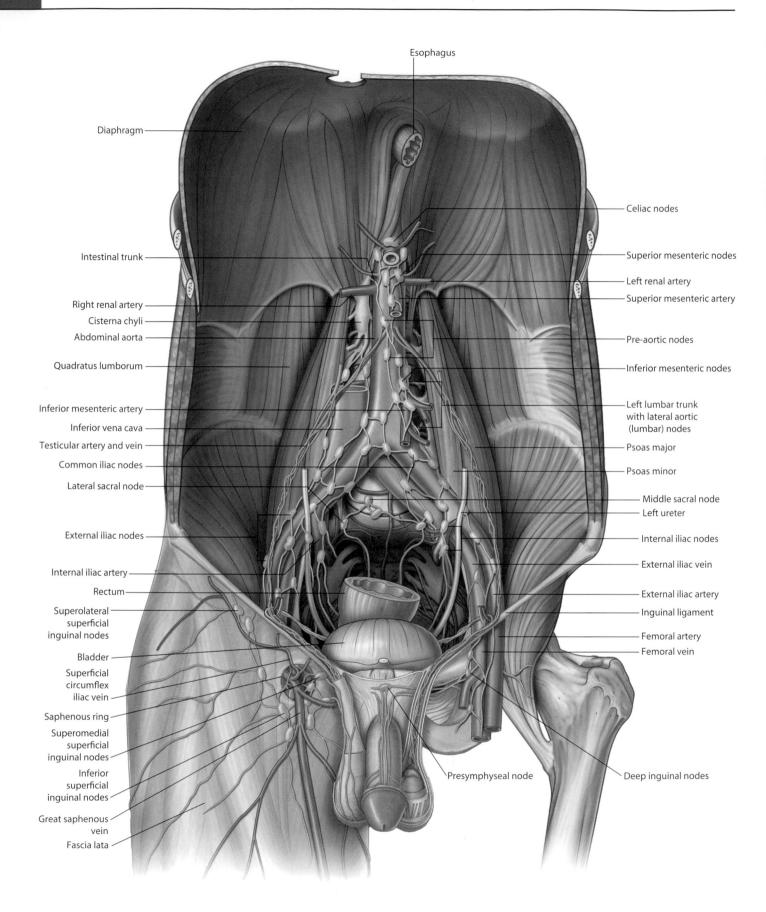

Esophagus

Diaphragm

Celiac nodes

Superior mesenteric nodes

Intestinal trunk

Left renal artery

Superior mesenteric artery

Right renal artery

Cisterna chyli

Abdominal aorta

Pre-aortic nodes

Inferior mesenteric nodes

Quadratus lumborum

Left lumbar trunk with lateral aortic (lumbar) nodes

Inferior mesenteric artery

Inferior vena cava

Psoas major

Testicular artery and vein

Psoas minor

Common iliac nodes

Lateral sacral node

Middle sacral node

Left ureter

Internal iliac nodes

External iliac nodes

External iliac vein

Internal iliac artery

External iliac artery

Rectum

Inguinal ligament

Superolateral superficial inguinal nodes

Femoral artery

Femoral vein

Bladder

Superficial circumflex iliac vein

Saphenous ring

Superomedial superficial inguinal nodes

Inferior superficial inguinal nodes

Presymphyseal node

Deep inguinal nodes

Great saphenous vein

Fascia lata

Lymphatics of pelvis and perineum in men

268

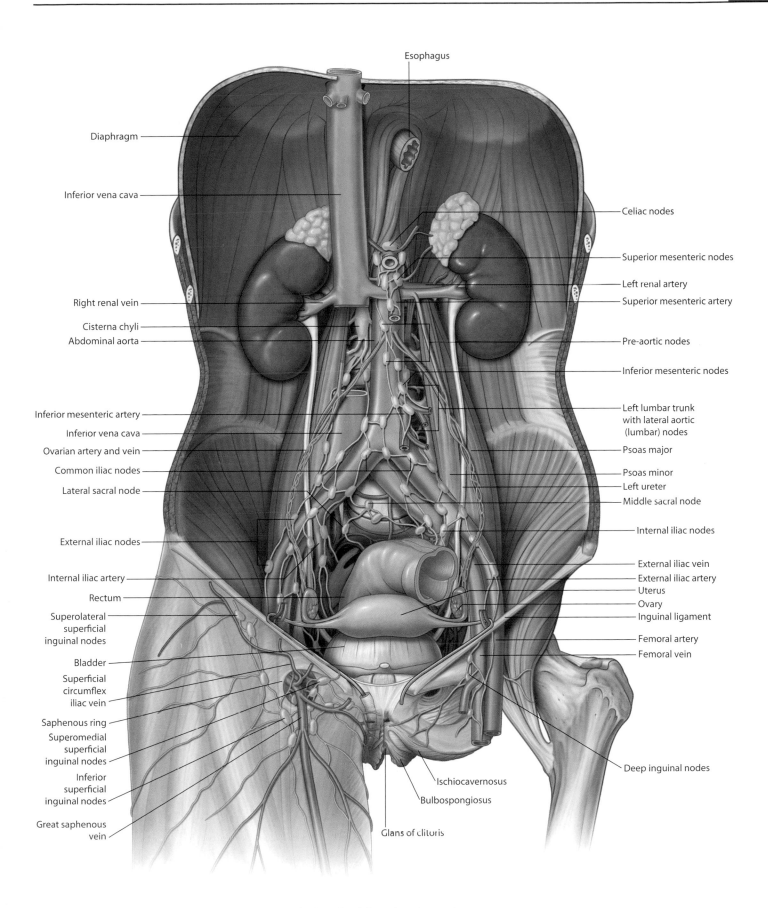

Esophagus

Diaphragm

Inferior vena cava

Right renal vein

Cisterna chyli

Abdominal aorta

Inferior mesenteric artery

Inferior vena cava

Ovarian artery and vein

Common iliac nodes

Lateral sacral node

External iliac nodes

Internal iliac artery

Rectum

Superolateral superficial inguinal nodes

Bladder

Superficial circumflex iliac vein

Saphenous ring

Superomedial superficial inguinal nodes

Inferior superficial inguinal nodes

Great saphenous vein

Celiac nodes

Superior mesenteric nodes

Left renal artery

Superior mesenteric artery

Pre-aortic nodes

Inferior mesenteric nodes

Left lumbar trunk with lateral aortic (lumbar) nodes

Psoas major

Psoas minor

Left ureter

Middle sacral node

Internal iliac nodes

External iliac vein

External iliac artery

Uterus

Ovary

Inguinal ligament

Femoral artery

Femoral vein

Deep inguinal nodes

Ischiocavernosus

Bulbospongiosus

Glans of clitoris

Lymphatics of pelvis and perineum in women

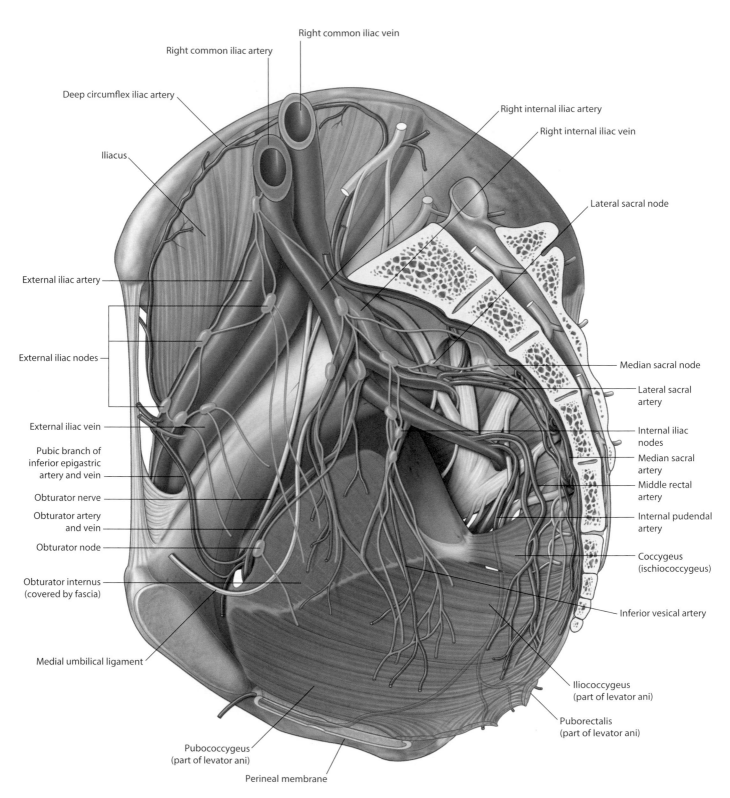

Right common iliac vein

Right common iliac artery

Deep circumflex iliac artery

Iliacus

Right internal iliac artery

Right internal iliac vein

Lateral sacral node

External iliac artery

External iliac nodes

External iliac vein

Pubic branch of inferior epigastric artery and vein

Obturator nerve

Obturator artery and vein

Obturator node

Obturator internus (covered by fascia)

Medial umbilical ligament

Median sacral node

Lateral sacral artery

Internal iliac nodes

Median sacral artery

Middle rectal artery

Internal pudendal artery

Coccygeus (ischiococcygeus)

Inferior vesical artery

Iliococcygeus (part of levator ani)

Puborectalis (part of levator ani)

Pubococcygeus (part of levator ani)

Perineal membrane

Lymphatics of pelvic cavity (sagittal view)

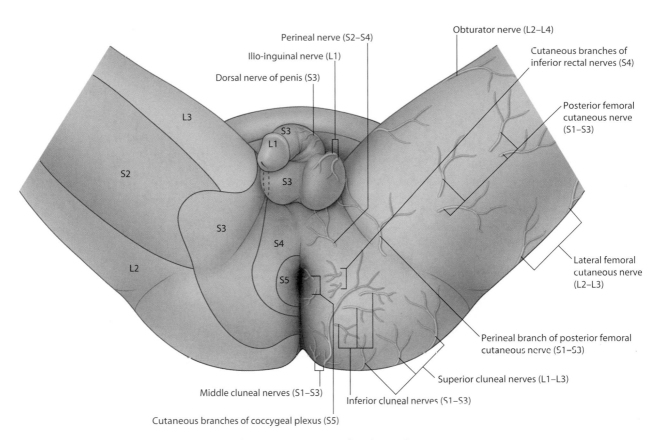

Perineal nerve (S2–S4)

Ilio-inguinal nerve (L1)

Dorsal nerve of penis (S3)

Obturator nerve (L2–L4)

Cutaneous branches of inferior rectal nerves (S4)

Posterior femoral cutaneous nerve (S1–S3)

Lateral femoral cutaneous nerve (L2–L3)

Perineal branch of posterior femoral cutaneous nerve (S1–S3)

Superior cluneal nerves (L1–L3)

Inferior cluneal nerves (S1–S3)

Middle cluneal nerves (S1–S3)

Cutaneous branches of coccygeal plexus (S5)

Dermatomes and cutaneous nerves of perineum in men

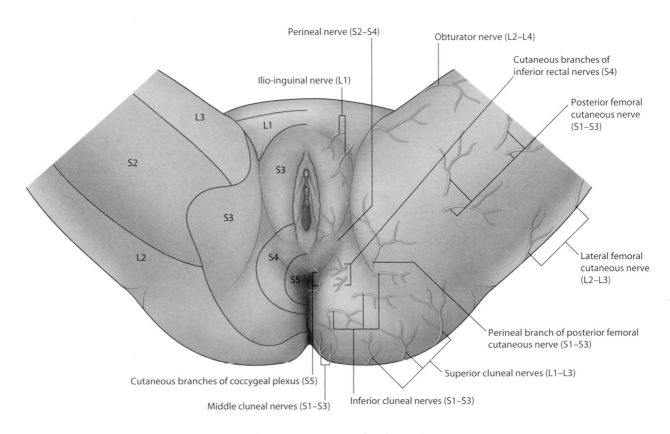

Perineal nerve (S2–S4)

Ilio-inguinal nerve (L1)

Obturator nerve (L2–L4)

Cutaneous branches of inferior rectal nerves (S4)

Posterior femoral cutaneous nerve (S1–S3)

Lateral femoral cutaneous nerve (L2–L3)

Perineal branch of posterior femoral cutaneous nerve (S1–S3)

Superior cluneal nerves (L1–L3)

Inferior cluneal nerves (S1–S3)

Cutaneous branches of coccygeal plexus (S5)

Middle cluneal nerves (S1–S3)

Dermatomes and cutaneous nerves of perineum in women

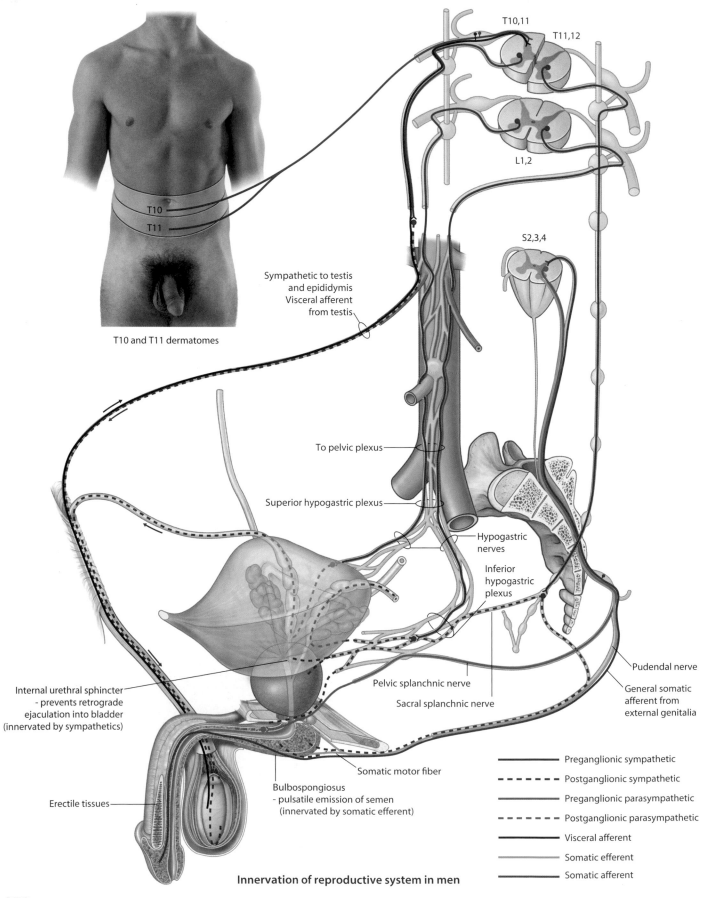

T10,11

T11,12

L1,2

S2,3,4

T10 and T11 dermatomes

Sympathetic to testis and epididymis
Visceral afferent from testis

To pelvic plexus

Superior hypogastric plexus

Hypogastric nerves

Inferior hypogastric plexus

Pudendal nerve

Pelvic splanchnic nerve

General somatic afferent from external genitalia

Sacral splanchnic nerve

Internal urethral sphincter
- prevents retrograde ejaculation into bladder
(innervated by sympathetics)

Somatic motor fiber

Bulbospongiosus
- pulsatile emission of semen
(innervated by somatic efferent)

Erectile tissues

———	Preganglionic sympathetic
- - - -	Postganglionic sympathetic
———	Preganglionic parasympathetic
- - - -	Postganglionic parasympathetic
———	Visceral afferent
———	Somatic efferent
———	Somatic afferent

Innervation of reproductive system in men

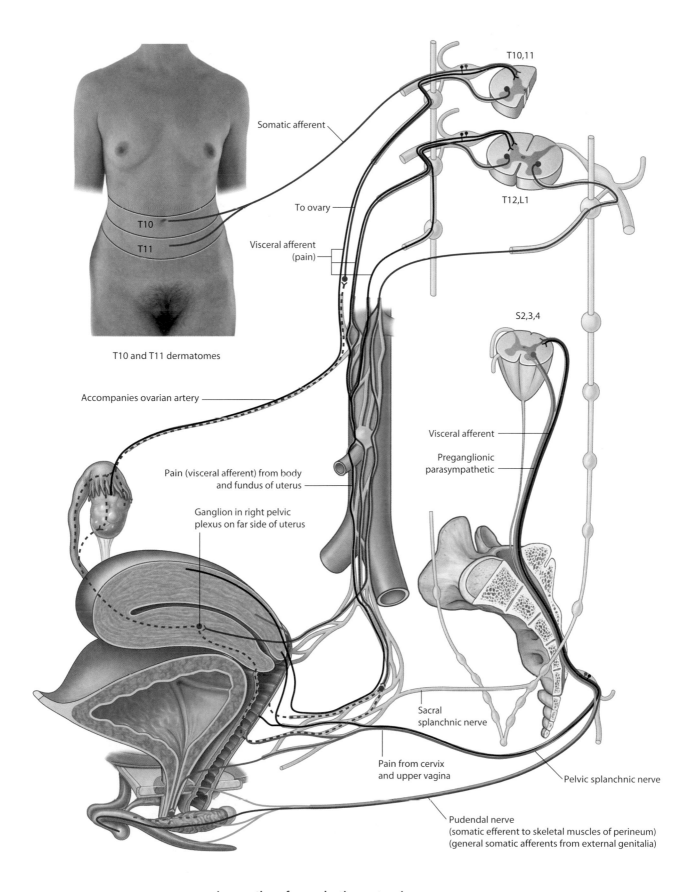

T10,11

Somatic afferent

To ovary

T12,L1

Visceral afferent
(pain)

S2,3,4

T10

T11

T10 and T11 dermatomes

Accompanies ovarian artery

Visceral afferent

Preganglionic
parasympathetic

Pain (visceral afferent) from body
and fundus of uterus

Ganglion in right pelvic
plexus on far side of uterus

Sacral
splanchnic nerve

Pain from cervix
and upper vagina

Pelvic splanchnic nerve

Pudendal nerve
(somatic efferent to skeletal muscles of perineum)
(general somatic afferents from external genitalia)

Innervation of reproductive system in women

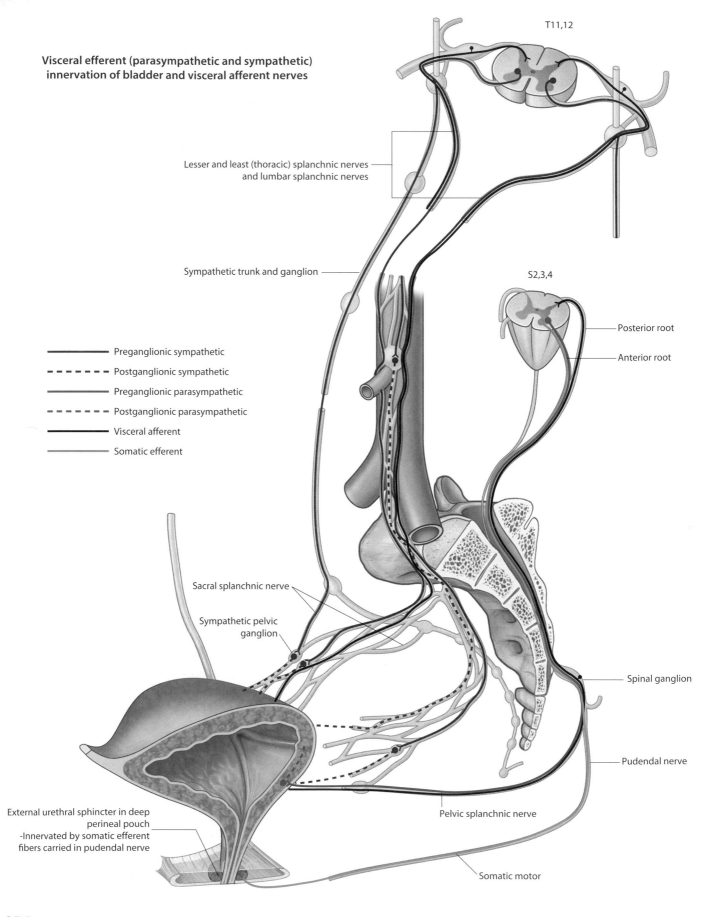

Visceral efferent (parasympathetic and sympathetic) innervation of bladder and visceral afferent nerves

T11,12

Lesser and least (thoracic) splanchnic nerves and lumbar splanchnic nerves

Sympathetic trunk and ganglion

S2,3,4

Posterior root

Anterior root

——— Preganglionic sympathetic

- - - - - Postganglionic sympathetic

——— Preganglionic parasympathetic

- - - - - Postganglionic parasympathetic

——— Visceral afferent

——— Somatic efferent

Sacral splanchnic nerve

Sympathetic pelvic ganglion

Spinal ganglion

Pudendal nerve

External urethral sphincter in deep perineal pouch -Innervated by somatic efferent fibers carried in pudendal nerve

Pelvic splanchnic nerve

Somatic motor

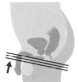

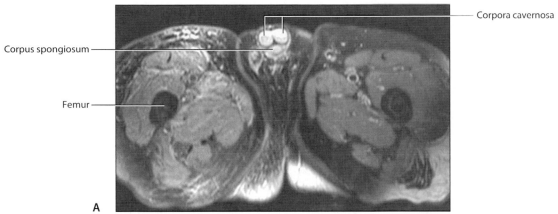

Corpora cavernosa

Corpus spongiosum —

Femur —

A

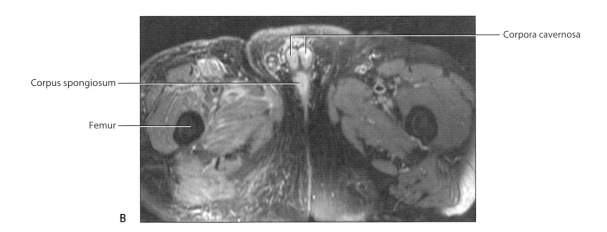

Corpora cavernosa

Corpus spongiosum —

Femur —

B

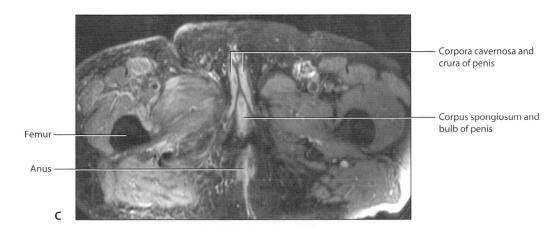

Corpora cavernosa and crura of penis

Corpus spongiosum and bulb of penis

Femur —

Anus —

C

A through C – Series of axial images that pass through the pelvic cavity and perineum from inferior to superior showing the various structures and their relationships with each other.
Fat-saturated T2-weighted MR images in axial plane

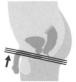

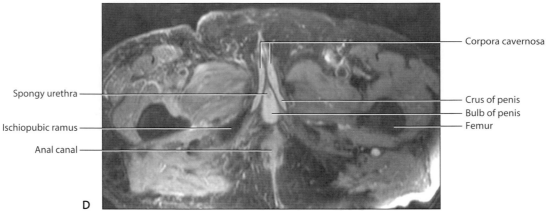

Corpora cavernosa

Spongy urethra

Crus of penis

Bulb of penis

Ischiopubic ramus

Femur

Anal canal

D

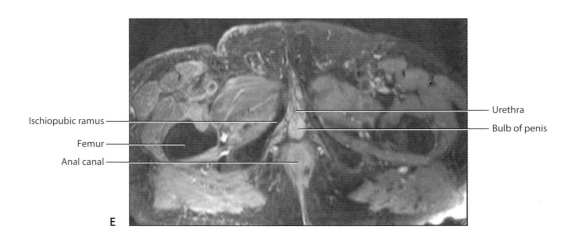

Ischiopubic ramus

Urethra

Bulb of penis

Femur

Anal canal

E

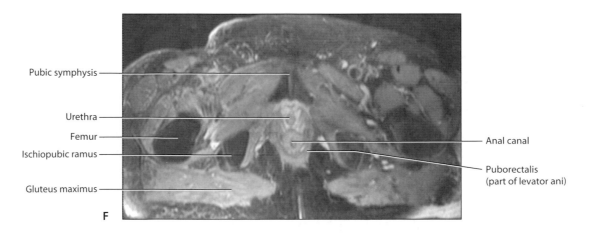

Pubic symphysis

Urethra

Femur

Ischiopubic ramus

Anal canal

Puborectalis
(part of levator ani)

Gluteus maximus

F

D through J – Series of axial images that pass through the pelvic cavity and perineum from inferior to superior showing the various structures and their relationships with each other.
Fat-saturated T2-weighted MR images in axial plane

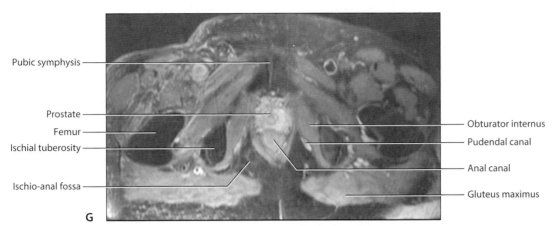

Pubic symphysis

Prostate

Femur

Ischial tuberosity

Ischio-anal fossa

Obturator internus

Pudendal canal

Anal canal

Gluteus maximus

G

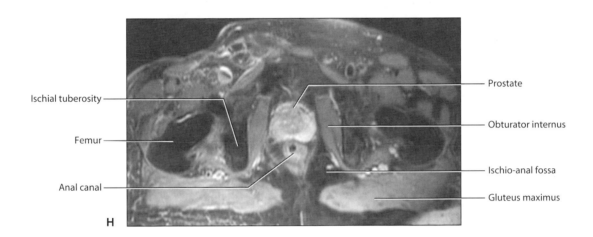

Ischial tuberosity

Femur

Anal canal

Prostate

Obturator internus

Ischio-anal fossa

Gluteus maximus

H

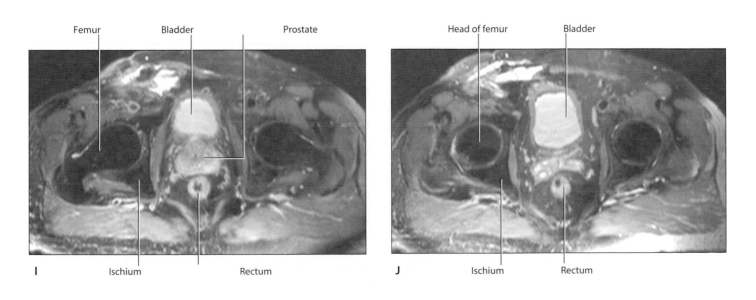

Femur　　Bladder　　Prostate

Head of femur　　Bladder

I　　Ischium　　Rectum

J　　Ischium　　Rectum

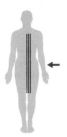

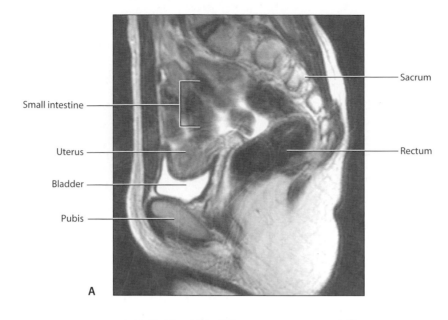

Small intestine

Uterus

Bladder

Pubis

Sacrum

Rectum

A

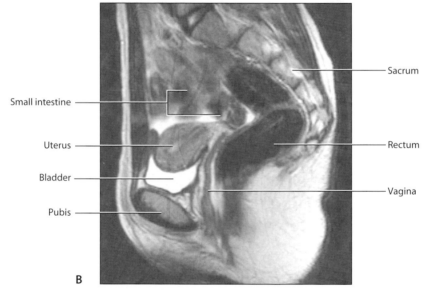

Small intestine

Uterus

Bladder

Pubis

Sacrum

Rectum

Vagina

B

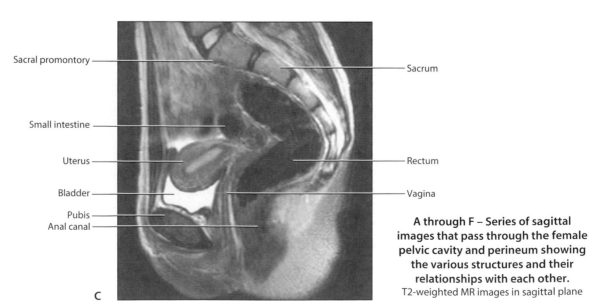

Sacral promontory

Small intestine

Uterus

Bladder

Pubis

Anal canal

Sacrum

Rectum

Vagina

A through F – Series of sagittal images that pass through the female pelvic cavity and perineum showing the various structures and their relationships with each other.
T2-weighted MR images in sagittal plane

C

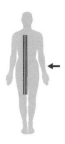

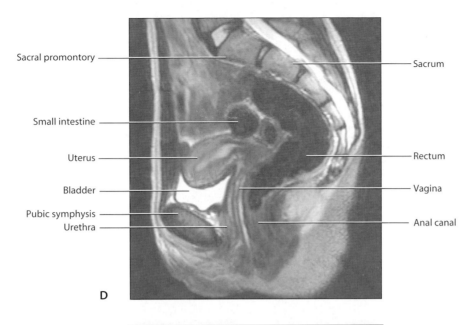

Sacral promontory — — Sacrum

Small intestine —

Uterus — — Rectum

Bladder — — Vagina

Pubic symphysis — — Anal canal
Urethra —

D

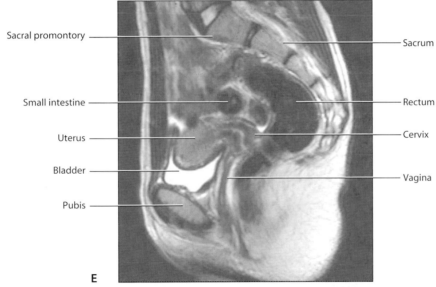

Sacral promontory — — Sacrum

Small intestine — — Rectum

Uterus — — Cervix

Bladder —

Pubis — — Vagina

E

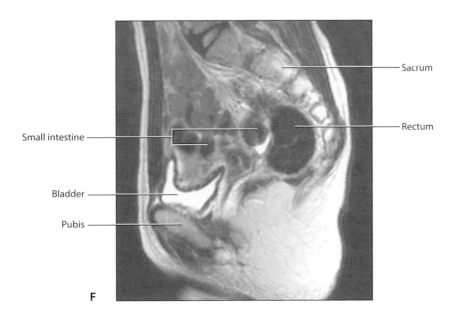

— Sacrum

Small intestine — — Rectum

Bladder —

Pubis —

F

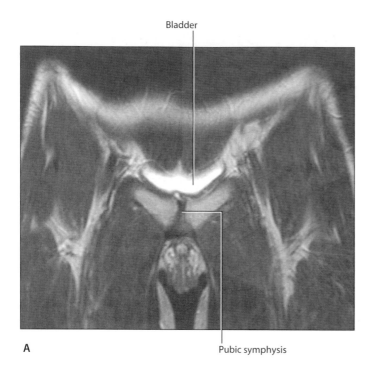

Bladder

Pubic symphysis

A

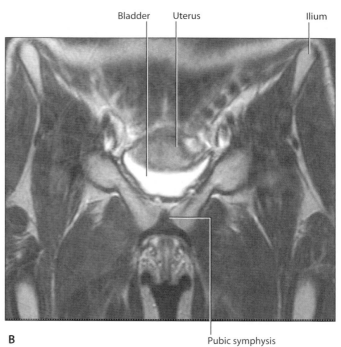

Bladder　Uterus　Ilium

Pubic symphysis

B

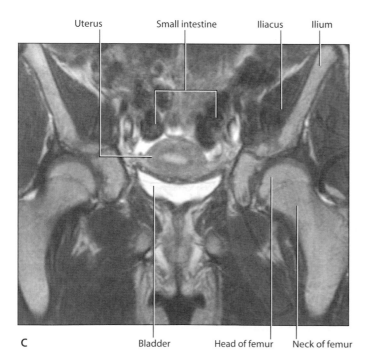

Uterus　Small intestine　Iliacus　Ilium

Bladder　Head of femur　Neck of femur

C

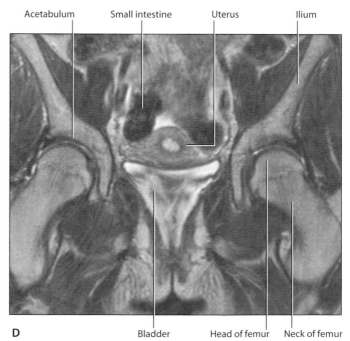

Acetabulum　Small intestine　Uterus　Ilium

Bladder　Head of femur　Neck of femur

D

A through G – Series of coronal images that pass through the pelvic cavity and perineum from anterior to posterior showing the various structures and their relationships with each other.
T2-weighted MR images in coronal plane

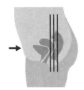

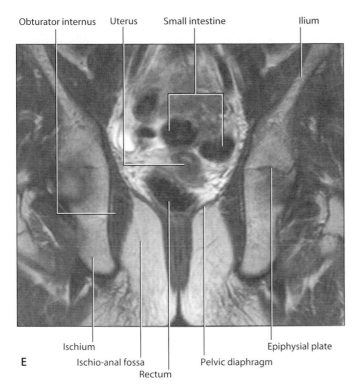

Obturator internus   Uterus   Small intestine   Ilium

Ischium
Ischio-anal fossa
Rectum
Pelvic diaphragm
Epiphysial plate

E

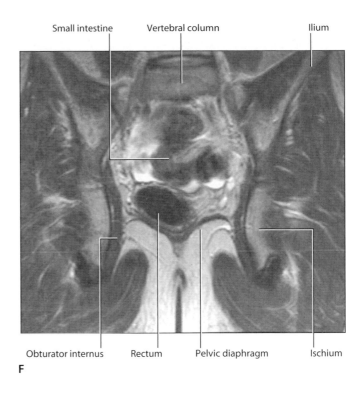

Small intestine   Vertebral column   Ilium

Obturator internus   Rectum   Pelvic diaphragm   Ischium

F

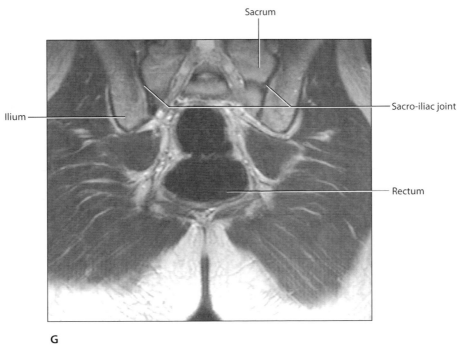

Sacrum

Ilium

Sacro-iliac joint

Rectum

G

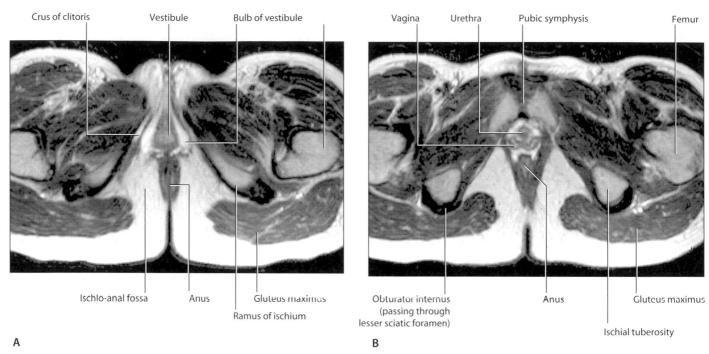

A

Crus of clitoris — Vestibule — Bulb of vestibule

Ischio-anal fossa — Anus — Gluteus maximus
Ramus of ischium

B

Vagina — Urethra — Pubic symphysis — Femur

Obturator internus
(passing through
lesser sciatic foramen) — Anus — Gluteus maximus

Ischial tuberosity

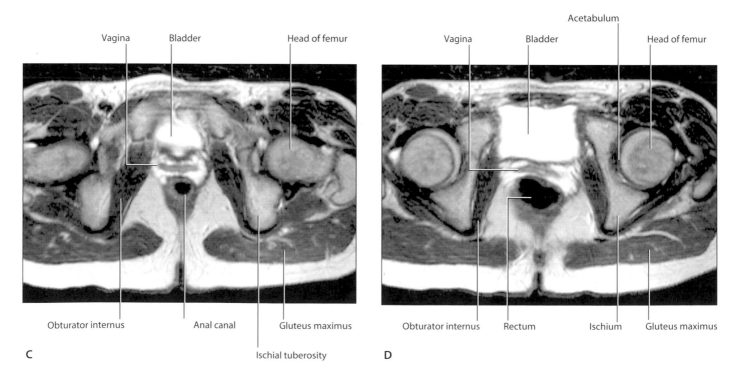

C

Vagina — Bladder — Head of femur

Obturator internus — Anal canal — Gluteus maximus

Ischial tuberosity

D

Acetabulum

Vagina — Bladder — Head of femur

Obturator internus — Rectum — Ischium — Gluteus maximus

A through H – Series of axial images that pass through the pelvic cavity and perineum from inferior to superior showing the various structures and their relationships with each other.
T2-weighted MR images in axial plane

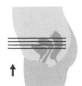

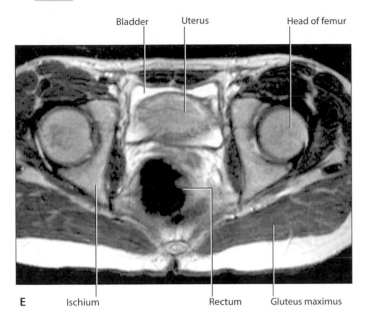

Bladder   Uterus   Head of femur

E   Ischium   Rectum   Gluteus maximus

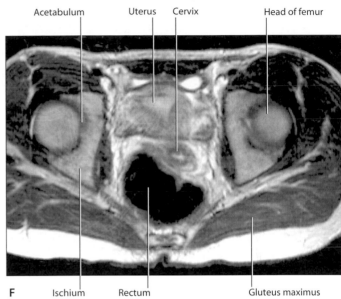

Acetabulum   Uterus   Cervix   Head of femur

F   Ischium   Rectum   Gluteus maximus

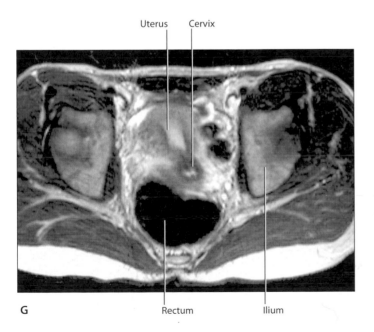

Uterus   Cervix

G   Rectum   Ilium

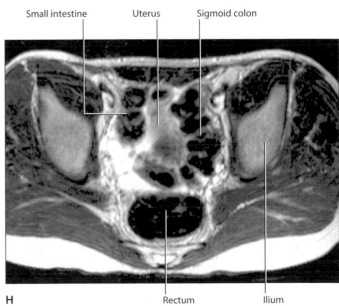

Small intestine   Uterus   Sigmoid colon

H   Rectum   Ilium

Branches of the sacral plexus

(spinal segments in parentheses do not consistently participate)

Branch		Spinal segments	Motor function	Sensory (cutaneous) function
Tibial part	1	L4 to S3	All muscles in the posterior or hamstring compartment of the thigh (including the hamstring part of the adductor magnus) except for the short head of the biceps All muscles in the posterior compartment of the leg All muscles in the sole of the foot	Skin on posterolateral and lateral surfaces of foot and sole of foot
Common fibular part	2	L4 to S2	Short head of biceps in the posterior compartment of the thigh All muscles in the anterior and lateral compartments of the leg Extensor digitorum brevis in the foot (also contributes to the supply of the first dorsal interosseous muscle)	Skin on the anterolateral surface of the leg and dorsal surface of the foot
Pudendal	3	S2 to S4	Skeletal muscles in the perineum including the external urethral and anal sphincters and levator ani (overlaps in supply of the levator ani and external sphincter with branches directly from ventral division of S4)	Most skin of the perineum, penis and clitoris
Superior gluteal	4	L4 to S1	Gluteus medius, gluteus minimus, and tensor fasciae latae	
Inferior gluteal	5	L5 to S2	Gluteus maximus	
Nerve to obturator internus and superior gemellus	6	L5 to S2	Obturator internus and superior gemellus	
Nerve to quadratus femoris and inferior gemellus	7	L4 to S1	Quadratus femoris and inferior gemellus	
Posterior femoral cutaneous (posterior cutaneous nerve of thigh)	8	S1, S3		Skin on the posterior aspect of the thigh
Perforating cutaneous	9	S2, S3		Skin over gluteal fold (overlaps with posterior femoral cutaneous)
Nerve to piriformis	10	(L5), S1, S2	Piriformis muscle	
Nerves to levator ani, coccygeus, and external anal sphincter	11	S4	Levator ani, coccygeus, and external anal sphincter (overlaps with pudendal nerve)	Small patch of skin between anus and coccyx

Branch		Spinal segments	Motor function	Sensory (cutaneous) function
Pelvic splanchnic nerves	12	S2, S3 (S4)	Visceral motor (preganglionic parasympathetic) to pelvic part of prevertebral plexus Stimulate erection, modulate mobility in gastrointestinal system distal to the left colic flexure, inhibitory to internal urethral sphincter	Visceral afferents from pelvic viscera and distal parts of colon. Pain from cervix and possibly from bladder and proximal urethra

Branches of the coccygeal plexus

Anococcygeal nerves	13	S4 to Co	Peri-anal skin	

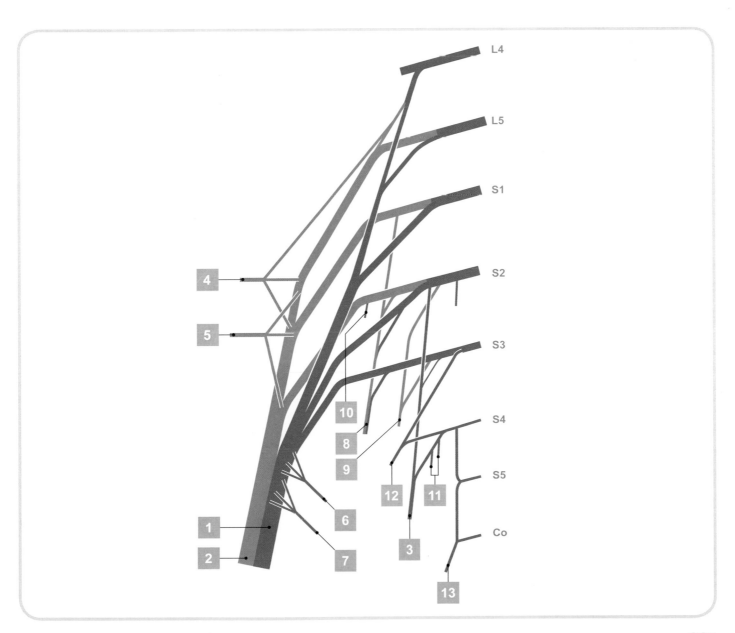

Muscles of the pelvic walls

(spinal segments in bold are the major segments innervating the muscle)

Muscle		Origin	Insertion	Innervation	Function
Obturator internus	1	Anterolateral wall of true pelvis (deep surface of obturator membrane and surrounding bone)	Medial surface of greater trochanter of femur	Nerve to obturator internus **L5, SI**	Lateral rotation of the extended hip joint; abduction of flexed hip
Piriformis	2	Anterior surface of sacrum between anterior sacral foramina	Medial side of superior border of greater trochanter of femur	Branches from L5, **SI**, and **S2**	Lateral rotation of the extended hip joint; abduction of flexed hip

Muscles of the pelvic diaphragm

Muscle		Origin	Insertion	Innervation	Function
Levator ani	3	In a line around the pelvic wall beginning on the posterior aspect of the pubic bone and extending across the obturator internus muscle as a tendinous arch (thickening of the obturator internus fascia) to the ischial spine	The anterior part is attached to the superior surface of the perineal membrane; the posterior part meets its partner on the other side at the perineal body, around the anal canal, and along the anococcygeal ligament	Branches direct from the anterior ramus of S4, and by the inferior rectal branch of the pudendal nerve (S2 to S4)	Contributes to the formation of the pelvic floor, which supports the pelvic viscera; maintains an angle between the rectum and anal canal. Reinforces the external anal sphincter and, in women, functions as a vaginal sphincter
Coccygeus	4	Ischial spine and pelvic surface of the sacrospinous ligament	Lateral margin of coccyx and related border of sacrum	Branches from the anterior rami of S3 and S4	Contributes to the formation of the pelvic floor, which supports the pelvic viscera; pulls coccyx forward after defecation

Muscles within the deep perineal pouch

Muscle		Origin	Insertion	Innervation	Function
External urethral sphincter	5	From the inferior ramus of the pubis on each side and adjacent walls of the deep perineal pouch	Surrounds membranous part of urethra	Perineal branches of the pudendal nerve (S2 to S4)	Compresses the membranous urethra; relaxes during micturition
Deep transverse perineal	6	Medial aspect of ischial ramus	Perineal body	Perineal branches of the pudendal nerve (S2 to S4)	Stabilizes the position of the perineal body
Compressor urethrae (in women only)	7	Ischiopubic ramus on each side	Blends with partner on other side anterior to the urethra	Perineal branches of the pudendal nerve (S2 to S4)	Functions as an accessory sphincter of the urethra
Sphincter urethrovaginalis (in women only)	8	Perineal body	Passes forward lateral to the vagina to blend with partner on other side anterior to the urethra	Perineal branches of the pudendal nerve (S2 to S4)	Functions as an accessory sphincter of the urethra (also may facilitate closing the vagina)

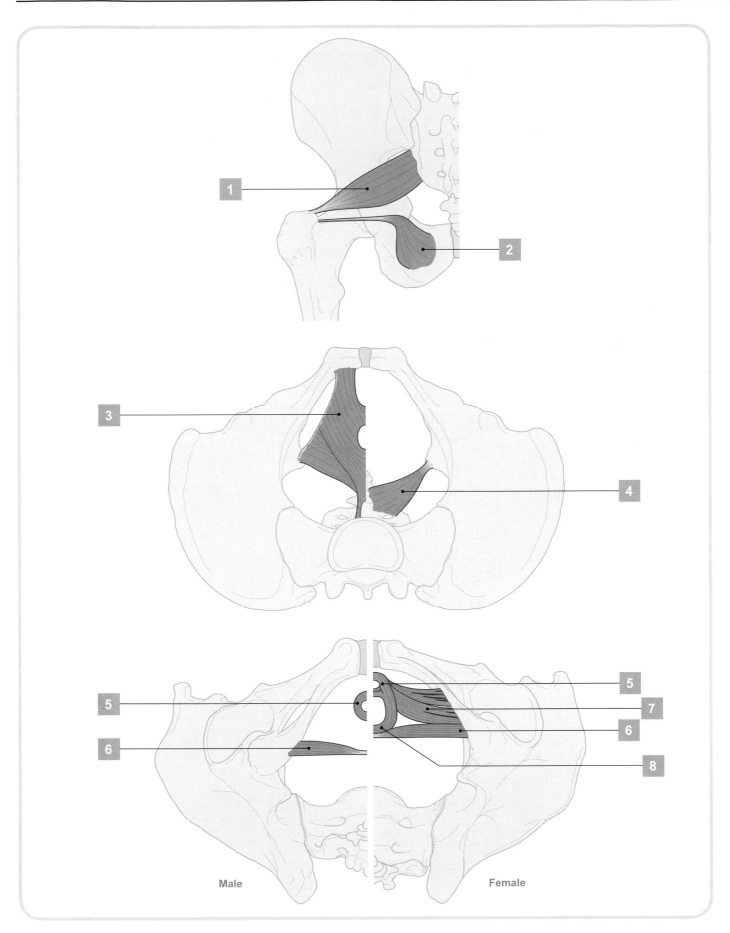

Male   Female

Muscles of the anal triangle

Muscle		Origin	Insertion	Innervation	Function
EXTERNAL ANAL SPHINCTER					
Deep part	1	Surrounds superior aspect of anal canal		Pudendal nerve (S2 and S3) and branches directly from S4	Closes anal canal
Superficial part	2	Surrounds lower part of anal canal	Anchored to perineal body and anococcygeal body		
Subcutaneous part	3	Surrounds anal aperture			

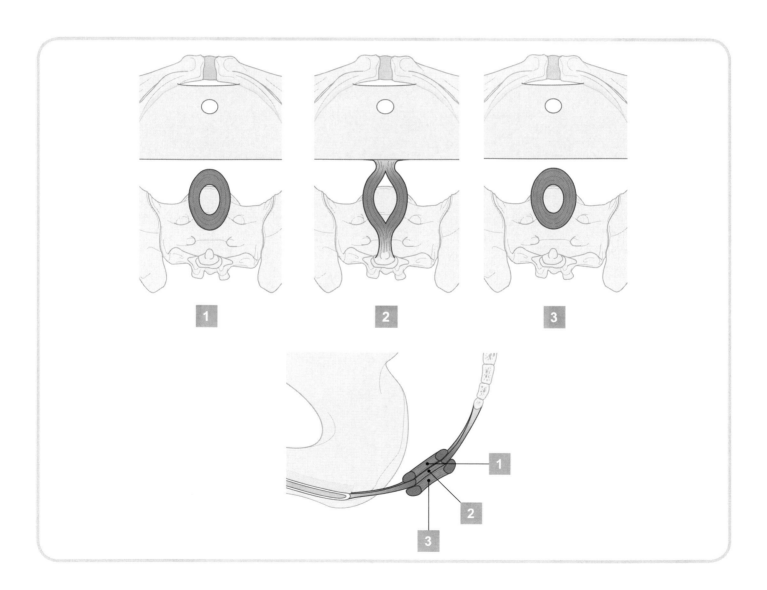

Muscles of the superficial perineal pouch

Muscle		Origin	Insertion	Innervation	Function
Ischiocavernosus	1	Ischial tuberosity and ramus	Crus of penis and clitoris	Pudendal nerve (S2 to S4)	Move blood from crura into the body of the erect penis and clitoris
Bulbospongiosus	2	In women: perineal body In men: perineal body, midline raphe	In women: bulb of vestibule, perineal membrane, body of clitoris, and corpus cavernosum In men: bulbospongiosus, perineal membrane, and corpus cavernosum	Pudendal nerve (S2 to S4)	Move blood from attached parts of the clitoris and penis into the glans In men: removal of residual urine from urethra after urination; pulsatile emission of semen during ejaculation
Superficial transverse perineal	3	Ischial tuberosity and ramus	Perineal body	Pudendal nerve (S2 to S4)	Stabilize the perineal body

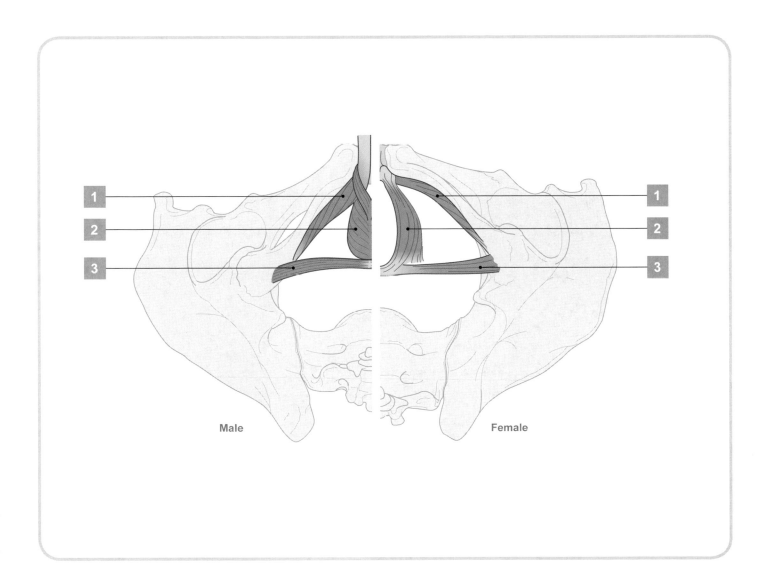

Male   Female

CONTENTS

LOWER LIMB

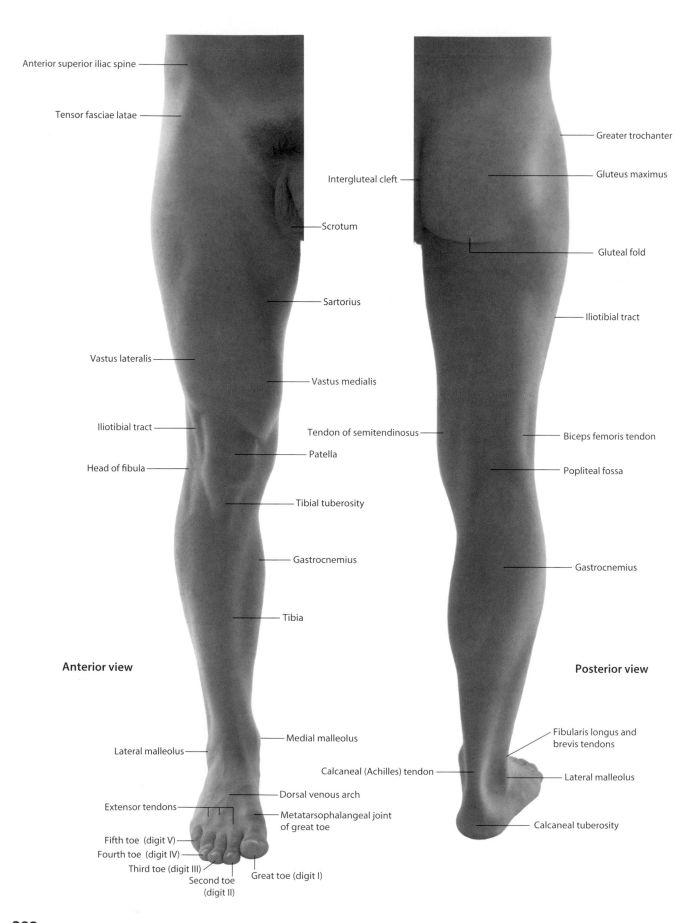

Anterior superior iliac spine

Tensor fasciae latae

Greater trochanter

Intergluteal cleft

Gluteus maximus

Scrotum

Gluteal fold

Sartorius

Iliotibial tract

Vastus lateralis

Vastus medialis

Iliotibial tract

Tendon of semitendinosus

Biceps femoris tendon

Patella

Head of fibula

Popliteal fossa

Tibial tuberosity

Gastrocnemius

Gastrocnemius

Tibia

Anterior view

Posterior view

Medial malleolus

Fibularis longus and brevis tendons

Lateral malleolus

Calcaneal (Achilles) tendon

Lateral malleolus

Dorsal venous arch

Extensor tendons

Metatarsophalangeal joint of great toe

Fifth toe (digit V)

Fourth toe (digit IV)

Third toe (digit III)

Calcaneal tuberosity

Great toe (digit I)

Second toe (digit II)

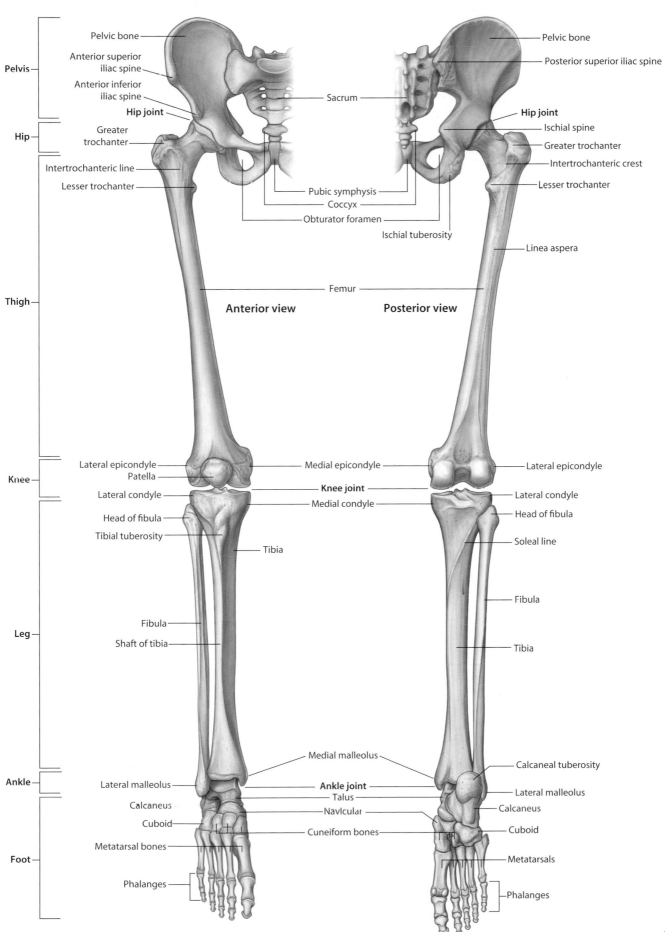

Pelvis

Pelvic bone

Anterior superior iliac spine

Anterior inferior iliac spine

Hip joint

Hip

Greater trochanter

Intertrochanteric line

Lesser trochanter

Thigh

Sacrum

Pubic symphysis

Coccyx

Obturator foramen

Ischial tuberosity

Femur

Anterior view

Pelvic bone

Posterior superior iliac spine

Hip joint

Ischial spine

Greater trochanter

Intertrochanteric crest

Lesser trochanter

Linea aspera

Posterior view

Knee

Lateral epicondyle

Patella

Lateral condyle

Head of fibula

Tibial tuberosity

Leg

Fibula

Shaft of tibia

Medial epicondyle

Knee joint

Medial condyle

Tibia

Lateral epicondyle

Lateral condyle

Head of fibula

Soleal line

Fibula

Tibia

Ankle

Lateral malleolus

Foot

Calcaneus

Cuboid

Metatarsal bones

Phalanges

Medial malleolus

Ankle joint

Talus

Navicular

Cuneiform bones

Calcaneal tuberosity

Lateral malleolus

Calcaneus

Cuboid

Metatarsals

Phalanges

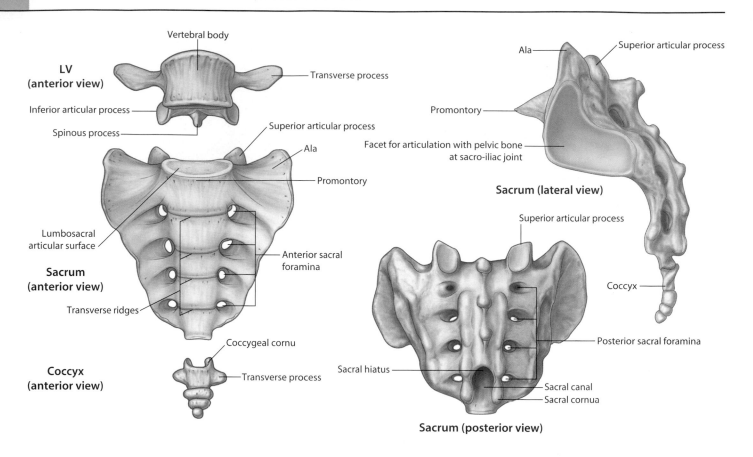

LV
(anterior view)

Vertebral body

Transverse process

Inferior articular process

Spinous process

Superior articular process

Ala

Promontory

Sacrum
(anterior view)

Lumbosacral
articular surface

Anterior sacral
foramina

Transverse ridges

Coccyx
(anterior view)

Coccygeal cornu

Transverse process

Ala

Superior articular process

Promontory

Facet for articulation with pelvic bone
at sacro-iliac joint

Sacrum (lateral view)

Superior articular process

Coccyx

Sacral hiatus

Posterior sacral foramina

Sacral canal

Sacral cornua

Sacrum (posterior view)

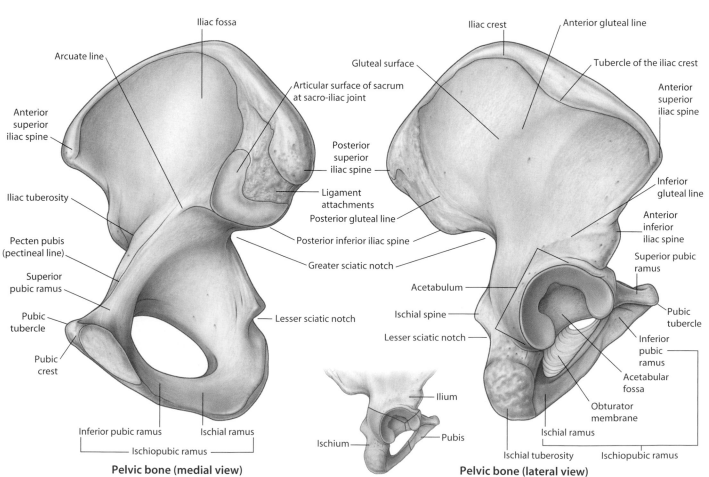

Iliac fossa

Arcuate line

Anterior
superior
iliac spine

Iliac tuberosity

Pecten pubis
(pectineal line)

Superior
pubic ramus

Pubic
tubercle

Pubic
crest

Inferior pubic ramus

Ischial ramus

Ischiopubic ramus

Pelvic bone (medial view)

Articular surface of sacrum
at sacro-iliac joint

Posterior
superior
iliac spine

Ligament
attachments

Posterior gluteal line

Posterior inferior iliac spine

Greater sciatic notch

Lesser sciatic notch

Iliac crest

Anterior gluteal line

Tubercle of the iliac crest

Anterior
superior
iliac spine

Gluteal surface

Inferior
gluteal line

Anterior
inferior
iliac spine

Superior pubic
ramus

Acetabulum

Ischial spine

Lesser sciatic notch

Pubic
tubercle

Inferior
pubic
ramus

Acetabular
fossa

Obturator
membrane

Ischial ramus

Ischial tuberosity

Ischiopubic ramus

Pelvic bone (lateral view)

Ilium

Ischium

Pubis

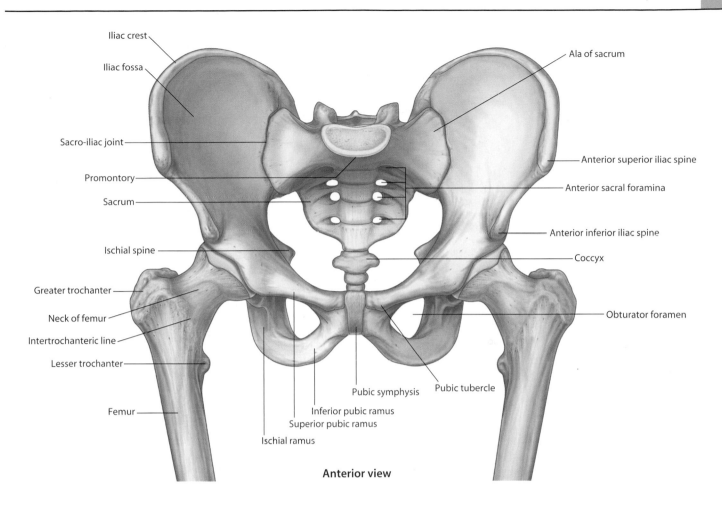

Iliac crest

Iliac fossa

Sacro-iliac joint

Promontory

Sacrum

Ischial spine

Greater trochanter

Neck of femur

Intertrochanteric line

Lesser trochanter

Femur

Ala of sacrum

Anterior superior iliac spine

Anterior sacral foramina

Anterior inferior iliac spine

Coccyx

Obturator foramen

Pubic symphysis

Pubic tubercle

Inferior pubic ramus

Superior pubic ramus

Ischial ramus

Anterior view

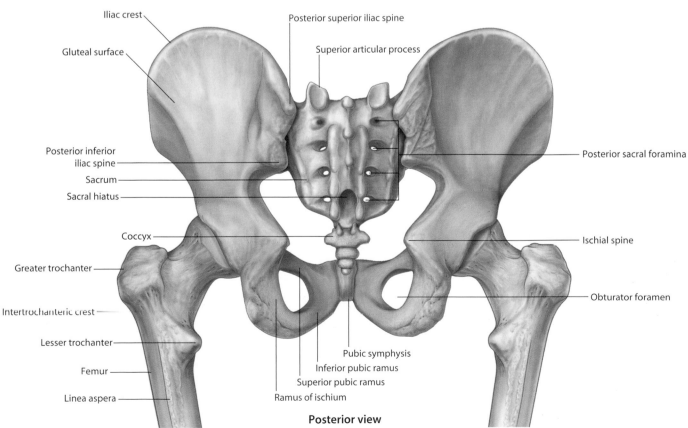

Iliac crest

Gluteal surface

Posterior superior iliac spine

Superior articular process

Posterior inferior iliac spine

Sacrum

Sacral hiatus

Coccyx

Greater trochanter

Intertrochanteric crest

Lesser trochanter

Femur

Linea aspera

Posterior sacral foramina

Ischial spine

Obturator foramen

Pubic symphysis

Inferior pubic ramus

Superior pubic ramus

Ramus of ischium

Posterior view

295

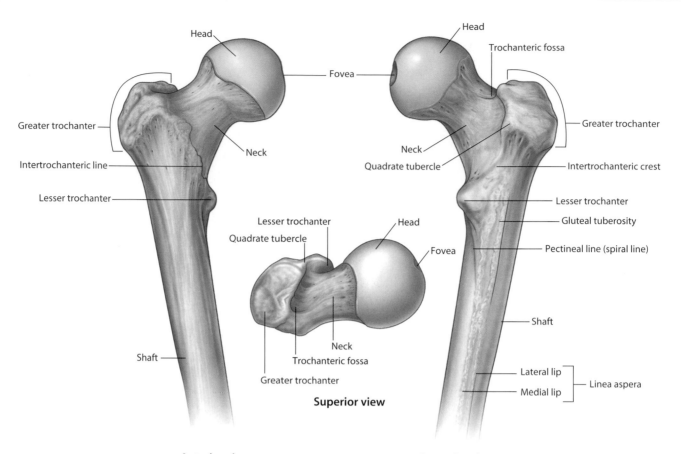

Head

Fovea

Greater trochanter

Intertrochanteric line

Lesser trochanter

Neck

Shaft

Head

Trochanteric fossa

Greater trochanter

Neck

Quadrate tubercle

Intertrochanteric crest

Lesser trochanter

Gluteal tuberosity

Pectineal line (spiral line)

Shaft

Lateral lip

Medial lip

Linea aspera

Lesser trochanter

Quadrate tubercle

Head

Fovea

Neck

Trochanteric fossa

Greater trochanter

Superior view

Anterior view

Posterior view

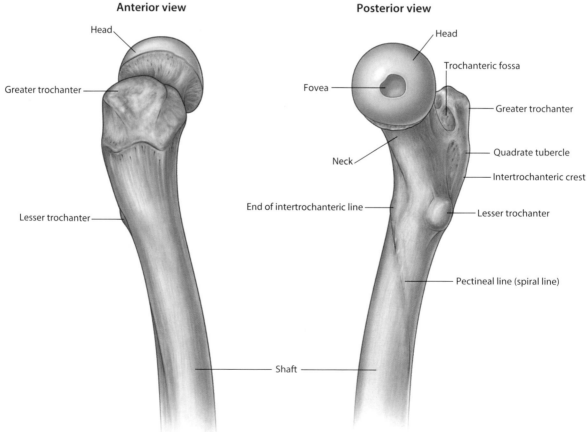

Head

Greater trochanter

Lesser trochanter

Shaft

Head

Fovea

Neck

End of intertrochanteric line

Trochanteric fossa

Greater trochanter

Quadrate tubercle

Intertrochanteric crest

Lesser trochanter

Pectineal line (spiral line)

Shaft

Lateral view

Medial view

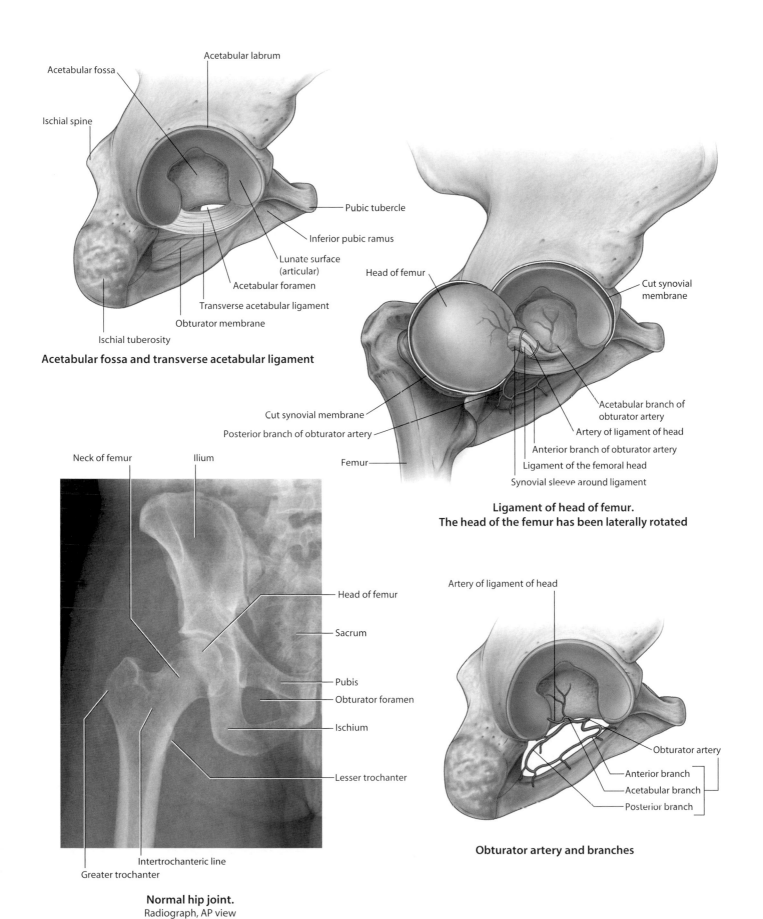

Acetabular fossa

Acetabular labrum

Ischial spine

Pubic tubercle

Inferior pubic ramus

Lunate surface (articular)

Acetabular foramen

Transverse acetabular ligament

Obturator membrane

Ischial tuberosity

Acetabular fossa and transverse acetabular ligament

Head of femur

Cut synovial membrane

Cut synovial membrane

Posterior branch of obturator artery

Femur

Acetabular branch of obturator artery

Artery of ligament of head

Anterior branch of obturator artery

Ligament of the femoral head

Synovial sleeve around ligament

Ligament of head of femur.
The head of the femur has been laterally rotated

Neck of femur

Ilium

Head of femur

Sacrum

Pubis

Obturator foramen

Ischium

Lesser trochanter

Intertrochanteric line

Greater trochanter

Normal hip joint.
Radiograph, AP view

Artery of ligament of head

Obturator artery

Anterior branch

Acetabular branch

Posterior branch

Obturator artery and branches

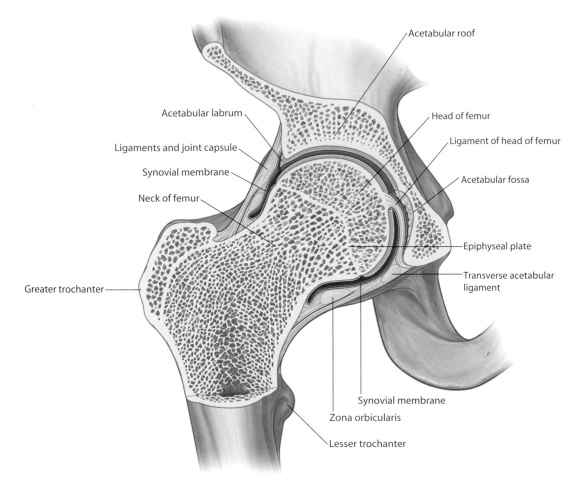

Acetabular roof

Acetabular labrum

Ligaments and joint capsule

Synovial membrane

Neck of femur

Greater trochanter

Head of femur

Ligament of head of femur

Acetabular fossa

Epiphyseal plate

Transverse acetabular ligament

Synovial membrane

Zona orbicularis

Lesser trochanter

Coronal section through hip joint

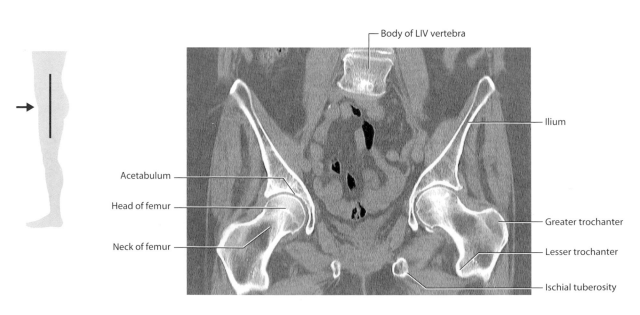

Body of LIV vertebra

Ilium

Acetabulum

Head of femur

Neck of femur

Greater trochanter

Lesser trochanter

Ischial tuberosity

Hip joints.
CT image in coronal plane

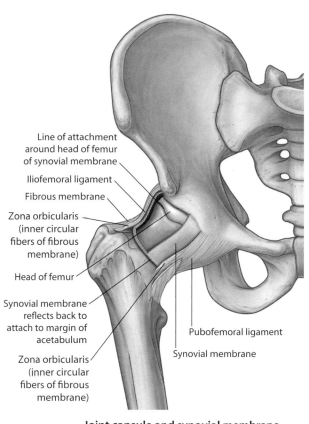

Line of attachment around head of femur of synovial membrane
Iliofemoral ligament
Fibrous membrane
Zona orbicularis (inner circular fibers of fibrous membrane)
Head of femur
Synovial membrane reflects back to attach to margin of acetabulum
Zona orbicularis (inner circular fibers of fibrous membrane)
Pubofemoral ligament
Synovial membrane

Joint capsule and synovial membrane

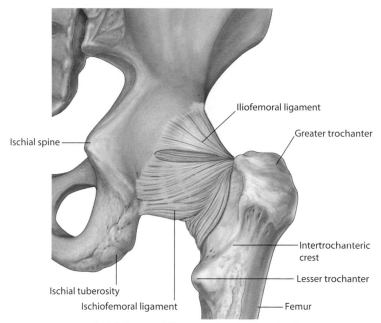

Ischial spine
Iliofemoral ligament
Greater trochanter
Intertrochanteric crest
Lesser trochanter
Ischial tuberosity
Ischiofemoral ligament
Femur

Ischiofemoral ligament (posterior view)

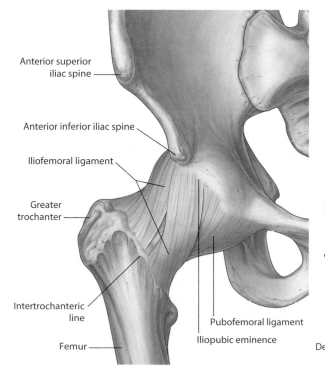

Anterior superior iliac spine
Anterior inferior iliac spine
Iliofemoral ligament
Greater trochanter
Intertrochanteric line
Femur
Pubofemoral ligament
Iliopubic eminence

Iliofemoral and pubofemoral ligaments (anterior view)

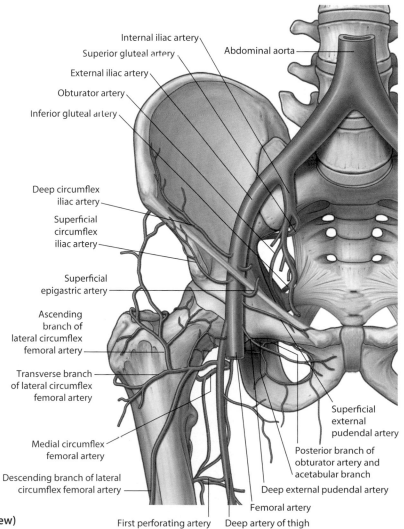

Internal iliac artery
Superior gluteal artery
External iliac artery
Obturator artery
Inferior gluteal artery
Abdominal aorta
Deep circumflex iliac artery
Superficial circumflex iliac artery
Superficial epigastric artery
Ascending branch of lateral circumflex femoral artery
Transverse branch of lateral circumflex femoral artery
Medial circumflex femoral artery
Descending branch of lateral circumflex femoral artery
Superficial external pudendal artery
Posterior branch of obturator artery and acetabular branch
Deep external pudendal artery
Femoral artery
First perforating artery
Deep artery of thigh

Arterial supply of the hip joint

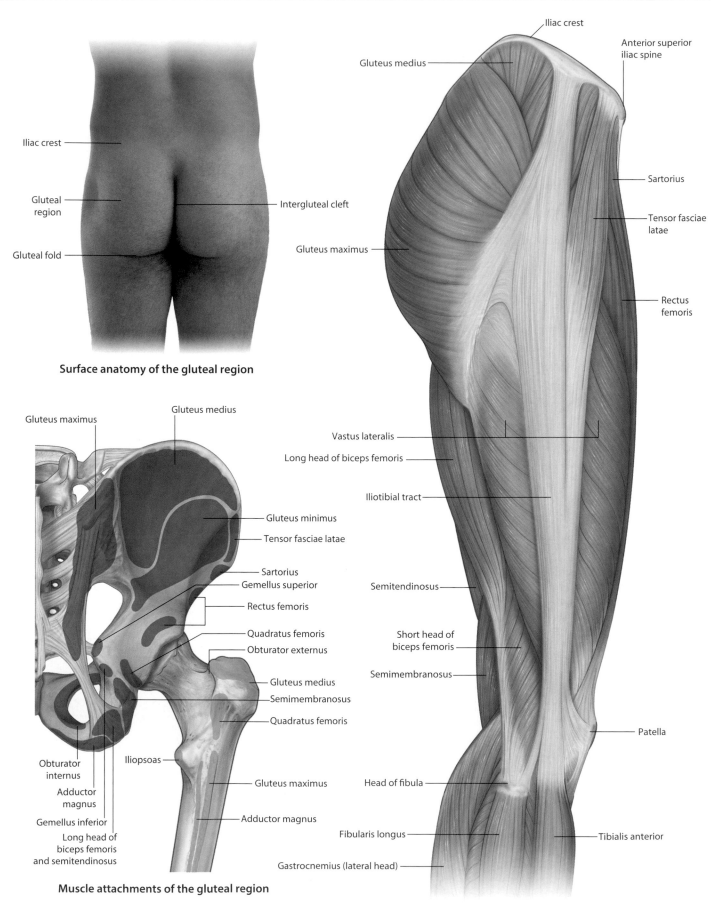

Iliac crest

Gluteus medius

Iliac crest

Anterior superior iliac spine

Gluteal region

Intergluteal cleft

Sartorius

Gluteus maximus

Tensor fasciae latae

Gluteal fold

Rectus femoris

Surface anatomy of the gluteal region

Gluteus maximus

Gluteus medius

Vastus lateralis

Long head of biceps femoris

Gluteus minimus

Iliotibial tract

Tensor fasciae latae

Sartorius

Gemellus superior

Rectus femoris

Semitendinosus

Quadratus femoris

Obturator externus

Short head of biceps femoris

Gluteus medius

Semimembranosus

Semimembranosus

Quadratus femoris

Obturator internus

Iliopsoas

Patella

Adductor magnus

Gluteus maximus

Head of fibula

Gemellus inferior

Adductor magnus

Fibularis longus

Tibialis anterior

Long head of biceps femoris and semitendinosus

Gastrocnemius (lateral head)

Muscle attachments of the gluteal region

Muscles of the hip and thigh (lateral view)

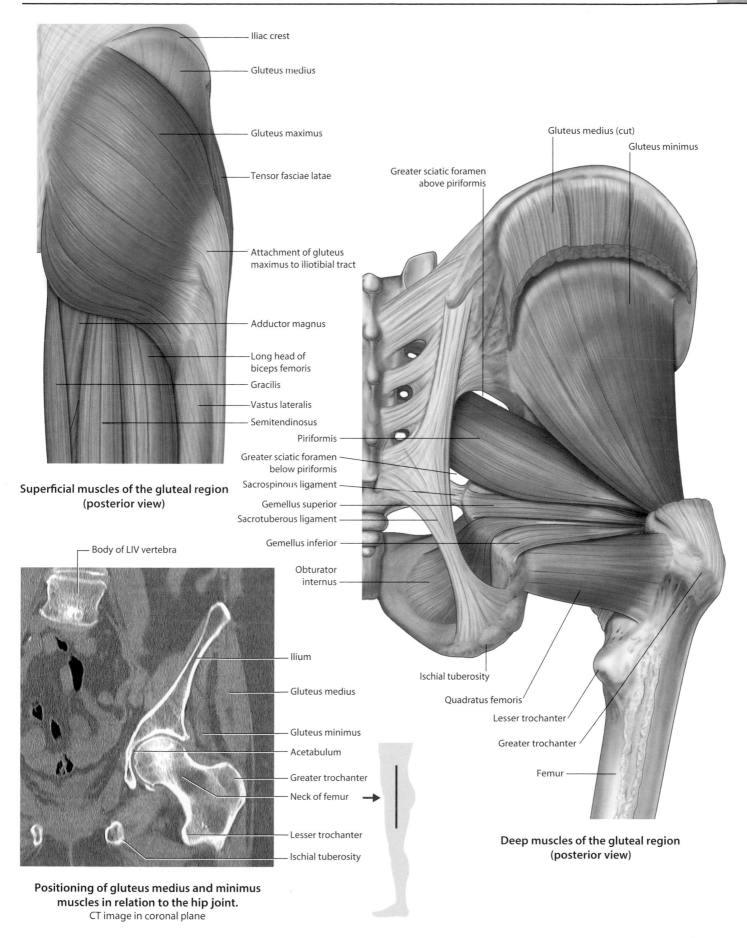

Iliac crest

Gluteus medius

Gluteus maximus

Tensor fasciae latae

Attachment of gluteus maximus to iliotibial tract

Adductor magnus

Long head of biceps femoris

Gracilis

Vastus lateralis

Semitendinosus

Superficial muscles of the gluteal region (posterior view)

Gluteus medius (cut)

Gluteus minimus

Greater sciatic foramen above piriformis

Piriformis

Greater sciatic foramen below piriformis

Sacrospinous ligament

Gemellus superior

Sacrotuberous ligament

Gemellus inferior

Obturator internus

Ischial tuberosity

Quadratus femoris

Lesser trochanter

Greater trochanter

Femur

Deep muscles of the gluteal region (posterior view)

Body of LIV vertebra

Ilium

Gluteus medius

Gluteus minimus

Acetabulum

Greater trochanter

Neck of femur

Lesser trochanter

Ischial tuberosity

Positioning of gluteus medius and minimus muscles in relation to the hip joint.
CT image in coronal plane

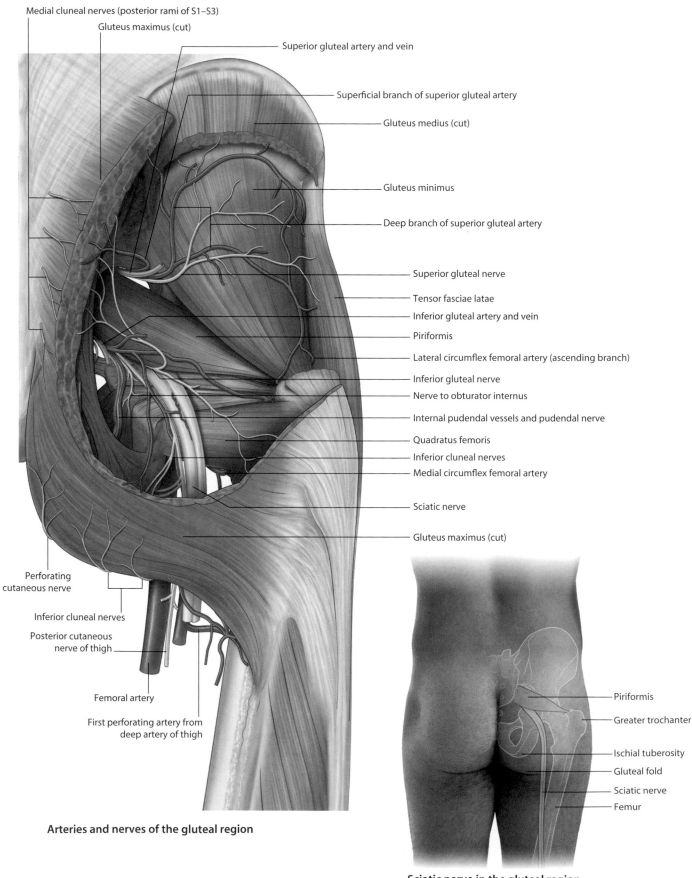

Medial cluneal nerves (posterior rami of S1–S3)

Gluteus maximus (cut)

Superior gluteal artery and vein

Superficial branch of superior gluteal artery

Gluteus medius (cut)

Gluteus minimus

Deep branch of superior gluteal artery

Superior gluteal nerve

Tensor fasciae latae

Inferior gluteal artery and vein

Piriformis

Lateral circumflex femoral artery (ascending branch)

Inferior gluteal nerve

Nerve to obturator internus

Internal pudendal vessels and pudendal nerve

Quadratus femoris

Inferior cluneal nerves

Medial circumflex femoral artery

Sciatic nerve

Gluteus maximus (cut)

Perforating cutaneous nerve

Inferior cluneal nerves

Posterior cutaneous nerve of thigh

Femoral artery

First perforating artery from deep artery of thigh

Arteries and nerves of the gluteal region

Piriformis

Greater trochanter

Ischial tuberosity

Gluteal fold

Sciatic nerve

Femur

Sciatic nerve in the gluteal region as it relates to the surface (posterior view)

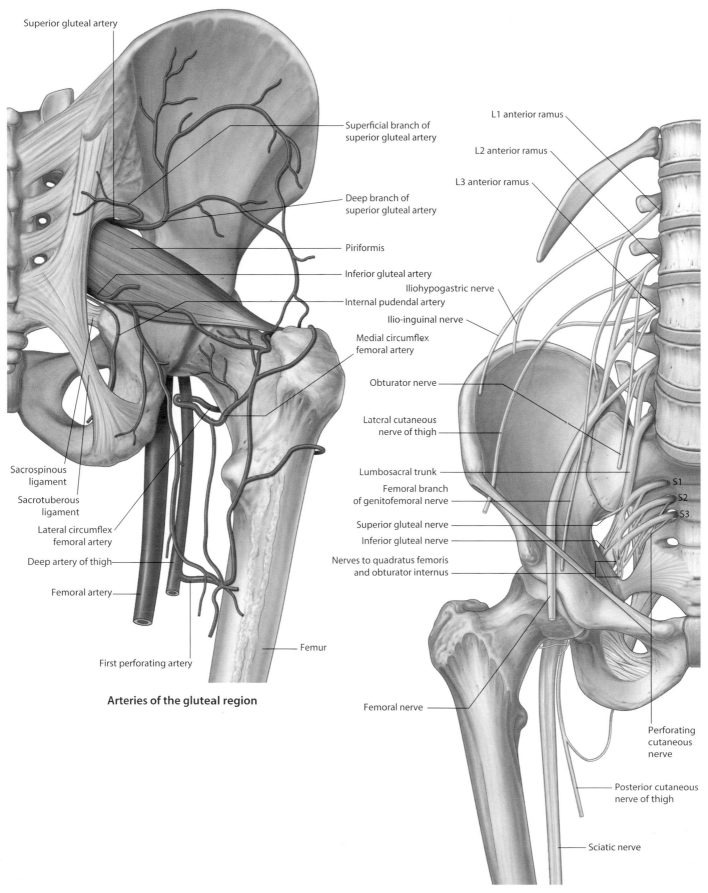

Superior gluteal artery

Superficial branch of superior gluteal artery

Deep branch of superior gluteal artery

Piriformis

Inferior gluteal artery

Internal pudendal artery

Medial circumflex femoral artery

Sacrospinous ligament

Sacrotuberous ligament

Lateral circumflex femoral artery

Deep artery of thigh

Femoral artery

First perforating artery

Femur

Arteries of the gluteal region

L1 anterior ramus

L2 anterior ramus

L3 anterior ramus

Iliohypogastric nerve

Ilio-inguinal nerve

Obturator nerve

Lateral cutaneous nerve of thigh

Lumbosacral trunk

Femoral branch of genitofemoral nerve

Superior gluteal nerve

Inferior gluteal nerve

Nerves to quadratus femoris and obturator internus

Femoral nerve

S1

S2

S3

Perforating cutaneous nerve

Posterior cutaneous nerve of thigh

Sciatic nerve

Branches of the lumbosacral plexus related to lower limb

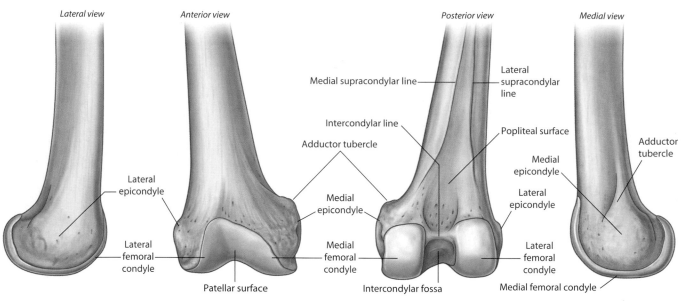

Lateral view

Anterior view

Posterior view

Medial view

Medial supracondylar line

Lateral supracondylar line

Intercondylar line

Popliteal surface

Adductor tubercle

Lateral epicondyle

Lateral femoral condyle

Medial epicondyle

Medial femoral condyle

Patellar surface

Intercondylar fossa

Adductor tubercle

Medial epicondyle

Lateral epicondyle

Lateral femoral condyle

Medial femoral condyle

Distal end of (right) femur

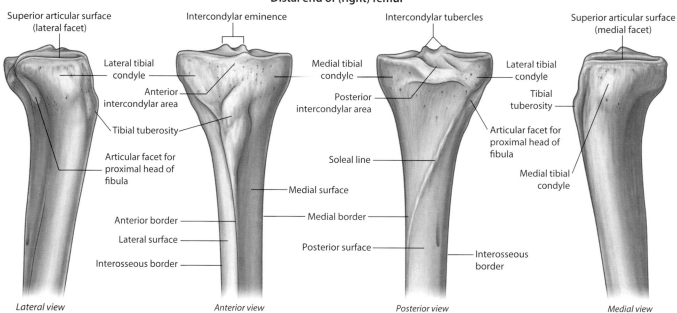

Superior articular surface (lateral facet)

Intercondylar eminence

Intercondylar tubercles

Superior articular surface (medial facet)

Lateral tibial condyle

Medial tibial condyle

Lateral tibial condyle

Anterior intercondylar area

Posterior intercondylar area

Tibial tuberosity

Tibial tuberosity

Articular facet for proximal head of fibula

Soleal line

Articular facet for proximal head of fibula

Medial tibial condyle

Medial surface

Medial border

Anterior border

Lateral surface

Posterior surface

Interosseous border

Interosseous border

Lateral view

Anterior view

Posterior view

Medial view

Proximal end of (right) tibia

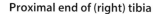

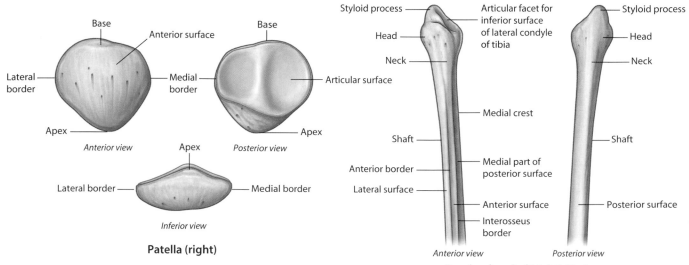

Base

Anterior surface

Base

Styloid process

Articular facet for inferior surface of lateral condyle of tibia

Styloid process

Lateral border

Medial border

Head

Head

Apex

Articular surface

Neck

Neck

Apex

Medial crest

Anterior view

Apex

Posterior view

Shaft

Shaft

Lateral border

Medial border

Medial part of posterior surface

Anterior border

Inferior view

Lateral surface

Anterior surface

Posterior surface

Patella (right)

Interosseus border

Anterior view

Posterior view

Proximal end of (right) fibula

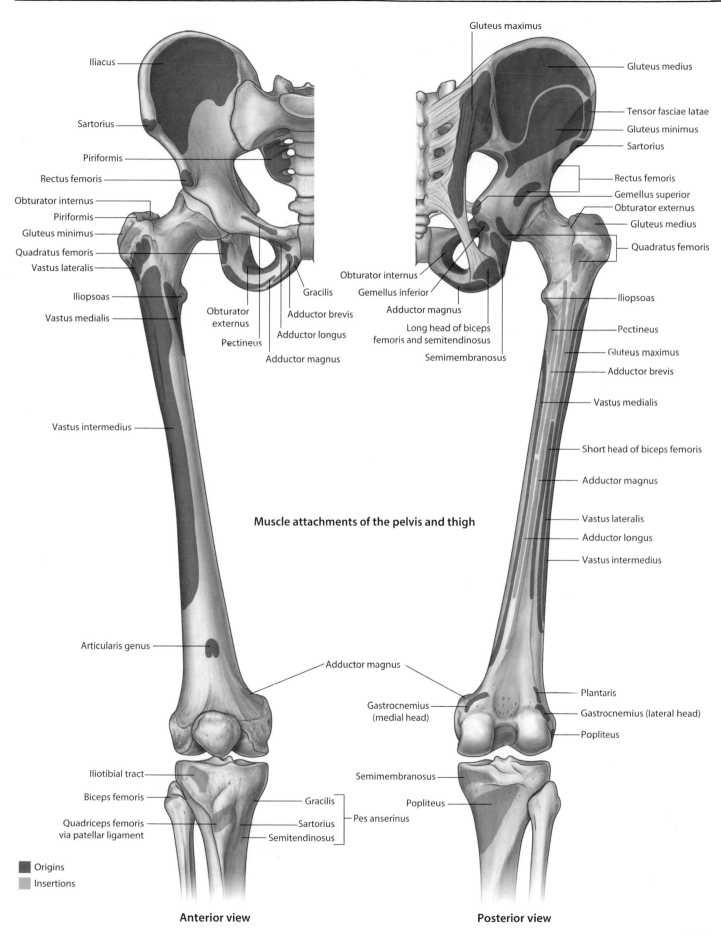

Iliacus

Sartorius

Piriformis

Rectus femoris

Obturator internus

Piriformis

Gluteus minimus

Quadratus femoris

Vastus lateralis

Iliopsoas

Vastus medialis

Vastus intermedius

Obturator externus

Pectineus

Gracilis

Adductor brevis

Adductor longus

Adductor magnus

Gluteus maximus

Gluteus medius

Tensor fasciae latae

Gluteus minimus

Sartorius

Rectus femoris

Gemellus superior

Obturator externus

Gluteus medius

Quadratus femoris

Obturator internus

Gemellus inferior

Adductor magnus

Long head of biceps femoris and semitendinosus

Semimembranosus

Iliopsoas

Pectineus

Gluteus maximus

Adductor brevis

Vastus medialis

Short head of biceps femoris

Adductor magnus

Vastus lateralis

Adductor longus

Vastus intermedius

Muscle attachments of the pelvis and thigh

Articularis genus

Adductor magnus

Gastrocnemius (medial head)

Plantaris

Gastrocnemius (lateral head)

Popliteus

Iliotibial tract

Biceps femoris

Quadriceps femoris via patellar ligament

Gracilis

Sartorius

Semitendinosus

Pes anserinus

Semimembranosus

Popliteus

■ Origins
■ Insertions

Anterior view

Posterior view

305

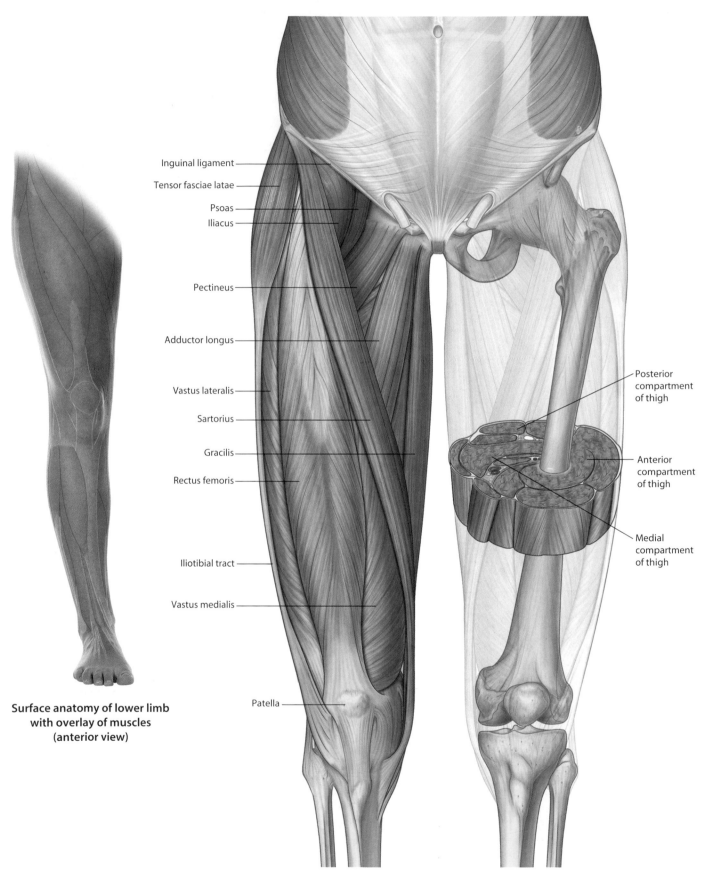

Inguinal ligament

Tensor fasciae latae

Psoas

Iliacus

Pectineus

Adductor longus

Vastus lateralis

Sartorius

Gracilis

Rectus femoris

Iliotibial tract

Vastus medialis

Patella

Posterior compartment of thigh

Anterior compartment of thigh

Medial compartment of thigh

Surface anatomy of lower limb with overlay of muscles (anterior view)

Superficial muscles of the thigh (anterior view)

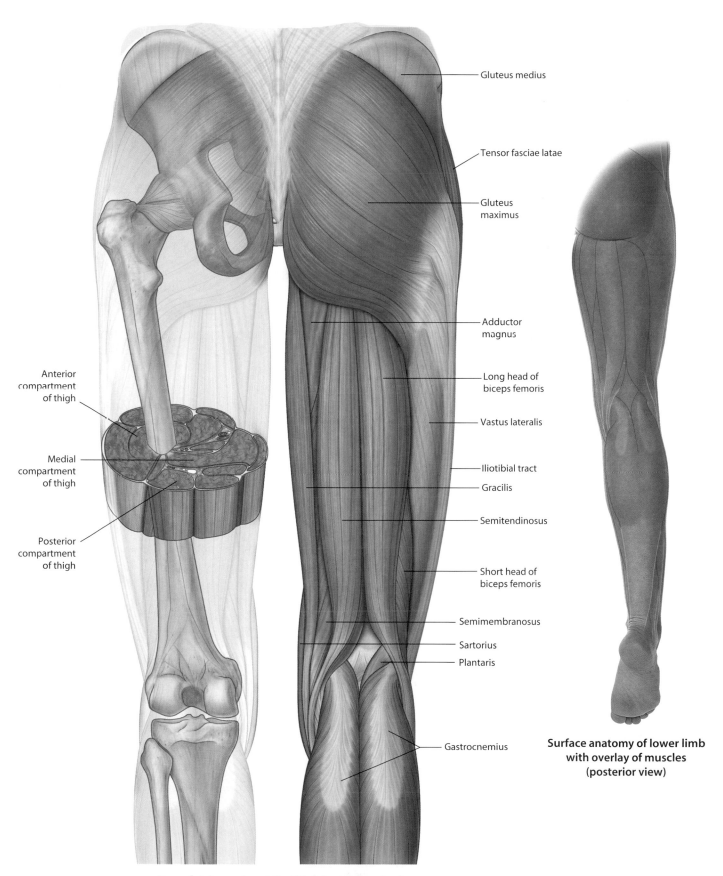

Gluteus medius

Tensor fasciae latae

Gluteus maximus

Adductor magnus

Long head of biceps femoris

Vastus lateralis

Iliotibial tract

Gracilis

Semitendinosus

Short head of biceps femoris

Semimembranosus

Sartorius

Plantaris

Gastrocnemius

Anterior compartment of thigh

Medial compartment of thigh

Posterior compartment of thigh

Surface anatomy of lower limb with overlay of muscles (posterior view)

Superficial muscles of the thigh (posterior view)

307

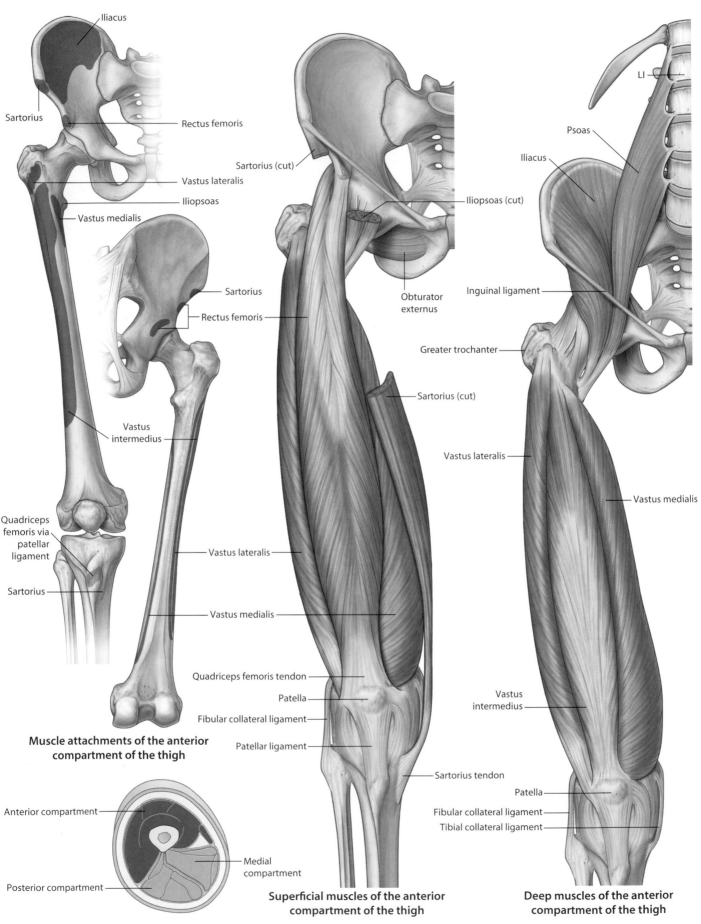

Iliacus

Sartorius

Rectus femoris

Vastus lateralis

Iliopsoas

Vastus medialis

Sartorius

Rectus femoris

Vastus intermedius

Quadriceps femoris via patellar ligament

Sartorius

Muscle attachments of the anterior compartment of the thigh

Anterior compartment

Posterior compartment

Medial compartment

Sartorius (cut)

Iliopsoas (cut)

Obturator externus

Quadriceps femoris tendon

Patella

Fibular collateral ligament

Patellar ligament

Vastus lateralis

Vastus medialis

Sartorius tendon

Superficial muscles of the anterior compartment of the thigh

L1

Psoas

Iliacus

Inguinal ligament

Greater trochanter

Sartorius (cut)

Vastus lateralis

Vastus medialis

Vastus intermedius

Patella

Fibular collateral ligament

Tibial collateral ligament

Deep muscles of the anterior compartment of the thigh

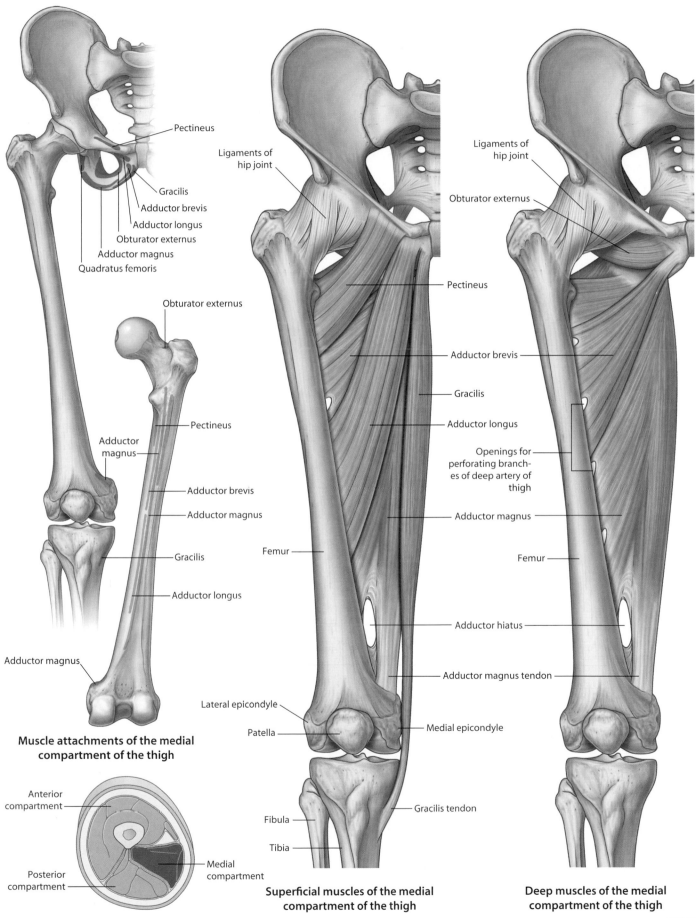

Pectineus
Gracilis
Adductor brevis
Adductor longus
Obturator externus
Adductor magnus
Quadratus femoris

Obturator externus
Pectineus
Adductor magnus
Adductor brevis
Adductor magnus
Gracilis
Adductor longus
Adductor magnus

Muscle attachments of the medial compartment of the thigh

Anterior compartment
Posterior compartment
Medial compartment

Ligaments of hip joint
Pectineus
Adductor brevis
Gracilis
Adductor longus
Femur
Lateral epicondyle
Patella
Medial epicondyle
Fibula
Tibia
Gracilis tendon

Superficial muscles of the medial compartment of the thigh

Ligaments of hip joint
Obturator externus
Adductor brevis
Openings for perforating branches of deep artery of thigh
Adductor magnus
Femur
Adductor hiatus
Adductor magnus tendon

Deep muscles of the medial compartment of the thigh

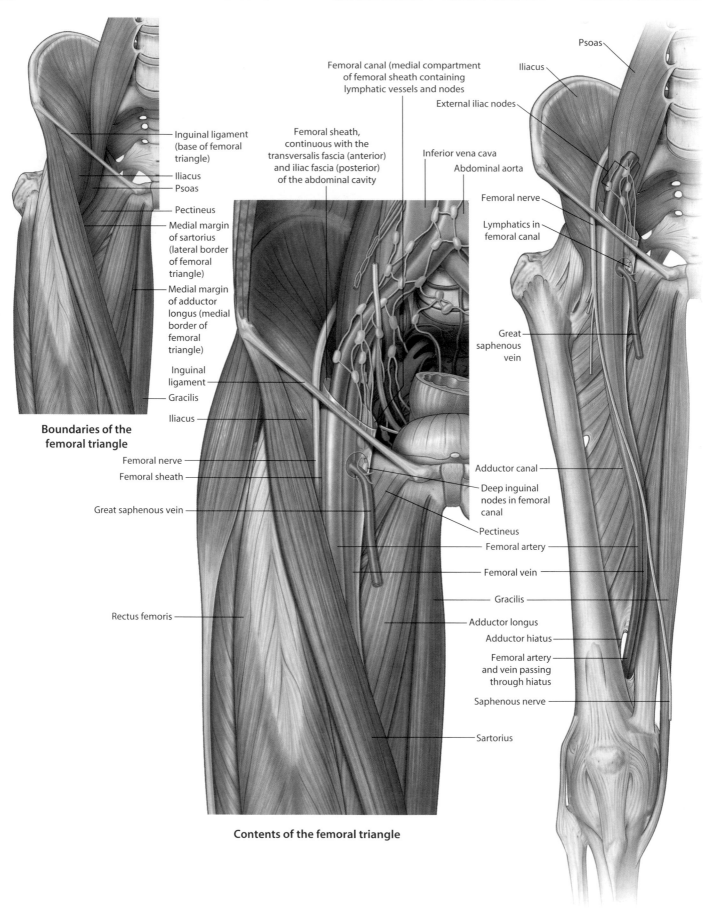

Inguinal ligament (base of femoral triangle)

Iliacus

Psoas

Pectineus

Medial margin of sartorius (lateral border of femoral triangle)

Medial margin of adductor longus (medial border of femoral triangle)

Inguinal ligament

Gracilis

Iliacus

Boundaries of the femoral triangle

Femoral canal (medial compartment of femoral sheath containing lymphatic vessels and nodes)

Femoral sheath, continuous with the transversalis fascia (anterior) and iliac fascia (posterior) of the abdominal cavity

Inferior vena cava

Femoral nerve

Femoral sheath

Great saphenous vein

Rectus femoris

Contents of the femoral triangle

Psoas

Iliacus

External iliac nodes

Inferior vena cava

Abdominal aorta

Femoral nerve

Lymphatics in femoral canal

Great saphenous vein

Adductor canal

Deep inguinal nodes in femoral canal

Pectineus

Femoral artery

Femoral vein

Gracilis

Adductor longus

Adductor hiatus

Femoral artery and vein passing through hiatus

Saphenous nerve

Sartorius

Adductor canal

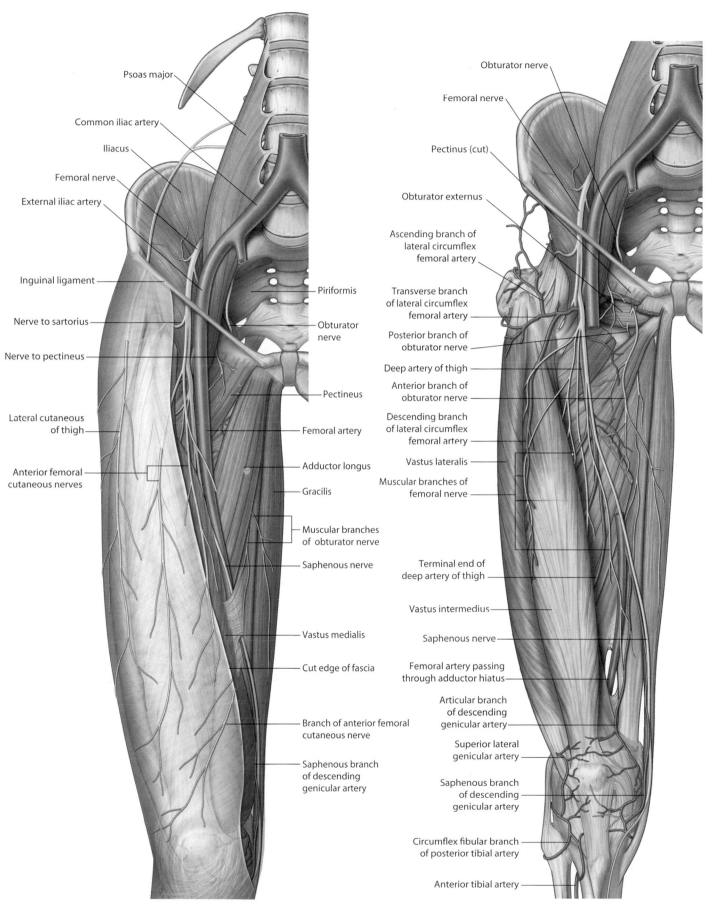

Psoas major

Common iliac artery

Iliacus

Femoral nerve

External iliac artery

Inguinal ligament

Nerve to sartorius

Nerve to pectineus

Lateral cutaneous of thigh

Anterior femoral cutaneous nerves

Piriformis

Obturator nerve

Pectineus

Femoral artery

Adductor longus

Gracilis

Muscular branches of obturator nerve

Saphenous nerve

Vastus medialis

Cut edge of fascia

Branch of anterior femoral cutaneous nerve

Saphenous branch of descending genicular artery

Obturator nerve

Femoral nerve

Pectinus (cut)

Obturator externus

Ascending branch of lateral circumflex femoral artery

Transverse branch of lateral circumflex femoral artery

Posterior branch of obturator nerve

Deep artery of thigh

Anterior branch of obturator nerve

Descending branch of lateral circumflex femoral artery

Vastus lateralis

Muscular branches of femoral nerve

Terminal end of deep artery of thigh

Vastus intermedius

Saphenous nerve

Femoral artery passing through adductor hiatus

Articular branch of descending genicular artery

Superior lateral genicular artery

Saphenous branch of descending genicular artery

Circumflex fibular branch of posterior tibial artery

Anterior tibial artery

Superficial arteries and nerves of the thigh (anterior view)

Deep arteries and nerves of the thigh (anterior view)

311

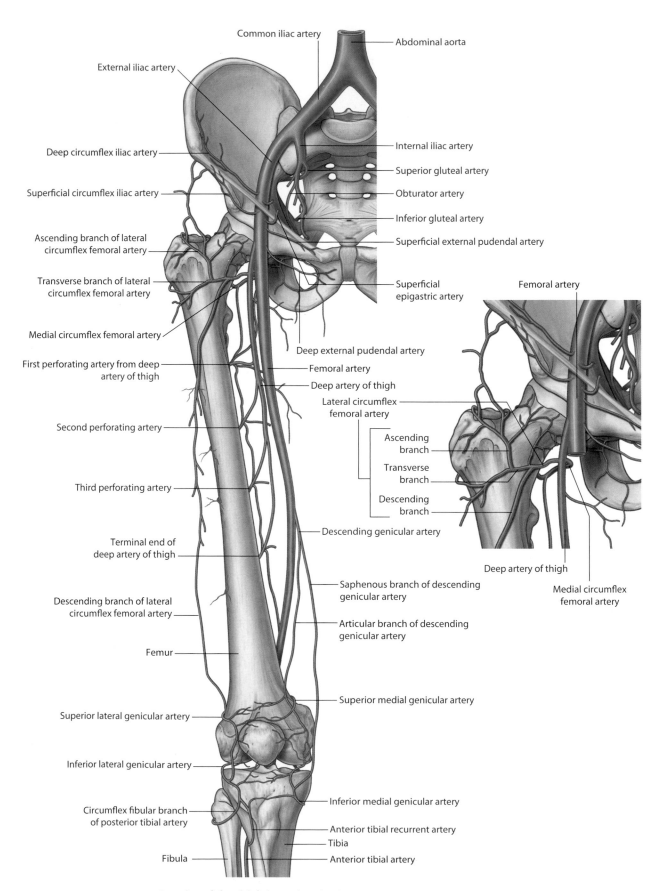

Common iliac artery

Abdominal aorta

External iliac artery

Deep circumflex iliac artery

Internal iliac artery

Superior gluteal artery

Superficial circumflex iliac artery

Obturator artery

Inferior gluteal artery

Ascending branch of lateral circumflex femoral artery

Superficial external pudendal artery

Transverse branch of lateral circumflex femoral artery

Femoral artery

Superficial epigastric artery

Medial circumflex femoral artery

First perforating artery from deep artery of thigh

Deep external pudendal artery

Femoral artery

Deep artery of thigh

Lateral circumflex femoral artery

Second perforating artery

Ascending branch

Transverse branch

Descending branch

Third perforating artery

Descending genicular artery

Terminal end of deep artery of thigh

Deep artery of thigh

Saphenous branch of descending genicular artery

Medial circumflex femoral artery

Descending branch of lateral circumflex femoral artery

Articular branch of descending genicular artery

Femur

Superior medial genicular artery

Superior lateral genicular artery

Inferior lateral genicular artery

Inferior medial genicular artery

Circumflex fibular branch of posterior tibial artery

Anterior tibial recurrent artery

Tibia

Fibula

Anterior tibial artery

Arteries of the thigh (anterior view)

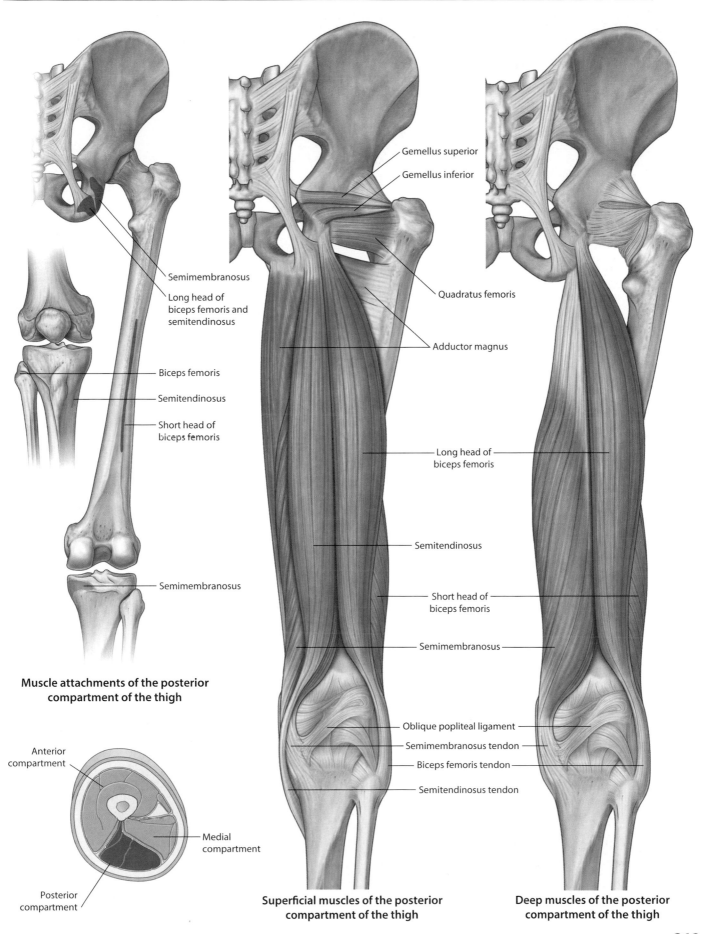

Semimembranosus

Long head of biceps femoris and semitendinosus

Biceps femoris

Semitendinosus

Short head of biceps femoris

Semimembranosus

Muscle attachments of the posterior compartment of the thigh

Anterior compartment

Medial compartment

Posterior compartment

Gemellus superior

Gemellus inferior

Quadratus femoris

Adductor magnus

Long head of biceps femoris

Semitendinosus

Short head of biceps femoris

Semimembranosus

Oblique popliteal ligament

Semimembranosus tendon

Biceps femoris tendon

Semitendinosus tendon

Superficial muscles of the posterior compartment of the thigh

Deep muscles of the posterior compartment of the thigh

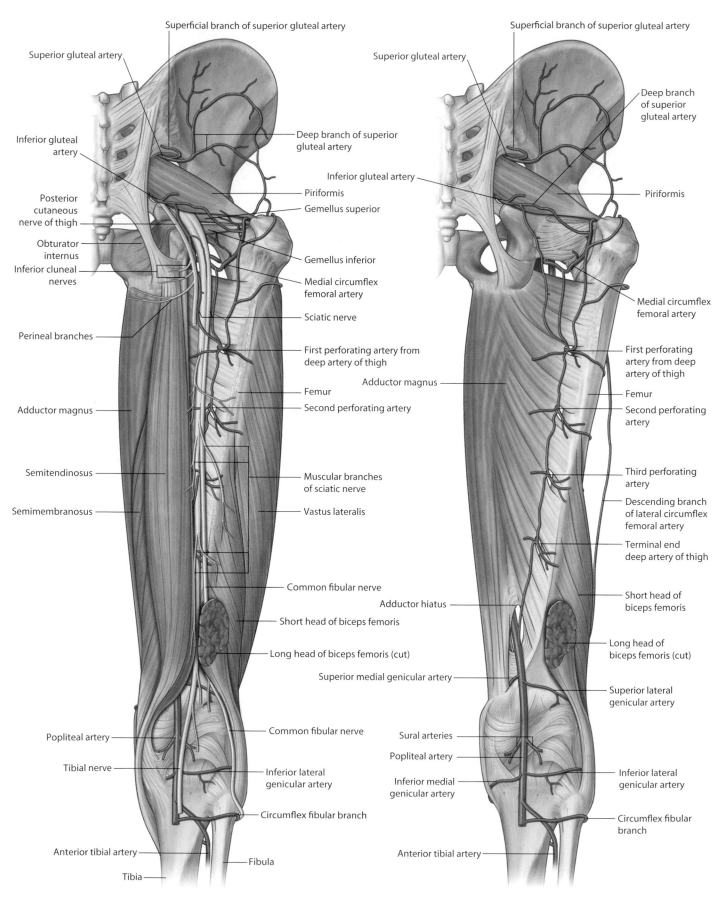

Superficial branch of superior gluteal artery

Superior gluteal artery

Inferior gluteal artery

Posterior cutaneous nerve of thigh

Obturator internus

Inferior cluneal nerves

Perineal branches

Adductor magnus

Semitendinosus

Semimembranosus

Popliteal artery

Tibial nerve

Anterior tibial artery

Tibia

Deep branch of superior gluteal artery

Piriformis

Gemellus superior

Gemellus inferior

Medial circumflex femoral artery

Sciatic nerve

First perforating artery from deep artery of thigh

Femur

Second perforating artery

Muscular branches of sciatic nerve

Vastus lateralis

Common fibular nerve

Short head of biceps femoris

Long head of biceps femoris (cut)

Superior medial genicular artery

Common fibular nerve

Inferior lateral genicular artery

Circumflex fibular branch

Fibula

Arteries and nerves of the thigh (posterior view)

Superficial branch of superior gluteal artery

Superior gluteal artery

Deep branch of superior gluteal artery

Inferior gluteal artery

Piriformis

Medial circumflex femoral artery

First perforating artery from deep artery of thigh

Femur

Second perforating artery

Adductor magnus

Third perforating artery

Descending branch of lateral circumflex femoral artery

Terminal end deep artery of thigh

Short head of biceps femoris

Long head of biceps femoris (cut)

Superior lateral genicular artery

Adductor hiatus

Sural arteries

Popliteal artery

Inferior medial genicular artery

Inferior lateral genicular artery

Circumflex fibular branch

Anterior tibial artery

Deep arteries of the thigh (posterior view)

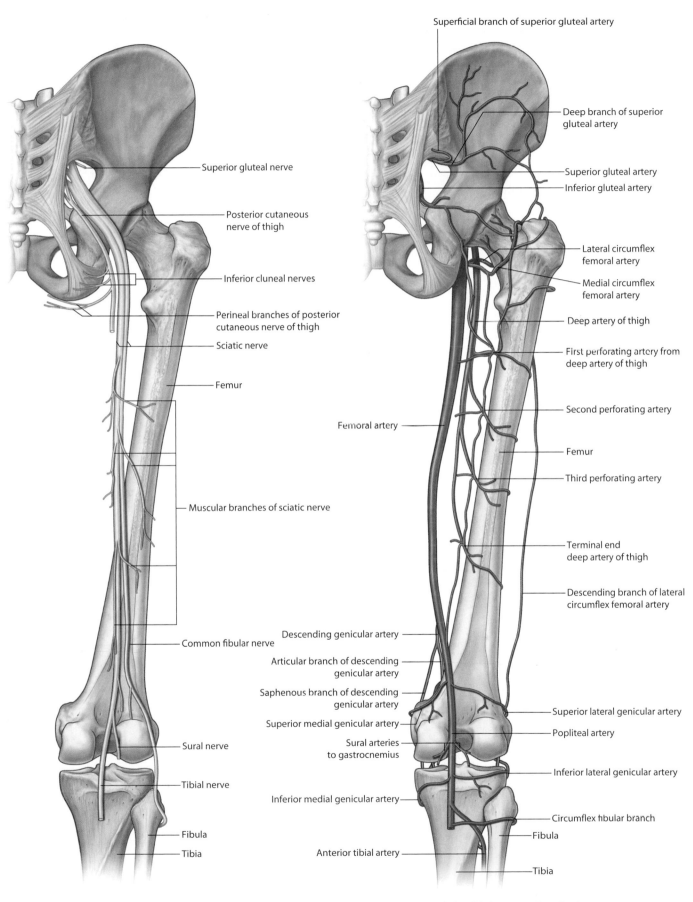

Superficial branch of superior gluteal artery

Deep branch of superior gluteal artery

Superior gluteal nerve

Superior gluteal artery

Inferior gluteal artery

Posterior cutaneous nerve of thigh

Lateral circumflex femoral artery

Inferior cluneal nerves

Medial circumflex femoral artery

Perineal branches of posterior cutaneous nerve of thigh

Deep artery of thigh

Sciatic nerve

First perforating artery from deep artery of thigh

Femur

Second perforating artery

Femoral artery

Femur

Third perforating artery

Muscular branches of sciatic nerve

Terminal end deep artery of thigh

Descending branch of lateral circumflex femoral artery

Common fibular nerve

Descending genicular artery

Articular branch of descending genicular artery

Saphenous branch of descending genicular artery

Superior lateral genicular artery

Superior medial genicular artery

Popliteal artery

Sural nerve

Sural arteries to gastrocnemius

Tibial nerve

Inferior lateral genicular artery

Inferior medial genicular artery

Circumflex fibular branch

Fibula

Fibula

Tibia

Anterior tibial artery

Tibia

Nerves of the thigh (posterior view)   **Arteries of the thigh (posterior view)**

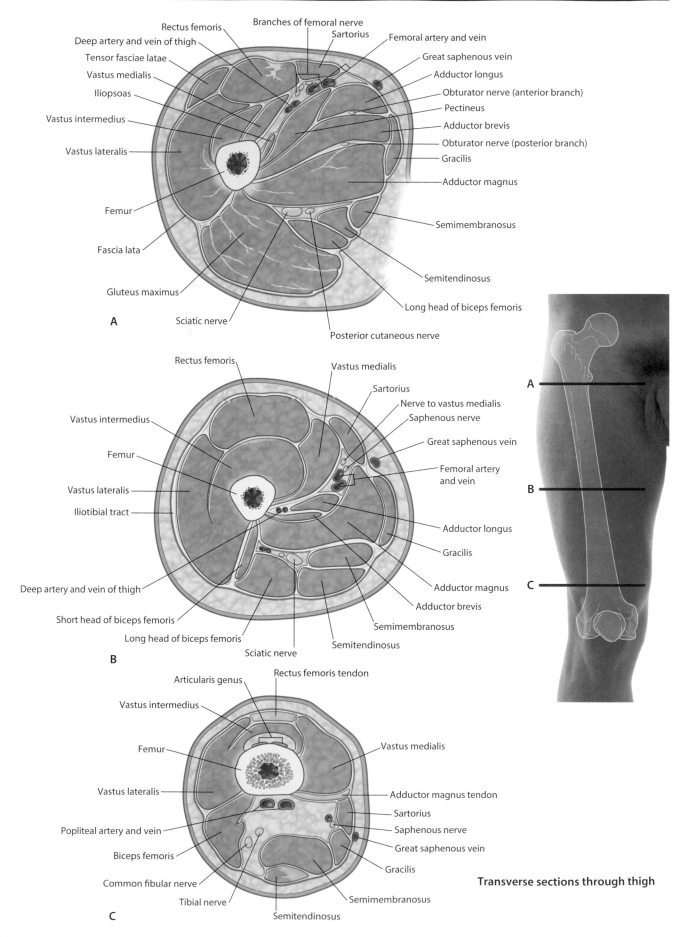

A

Rectus femoris
Deep artery and vein of thigh
Tensor fasciae latae
Vastus medialis
Iliopsoas
Vastus intermedius
Vastus lateralis
Femur
Fascia lata
Gluteus maximus
Sciatic nerve

Branches of femoral nerve
Sartorius
Femoral artery and vein
Great saphenous vein
Adductor longus
Obturator nerve (anterior branch)
Pectineus
Adductor brevis
Obturator nerve (posterior branch)
Gracilis
Adductor magnus
Semimembranosus
Semitendinosus
Long head of biceps femoris
Posterior cutaneous nerve

B

Rectus femoris
Vastus intermedius
Femur
Vastus lateralis
Iliotibial tract
Deep artery and vein of thigh
Short head of biceps femoris
Long head of biceps femoris
Sciatic nerve

Vastus medialis
Sartorius
Nerve to vastus medialis
Saphenous nerve
Great saphenous vein
Femoral artery and vein
Adductor longus
Gracilis
Adductor magnus
Adductor brevis
Semimembranosus
Semitendinosus

C

Articularis genus
Vastus intermedius
Femur
Vastus lateralis
Popliteal artery and vein
Biceps femoris
Common fibular nerve
Tibial nerve
Semitendinosus

Rectus femoris tendon
Vastus medialis
Adductor magnus tendon
Sartorius
Saphenous nerve
Great saphenous vein
Gracilis
Semimembranosus

Transverse sections through thigh

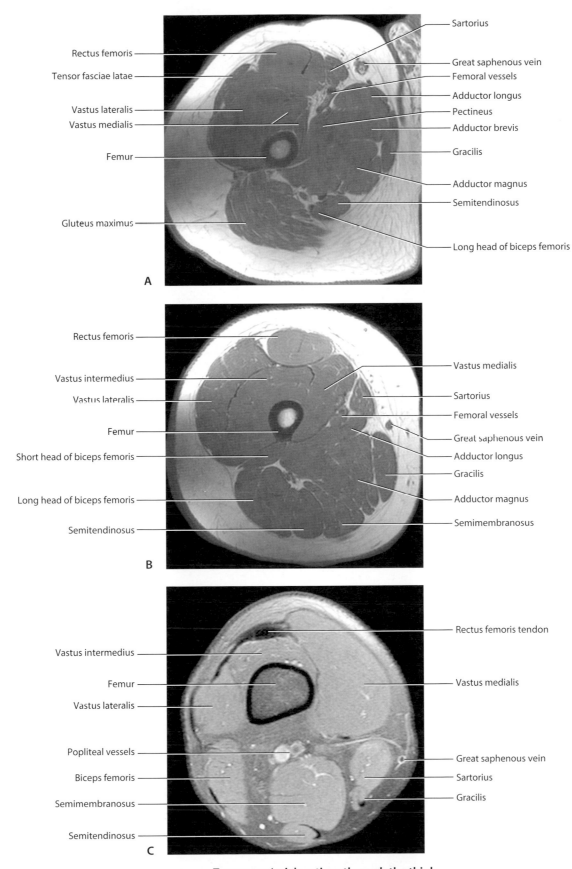

Rectus femoris

Tensor fasciae latae

Vastus lateralis
Vastus medialis

Femur

Gluteus maximus

Sartorius

Great saphenous vein
Femoral vessels
Adductor longus
Pectineus
Adductor brevis
Gracilis
Adductor magnus
Semitendinosus
Long head of biceps femoris

A

Rectus femoris

Vastus intermedius

Vastus lateralis

Femur

Short head of biceps femoris

Long head of biceps femoris

Semitendinosus

Vastus medialis
Sartorius
Femoral vessels
Great saphenous vein
Adductor longus
Gracilis
Adductor magnus
Semimembranosus

B

Vastus intermedius

Femur

Vastus lateralis

Popliteal vessels

Biceps femoris

Semimembranosus

Semitendinosus

Rectus femoris tendon
Vastus medialis
Great saphenous vein
Sartorius
Gracilis

C

Transverse/axial sections through the thigh.
A. Proximal/upper thigh. T1-weighted MR image in axial plane
B. Middle thigh. T1-weighted MR image in axial plane
C. Distal/lower thigh. Fat-saturated T2-weighted MR image in axial plane

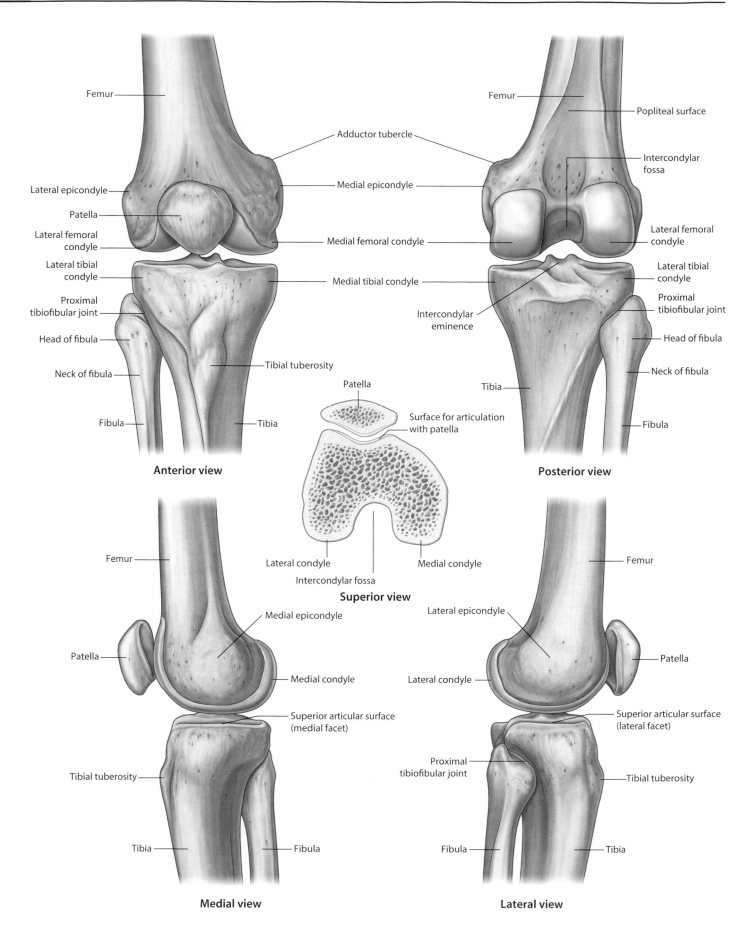

Femur

Adductor tubercle

Medial epicondyle

Lateral epicondyle

Patella

Lateral femoral condyle

Medial femoral condyle

Lateral tibial condyle

Medial tibial condyle

Proximal tibiofibular joint

Head of fibula

Neck of fibula

Tibial tuberosity

Fibula

Tibia

Anterior view

Femur

Popliteal surface

Intercondylar fossa

Lateral femoral condyle

Lateral tibial condyle

Proximal tibiofibular joint

Intercondylar eminence

Head of fibula

Neck of fibula

Tibia

Fibula

Posterior view

Patella

Surface for articulation with patella

Lateral condyle

Medial condyle

Intercondylar fossa

Superior view

Femur

Patella

Tibial tuberosity

Tibia

Medial epicondyle

Medial condyle

Superior articular surface (medial facet)

Fibula

Medial view

Lateral epicondyle

Lateral condyle

Femur

Patella

Superior articular surface (lateral facet)

Proximal tibiofibular joint

Tibial tuberosity

Fibula

Tibia

Lateral view

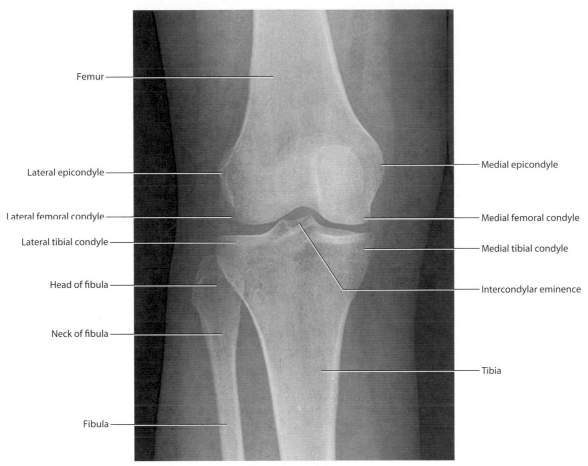

Femur

Lateral epicondyle

Lateral femoral condyle

Lateral tibial condyle

Head of fibula

Neck of fibula

Fibula

Medial epicondyle

Medial femoral condyle

Medial tibial condyle

Intercondylar eminence

Tibia

Normal knee joint.
Radiograph, AP view

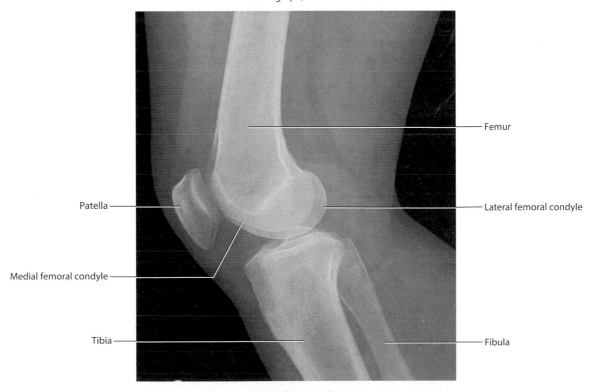

Patella

Medial femoral condyle

Tibia

Femur

Lateral femoral condyle

Fibula

Normal knee joint.
Radiograph, lateral view

319

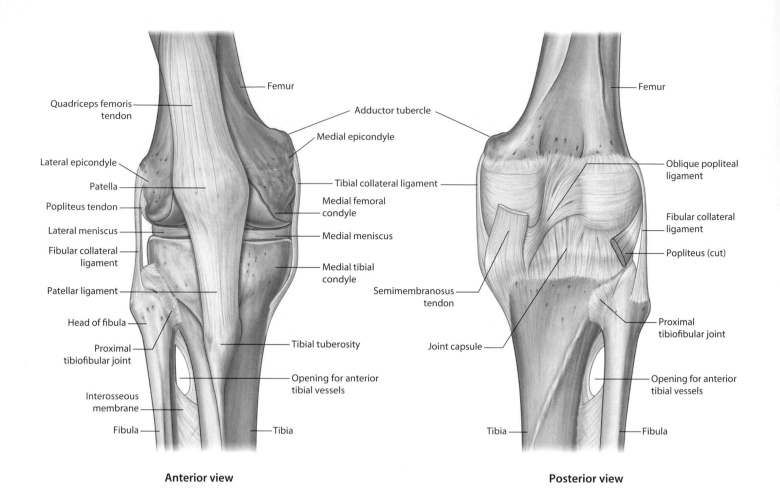

Anterior view

Posterior view

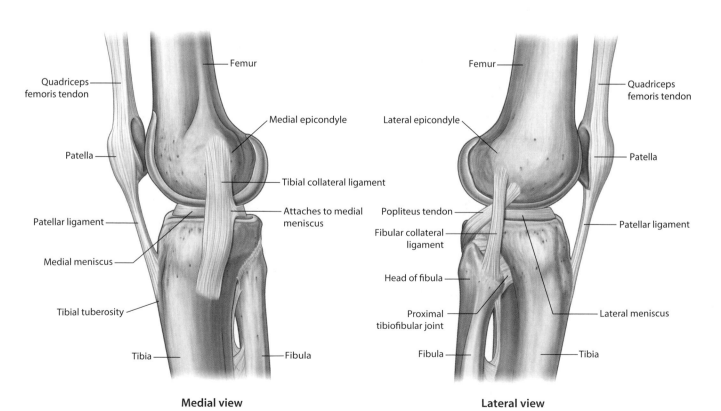

Medial view

Lateral view

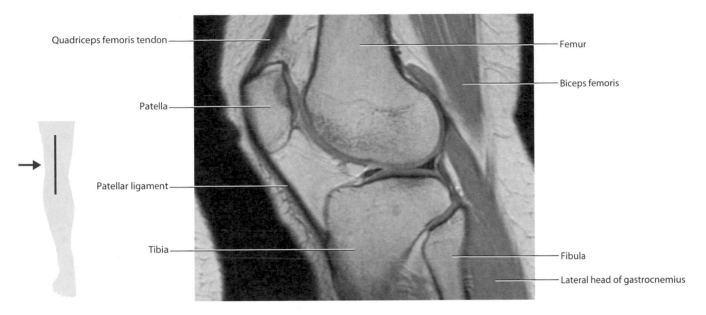

Quadriceps femoris tendon

Patella

Patellar ligament

Tibia

Femur

Biceps femoris

Fibula

Lateral head of gastrocnemius

Normal knee joint.
T2-weighted MR image in sagittal plane

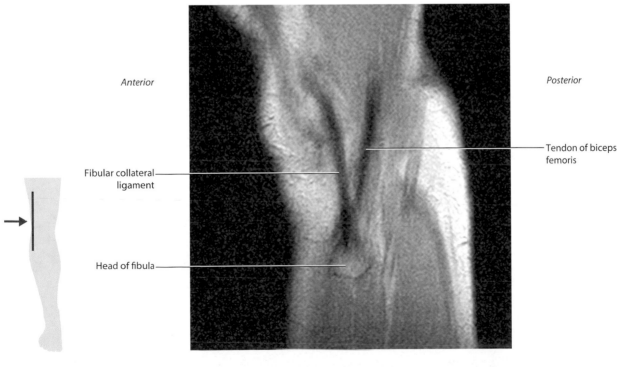

Anterior

Posterior

Fibular collateral ligament

Head of fibula

Tendon of biceps femoris

**Unique view showing the fibular collateral ligament and the
tendon of the biceps femoris muscle attaching to the head of the fibula.**
T2-weighted MR image in sagittal plane

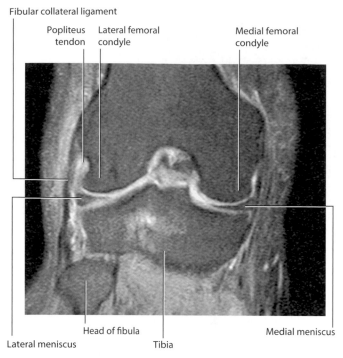

Fibular collateral ligament
Popliteus tendon
Lateral femoral condyle
Medial femoral condyle
Lateral meniscus
Head of fibula
Tibia
Medial meniscus

Coronal view of knee joint showing the fibular collateral ligament and its relationship to surrounding structures.
Fat-saturated T2-weighted MR image in coronal plane

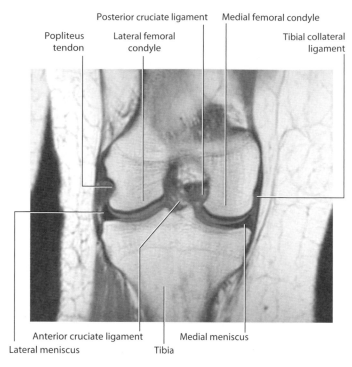

Posterior cruciate ligament
Medial femoral condyle
Popliteus tendon
Lateral femoral condyle
Tibial collateral ligament
Anterior cruciate ligament
Lateral meniscus
Medial meniscus
Tibia

Anterior view of knee joint showing the relationship between the tibial collateral ligament and the medial meniscus.
T1-weighted MR image in coronal plane

Anterior cruciate ligament
Posterior cruciate ligament
Lateral femoral condyle
Medial femoral condyle
Lateral meniscus
Medial meniscus
Lateral tibial condyle
Medial tibial condyle
Transverse ligament
Fibula
Tibia

Anterior view (flexed)

Femur
Intercondylar fossa
Anterior cruciate ligament
Lateral femoral condyle
Lateral meniscus
Medial femoral condyle
Medial meniscus
Posterior meniscofemoral ligament
Posterior cruciate ligament
Tibia
Fibula

Posterior view

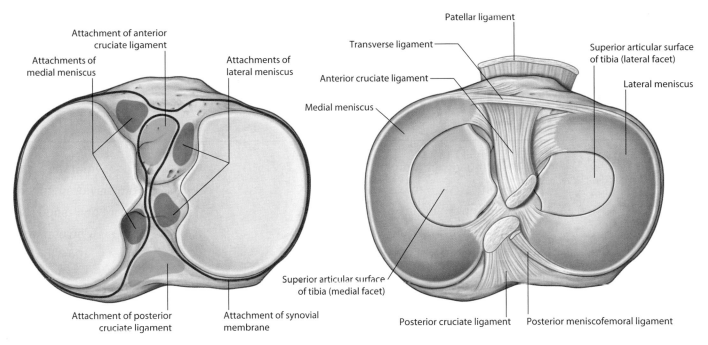

Attachment of anterior cruciate ligament

Attachments of medial meniscus

Attachments of lateral meniscus

Attachment of posterior cruciate ligament

Attachment of synovial membrane

**Attachments of menisci, cruciate ligaments, and synovial membrane of the right tibia.
(superior view)**

Patellar ligament

Transverse ligament

Anterior cruciate ligament

Medial meniscus

Superior articular surface of tibia (lateral facet)

Lateral meniscus

Superior articular surface of tibia (medial facet)

Posterior cruciate ligament

Posterior meniscofemoral ligament

**Menisci of the right knee joint.
(superior view)**

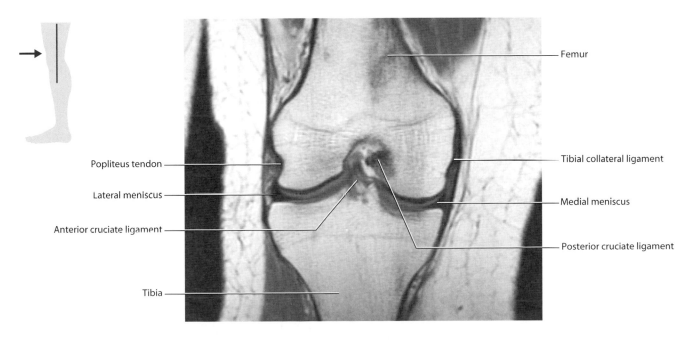

Femur

Popliteus tendon

Lateral meniscus

Anterior cruciate ligament

Tibia

Tibial collateral ligament

Medial meniscus

Posterior cruciate ligament

Anterior view of knee joint showing the anterior and posterior cruciate ligaments.
T2-weighted MR image in coronal plane

323

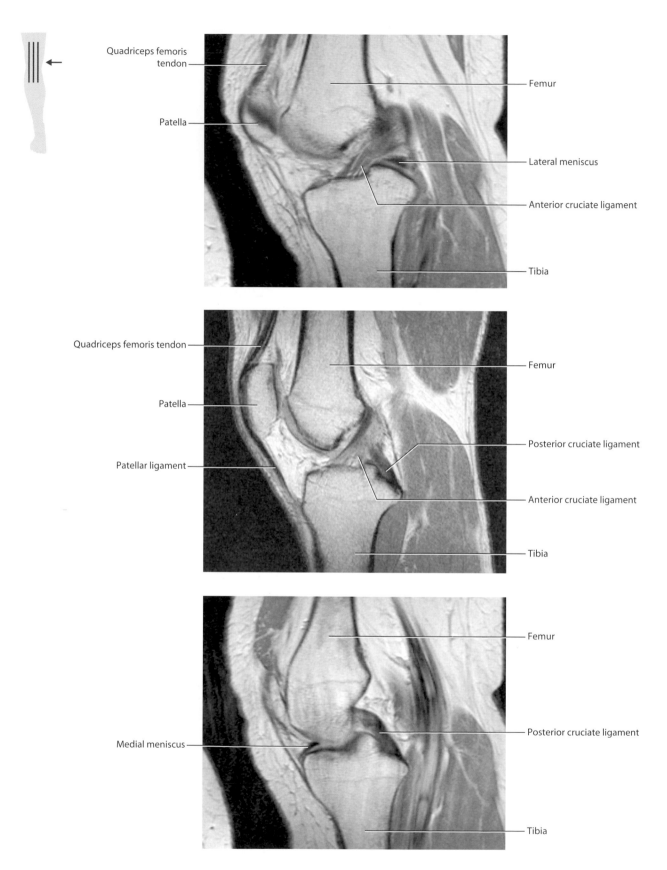

Quadriceps femoris tendon

Patella

Femur

Lateral meniscus

Anterior cruciate ligament

Tibia

Quadriceps femoris tendon

Patella

Patellar ligament

Femur

Posterior cruciate ligament

Anterior cruciate ligament

Tibia

Femur

Medial meniscus

Posterior cruciate ligament

Tibia

**A series of images moving from medial to lateral showing the relationship
between anterior and posterior cruciate ligaments.**
T2-weighted MR images in sagittal plane

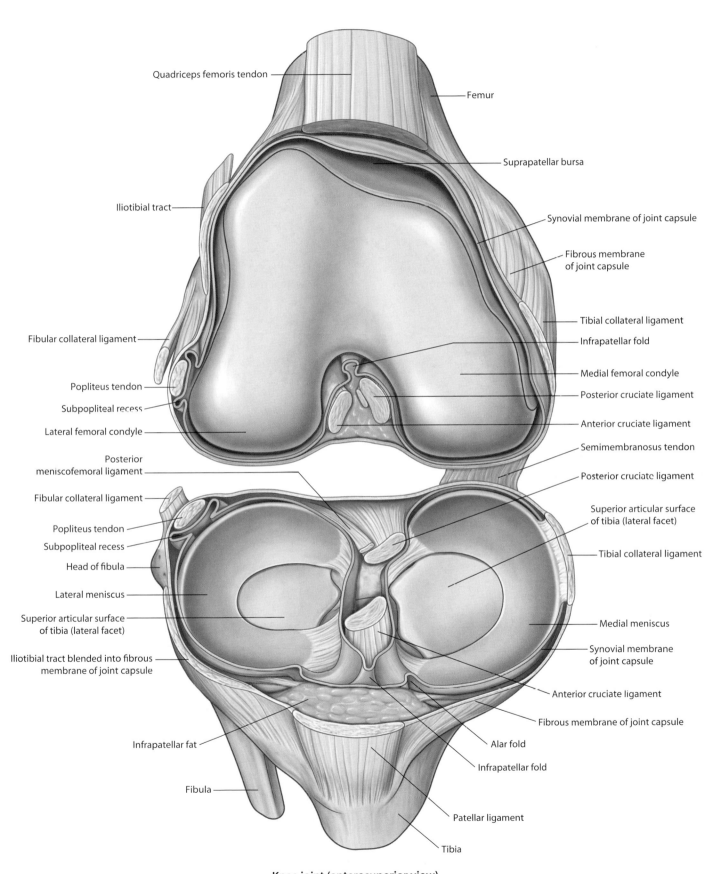

Quadriceps femoris tendon

Femur

Suprapatellar bursa

Iliotibial tract

Synovial membrane of joint capsule

Fibrous membrane
of joint capsule

Tibial collateral ligament

Infrapatellar fold

Fibular collateral ligament

Medial femoral condyle

Popliteus tendon

Posterior cruciate ligament

Subpopliteal recess

Anterior cruciate ligament

Lateral femoral condyle

Semimembranosus tendon

Posterior
meniscofemoral ligament

Posterior cruciate ligament

Fibular collateral ligament

Superior articular surface
of tibia (lateral facet)

Popliteus tendon

Subpopliteal recess

Tibial collateral ligament

Head of fibula

Lateral meniscus

Superior articular surface
of tibia (lateral facet)

Medial meniscus

Iliotibial tract blended into fibrous
membrane of joint capsule

Synovial membrane
of joint capsule

Anterior cruciate ligament

Fibrous membrane of joint capsule

Infrapatellar fat

Alar fold

Infrapatellar fold

Fibula

Patellar ligament

Tibia

Knee joint (anterosuperior view)

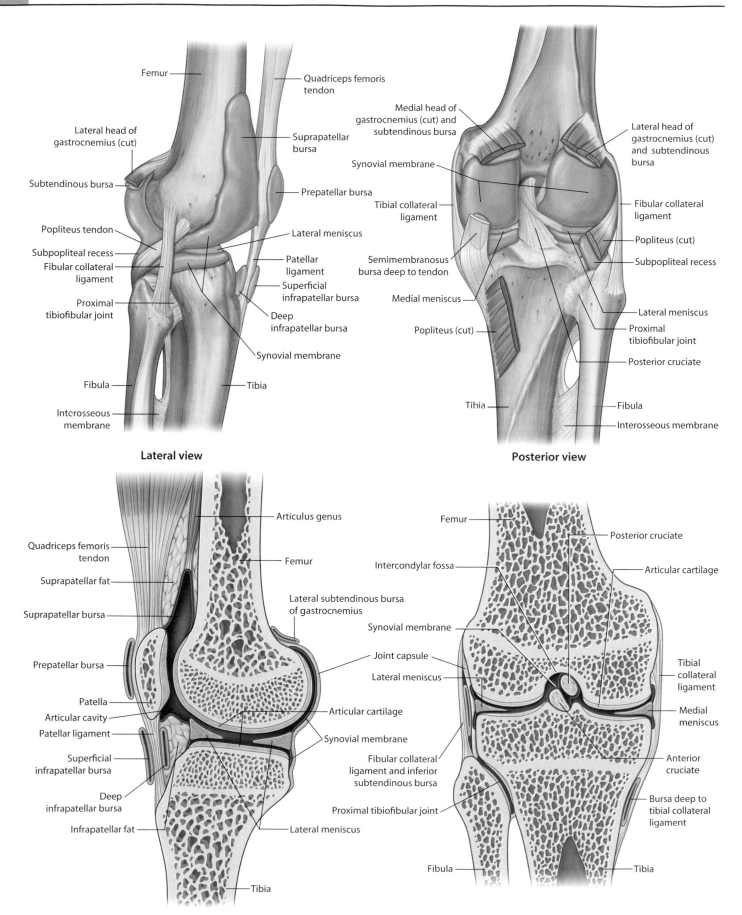

Femur

Quadriceps femoris
tendon

Lateral head of
gastrocnemius (cut)

Suprapatellar
bursa

Subtendinous bursa

Prepatellar bursa

Popliteus tendon

Lateral meniscus

Subpopliteal recess

Patellar
ligament

Fibular collateral
ligament

Superficial
infrapatellar bursa

Proximal
tibiofibular joint

Deep
infrapatellar bursa

Synovial membrane

Fibula

Tibia

Interosseous
membrane

Lateral view

Medial head of
gastrocnemius (cut) and
subtendinous bursa

Lateral head of
gastrocnemius (cut)
and subtendinous
bursa

Synovial membrane

Tibial collateral
ligament

Fibular collateral
ligament

Popliteus (cut)

Semimembranosus
bursa deep to tendon

Subpopliteal recess

Medial meniscus

Lateral meniscus

Popliteus (cut)

Proximal
tibiofibular joint

Posterior cruciate

Tibia

Fibula

Interosseous membrane

Posterior view

Quadriceps femoris
tendon

Articulus genus

Suprapatellar fat

Femur

Suprapatellar bursa

Lateral subtendinous bursa
of gastrocnemius

Prepatellar bursa

Patella

Articular cavity

Articular cartilage

Patellar ligament

Synovial membrane

Superficial
infrapatellar bursa

Deep
infrapatellar bursa

Infrapatellar fat

Lateral meniscus

Tibia

Paramedian section through knee joint

Femur

Posterior cruciate

Intercondylar fossa

Articular cartilage

Synovial membrane

Joint capsule

Tibial
collateral
ligament

Lateral meniscus

Medial
meniscus

Fibular collateral
ligament and inferior
subtendinous bursa

Anterior
cruciate

Proximal tibiofibular joint

Bursa deep to
tibial collateral
ligament

Fibula

Tibia

Coronal section through knee joint (anterior view)

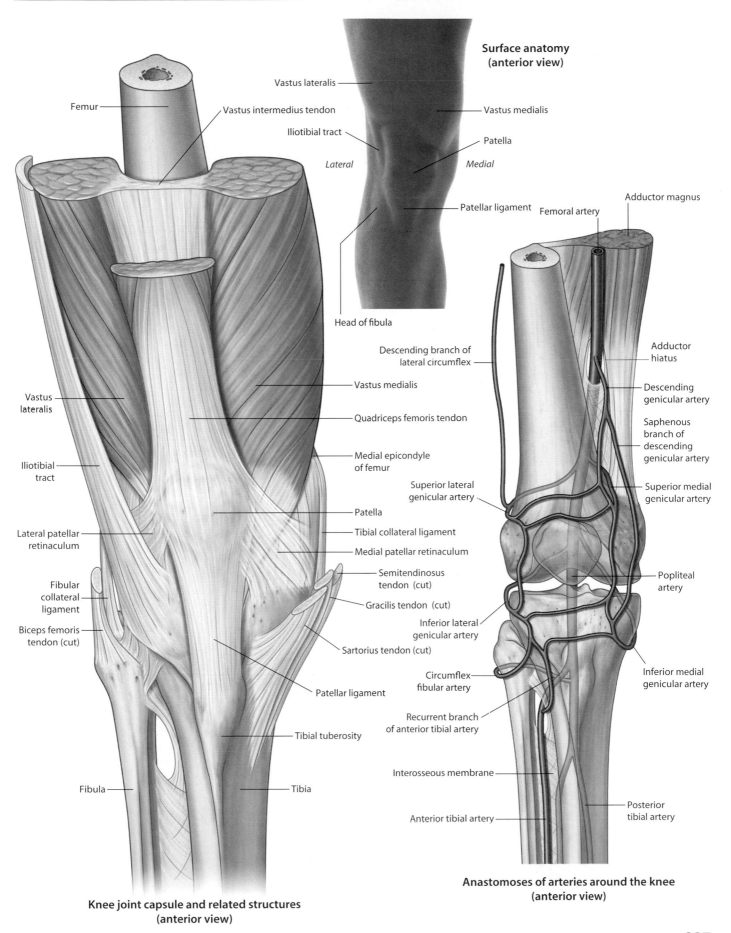

**Surface anatomy
(anterior view)**

Vastus lateralis

Vastus intermedius tendon

Iliotibial tract

Femur

Vastus medialis

Patella

Lateral

Medial

Patellar ligament

Femoral artery

Adductor magnus

Head of fibula

Descending branch of
lateral circumflex

Adductor
hiatus

Descending
genicular artery

Saphenous
branch of
descending
genicular artery

Superior medial
genicular artery

Vastus
lateralis

Vastus medialis

Quadriceps femoris tendon

Medial epicondyle
of femur

Iliotibial
tract

Patella

Tibial collateral ligament

Superior lateral
genicular artery

Popliteal
artery

Lateral patellar
retinaculum

Medial patellar retinaculum

Semitendinosus
tendon (cut)

Fibular
collateral
ligament

Gracilis tendon (cut)

Inferior lateral
genicular artery

Biceps femoris
tendon (cut)

Sartorius tendon (cut)

Inferior medial
genicular artery

Patellar ligament

Circumflex
fibular artery

Recurrent branch
of anterior tibial artery

Tibial tuberosity

Interosseous membrane

Fibula

Tibia

Posterior
tibial artery

Anterior tibial artery

**Anastomoses of arteries around the knee
(anterior view)**

**Knee joint capsule and related structures
(anterior view)**

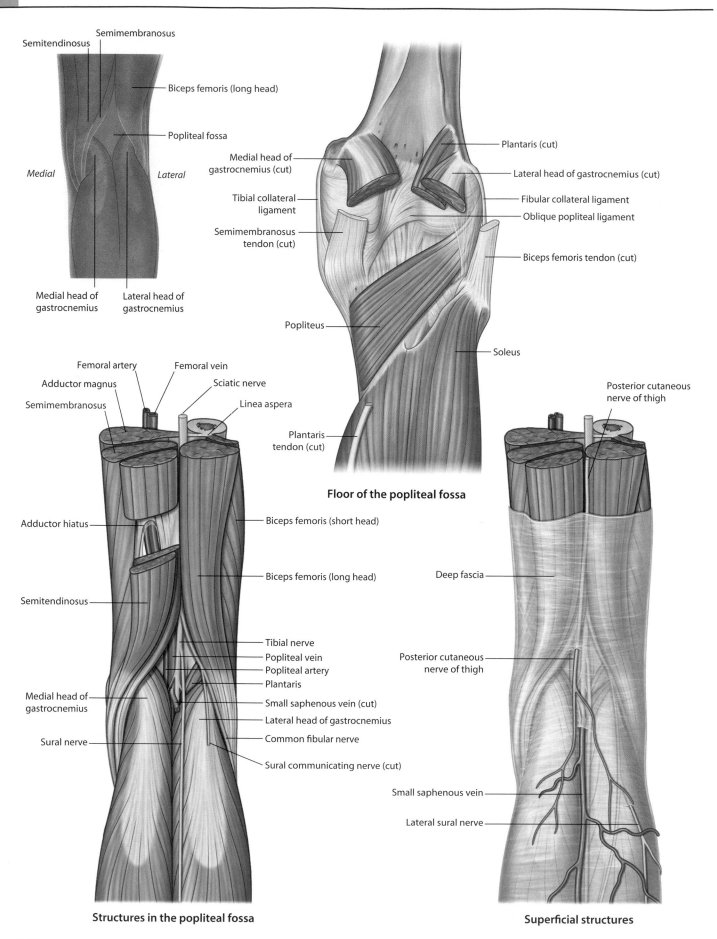

Semitendinosus

Semimembranosus

Biceps femoris (long head)

Popliteal fossa

Medial

Lateral

Medial head of gastrocnemius

Lateral head of gastrocnemius

Medial head of gastrocnemius (cut)

Plantaris (cut)

Lateral head of gastrocnemius (cut)

Tibial collateral ligament

Fibular collateral ligament

Oblique popliteal ligament

Semimembranosus tendon (cut)

Biceps femoris tendon (cut)

Popliteus

Soleus

Plantaris tendon (cut)

Floor of the popliteal fossa

Femoral artery

Femoral vein

Adductor magnus

Sciatic nerve

Semimembranosus

Linea aspera

Posterior cutaneous nerve of thigh

Adductor hiatus

Biceps femoris (short head)

Biceps femoris (long head)

Deep fascia

Semitendinosus

Tibial nerve

Popliteal vein

Popliteal artery

Plantaris

Posterior cutaneous nerve of thigh

Medial head of gastrocnemius

Small saphenous vein (cut)

Lateral head of gastrocnemius

Common fibular nerve

Sural nerve

Sural communicating nerve (cut)

Small saphenous vein

Lateral sural nerve

Structures in the popliteal fossa

Superficial structures

328

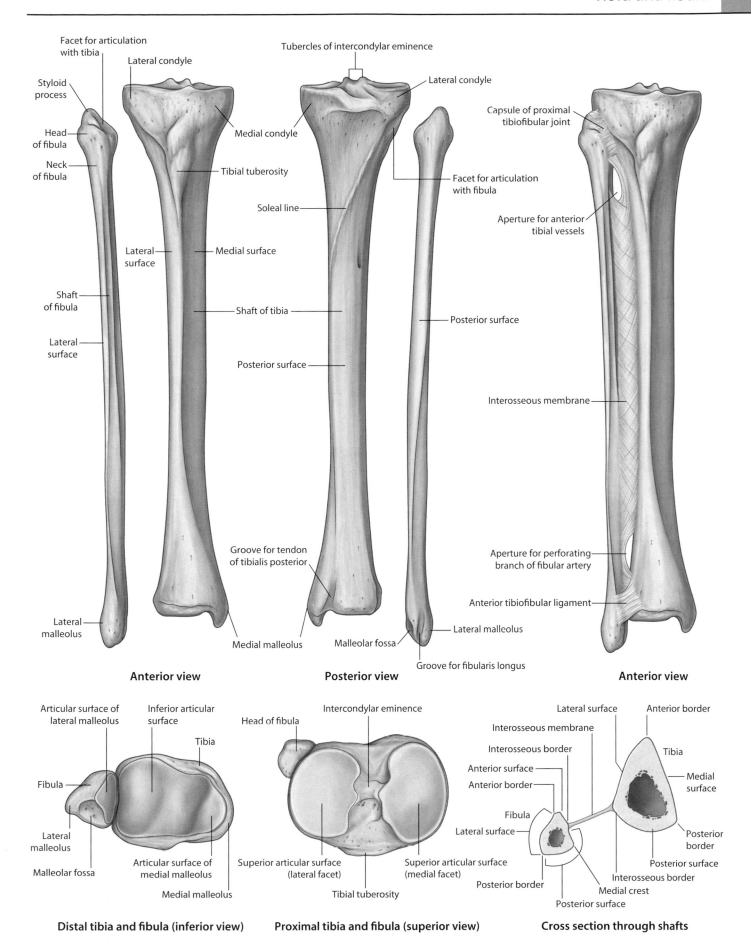

Facet for articulation with tibia

Lateral condyle

Styloid process

Head of fibula

Neck of fibula

Medial condyle

Tibial tuberosity

Lateral surface

Medial surface

Shaft of fibula

Shaft of tibia

Lateral surface

Posterior surface

Lateral malleolus

Medial malleolus

Anterior view

Tubercles of intercondylar eminence

Lateral condyle

Facet for articulation with fibula

Soleal line

Posterior surface

Groove for tendon of tibialis posterior

Malleolar fossa

Lateral malleolus

Groove for fibularis longus

Posterior view

Capsule of proximal tibiofibular joint

Aperture for anterior tibial vessels

Interosseous membrane

Aperture for perforating branch of fibular artery

Anterior tibiofibular ligament

Anterior view

Articular surface of lateral malleolus

Inferior articular surface

Tibia

Fibula

Lateral malleolus

Malleolar fossa

Articular surface of medial malleolus

Medial malleolus

Distal tibia and fibula (inferior view)

Head of fibula

Intercondylar eminence

Superior articular surface (lateral facet)

Tibial tuberosity

Superior articular surface (medial facet)

Proximal tibia and fibula (superior view)

Lateral surface

Anterior border

Interosseous membrane

Interosseous border

Anterior surface

Anterior border

Tibia

Medial surface

Fibula

Lateral surface

Posterior border

Posterior surface

Interosseous border

Posterior surface

Medial crest

Posterior border

Cross section through shafts

329

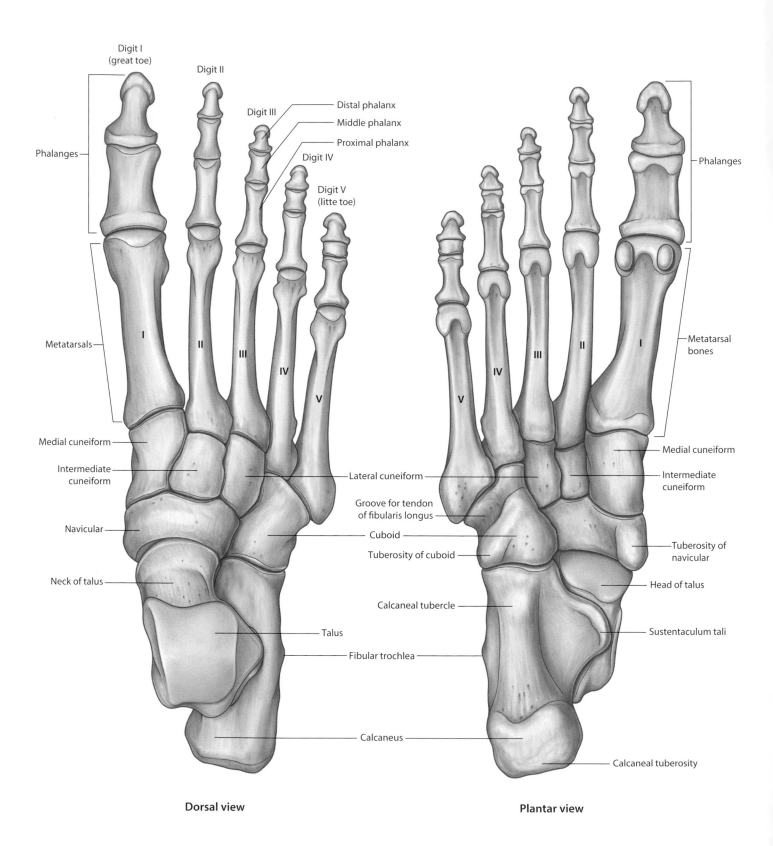

Digit I
(great toe)

Digit II

Digit III

Distal phalanx

Middle phalanx

Proximal phalanx

Digit IV

Phalanges

Digit V
(litte toe)

Phalanges

Metatarsals

Metatarsal
bones

Medial cuneiform

Intermediate
cuneiform

Medial cuneiform

Intermediate
cuneiform

Navicular

Lateral cuneiform

Groove for tendon
of fibularis longus

Cuboid

Tuberosity of cuboid

Tuberosity of
navicular

Neck of talus

Head of talus

Talus

Calcaneal tubercle

Sustentaculum tali

Fibular trochlea

Calcaneus

Calcaneal tuberosity

Dorsal view

Plantar view

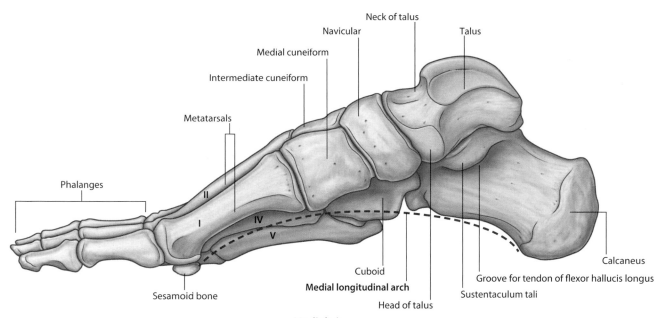

Medial cuneiform
Intermediate cuneiform
Metatarsals
Navicular
Neck of talus
Talus
Phalanges
II
I
IV
V
Sesamoid bone
Cuboid
Medial longitudinal arch
Head of talus
Groove for tendon of flexor hallucis longus
Sustentaculum tali
Calcaneus

Medial view

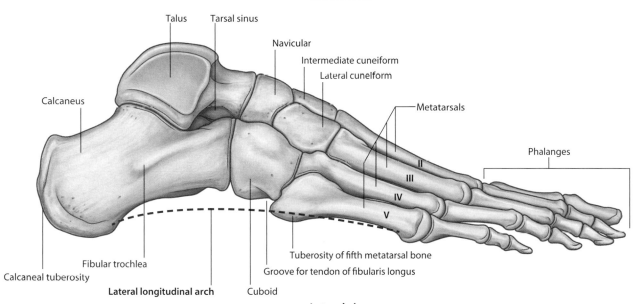

Talus
Tarsal sinus
Navicular
Intermediate cuneiform
Lateral cunelform
Metatarsals
Calcaneus
Phalanges
II
III
IV
V
Calcaneal tuberosity
Fibular trochlea
Lateral longitudinal arch
Cuboid
Groove for tendon of fibularis longus
Tuberosity of fifth metatarsal bone

Lateral view

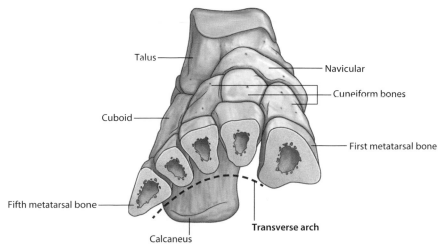

Talus
Navicular
Cuneiform bones
First metatarsal bone
Cuboid
Fifth metatarsal bone
Calcaneus
Transverse arch

Cross section through the foot bones

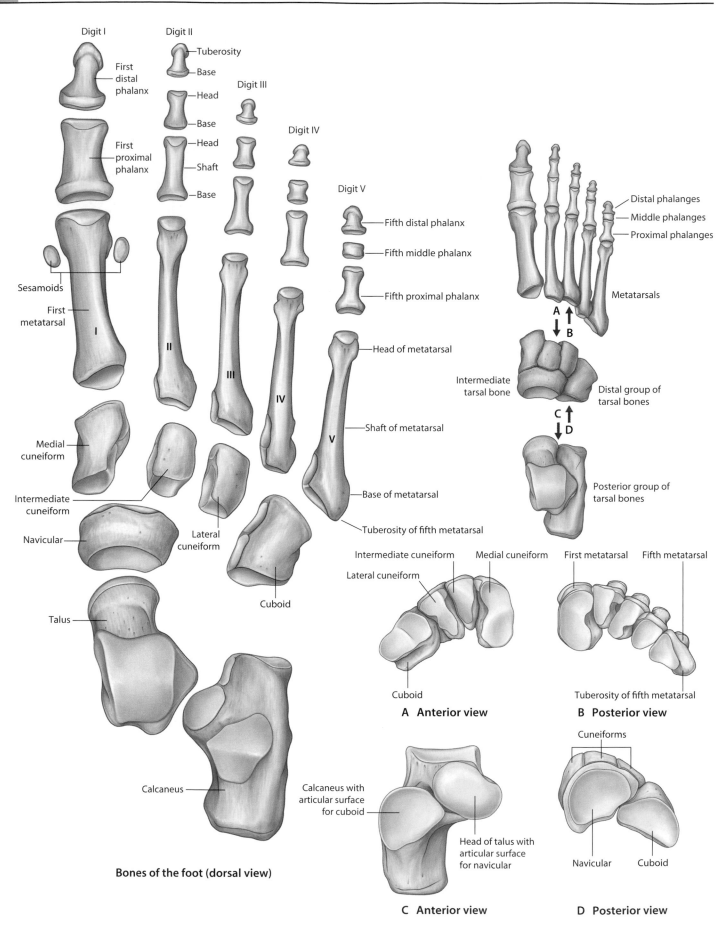

Digit I

First distal phalanx

First proximal phalanx

Sesamoids

First metatarsal

I

Medial cuneiform

Intermediate cuneiform

Navicular

Talus

Calcaneus

Digit II
Tuberosity
Base
Head
Base
Head
Shaft
Base

II

Digit III
Head

III

Lateral cuneiform

Cuboid

Digit IV

IV

Digit V
Fifth distal phalanx
Fifth middle phalanx
Fifth proximal phalanx

V

Head of metatarsal

Shaft of metatarsal

Base of metatarsal

Tuberosity of fifth metatarsal

Distal phalanges
Middle phalanges
Proximal phalanges

Metatarsals

A
B

Intermediate tarsal bone

Distal group of tarsal bones

C
D

Posterior group of tarsal bones

Bones of the foot (dorsal view)

Intermediate cuneiform   Medial cuneiform   First metatarsal   Fifth metatarsal

Lateral cuneiform

Cuboid

A Anterior view

Tuberosity of fifth metatarsal

B Posterior view

Calcaneus with articular surface for cuboid

Head of talus with articular surface for navicular

C Anterior view

Cuneiforms

Navicular   Cuboid

D Posterior view

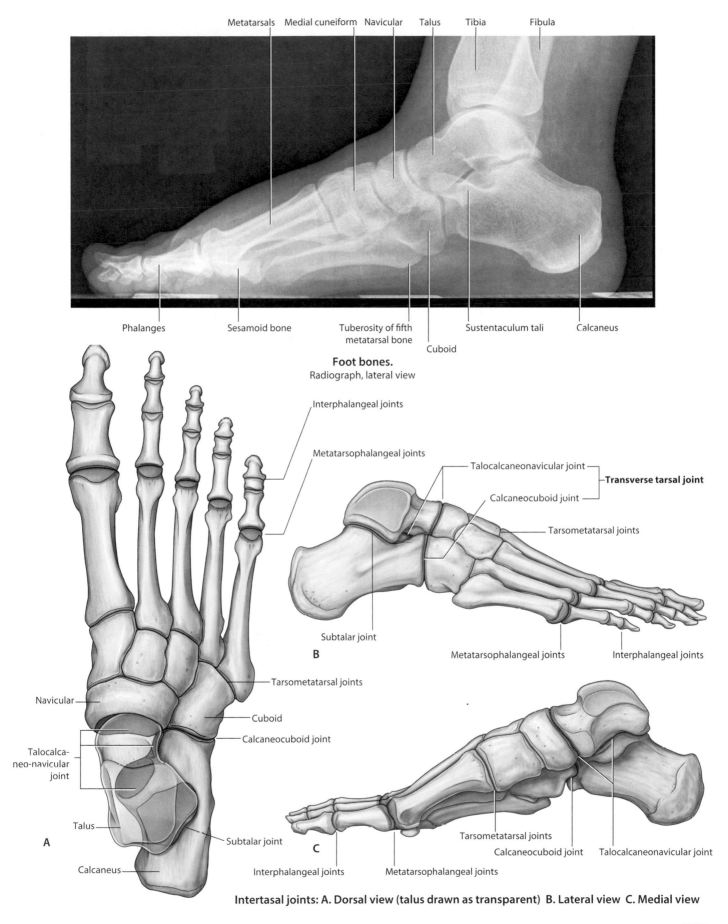

Metatarsals Medial cuneiform Navicular Talus Tibia Fibula

Phalanges Sesamoid bone Tuberosity of fifth metatarsal bone Cuboid Sustentaculum tali Calcaneus

Foot bones.
Radiograph, lateral view

Interphalangeal joints

Metatarsophalangeal joints

Talocalcaneonavicular joint —
Calcaneocuboid joint —
Transverse tarsal joint
Tarsometatarsal joints

Subtalar joint

B

Metatarsophalangeal joints   Interphalangeal joints

Navicular

Tarsometatarsal joints

Cuboid

Calcaneocuboid joint

Talocalca-
neo-navicular
joint

Talus

Subtalar joint

A

Calcaneus

C

Interphalangeal joints   Metatarsophalangeal joints

Tarsometatarsal joints

Calcaneocuboid joint   Talocalcaneonavicular joint

Intertasal joints: A. Dorsal view (talus drawn as transparent) B. Lateral view C. Medial view

333

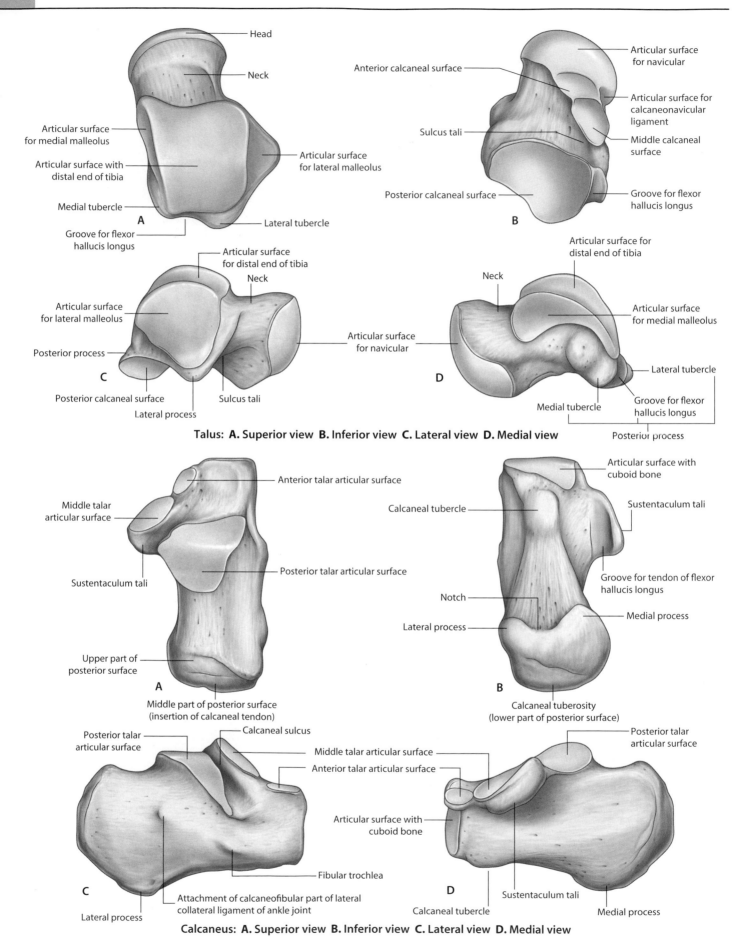

Head

Neck

Articular surface for medial malleolus

Articular surface with distal end of tibia

Medial tubercle

A

Groove for flexor hallucis longus

Articular surface for lateral malleolus

Lateral tubercle

Anterior calcaneal surface

Sulcus tali

Posterior calcaneal surface

B

Articular surface for navicular

Articular surface for calcaneonavicular ligament

Middle calcaneal surface

Groove for flexor hallucis longus

Articular surface for distal end of tibia

Neck

Articular surface for lateral malleolus

Posterior process

C

Posterior calcaneal surface

Lateral process

Sulcus tali

Articular surface for navicular

Articular surface for distal end of tibia

Neck

Articular surface for medial malleolus

Lateral tubercle

Groove for flexor hallucis longus

D

Medial tubercle

Posterior process

Talus: A. Superior view B. Inferior view C. Lateral view D. Medial view

Middle talar articular surface

Sustentaculum tali

Upper part of posterior surface

A

Middle part of posterior surface (insertion of calcaneal tendon)

Anterior talar articular surface

Posterior talar articular surface

Calcaneal tubercle

Notch

Lateral process

B

Calcaneal tuberosity (lower part of posterior surface)

Articular surface with cuboid bone

Sustentaculum tali

Groove for tendon of flexor hallucis longus

Medial process

Posterior talar articular surface

Calcaneal sulcus

Middle talar articular surface

Anterior talar articular surface

Articular surface with cuboid bone

C

Lateral process

Fibular trochlea

Attachment of calcaneofibular part of lateral collateral ligament of ankle joint

Posterior talar articular surface

D

Calcaneal tubercle

Sustentaculum tali

Medial process

Calcaneus: A. Superior view B. Inferior view C. Lateral view D. Medial view

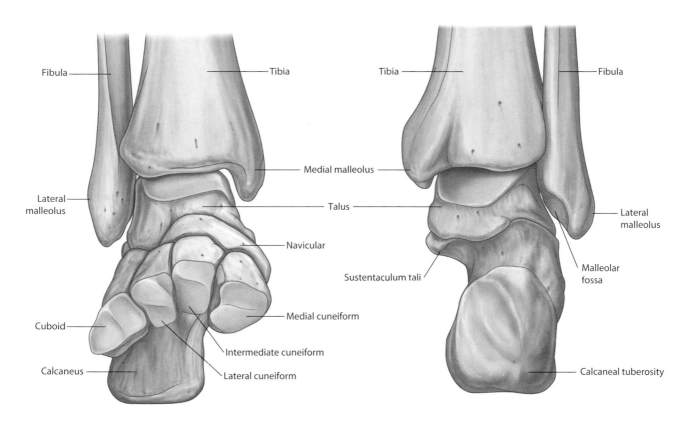

Fibula

Tibia

Medial malleolus

Lateral malleolus

Talus

Navicular

Cuboid

Medial cuneiform

Calcaneus

Intermediate cuneiform

Lateral cuneiform

Anterior view
(metatarsals and phalanges removed)

Tibia

Fibula

Medial malleolus

Talus

Lateral malleolus

Sustentaculum tali

Malleolar fossa

Calcaneal tuberosity

Posterior view

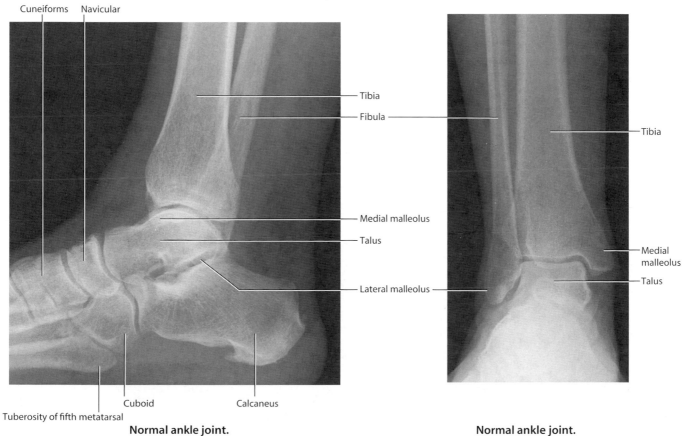

Cuneiforms   Navicular

Tibia

Fibula

Medial malleolus

Talus

Lateral malleolus

Tibia

Medial malleolus

Talus

Tuberosity of fifth metatarsal

Cuboid

Calcaneus

Normal ankle joint.
Radiograph, lateral view

Normal ankle joint.
Radiograph, AP view

335

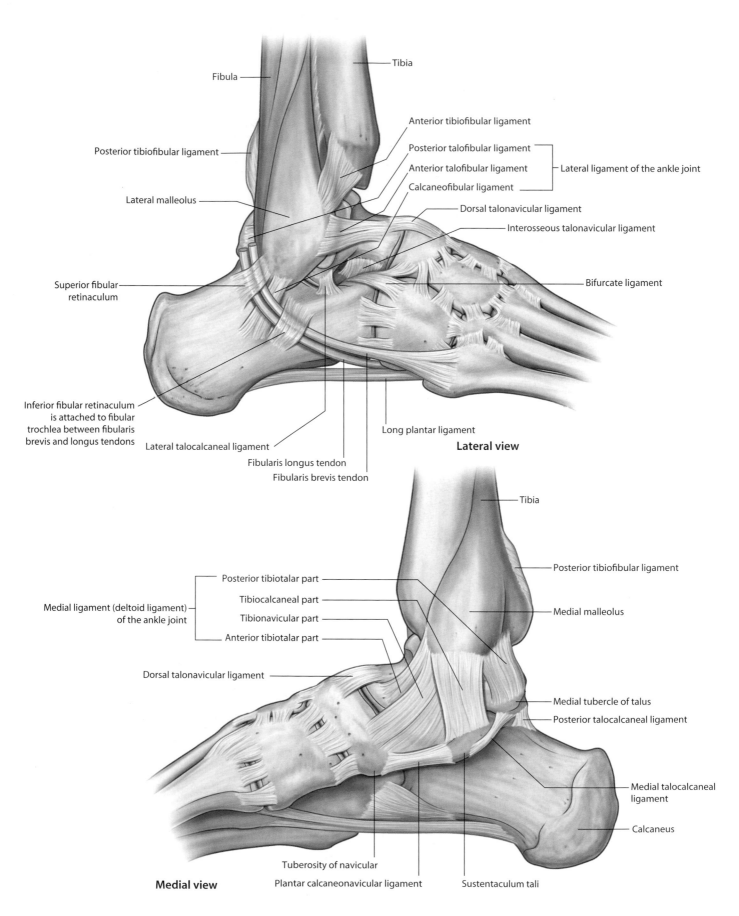

Fibula

Tibia

Posterior tibiofibular ligament

Anterior tibiofibular ligament

Posterior talofibular ligament

Anterior talofibular ligament

Calcaneofibular ligament

Lateral ligament of the ankle joint

Lateral malleolus

Dorsal talonavicular ligament

Interosseous talonavicular ligament

Superior fibular retinaculum

Bifurcate ligament

Inferior fibular retinaculum is attached to fibular trochlea between fibularis brevis and longus tendons

Lateral talocalcaneal ligament

Fibularis longus tendon

Fibularis brevis tendon

Long plantar ligament

Lateral view

Tibia

Posterior tibiofibular ligament

Posterior tibiotalar part

Tibiocalcaneal part

Tibionavicular part

Anterior tibiotalar part

Medial ligament (deltoid ligament) of the ankle joint

Medial malleolus

Dorsal talonavicular ligament

Medial tubercle of talus

Posterior talocalcaneal ligament

Medial talocalcaneal ligament

Calcaneus

Medial view

Tuberosity of navicular

Plantar calcaneonavicular ligament

Sustentaculum tali

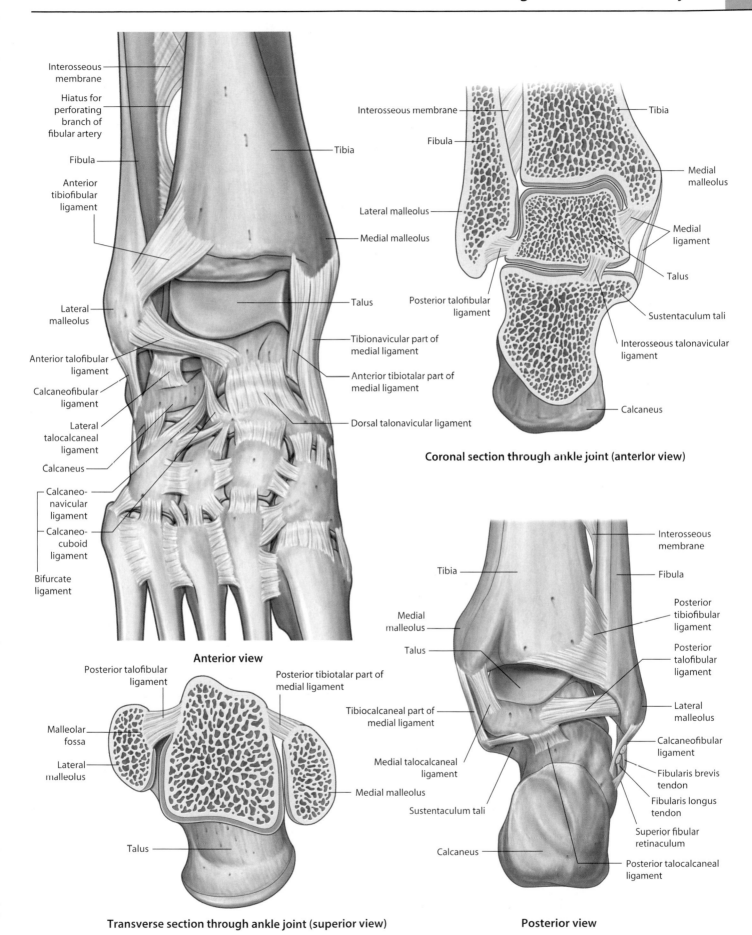

Interosseous membrane

Hiatus for perforating branch of fibular artery

Fibula

Anterior tibiofibular ligament

Lateral malleolus

Anterior talofibular ligament

Calcaneofibular ligament

Lateral talocalcaneal ligament

Calcaneus

Calcaneonavicular ligament

Calcaneocuboid ligament

Bifurcate ligament

Tibia

Talus

Tibionavicular part of medial ligament

Anterior tibiotalar part of medial ligament

Dorsal talonavicular ligament

Anterior view

Interosseous membrane

Fibula

Lateral malleolus

Posterior talofibular ligament

Tibia

Medial malleolus

Medial ligament

Talus

Sustentaculum tali

Interosseous talonavicular ligament

Calcaneus

Coronal section through ankle joint (anterior view)

Posterior talofibular ligament

Malleolar fossa

Lateral malleolus

Talus

Posterior tibiotalar part of medial ligament

Medial malleolus

Transverse section through ankle joint (superior view)

Tibia

Medial malleolus

Talus

Tibiocalcaneal part of medial ligament

Medial talocalcaneal ligament

Sustentaculum tali

Calcaneus

Interosseous membrane

Fibula

Posterior tibiofibular ligament

Posterior talofibular ligament

Lateral malleolus

Calcaneofibular ligament

Fibularis brevis tendon

Fibularis longus tendon

Superior fibular retinaculum

Posterior talocalcaneal ligament

Posterior view

337

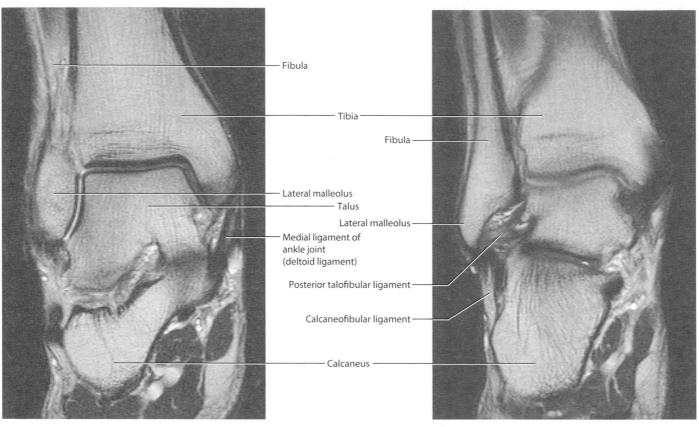

Fibula

Tibia

Fibula

Lateral malleolus

Talus

Lateral malleolus

Medial ligament of
ankle joint
(deltoid ligament)

Posterior talofibular ligament

Calcaneofibular ligament

Calcaneus

**Coronal view of the ankle joint showing the medial
ligament of the ankle joint (deltoid ligament).**
T2-weighted MR image in coronal plane

**Coronal view of the ankle joint showing the
posterior talofibular and calcaneofibular ligaments.**
T2-weighted MR image in coronal plane

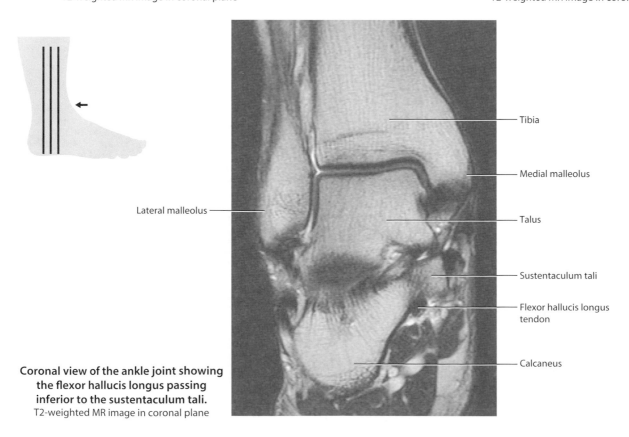

Tibia

Medial malleolus

Lateral malleolus

Talus

Sustentaculum tali

Flexor hallucis longus
tendon

Calcaneus

**Coronal view of the ankle joint showing
the flexor hallucis longus passing
inferior to the sustentaculum tali.**
T2-weighted MR image in coronal plane

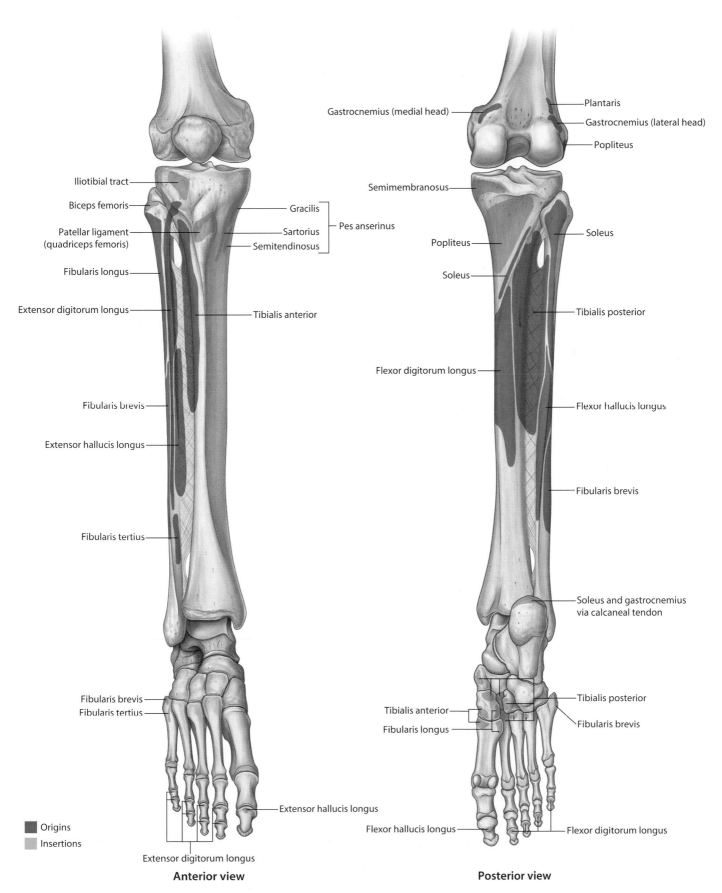

Gastrocnemius (medial head)
Plantaris
Gastrocnemius (lateral head)
Popliteus
Semimembranosus
Soleus
Popliteus
Soleus
Tibialis posterior
Flexor digitorum longus
Flexor hallucis longus
Fibularis brevis
Soleus and gastrocnemius via calcaneal tendon
Tibialis posterior
Tibialis anterior
Fibularis longus
Fibularis brevis
Flexor hallucis longus
Flexor digitorum longus

Iliotibial tract
Biceps femoris
Gracilis
Patellar ligament (quadriceps femoris)
Sartorius
Pes anserinus
Semitendinosus
Fibularis longus
Extensor digitorum longus
Tibialis anterior
Fibularis brevis
Extensor hallucis longus
Fibularis tertius
Fibularis brevis
Fibularis tertius
Extensor hallucis longus
Extensor digitorum longus

■ Origins
■ Insertions

Anterior view

Posterior view

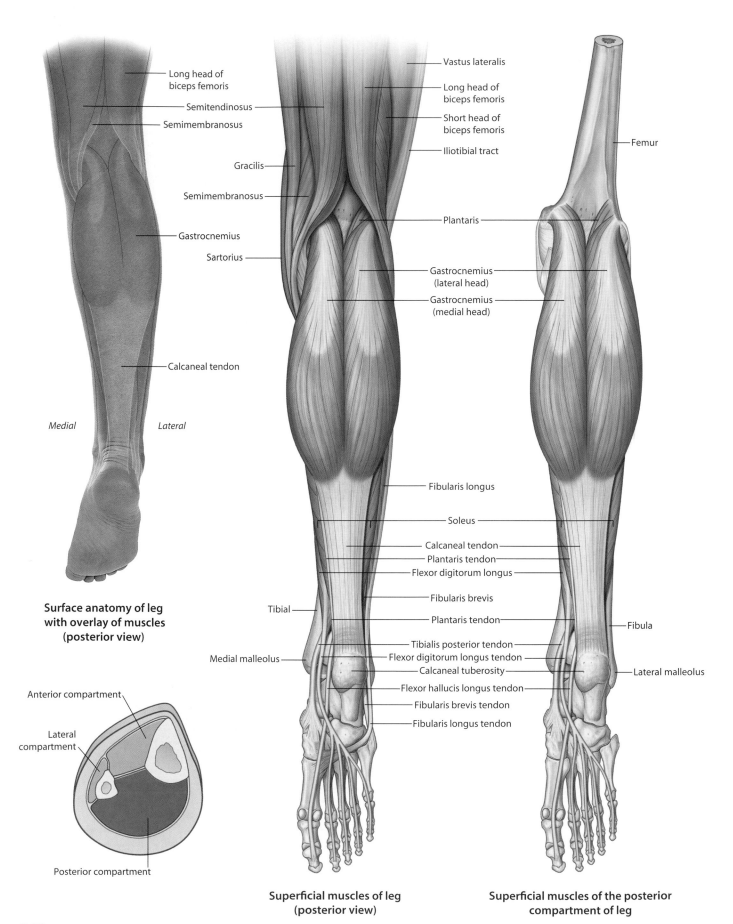

Long head of
biceps femoris

Semitendinosus

Semimembranosus

Gracilis

Semimembranosus

Gastrocnemius

Sartorius

Calcaneal tendon

Medial　　*Lateral*

**Surface anatomy of leg
with overlay of muscles
(posterior view)**

Anterior compartment

Lateral
compartment

Posterior compartment

Vastus lateralis

Long head of
biceps femoris

Short head of
biceps femoris

Iliotibial tract

Plantaris

Gastrocnemius
(lateral head)

Gastrocnemius
(medial head)

Fibularis longus

Soleus

Calcaneal tendon

Plantaris tendon

Flexor digitorum longus

Fibularis brevis

Tibial

Plantaris tendon

Tibialis posterior tendon

Medial malleolus

Flexor digitorum longus tendon

Calcaneal tuberosity

Flexor hallucis longus tendon

Fibularis brevis tendon

Fibularis longus tendon

**Superficial muscles of leg
(posterior view)**

Femur

Fibula

Lateral malleolus

**Superficial muscles of the posterior
compartment of leg**

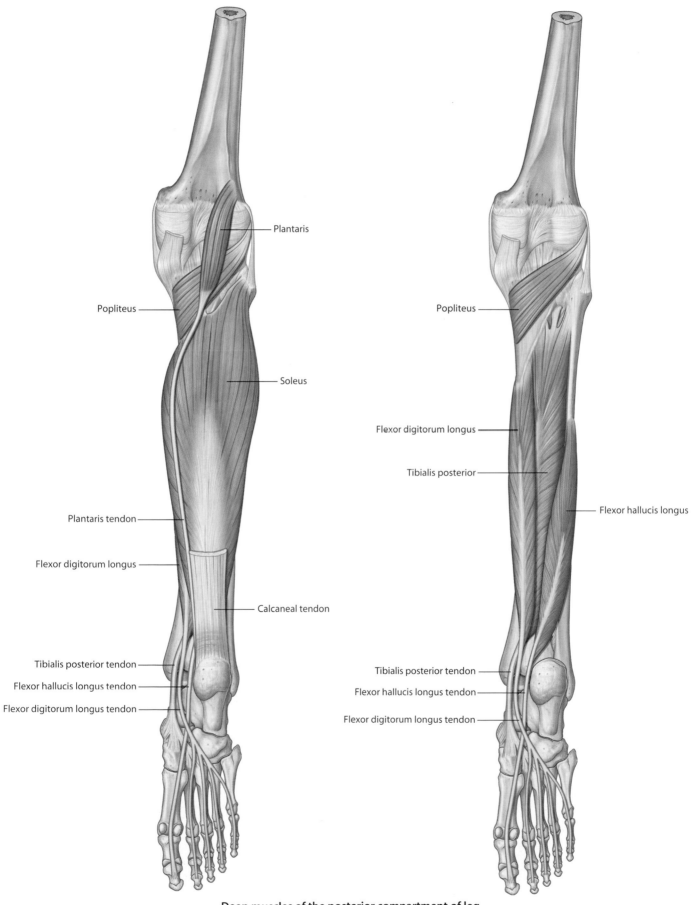

Plantaris

Popliteus

Soleus

Popliteus

Flexor digitorum longus

Tibialis posterior

Flexor hallucis longus

Plantaris tendon

Flexor digitorum longus

Calcaneal tendon

Tibialis posterior tendon

Flexor hallucis longus tendon

Flexor digitorum longus tendon

Tibialis posterior tendon

Flexor hallucis longus tendon

Flexor digitorum longus tendon

Deep muscles of the posterior compartment of leg

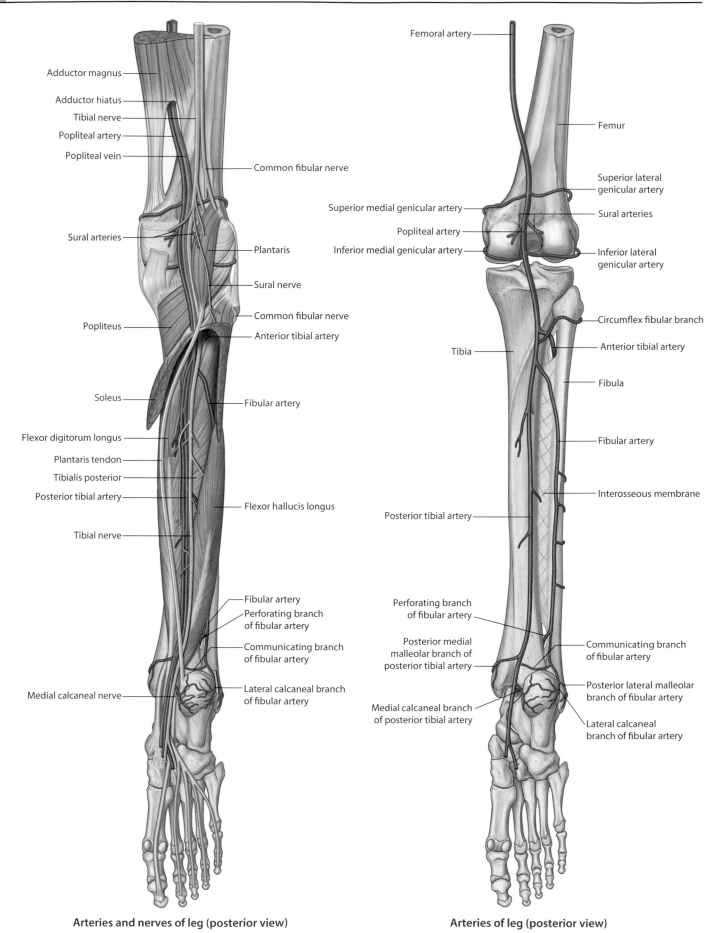

Adductor magnus

Adductor hiatus

Tibial nerve

Popliteal artery

Popliteal vein

Common fibular nerve

Sural arteries

Plantaris

Sural nerve

Common fibular nerve

Popliteus

Anterior tibial artery

Soleus

Fibular artery

Flexor digitorum longus

Plantaris tendon

Tibialis posterior

Posterior tibial artery

Flexor hallucis longus

Tibial nerve

Fibular artery

Perforating branch
of fibular artery

Communicating branch
of fibular artery

Medial calcaneal nerve

Lateral calcaneal branch
of fibular artery

Femoral artery

Femur

Superior lateral
genicular artery

Superior medial genicular artery

Sural arteries

Popliteal artery

Inferior medial genicular artery

Inferior lateral
genicular artery

Circumflex fibular branch

Anterior tibial artery

Tibia

Fibula

Fibular artery

Interosseous membrane

Posterior tibial artery

Perforating branch
of fibular artery

Communicating branch
of fibular artery

Posterior medial
malleolar branch of
posterior tibial artery

Medial calcaneal branch
of posterior tibial artery

Posterior lateral malleolar
branch of fibular artery

Lateral calcaneal
branch of fibular artery

Arteries and nerves of leg (posterior view)

Arteries of leg (posterior view)

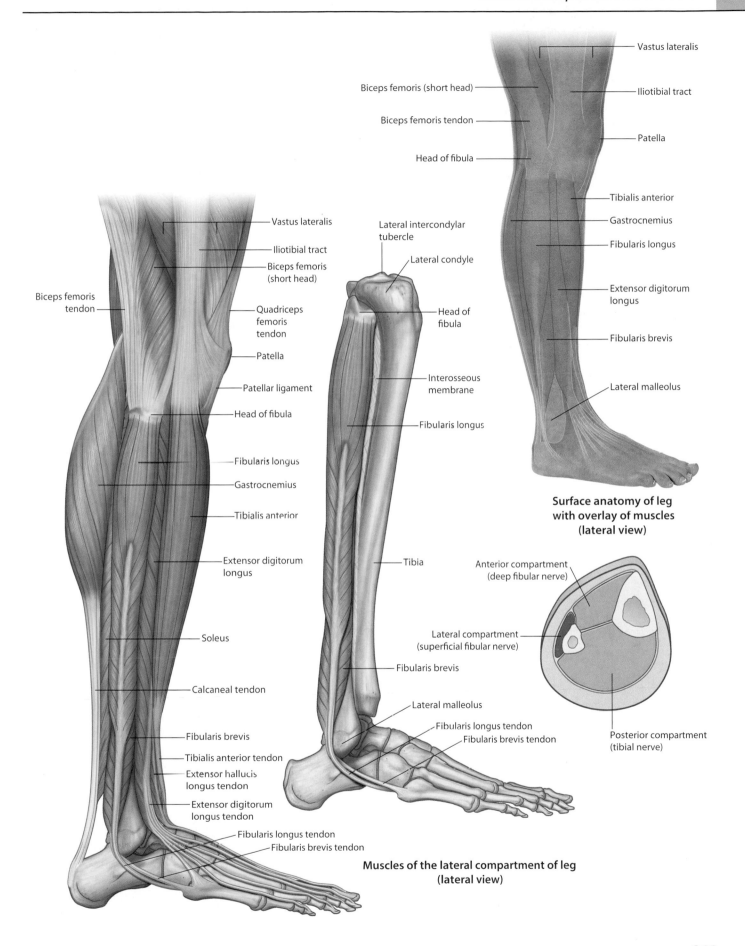

Vastus lateralis

Biceps femoris (short head)

Iliotibial tract

Biceps femoris tendon

Patella

Head of fibula

Tibialis anterior

Gastrocnemius

Fibularis longus

Extensor digitorum longus

Fibularis brevis

Lateral malleolus

**Surface anatomy of leg
with overlay of muscles
(lateral view)**

Vastus lateralis

Iliotibial tract

Biceps femoris
(short head)

Biceps femoris
tendon

Quadriceps
femoris
tendon

Patella

Patellar ligament

Head of fibula

Fibularis longus

Gastrocnemius

Tibialis anterior

Extensor digitorum
longus

Soleus

Calcaneal tendon

Fibularis brevis

Tibialis anterior tendon

Extensor hallucis
longus tendon

Extensor digitorum
longus tendon

Fibularis longus tendon
Fibularis brevis tendon

Lateral intercondylar
tubercle

Lateral condyle

Head of
fibula

Interosseous
membrane

Fibularis longus

Tibia

Fibularis brevis

Lateral malleolus

Fibularis longus tendon
Fibularis brevis tendon

**Muscles of the lateral compartment of leg
(lateral view)**

Anterior compartment
(deep fibular nerve)

Lateral compartment
(superficial fibular nerve)

Posterior compartment
(tibial nerve)

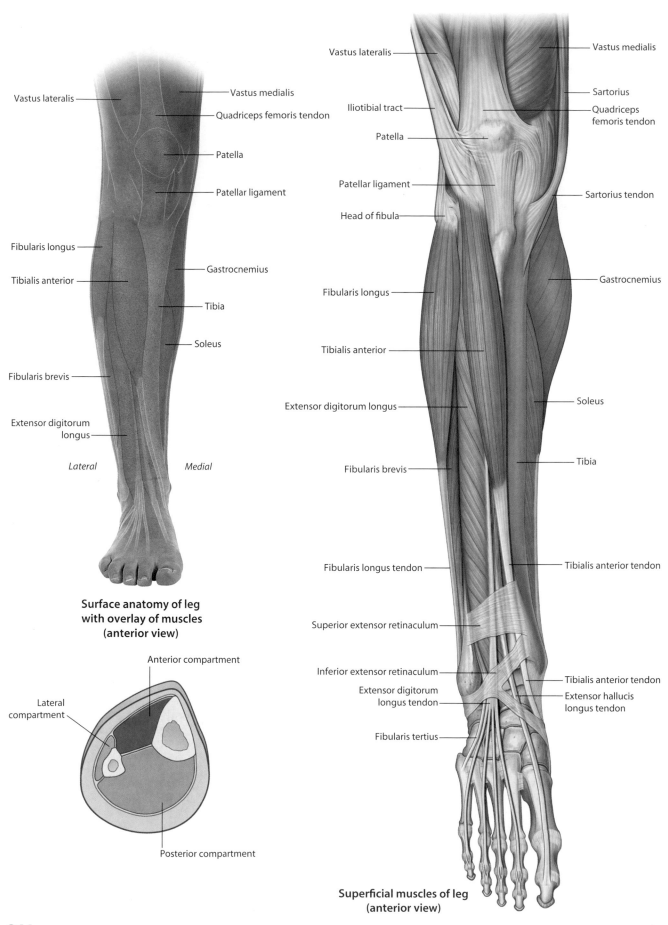

Vastus lateralis

Vastus medialis

Quadriceps femoris tendon

Patella

Patellar ligament

Fibularis longus

Tibialis anterior

Gastrocnemius

Tibia

Soleus

Fibularis brevis

Extensor digitorum longus

Lateral

Medial

Surface anatomy of leg with overlay of muscles (anterior view)

Anterior compartment

Lateral compartment

Posterior compartment

Vastus lateralis

Vastus medialis

Iliotibial tract

Sartorius

Patella

Quadriceps femoris tendon

Patellar ligament

Head of fibula

Sartorius tendon

Fibularis longus

Gastrocnemius

Tibialis anterior

Extensor digitorum longus

Soleus

Fibularis brevis

Tibia

Fibularis longus tendon

Tibialis anterior tendon

Superior extensor retinaculum

Inferior extensor retinaculum

Extensor digitorum longus tendon

Tibialis anterior tendon

Extensor hallucis longus tendon

Fibularis tertius

Superficial muscles of leg (anterior view)

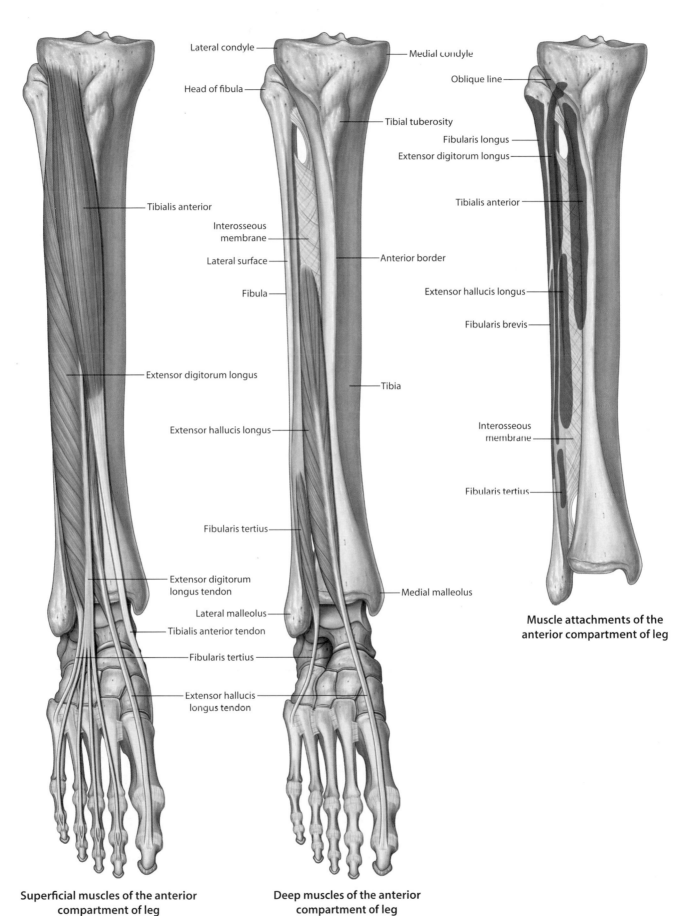

Lateral condyle

Head of fibula

Medial condyle

Oblique line

Tibial tuberosity

Fibularis longus

Extensor digitorum longus

Tibialis anterior

Tibialis anterior

Interosseous membrane

Lateral surface

Anterior border

Extensor hallucis longus

Fibula

Fibularis brevis

Extensor digitorum longus

Tibia

Extensor hallucis longus

Interosseous membrane

Fibularis tertius

Fibularis tertius

Extensor digitorum longus tendon

Medial malleolus

Lateral malleolus

Tibialis anterior tendon

Fibularis tertius

Extensor hallucis longus tendon

Muscle attachments of the anterior compartment of leg

Superficial muscles of the anterior compartment of leg

Deep muscles of the anterior compartment of leg

345

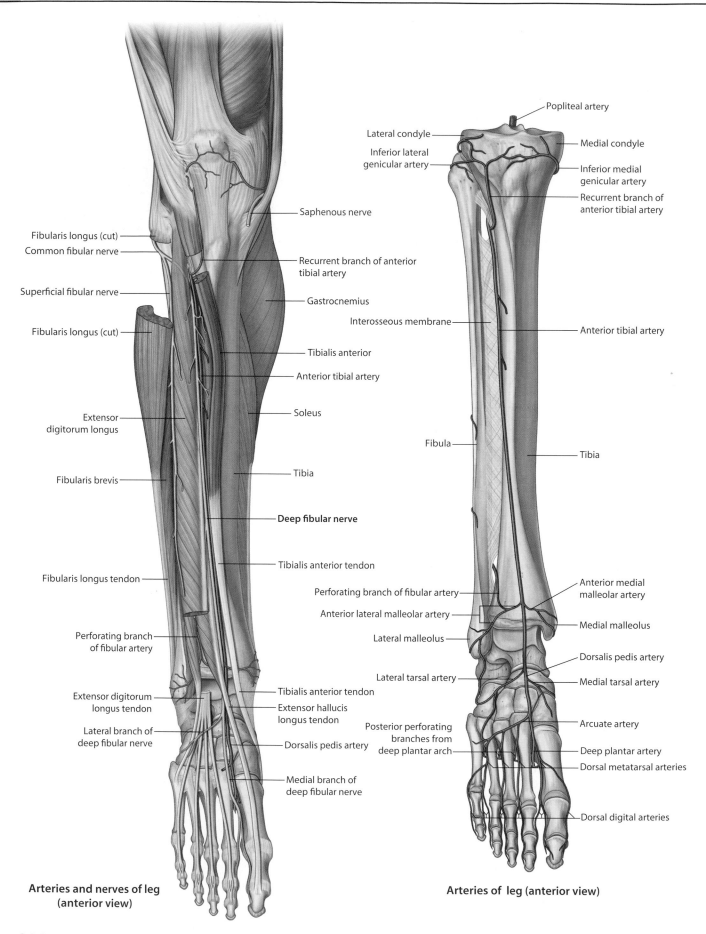

Fibularis longus (cut)

Common fibular nerve

Superficial fibular nerve

Fibularis longus (cut)

Extensor digitorum longus

Fibularis brevis

Fibularis longus tendon

Perforating branch of fibular artery

Extensor digitorum longus tendon

Lateral branch of deep fibular nerve

Saphenous nerve

Recurrent branch of anterior tibial artery

Gastrocnemius

Tibialis anterior

Anterior tibial artery

Soleus

Tibia

Deep fibular nerve

Tibialis anterior tendon

Tibialis anterior tendon

Extensor hallucis longus tendon

Dorsalis pedis artery

Medial branch of deep fibular nerve

Arteries and nerves of leg (anterior view)

Popliteal artery

Lateral condyle

Inferior lateral genicular artery

Medial condyle

Inferior medial genicular artery

Recurrent branch of anterior tibial artery

Interosseous membrane

Anterior tibial artery

Fibula

Tibia

Perforating branch of fibular artery

Anterior lateral malleolar artery

Lateral malleolus

Lateral tarsal artery

Posterior perforating branches from deep plantar arch

Anterior medial malleolar artery

Medial malleolus

Dorsalis pedis artery

Medial tarsal artery

Arcuate artery

Deep plantar artery

Dorsal metatarsal arteries

Dorsal digital arteries

Arteries of leg (anterior view)

346

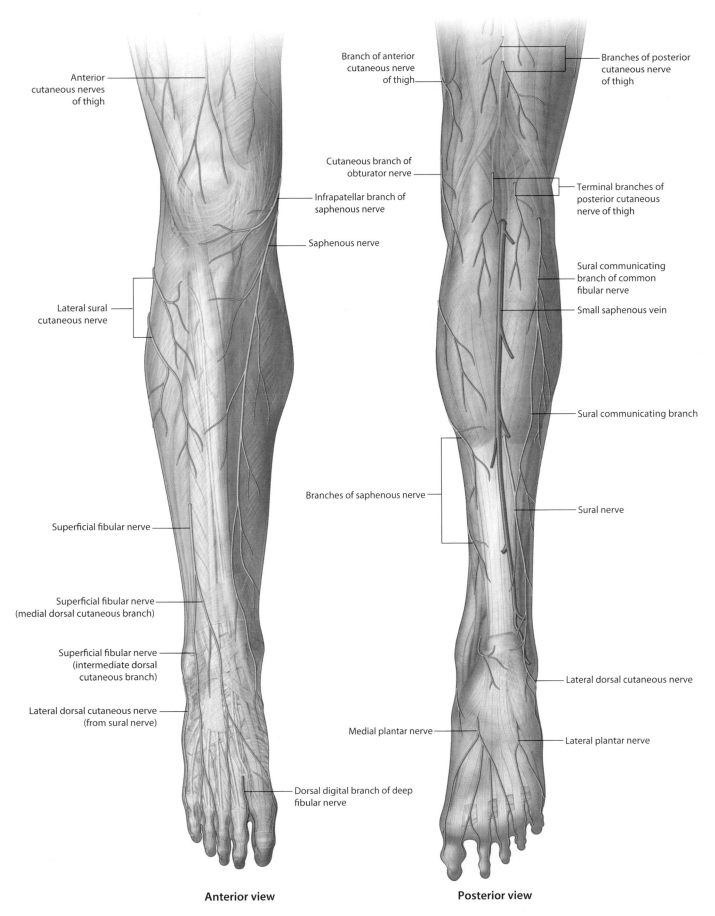

Anterior cutaneous nerves of thigh

Lateral sural cutaneous nerve

Superficial fibular nerve

Superficial fibular nerve (medial dorsal cutaneous branch)

Superficial fibular nerve (intermediate dorsal cutaneous branch)

Lateral dorsal cutaneous nerve (from sural nerve)

Branch of anterior cutaneous nerve of thigh

Cutaneous branch of obturator nerve

Infrapatellar branch of saphenous nerve

Saphenous nerve

Branches of saphenous nerve

Dorsal digital branch of deep fibular nerve

Branches of posterior cutaneous nerve of thigh

Terminal branches of posterior cutaneous nerve of thigh

Sural communicating branch of common fibular nerve

Small saphenous vein

Sural communicating branch

Sural nerve

Lateral dorsal cutaneous nerve

Medial plantar nerve

Lateral plantar nerve

Anterior view

Posterior view

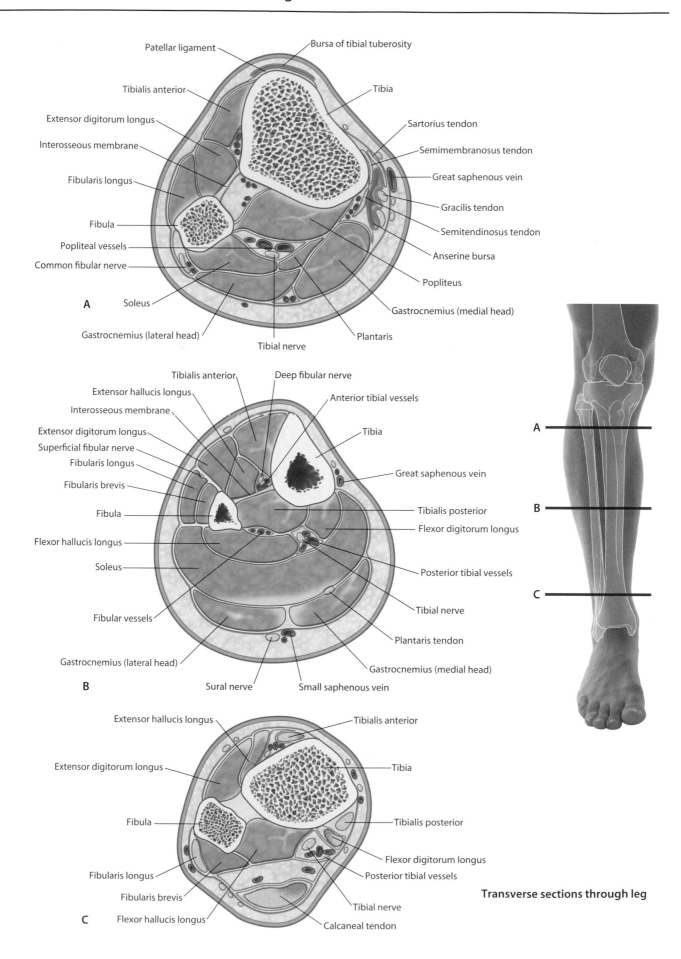

A

Patellar ligament
Bursa of tibial tuberosity
Tibialis anterior
Tibia
Extensor digitorum longus
Sartorius tendon
Interosseous membrane
Semimembranosus tendon
Fibularis longus
Great saphenous vein
Fibula
Gracilis tendon
Popliteal vessels
Semitendinosus tendon
Common fibular nerve
Anserine bursa
Soleus
Popliteus
Gastrocnemius (lateral head)
Gastrocnemius (medial head)
Tibial nerve
Plantaris

B

Tibialis anterior
Deep fibular nerve
Extensor hallucis longus
Anterior tibial vessels
Interosseous membrane
Extensor digitorum longus
Tibia
Superficial fibular nerve
Fibularis longus
Great saphenous vein
Fibularis brevis
Tibialis posterior
Fibula
Flexor digitorum longus
Flexor hallucis longus
Soleus
Posterior tibial vessels
Fibular vessels
Tibial nerve
Gastrocnemius (lateral head)
Plantaris tendon
Gastrocnemius (medial head)
Sural nerve
Small saphenous vein

C

Extensor hallucis longus
Tibialis anterior
Extensor digitorum longus
Tibia
Fibula
Tibialis posterior
Flexor digitorum longus
Posterior tibial vessels
Fibularis longus
Tibial nerve
Fibularis brevis
Calcaneal tendon
Flexor hallucis longus

A

B

C

Transverse sections through leg

348

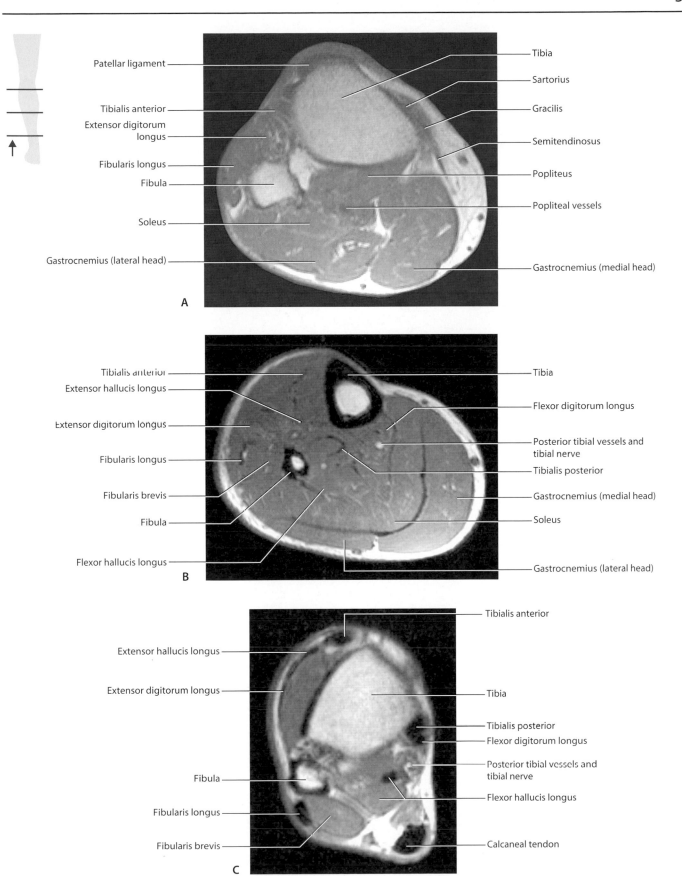

Patellar ligament

Tibialis anterior

Extensor digitorum longus

Fibularis longus

Fibula

Soleus

Gastrocnemius (lateral head)

Tibia

Sartorius

Gracilis

Semitendinosus

Popliteus

Popliteal vessels

Gastrocnemius (medial head)

A

Tibialis anterior

Extensor hallucis longus

Extensor digitorum longus

Fibularis longus

Fibularis brevis

Fibula

Flexor hallucis longus

Tibia

Flexor digitorum longus

Posterior tibial vessels and tibial nerve

Tibialis posterior

Gastrocnemius (medial head)

Soleus

Gastrocnemius (lateral head)

B

Extensor hallucis longus

Extensor digitorum longus

Fibula

Fibularis longus

Fibularis brevis

Tibialis anterior

Tibia

Tibialis posterior

Flexor digitorum longus

Posterior tibial vessels and tibial nerve

Flexor hallucis longus

Calcaneal tendon

C

Transverse/axial sections through the leg.

A. Proximal/upper leg. T1-weighted MR image in axial plane
B. Middle leg. T1-weighted MR image in axial plane
C. Distal/lower leg. T1-weighted MR image in axial plane

Muscle attachments of the foot

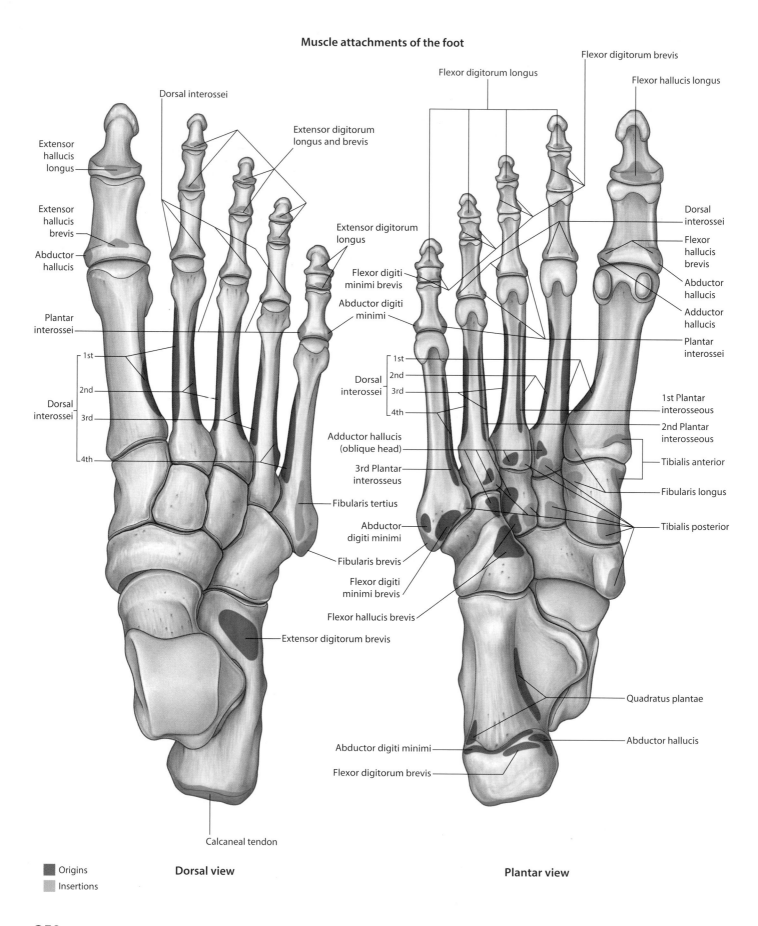

Flexor digitorum longus

Flexor digitorum brevis

Flexor hallucis longus

Dorsal interossei

Extensor digitorum longus and brevis

Extensor hallucis longus

Extensor hallucis brevis

Abductor hallucis

Extensor digitorum longus

Flexor digiti minimi brevis

Abductor digiti minimi

Dorsal interossei

Plantar interossei

1st
2nd
3rd
4th

Dorsal interossei

Adductor hallucis (oblique head)

3rd Plantar interosseus

Fibularis tertius

Abductor digiti minimi

Fibularis brevis

Flexor digiti minimi brevis

Flexor hallucis brevis

Extensor digitorum brevis

Dorsal interossei

1st
2nd
3rd
4th

Flexor hallucis brevis

Abductor hallucis

Adductor hallucis

Plantar interossei

1st Plantar interosseous

2nd Plantar interosseous

Tibialis anterior

Fibularis longus

Tibialis posterior

Quadratus plantae

Abductor hallucis

Abductor digiti minimi

Flexor digitorum brevis

Calcaneal tendon

Origins

Insertions

Dorsal view

Plantar view

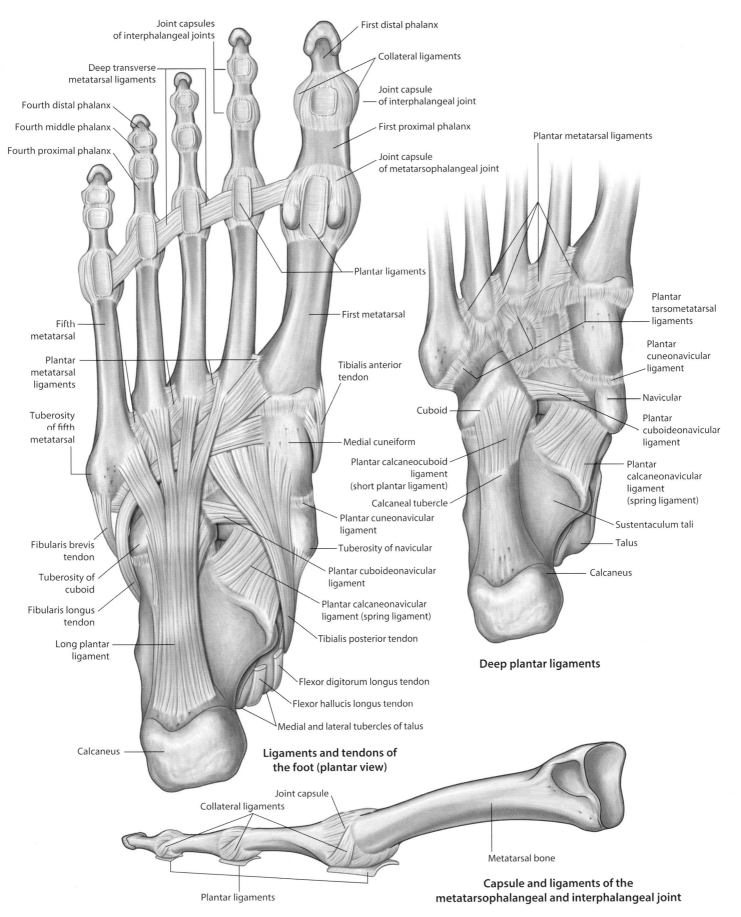

Joint capsules of interphalangeal joints

First distal phalanx

Deep transverse metatarsal ligaments

Collateral ligaments

Fourth distal phalanx

Joint capsule of interphalangeal joint

Fourth middle phalanx

First proximal phalanx

Fourth proximal phalanx

Joint capsule of metatarsophalangeal joint

Plantar metatarsal ligaments

Fifth metatarsal

Plantar ligaments

First metatarsal

Plantar metatarsal ligaments

Tibialis anterior tendon

Plantar tarsometatarsal ligaments

Tuberosity of fifth metatarsal

Medial cuneiform

Plantar cuneonavicular ligament

Plantar calcaneocuboid ligament (short plantar ligament)

Cuboid

Navicular

Fibularis brevis tendon

Calcaneal tubercle

Plantar cuboideonavicular ligament

Tuberosity of cuboid

Plantar cuneonavicular ligament

Plantar calcaneonavicular ligament (spring ligament)

Fibularis longus tendon

Tuberosity of navicular

Sustentaculum tali

Long plantar ligament

Plantar cuboideonavicular ligament

Talus

Plantar calcaneonavicular ligament (spring ligament)

Calcaneus

Flexor digitorum longus tendon

Tibialis posterior tendon

Flexor hallucis longus tendon

Medial and lateral tubercles of talus

Calcaneus

Ligaments and tendons of the foot (plantar view)

Deep plantar ligaments

Joint capsule

Collateral ligaments

Metatarsal bone

Plantar ligaments

Capsule and ligaments of the metatarsophalangeal and interphalangeal joint

351

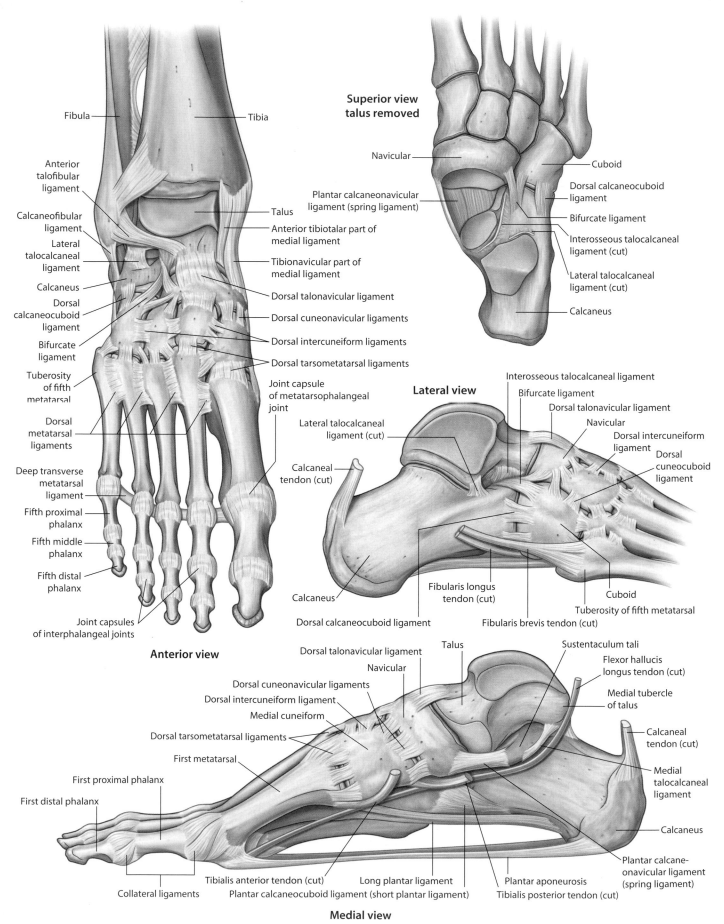

Fibula

Tibia

Anterior talofibular ligament

Calcaneofibular ligament

Lateral talocalcaneal ligament

Calcaneus

Dorsal calcaneocuboid ligament

Bifurcate ligament

Tuberosity of fifth metatarsal

Dorsal metatarsal ligaments

Deep transverse metatarsal ligament

Fifth proximal phalanx

Fifth middle phalanx

Fifth distal phalanx

Joint capsules of interphalangeal joints

Talus

Anterior tibiotalar part of medial ligament

Tibionavicular part of medial ligament

Dorsal talonavicular ligament

Dorsal cuneonavicular ligaments

Dorsal intercuneiform ligaments

Dorsal tarsometatarsal ligaments

Joint capsule of metatarsophalangeal joint

Anterior view

Superior view talus removed

Navicular

Cuboid

Dorsal calcaneocuboid ligament

Plantar calcaneonavicular ligament (spring ligament)

Bifurcate ligament

Interosseous talocalcaneal ligament (cut)

Lateral talocalcaneal ligament (cut)

Calcaneus

Lateral view

Interosseous talocalcaneal ligament

Bifurcate ligament

Dorsal talonavicular ligament

Navicular

Dorsal intercuneiform ligament

Dorsal cuneocuboid ligament

Lateral talocalcaneal ligament (cut)

Calcaneal tendon (cut)

Calcaneus

Dorsal calcaneocuboid ligament

Fibularis longus tendon (cut)

Fibularis brevis tendon (cut)

Cuboid

Tuberosity of fifth metatarsal

Dorsal talonavicular ligament

Navicular

Dorsal cuneonavicular ligaments

Dorsal intercuneiform ligament

Medial cuneiform

Dorsal tarsometatarsal ligaments

First metatarsal

First proximal phalanx

First distal phalanx

Collateral ligaments

Tibialis anterior tendon (cut)

Plantar calcaneocuboid ligament (short plantar ligament)

Long plantar ligament

Plantar aponeurosis

Tibialis posterior tendon (cut)

Talus

Sustentaculum tali

Flexor hallucis longus tendon (cut)

Medial tubercle of talus

Calcaneal tendon (cut)

Medial talocalcaneal ligament

Calcaneus

Plantar calcaneo-navicular ligament (spring ligament)

Medial view

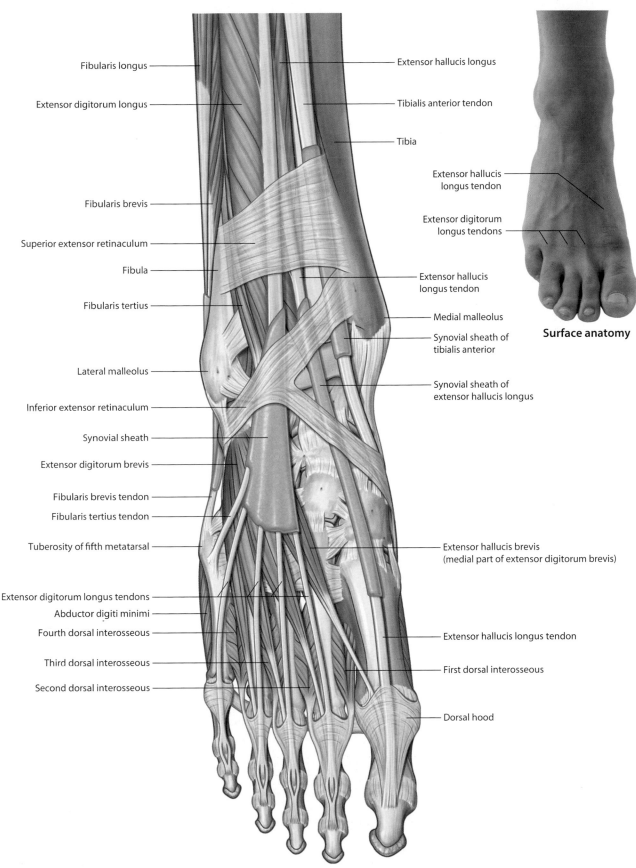

Fibularis longus

Extensor digitorum longus

Fibularis brevis

Superior extensor retinaculum

Fibula

Fibularis tertius

Lateral malleolus

Inferior extensor retinaculum

Synovial sheath

Extensor digitorum brevis

Fibularis brevis tendon

Fibularis tertius tendon

Tuberosity of fifth metatarsal

Extensor digitorum longus tendons

Abductor digiti minimi

Fourth dorsal interosseous

Third dorsal interosseous

Second dorsal interosseous

Extensor hallucis longus

Tibialis anterior tendon

Tibia

Extensor hallucis longus tendon

Extensor digitorum longus tendons

Extensor hallucis longus tendon

Medial malleolus

Synovial sheath of tibialis anterior

Synovial sheath of extensor hallucis longus

Surface anatomy

Extensor hallucis brevis (medial part of extensor digitorum brevis)

Extensor hallucis longus tendon

First dorsal interosseous

Dorsal hood

Superficial structures of the foot (dorsal view)

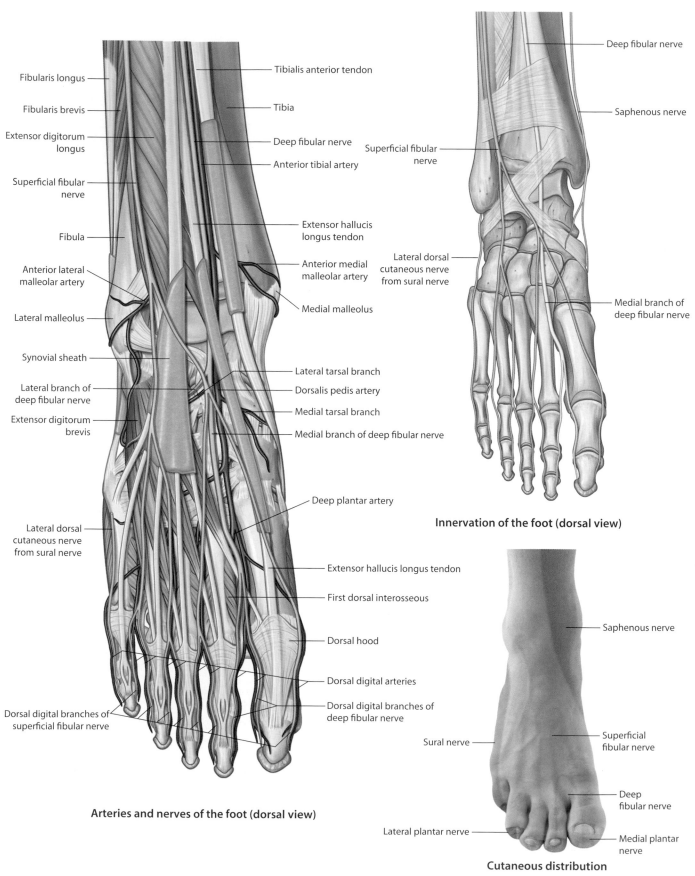

Fibularis longus

Fibularis brevis

Extensor digitorum longus

Superficial fibular nerve

Fibula

Anterior lateral malleolar artery

Lateral malleolus

Synovial sheath

Lateral branch of deep fibular nerve

Extensor digitorum brevis

Lateral dorsal cutaneous nerve from sural nerve

Dorsal digital branches of superficial fibular nerve

Tibialis anterior tendon

Tibia

Deep fibular nerve

Anterior tibial artery

Extensor hallucis longus tendon

Anterior medial malleolar artery

Medial malleolus

Lateral tarsal branch

Dorsalis pedis artery

Medial tarsal branch

Medial branch of deep fibular nerve

Deep plantar artery

Extensor hallucis longus tendon

First dorsal interosseous

Dorsal hood

Dorsal digital arteries

Dorsal digital branches of deep fibular nerve

Arteries and nerves of the foot (dorsal view)

Deep fibular nerve

Saphenous nerve

Superficial fibular nerve

Lateral dorsal cutaneous nerve from sural nerve

Medial branch of deep fibular nerve

Innervation of the foot (dorsal view)

Saphenous nerve

Sural nerve

Superficial fibular nerve

Deep fibular nerve

Lateral plantar nerve

Medial plantar nerve

Cutaneous distribution

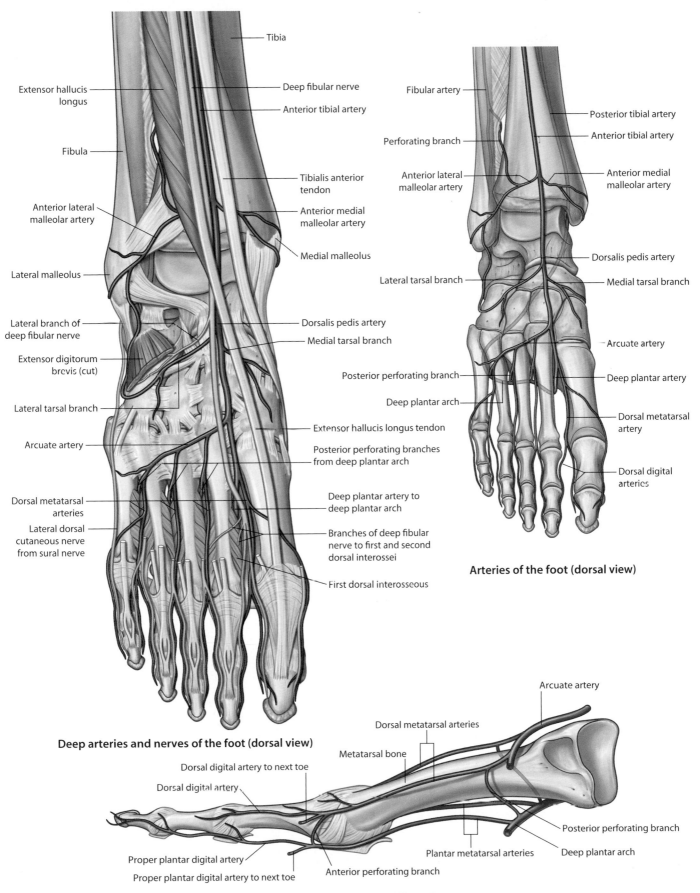

Tibia

Extensor hallucis longus

Deep fibular nerve

Anterior tibial artery

Fibula

Tibialis anterior tendon

Anterior lateral malleolar artery

Anterior medial malleolar artery

Medial malleolus

Lateral malleolus

Lateral branch of deep fibular nerve

Dorsalis pedis artery

Medial tarsal branch

Extensor digitorum brevis (cut)

Lateral tarsal branch

Arcuate artery

Dorsal metatarsal arteries

Lateral dorsal cutaneous nerve from sural nerve

Extensor hallucis longus tendon

Posterior perforating branches from deep plantar arch

Deep plantar artery to deep plantar arch

Branches of deep fibular nerve to first and second dorsal interossei

First dorsal interosseous

Deep arteries and nerves of the foot (dorsal view)

Fibular artery

Posterior tibial artery

Perforating branch

Anterior tibial artery

Anterior lateral malleolar artery

Anterior medial malleolar artery

Dorsalis pedis artery

Lateral tarsal branch

Medial tarsal branch

Arcuate artery

Posterior perforating branch

Deep plantar artery

Deep plantar arch

Dorsal metatarsal artery

Dorsal digital arteries

Arteries of the foot (dorsal view)

Arcuate artery

Dorsal metatarsal arteries

Metatarsal bone

Dorsal digital artery to next toe

Dorsal digital artery

Posterior perforating branch

Deep plantar arch

Proper plantar digital artery

Plantar metatarsal arteries

Proper plantar digital artery to next toe

Anterior perforating branch

Arteries of digit III (middle toe)

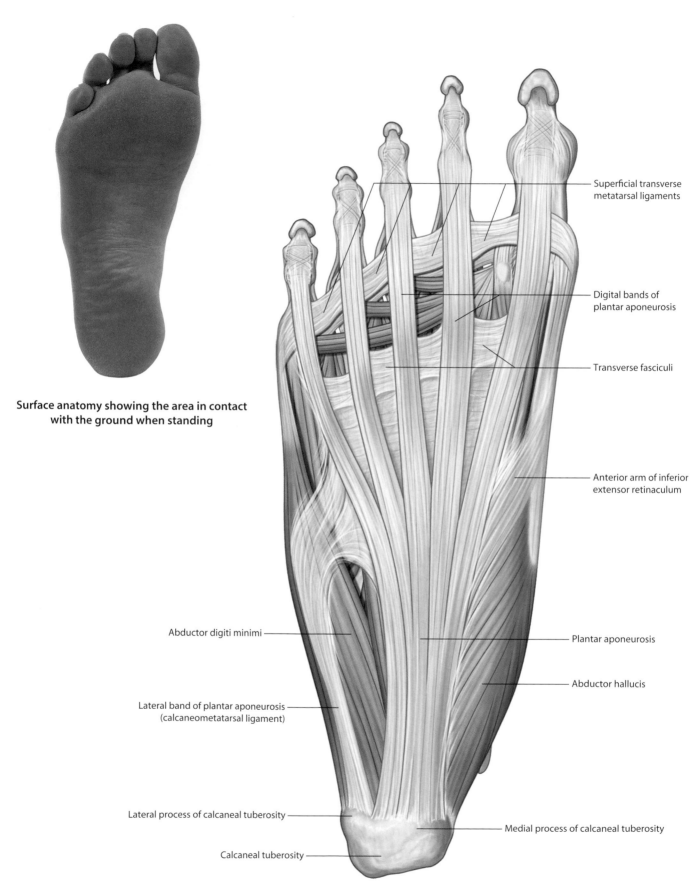

Surface anatomy showing the area in contact with the ground when standing

Superficial transverse metatarsal ligaments

Digital bands of plantar aponeurosis

Transverse fasciculi

Anterior arm of inferior extensor retinaculum

Plantar aponeurosis

Abductor hallucis

Abductor digiti minimi

Lateral band of plantar aponeurosis (calcaneometatarsal ligament)

Lateral process of calcaneal tuberosity

Medial process of calcaneal tuberosity

Calcaneal tuberosity

Superficial structures of the foot (plantar view)

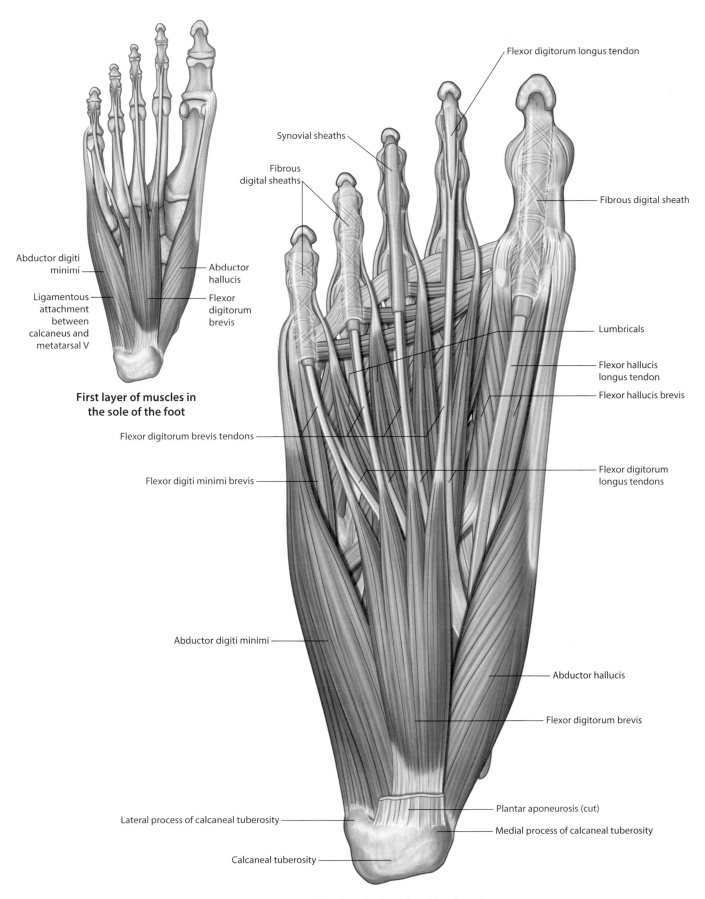

Flexor digitorum longus tendon

Synovial sheaths

Fibrous digital sheaths

Fibrous digital sheath

Abductor digiti minimi

Abductor hallucis

Ligamentous attachment between calcaneus and metatarsal V

Flexor digitorum brevis

Lumbricals

Flexor hallucis longus tendon

Flexor hallucis brevis

First layer of muscles in the sole of the foot

Flexor digitorum brevis tendons

Flexor digitorum longus tendons

Flexor digiti minimi brevis

Abductor digiti minimi

Abductor hallucis

Flexor digitorum brevis

Plantar aponeurosis (cut)

Lateral process of calcaneal tuberosity

Medial process of calcaneal tuberosity

Calcaneal tuberosity

Muscles of sole of foot (first layer)

357

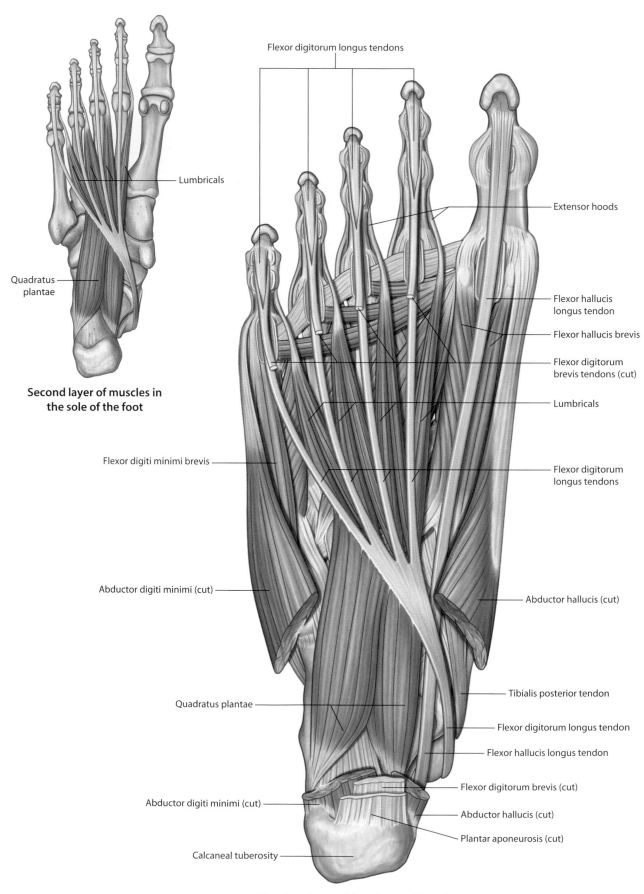

Flexor digitorum longus tendons

Extensor hoods

Lumbricals

Flexor hallucis longus tendon

Flexor hallucis brevis

Quadratus plantae

Flexor digitorum brevis tendons (cut)

Lumbricals

Second layer of muscles in the sole of the foot

Flexor digiti minimi brevis

Flexor digitorum longus tendons

Abductor digiti minimi (cut)

Abductor hallucis (cut)

Tibialis posterior tendon

Quadratus plantae

Flexor digitorum longus tendon

Flexor hallucis longus tendon

Flexor digitorum brevis (cut)

Abductor digiti minimi (cut)

Abductor hallucis (cut)

Plantar aponeurosis (cut)

Calcaneal tuberosity

Muscles of sole of foot (second layer)

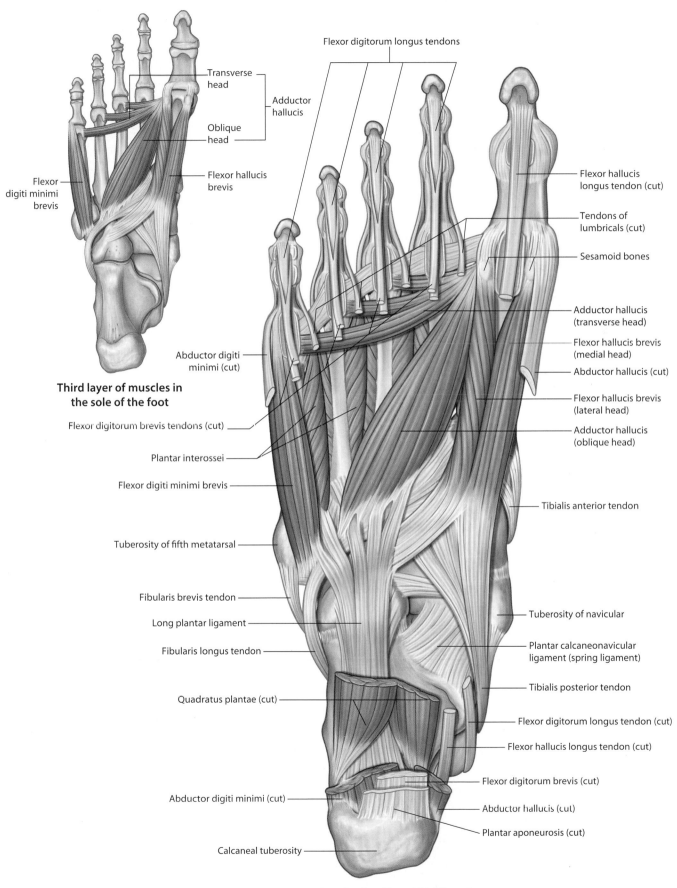

Transverse head

Adductor hallucis

Oblique head

Flexor digiti minimi brevis

Flexor hallucis brevis

Third layer of muscles in the sole of the foot

Flexor digitorum longus tendons

Flexor hallucis longus tendon (cut)

Tendons of lumbricals (cut)

Sesamoid bones

Adductor hallucis (transverse head)

Flexor hallucis brevis (medial head)

Abductor hallucis (cut)

Flexor hallucis brevis (lateral head)

Adductor hallucis (oblique head)

Abductor digiti minimi (cut)

Flexor digitorum brevis tendons (cut)

Plantar interossei

Flexor digiti minimi brevis

Tuberosity of fifth metatarsal

Fibularis brevis tendon

Long plantar ligament

Fibularis longus tendon

Quadratus plantae (cut)

Abductor digiti minimi (cut)

Calcaneal tuberosity

Tibialis anterior tendon

Tuberosity of navicular

Plantar calcaneonavicular ligament (spring ligament)

Tibialis posterior tendon

Flexor digitorum longus tendon (cut)

Flexor hallucis longus tendon (cut)

Flexor digitorum brevis (cut)

Abductor hallucis (cut)

Plantar aponeurosis (cut)

Muscles of sole of foot (third layer)

359

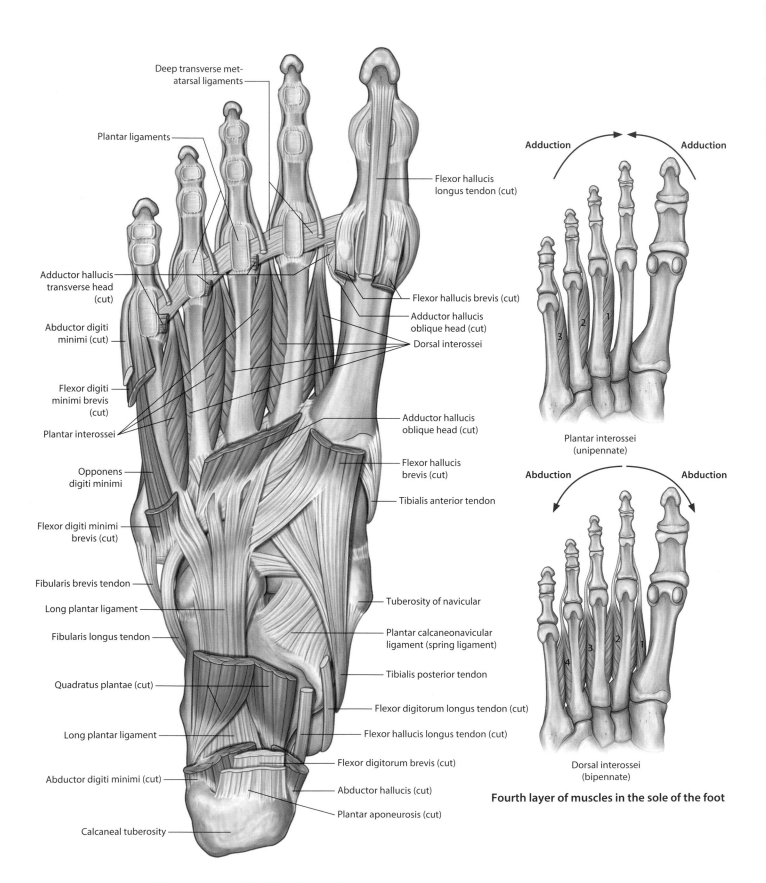

Deep transverse met-
atarsal ligaments

Plantar ligaments

Flexor hallucis
longus tendon (cut)

Adductor hallucis
transverse head
(cut)

Abductor digiti
minimi (cut)

Flexor digiti
minimi brevis
(cut)

Plantar interossei

Opponens
digiti minimi

Flexor digiti minimi
brevis (cut)

Fibularis brevis tendon

Long plantar ligament

Fibularis longus tendon

Quadratus plantae (cut)

Long plantar ligament

Abductor digiti minimi (cut)

Calcaneal tuberosity

Flexor hallucis brevis (cut)

Adductor hallucis
oblique head (cut)

Dorsal interossei

Adductor hallucis
oblique head (cut)

Flexor hallucis
brevis (cut)

Tibialis anterior tendon

Tuberosity of navicular

Plantar calcaneonavicular
ligament (spring ligament)

Tibialis posterior tendon

Flexor digitorum longus tendon (cut)

Flexor hallucis longus tendon (cut)

Flexor digitorum brevis (cut)

Abductor hallucis (cut)

Plantar aponeurosis (cut)

Muscles of sole of foot (fourth layer)

Adduction — Adduction

Plantar interossei
(unipennate)

Abduction — Abduction

Dorsal interossei
(bipennate)

Fourth layer of muscles in the sole of the foot

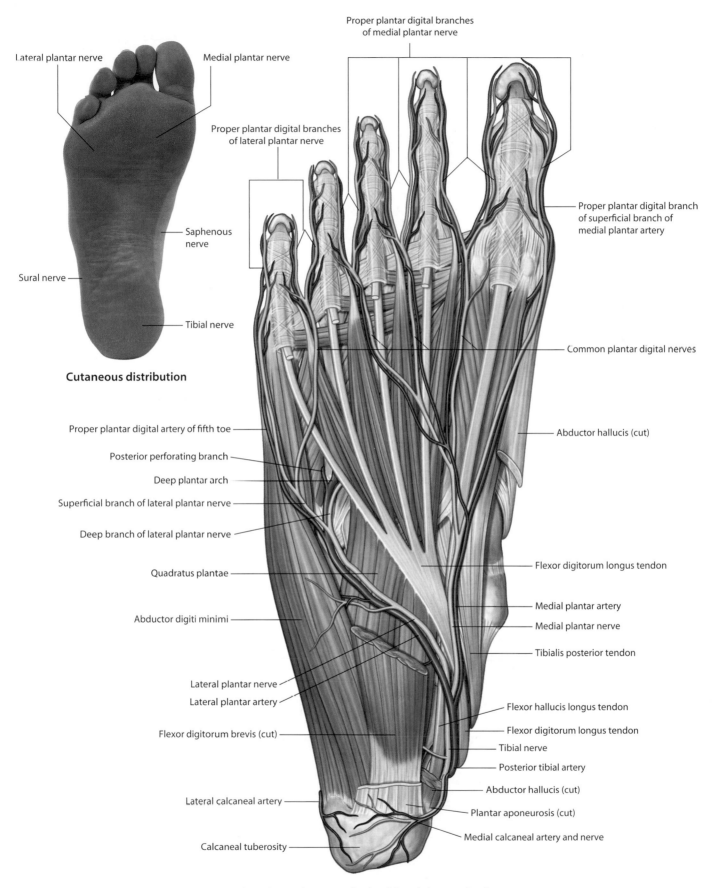

Proper plantar digital branches
of medial plantar nerve

Lateral plantar nerve

Medial plantar nerve

Proper plantar digital branches
of lateral plantar nerve

Proper plantar digital branch
of superficial branch of
medial plantar nerve

Saphenous
nerve

Sural nerve

Tibial nerve

Common plantar digital nerves

Cutaneous distribution

Proper plantar digital artery of fifth toe

Posterior perforating branch

Deep plantar arch

Superficial branch of lateral plantar nerve

Deep branch of lateral plantar nerve

Quadratus plantae

Abductor digiti minimi

Lateral plantar nerve

Lateral plantar artery

Flexor digitorum brevis (cut)

Lateral calcaneal artery

Calcaneal tuberosity

Abductor hallucis (cut)

Flexor digitorum longus tendon

Medial plantar artery

Medial plantar nerve

Tibialis posterior tendon

Flexor hallucis longus tendon

Flexor digitorum longus tendon

Tibial nerve

Posterior tibial artery

Abductor hallucis (cut)

Plantar aponeurosis (cut)

Medial calcaneal artery and nerve

Arteries and nerves of sole of foot (plantar view)

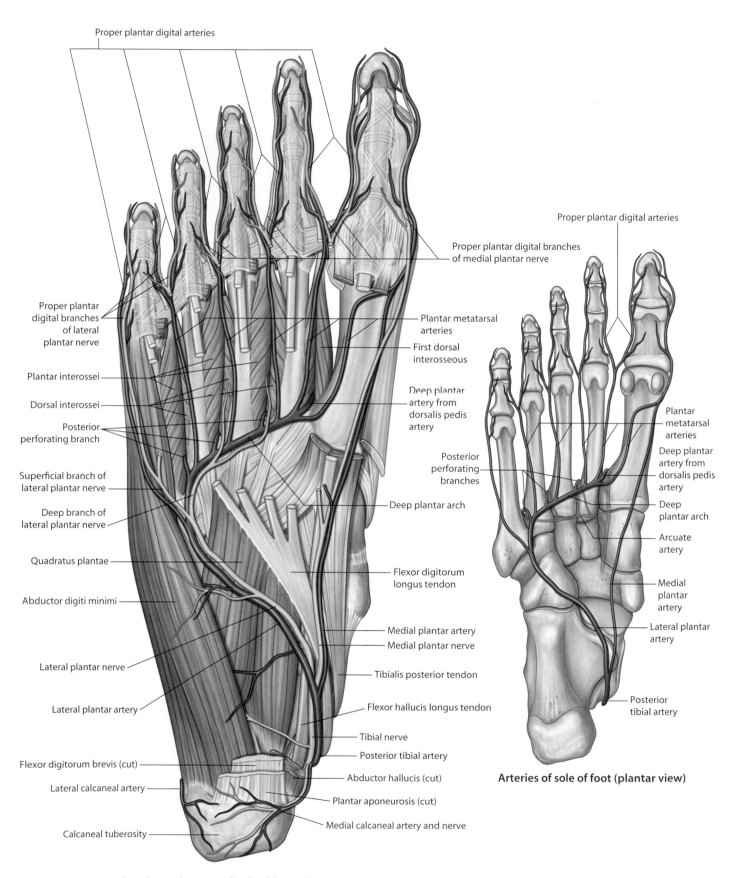

Proper plantar digital arteries

Proper plantar digital branches
of medial plantar nerve

Proper plantar
digital branches
of lateral
plantar nerve

Plantar metatarsal
arteries

First dorsal
interosseous

Plantar interossei

Dorsal interossei

Posterior
perforating branch

Deep plantar
artery from
dorsalis pedis
artery

Superficial branch of
lateral plantar nerve

Posterior
perforating
branches

Deep branch of
lateral plantar nerve

Deep plantar arch

Quadratus plantae

Flexor digitorum
longus tendon

Abductor digiti minimi

Medial plantar artery

Medial plantar nerve

Lateral plantar nerve

Tibialis posterior tendon

Lateral plantar artery

Flexor hallucis longus tendon

Tibial nerve

Posterior tibial artery

Flexor digitorum brevis (cut)

Abductor hallucis (cut)

Lateral calcaneal artery

Plantar aponeurosis (cut)

Medial calcaneal artery and nerve

Calcaneal tuberosity

Proper plantar digital arteries

Plantar
metatarsal
arteries

Deep plantar
artery from
dorsalis pedis
artery

Deep
plantar arch

Arcuate
artery

Medial
plantar
artery

Lateral plantar
artery

Posterior
tibial artery

Arteries of sole of foot (plantar view)

Arteries and nerves of sole of foot (plantar view)

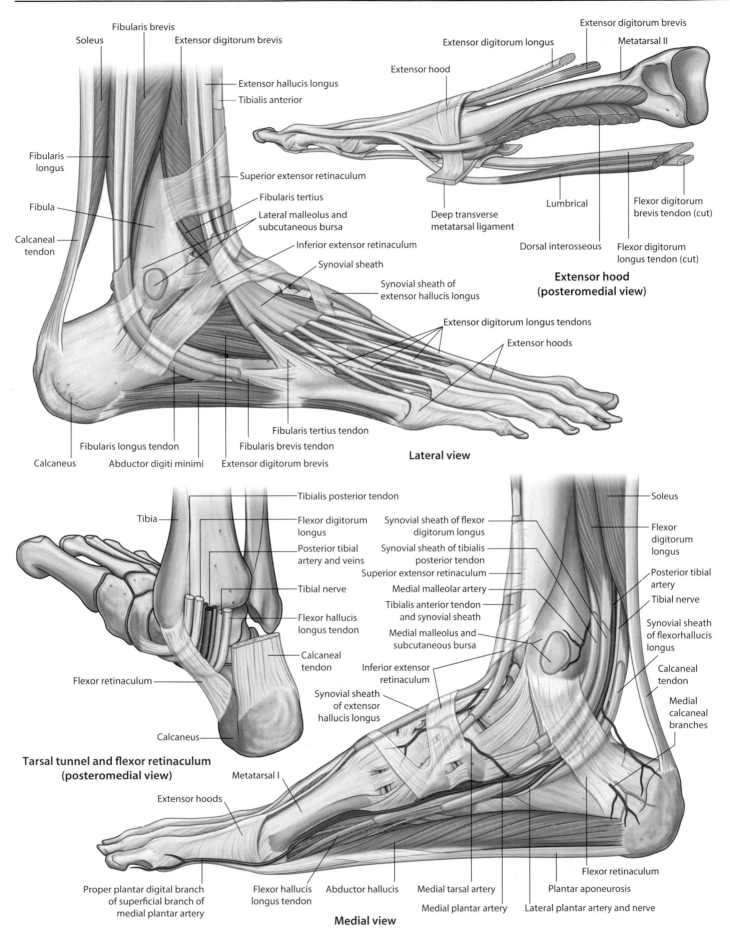

Lateral view

Soleus
Fibularis brevis
Extensor digitorum brevis
Extensor hallucis longus
Tibialis anterior
Fibularis longus
Fibula
Calcaneal tendon
Superior extensor retinaculum
Fibularis tertius
Lateral malleolus and subcutaneous bursa
Inferior extensor retinaculum
Synovial sheath
Synovial sheath of extensor hallucis longus
Extensor digitorum longus tendons
Extensor hoods
Fibularis tertius tendon
Fibularis brevis tendon
Extensor digitorum brevis
Calcaneus
Fibularis longus tendon
Abductor digiti minimi
Extensor digitorum brevis

Extensor hood (posteromedial view)

Extensor digitorum longus
Extensor hood
Extensor digitorum brevis
Metatarsal II
Deep transverse metatarsal ligament
Lumbrical
Dorsal interosseous
Flexor digitorum brevis tendon (cut)
Flexor digitorum longus tendon (cut)

Tarsal tunnel and flexor retinaculum (posteromedial view)

Tibia
Tibialis posterior tendon
Flexor digitorum longus
Posterior tibial artery and veins
Tibial nerve
Flexor hallucis longus tendon
Calcaneal tendon
Flexor retinaculum
Calcaneus

Medial view

Soleus
Flexor digitorum longus
Posterior tibial artery
Tibial nerve
Synovial sheath of flexor hallucis longus
Calcaneal tendon
Medial calcaneal branches
Synovial sheath of flexor digitorum longus
Synovial sheath of tibialis posterior tendon
Superior extensor retinaculum
Medial malleolar artery
Tibialis anterior tendon and synovial sheath
Medial malleolus and subcutaneous bursa
Inferior extensor retinaculum
Synovial sheath of extensor hallucis longus
Metatarsal I
Extensor hoods
Proper plantar digital branch of superficial branch of medial plantar artery
Flexor hallucis longus tendon
Abductor hallucis
Medial tarsal artery
Medial plantar artery
Lateral plantar artery and nerve
Plantar aponeurosis
Flexor retinaculum

363

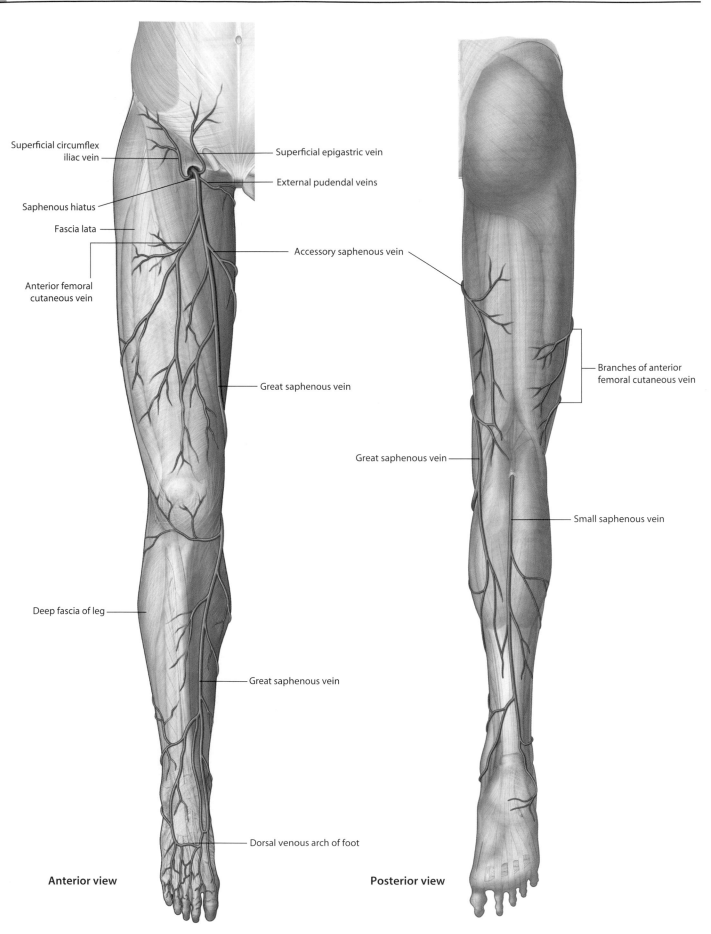

Superficial circumflex iliac vein

Superficial epigastric vein

Saphenous hiatus

External pudendal veins

Fascia lata

Accessory saphenous vein

Anterior femoral cutaneous vein

Branches of anterior femoral cutaneous vein

Great saphenous vein

Great saphenous vein

Small saphenous vein

Deep fascia of leg

Great saphenous vein

Dorsal venous arch of foot

Anterior view

Posterior view

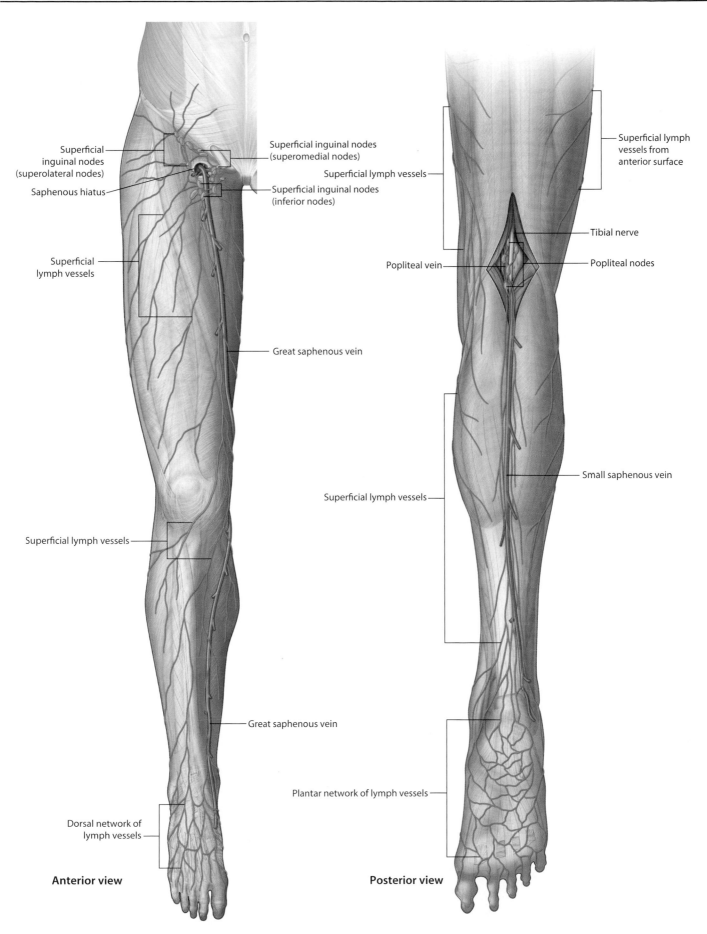

Superficial
inguinal nodes
(superolateral nodes)

Saphenous hiatus

Superficial
lymph vessels

Superficial lymph vessels

Great saphenous vein

Dorsal network of
lymph vessels

Anterior view

Superficial inguinal nodes
(superomedial nodes)

Superficial lymph vessels

Superficial inguinal nodes
(inferior nodes)

Great saphenous vein

Superficial lymph
vessels from
anterior surface

Tibial nerve

Popliteal vein

Popliteal nodes

Small saphenous vein

Superficial lymph vessels

Plantar network of lymph vessels

Posterior view

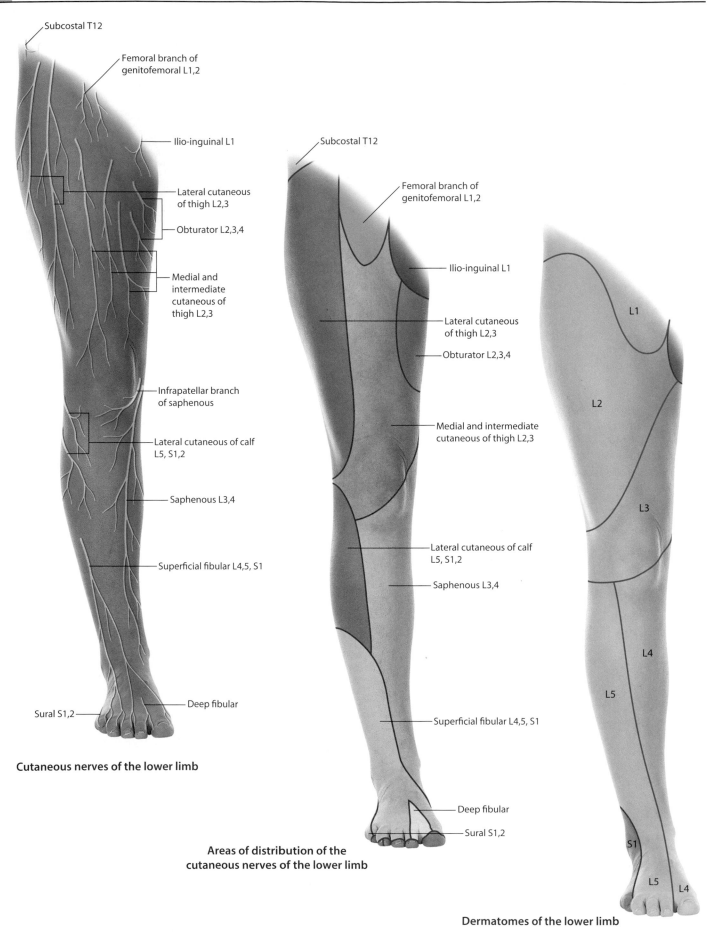

Subcostal T12

Femoral branch of
genitofemoral L1,2

Ilio-inguinal L1

Lateral cutaneous
of thigh L2,3

Obturator L2,3,4

Medial and
intermediate
cutaneous of
thigh L2,3

Infrapatellar branch
of saphenous

Lateral cutaneous of calf
L5, S1,2

Saphenous L3,4

Superficial fibular L4,5, S1

Sural S1,2

Deep fibular

Cutaneous nerves of the lower limb

Subcostal T12

Femoral branch of
genitofemoral L1,2

Ilio-inguinal L1

Lateral cutaneous
of thigh L2,3

Obturator L2,3,4

Medial and intermediate
cutaneous of thigh L2,3

Lateral cutaneous of calf
L5, S1,2

Saphenous L3,4

Superficial fibular L4,5, S1

Deep fibular

Sural S1,2

**Areas of distribution of the
cutaneous nerves of the lower limb**

L1

L2

L3

L4

L5

S1

L5

L4

Dermatomes of the lower limb

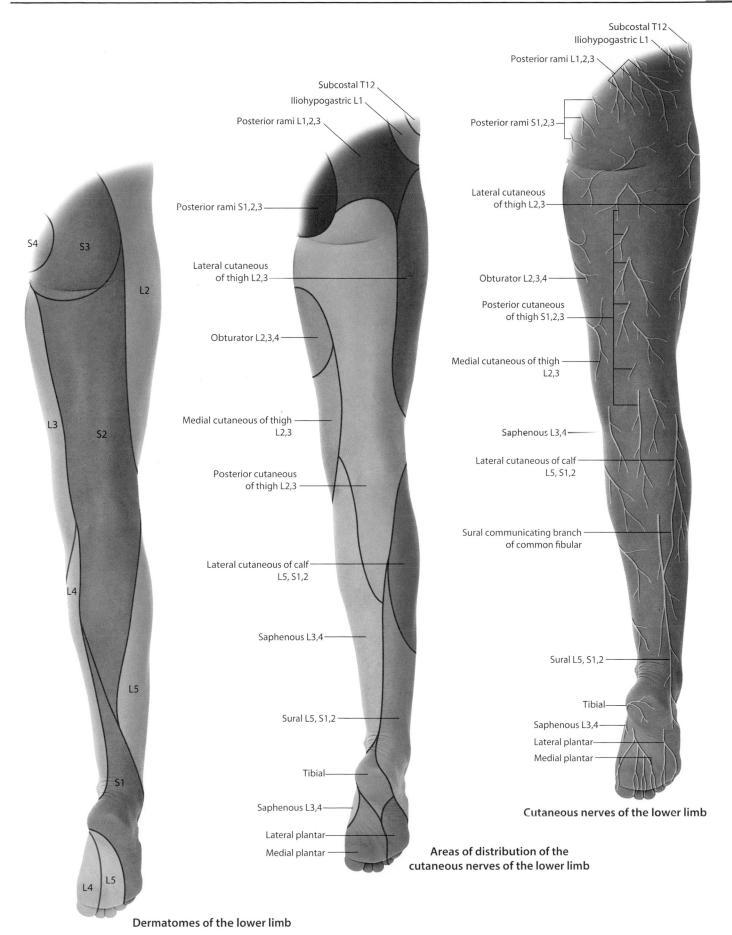

Subcostal T12

Iliohypogastric L1

Posterior rami L1,2,3

Posterior rami S1,2,3

Lateral cutaneous
of thigh L2,3

Obturator L2,3,4

Posterior cutaneous
of thigh S1,2,3

Medial cutaneous of thigh
L2,3

Saphenous L3,4

Lateral cutaneous of calf
L5, S1,2

Sural communicating branch
of common fibular

Sural L5, S1,2

Tibial

Saphenous L3,4

Lateral plantar

Medial plantar

Cutaneous nerves of the lower limb

Subcostal T12

Iliohypogastric L1

Posterior rami L1,2,3

Posterior rami S1,2,3

Lateral cutaneous
of thigh L2,3

Obturator L2,3,4

Medial cutaneous of thigh
L2,3

Posterior cutaneous
of thigh L2,3

Lateral cutaneous of calf
L5, S1,2

Saphenous L3,4

Sural L5, S1,2

Tibial

Saphenous L3,4

Lateral plantar

Medial plantar

**Areas of distribution of the
cutaneous nerves of the lower limb**

S4 S3

L2

L3 S2

L4

L5

S1

L4 L5

Dermatomes of the lower limb

Branches of the lumbosacral plexus associated with the lower limb

Branch		Spinal segments	Function: motor	Function: sensory (cutaneous)
Ilio-inguinal	1	L1	No motor function in lower limb, but innervates muscles of the abdominal wall	Skin over anteromedial part of upper thigh and adjacent skin of perineum
Genitofemoral	2	L1, L2	No motor function in lower limb, but genital branch innervates cremaster muscle in the wall of the spermatic cord in men	Femoral branch innervates skin on anterior central part of upper thigh; the genital branch innervates skin in anterior part of perineum (anterior scrotum in men, and mons pubis and anterior labia majora in women)
Femoral	3	L2 to L4	All muscles in the anterior compartment of thigh; in the abdomen, also gives rise to branches that supply iliacus and pectineus	Skin over the anterior thigh, anteromedial knee, medial side of the leg, and the medial side of the foot
Obturator	4	L2 to L4	All muscles in the medial compartment of thigh (except pectineus and the part of adductor magnus attached to the ischium); also innervates obturator externus	Skin over upper medial aspect of thigh
Sciatic	5	L4 to S3	All muscles in the posterior compartment of thigh and the part of adductor magnus attached to the ischium; all muscles in the leg and foot	Skin over lateral side of leg and foot, and over the sole and dorsal surface of foot
Superior gluteal	6	L4 to S1	Muscles of the gluteal region (gluteus medius, gluteus minimus, tensor fasciae latae)	
Inferior gluteal	7	L5 to S2	Muscle of the gluteal region (gluteus maximus)	
Lateral cutaneous nerve of thigh	8	L2, L3		Parietal peritoneum in iliac fossa; skin over anterolateral thigh
Posterior cutaneous nerve of thigh	9	S1 to S3		Skin over gluteal fold and upper medial aspect of thigh and adjacent perineum, posterior aspect of thigh, and upper posterior leg
Nerve to quadratus femoris	10	L4 to S1	Muscles of gluteal region (quadratus femoris and gemellus inferior)	
Nerve to obturator internus	11	L5 to S2	Muscles of gluteal region (obturator internus and gemellus superior)	
Perforating cutaneous nerve	12	S2, S3		Skin over medial aspect of gluteal fold

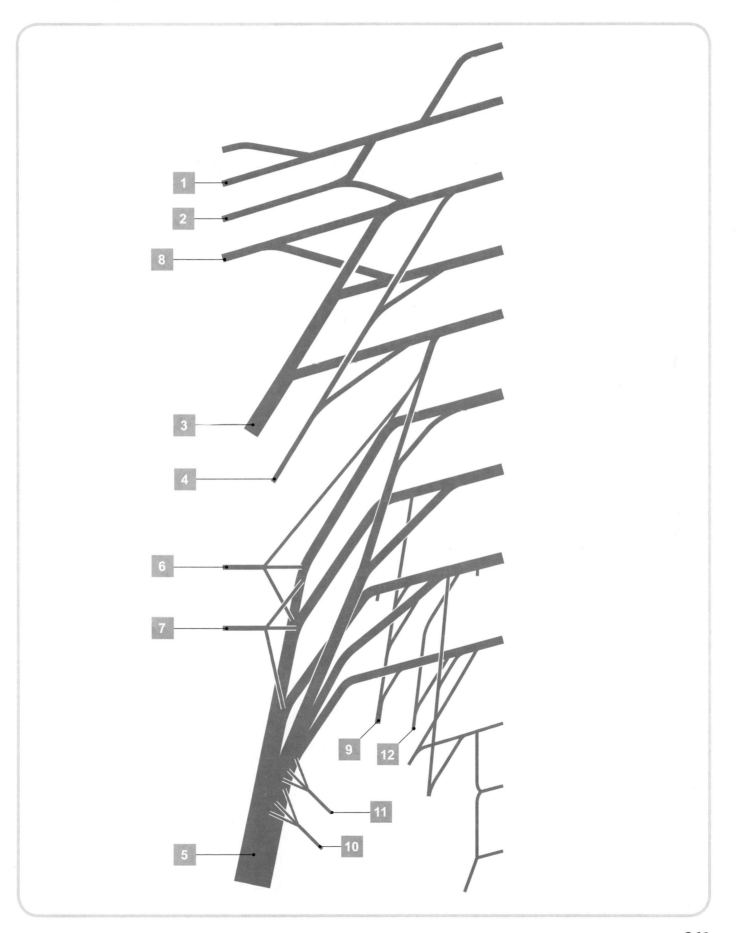

Muscles of the gluteal region
(spinal segments in bold are the major segments innervating the muscle)

Muscle		Origin	Insertion	Innervation	Function
Piriformis	1	Anterior surface of sacrum between anterior sacral foramina	Medial side of superior border of greater trochanter of femur	Branches from **L5, S1, S2**	Laterally rotates the extended femur at hip joint; abducts flexed femur at hip joint
Obturator internus	2	Anterolateral wall of true pelvis; deep surface of obturator membrane and surrounding bone	Medial side of greater trochanter of femur	Nerve to obturator internus (L5, **S1**)	Laterally rotates the extended femur at hip joint; abducts flexed femur at hip joint
Gemellus superior	3	External surface of ischial spine	Along length of superior surface of the obturator internus tendon and into the medial side of greater trochanter of femur with obturator internus tendon	Nerve to obturator internus (L5, **S1**)	Laterally rotates the extended femur at hip joint; abducts flexed femur at hip joint
Gemellus inferior	4	Upper aspect of ischial tuberosity	Along length of inferior surface of the obturator internus tendon and into the medial side of greater trochanter of femur with obturator internus tendon	Nerve to quadratus femoris (**L5, S1**)	Laterally rotates the extended femur at hip joint; abducts flexed femur at hip joint
Quadratus femoris	5	Lateral aspect of the ischium just anterior to the ischial tuberosity	Quadrate tubercle on the intertrochanteric crest of the proximal femur	Nerve to quadratus femoris (**L5, S1**)	Laterally rotates femur at hip joint
Gluteus minimus	6	External surface of ilium between inferior and anterior gluteal lines	Linear facet on the anterolateral aspect of the greater trochanter	Superior gluteal nerve (**L4, L5**, S1)	Abducts femur at hip joint; holds pelvis secure over stance leg and prevents pelvic drop on the opposite swing side during walking; medially rotates thigh
Gluteus medius	7	External surface of ilium between anterior and posterior gluteal lines	Elongate facet on the lateral surface of the greater trochanter	Superior gluteal nerve (**L4, L5**, S1)	Abducts femur at hip joint; holds pelvis secure over stance leg and prevents pelvic drop on the opposite swing side during walking; medially rotates thigh
Gluteus maximus	8	Fascia covering gluteus medius, external surface of ilium behind posterior gluteal line, fascia of erector spinae, dorsal surface of lower sacrum, lateral margin of coccyx, external surface of sacrotuberous ligament	Posterior aspect of iliotibial tract of fascia lata and gluteal tuberosity of proximal femur	Inferior gluteal nerve (**L5, S1**, S2)	Powerful extensor of flexed femur at hip joint; lateral stabilizer of hip joint and knee joint; laterally rotates and abducts thigh
Tensor fasciae latae	9	Lateral aspect of crest of ilium between anterior superior iliac spine and tubercle of the crest	Iliotibial tract of fascia lata	Superior gluteal nerve (**L4, L5**, S1)	Stabilizes the knee in extension

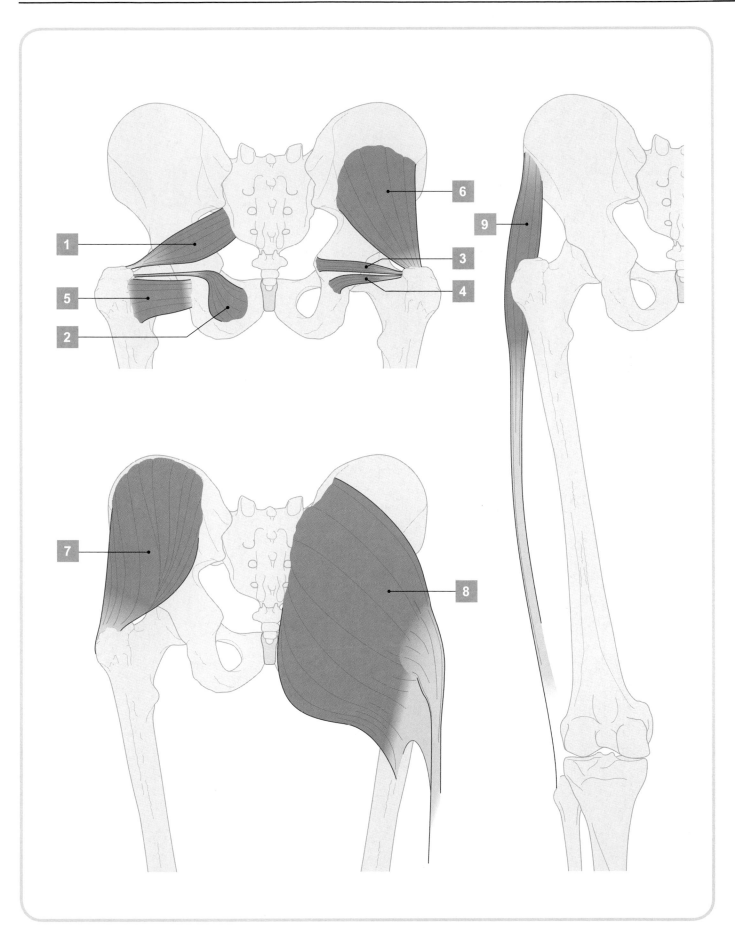

Muscles of the anterior compartment of thigh

(spinal segments in bold are the major segments innervating the muscle)

Muscle		Origin	Insertion	Innervation	Function
Psoas major	1	Posterior abdominal wall (lumbar transverse processes, intervertebral discs, and adjacent bodies from TXII to LV and tendinous arches between these points)	Lesser trochanter of femur	Anterior rami [**L1**, **L2**, L3]	Flexes the thigh at the hip joint
Iliacus	2	Posterior abdominal wall (iliac fossa)	Lesser trochanter of femur	Femoral nerve [**L2**, L3]	Flexes the thigh at the hip joint
Vastus medialis	3	Femur—medial part of intertrochanteric line, pectineal line, medial lip of the linea aspera, medial supracondylar line	Quadriceps femoris tendon and medial border of patella	Femoral nerve [L2, **L3**, **L4**]	Extends the leg at the knee joint
Vastus intermedius	4	Femur—upper two thirds of anterior and lateral surfaces	Quadriceps femoris tendon and lateral margin of patella	Femoral nerve [L2, **L3**, **L4**]	Extends the leg at the knee joint
Vastus lateralis	5	Femur—lateral part of intertrochanteric line, margin of greater trochanter, lateral margin of gluteal tuberosity, lateral lip of the linea aspera	Quadriceps femoris tendon	Femoral nerve [L2, **L3**, **L4**]	Extends the leg at the knee joint
Rectus femoris	6	Straight head originates from the anterior inferior iliac spine; reflected head originates from the ilium just superior to the acetabulum	Quadriceps femoris tendon	Femoral nerve [L2, **L3**, **L4**]	Flexes the thigh at the hip joint and extends the leg at the knee joint
Sartorius	7	Anterior superior iliac spine	Medial surface of tibia just inferomedial to tibial tuberosity	Femoral nerve [**L2**, **L3**]	Flexes the thigh at the hip joint and flexes the leg at the knee joint

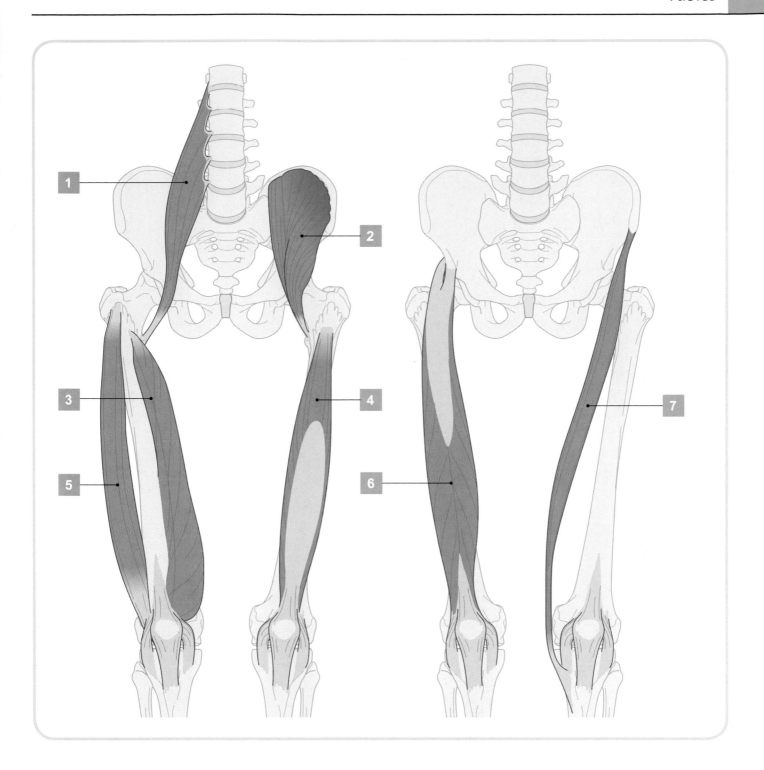

Muscles of the medial compartment of thigh

(spinal segments in bold are the major segments innervating the muscle)

Muscle		Origin	Insertion	Innervation	Function
Gracilis	1	A line on the external surfaces of the body of the pubis, the inferior pubic ramus, and the ramus of the ischium	Medial surface of proximal shaft of tibia	Obturator nerve [**L2**, L3]	Adducts thigh at hip joint and flexes leg at knee joint
Pectineus	2	Pectineal line (pecten pubis) and adjacent bone of pelvis	Oblique line extending from base of lesser trochanter to linea aspera on posterior surface of proximal femur	Femoral nerve [**L2**, L3]	Adducts and flexes thigh at hip joint
Adductor longus	3	External surface of body of pubis (triangular depression inferior to pubic crest and lateral to pubic symphysis)	Linea aspera on middle one third of shaft of femur	Obturator nerve (anterior division) [L2, **L3**, L4]	Adducts and medially rotates thigh at hip joint
Adductor brevis	4	External surface of body of pubis and inferior pubic ramus	Posterior surface of proximal femur and upper one third of linea aspera	Obturator nerve [**L2, L3**]	Adducts and medially rotates thigh at hip joint
Adductor magnus	5	Adductor part—ischiopubic ramus Hamstring part—ischial tuberosity	Posterior surface of proximal femur, linea aspera, medial supracondylar line Adductor tubercle and supracondylar line	Obturator nerve [**L2, L3**, L4] Sciatic nerve (tibial division) [**L2, L3**, L4]	Adducts and medially rotates thigh at hip joint
Obturator externus	6	External surface of obturator membrane and adjacent bone	Trochanteric fossa	Obturator nerve (posterior division) [L3, **L4**]	Laterally rotates thigh at hip joint

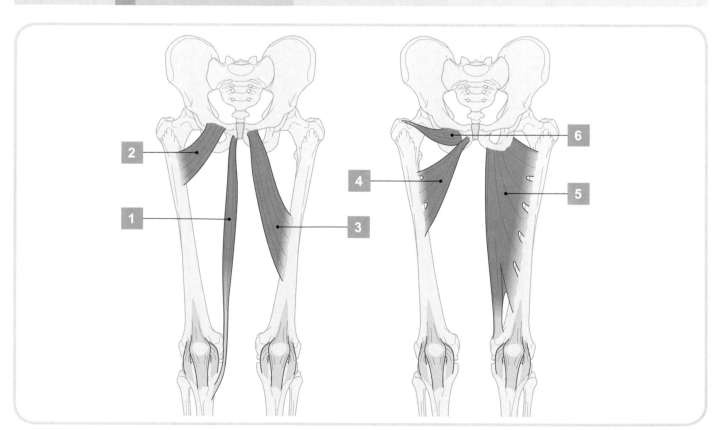

Muscles of the posterior compartment of thigh

(spinal segments in bold are the major segments innervating the muscle)

Muscle		Origin	Insertion	Innervation	Function
Biceps femoris	1	Long head—inferomedial part of the upper area of the ischial tuberosity; short head—lateral lip of linea aspera	Head of fibula	Sciatic nerve [L5, **S1**, S2]	Flexes leg at knee joint; extends and laterally rotates thigh at hip joint and laterally rotates leg at knee joint
Semitendinosus	2	Inferomedial part of the upper area of the ischial tuberosity	Medial surface of proximal tibia	Sciatic nerve [L5, **S1**, S2]	Flexes leg at knee joint and extends thigh at hip joint; medially rotates thigh at hip joint and leg at knee joint
Semimembranosus	3	Superolateral impression on the ischial tuberosity	Groove and adjacent bone on medial and posterior surface of medial tibial condyle	Sciatic nerve [L5, **S1**, S2]	Flexes leg at knee joint and extends thigh at hip joint; medially rotates thigh at hip joint and leg at knee joint

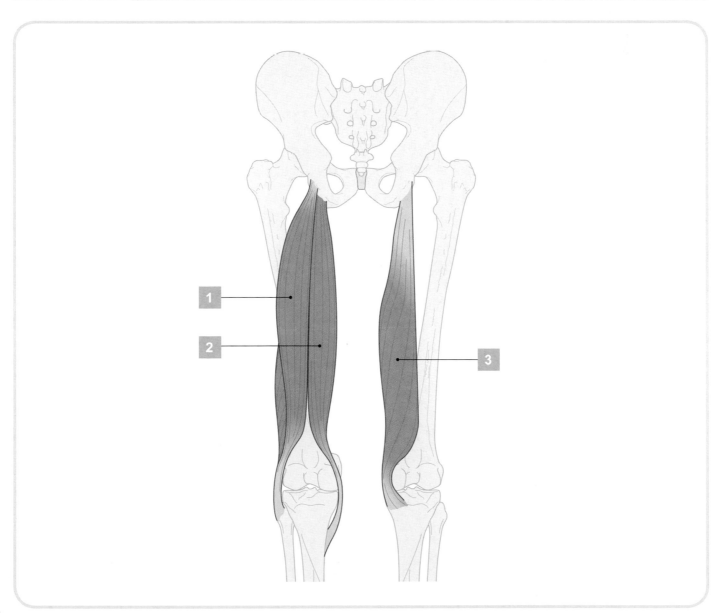

Superficial group of muscles in the posterior compartment of leg

(spinal segments in bold are the major segments innervating the muscle)

Muscle		Origin	Insertion	Innervation	Function
Gastrocnemius	1	Medial head—posterior surface of distal femur just superior to medial condyle; lateral head—upper posterolateral surface of lateral femoral condyle	Via calcaneal tendon, to posterior surface of calcaneus	Tibial nerve **[S1, S2]**	Plantarflexes foot and flexes knee
Plantaris	2	Inferior part of lateral supracondylar line of femur and oblique popliteal ligament of knee	Via calcaneal tendon, to posterior surface of calcaneus	Tibial nerve **[S1, S2]**	Plantarflexes foot and flexes knee
Soleus	3	Soleal line and medial border of tibia; posterior aspect of fibular head and adjacent surfaces of neck and proximal shaft; tendinous arch between tibial and fibular attachments	Via calcaneal tendon, to posterior surface of calcaneus	Tibial nerve **[S1, S2]**	Plantarflexes the foot

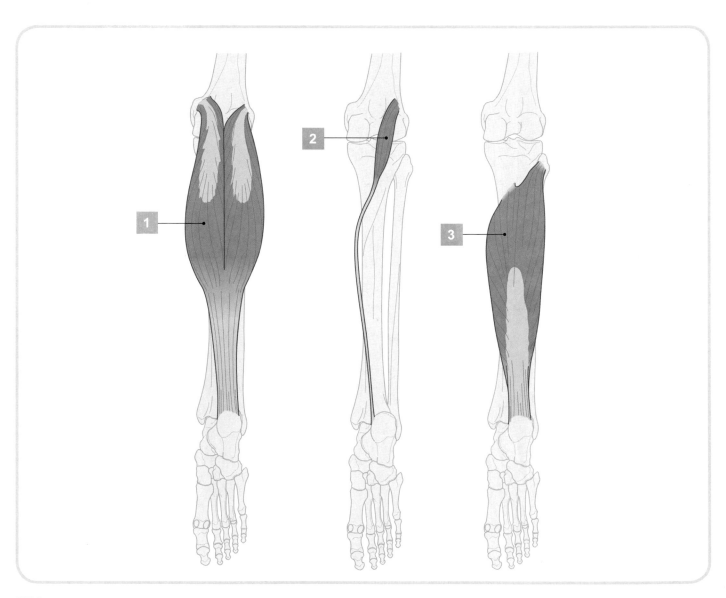

Deep group of muscles in the posterior compartment of leg

(spinal segments in bold are the major segments innervating the muscle)

Muscle		Origin	Insertion	Innervation	Function
Popliteus	1	Lateral femoral condyle	Posterior surface of proximal tibia	Tibial nerve [L4 to S1]	Stabilizes knee joint (resists lateral rotation of tibia on femur) Unlocks knee joint (laterally rotates femur on fixed tibia)
Flexor hallucis longus	2	Posterior surface of fibula and adjacent interosseous membrane	Plantar surface of distal phalanx of great toe	Tibial nerve [**S2**, S3]	Flexes great toe
Flexor digitorum longus	3	Medial side of posterior surface of the tibia	Plantar surfaces of bases of distal phalanges of the lateral four toes	Tibial nerve [**S2**, S3]	Flexes lateral four toes
Tibialis posterior	4	Posterior surfaces of interosseous membrane and adjacent regions of tibia and fibula	Mainly to tuberosity of navicular and adjacent region of medial cuneiform	Tibial nerve [L4, L5]	Inversion and plantarflexion of foot; support of medial arch of foot during walking

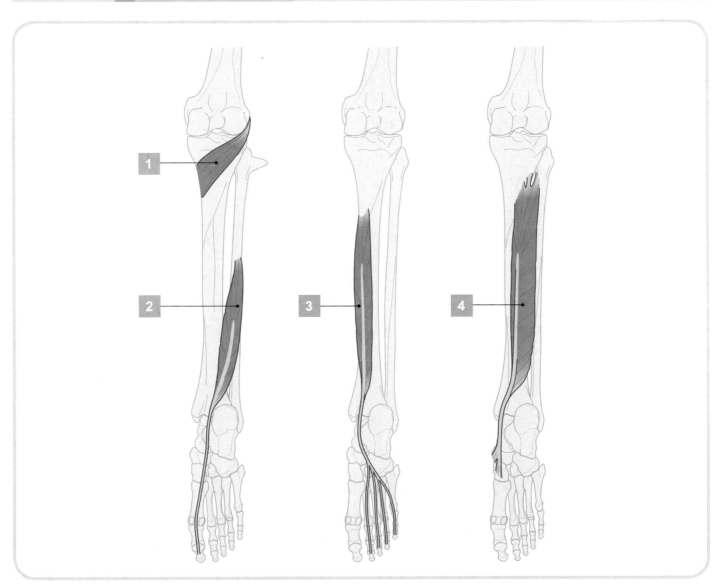

Muscles of the lateral compartment of leg
(spinal segments in bold are the major segments innervating the muscle)

Muscle		Origin	Insertion	Innervation	Function
Fibularis longus	1	Upper lateral surface of fibula, head of fibula, and occasionally the lateral tibial condyle	Undersurface of lateral sides of distal end of medial cuneiform and base of metatarsal I	Superficial fibular nerve [**L5**, **S1**, S2]	Eversion and plantarflexion of foot; supports arches of foot
Fibularis brevis	2	Lower two thirds of lateral surface of shaft of fibula	Lateral tubercle at base of metatarsal V	Superficial fibular nerve [**L5**, **S1**, S2]	Eversion of foot

Muscles of the anterior compartment of leg

Muscle		Origin	Insertion	Innervation	Function
Tibialis anterior	3	Lateral surface of tibia and adjacent interosseous membrane	Medial and inferior surfaces of medial cuneiform and adjacent surfaces on base of metatarsal I	Deep fibular nerve [**L4**, L5]	Dorsiflexion of foot at ankle joint; inversion of foot; dynamic support of medial arch of foot
Extensor hallucis longus	4	Middle one half of medial surface of fibula and adjacent surface of interosseous membrane	Dorsal surface of base of distal phalanx of great toe	Deep fibular nerve [**L5**, **S1**]	Extension of great toe and dorsiflexion of foot
Extensor digitorum longus	5	Proximal one half of medial surface of fibula and related surface of lateral tibial condyle	Via dorsal digital expansions into bases of distal and middle phalanges of lateral four toes	Deep fibular nerve [**L5**, **S1**]	Extension of lateral four toes and dorsiflexion of foot
Fibularis tertius	6	Distal part of medial surface of fibula	Dorsomedial surface of base of metatarsal V	Deep fibular nerve [**L5**, **S1**]	Dorsiflexion and eversion of foot

Muscles of the dorsal aspect of the foot

Muscle		Origin	Insertion	Innervation	Function
Extensor digitorum brevis	7	Superolateral surface of the calcaneus	Lateral sides of the tendons of extensor digitorum longus of toes II to IV	Deep fibular nerve [**S1**, **S2**]	Extension of metatarsophalangeal joints of toes II to IV
Extensor hallucis brevis	8	Superolateral surface of calcaneus	Base of proximal phalanx of great toe	Deep fibular nerve [S1, S2]	Extension of metatarsophalangeal joint of great toe

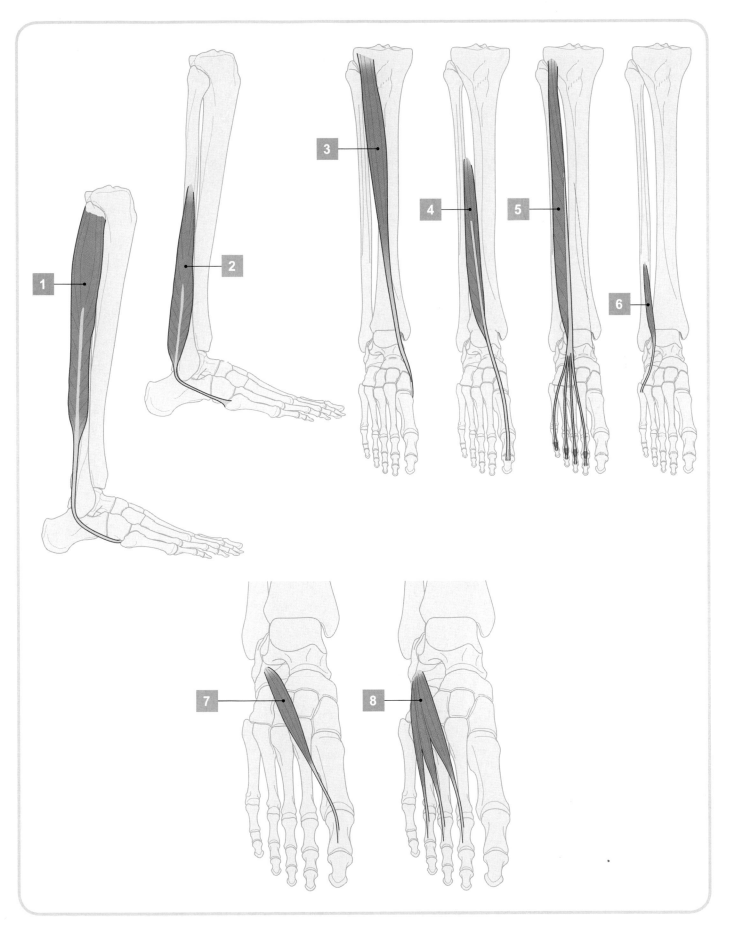

First layer of muscles in the sole of the foot
(spinal segments in bold are the major segments innervating the muscle)

Muscle		Origin	Insertion	Innervation	Function
Abductor hallucis	1	Medial process of calcaneal tuberosity	Medial side of base of proximal phalanx of great toe	Medial plantar nerve from the tibial nerve [**S1**, **S2**, **S3**]	Abducts and flexes great toe at metatarsophalangeal joint
Flexor digitorum brevis	2	Medial process of calcaneal tuberosity and plantar aponeurosis	Sides of plantar surface of middle phalanges of lateral four toes	Medial plantar nerve from the tibial nerve [**S1**, **S2**, **S3**]	Flexes lateral four toes at proximal interphalangeal joint
Abductor digiti minimi	3	Lateral and medial processes of calcaneal tuberosity, and band of connective tissue connecting calcaneus with base of metatarsal V	Lateral side of base of proximal phalanx of little toe	Lateral plantar nerve from the tibial nerve [**S1**, **S2**, **S3**]	Abducts little toe at the metatarsophalangeal joint

Second layer of muscles in the sole of the foot

Quadratus plantae	4	Medial surface of calcaneus and lateral process of calcaneal tuberosity	Lateral side of tendon of flexor digitorum longus in proximal sole of the foot	Lateral plantar nerve from tibial nerve [**S1**, **S2**, **S3**]	Assists flexor digitorum longus tendon in flexing toes II to V
Lumbricals	5	First lumbrical—medial side of tendon of flexor digitorum longus associated with toe II; second, third, and fourth lumbricals—adjacent surfaces of adjacent tendons of flexor digitorum longus	Medial free margins of extensor hoods of toes II to V	First lumbrical—medial plantar nerve from the tibial nerve; second, third, and fourth lumbricals—lateral plantar nerve from the tibial nerve [**S2**, **S3**]	Flexion of metatarsophalangeal joint and extension of interphalangeal joints

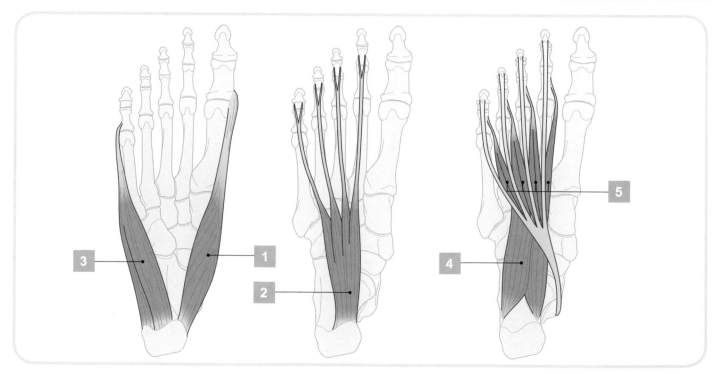

Third layer of muscles in the sole of the foot
(spinal segments in bold are the major segments innervating the muscle)

Muscle		Origin	Insertion	Innervation	Function
Flexor digiti minimi brevis	1	Base of metatarsal V and related sheath of fibularis longus tendon	Lateral side of base of proximal phalanx of little toe	Lateral plantar nerve from tibial nerve [S2, S3]	Flexes little toe at metatarsophalangeal joint
Flexor hallucis brevis	2	Plantar surface of cuboid and lateral cuneiform; tendon of tibialis posterior	Lateral and medial sides of base of proximal phalanx of the great toe	Medial plantar nerve from tibial nerve [S1, S2]	Flexes metatarsophalangeal joint of the great toe
Adductor hallucis	3	Transverse head—ligaments associated with metatarsophalangeal joints of lateral three toes; oblique head—bases of metatarsals II to IV and from sheath covering fibularis longus	Lateral side of base of proximal phalanx of great toe	Lateral plantar nerve from tibial nerve [S2, S3]	Adducts great toe at metatarsophalangeal joint

Fourth layer of muscles in the sole of the foot

Muscle		Origin	Insertion	Innervation	Function
Dorsal interossei	4	Sides of adjacent metatarsals	Extensor hoods and bases of proximal phalanges of toes II to IV	Lateral plantar nerve from tibial nerve; first and second dorsal interossei also innervated by deep fibular nerve [S2, S3]	Abduction of toes II to IV at metatarsophalangeal joints; resist extension of metatarsophalangeal joints and flexion of interphalangeal joints
Plantar interossei	5	Medial sides of metatarsals of toes III to V	Extensor hoods and bases of proximal phalanges of toes III to V	Lateral plantar nerve from tibial nerve [S2, S3]	Adduction of toes III to V at metatarsophalangeal joints; resist extension of the metatarsophalangeal joints and flexion of the interphalangeal joints

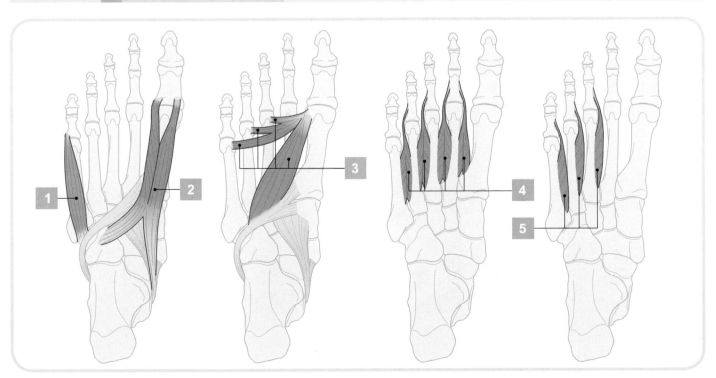

CONTENTS

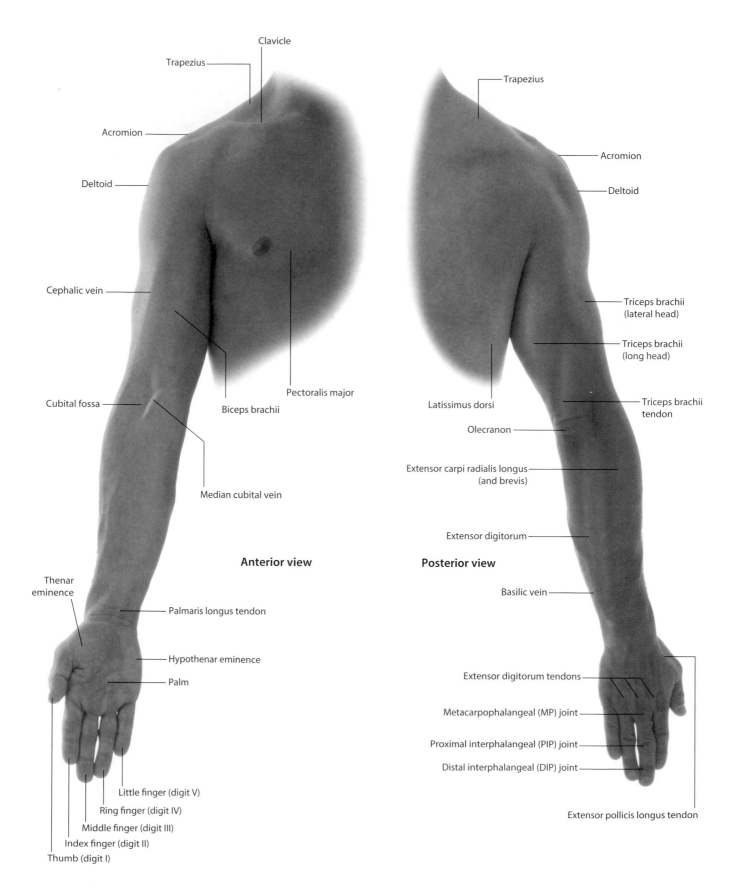

Clavicle

Trapezius

Acromion

Deltoid

Cephalic vein

Cubital fossa

Pectoralis major

Biceps brachii

Median cubital vein

Anterior view

Thenar eminence

Palmaris longus tendon

Hypothenar eminence

Palm

Little finger (digit V)

Ring finger (digit IV)

Middle finger (digit III)

Index finger (digit II)

Thumb (digit I)

Trapezius

Acromion

Deltoid

Triceps brachii (lateral head)

Triceps brachii (long head)

Triceps brachii tendon

Latissimus dorsi

Olecranon

Extensor carpi radialis longus (and brevis)

Extensor digitorum

Posterior view

Basilic vein

Extensor digitorum tendons

Metacarpophalangeal (MP) joint

Proximal interphalangeal (PIP) joint

Distal interphalangeal (DIP) joint

Extensor pollicis longus tendon

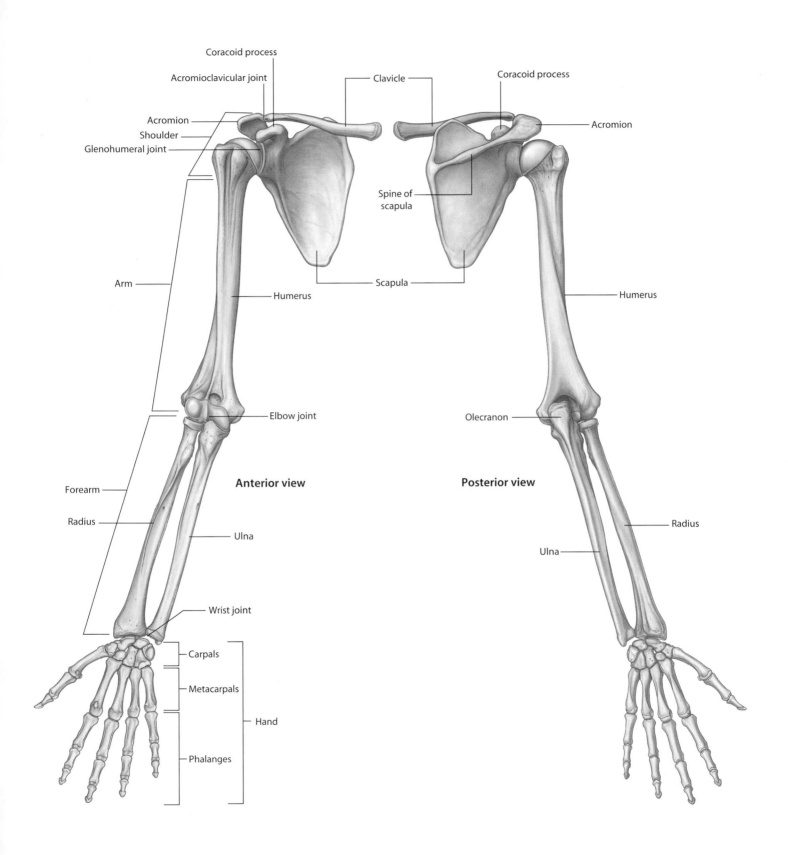

Coracoid process

Acromioclavicular joint

Clavicle

Coracoid process

Acromion

Shoulder

Acromion

Glenohumeral joint

Spine of scapula

Arm

Humerus

Scapula

Humerus

Anterior view

Elbow joint

Olecranon

Posterior view

Forearm

Radius

Radius

Ulna

Ulna

Wrist joint

Carpals

Metacarpals

Hand

Phalanges

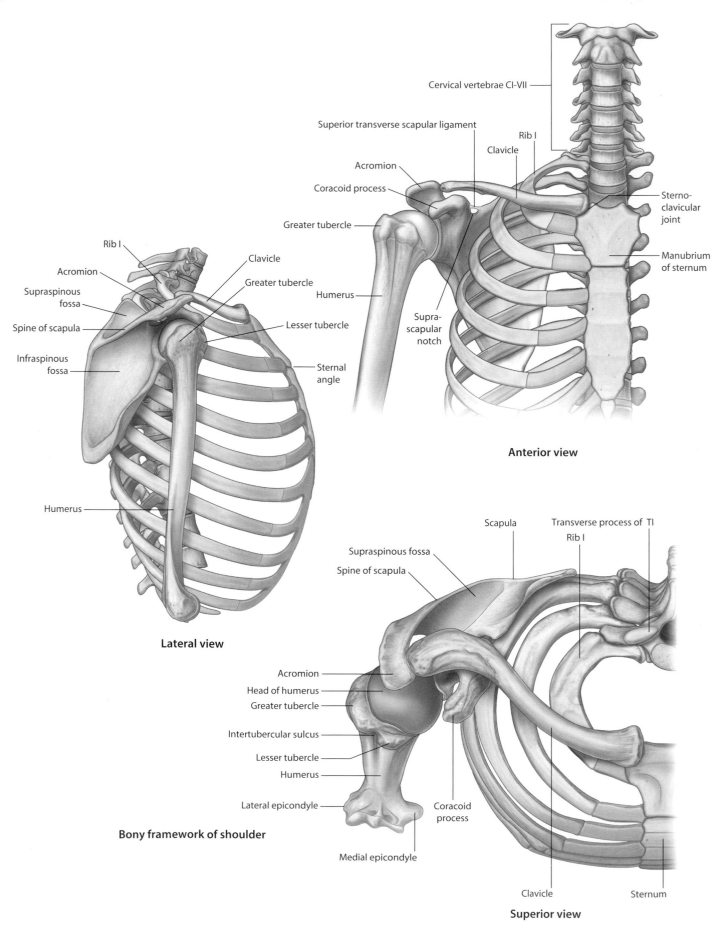

Cervical vertebrae CI–VII

Superior transverse scapular ligament

Rib I

Clavicle

Acromion

Coracoid process

Greater tubercle

Sterno-clavicular joint

Humerus

Supra-scapular notch

Manubrium of sternum

Anterior view

Rib I

Acromion

Clavicle

Supraspinous fossa

Greater tubercle

Spine of scapula

Lesser tubercle

Infraspinous fossa

Sternal angle

Humerus

Lateral view

Scapula

Transverse process of TI

Supraspinous fossa

Rib I

Spine of scapula

Acromion

Head of humerus

Greater tubercle

Intertubercular sulcus

Lesser tubercle

Humerus

Lateral epicondyle

Coracoid process

Bony framework of shoulder

Medial epicondyle

Clavicle

Sternum

Superior view

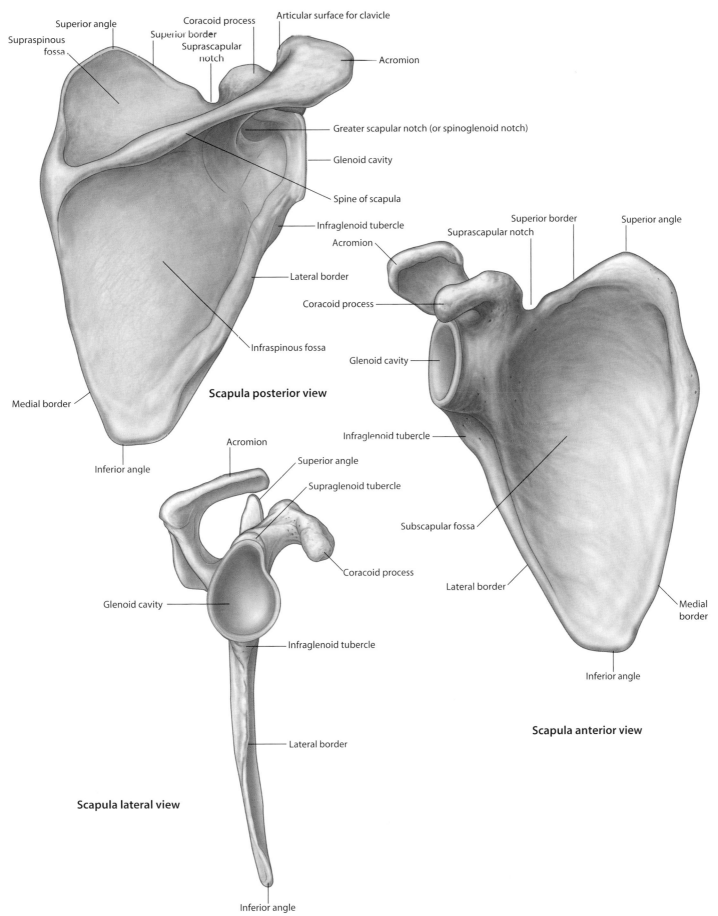

Superior angle

Supraspinous fossa

Superior border

Coracoid process

Suprascapular notch

Articular surface for clavicle

Acromion

Greater scapular notch (or spinoglenoid notch)

Glenoid cavity

Spine of scapula

Infraglenoid tubercle

Lateral border

Infraspinous fossa

Medial border

Inferior angle

Scapula posterior view

Superior border

Superior angle

Suprascapular notch

Acromion

Coracoid process

Glenoid cavity

Infraglenoid tubercle

Subscapular fossa

Lateral border

Medial border

Inferior angle

Scapula anterior view

Acromion

Superior angle

Supraglenoid tubercle

Coracoid process

Glenoid cavity

Infraglenoid tubercle

Lateral border

Inferior angle

Scapula lateral view

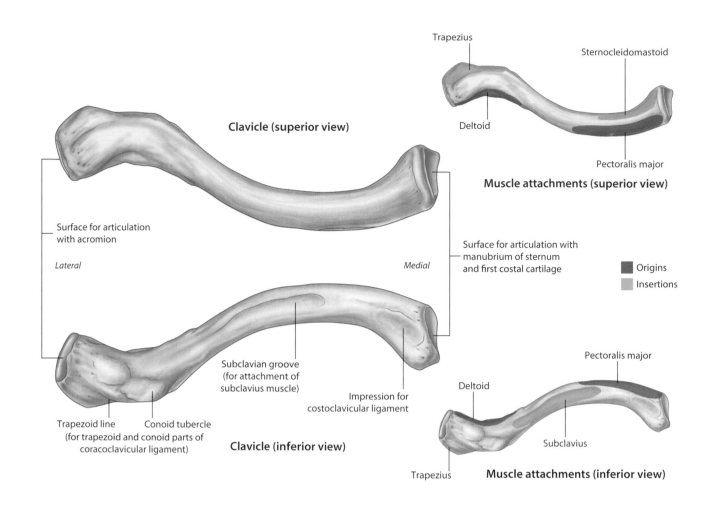

Clavicle (superior view)

Trapezius

Sternocleidomastoid

Deltoid

Pectoralis major

Muscle attachments (superior view)

Surface for articulation with acromion

Lateral

Surface for articulation with manubrium of sternum and first costal cartilage

■ Origins
■ Insertions

Medial

Subclavian groove (for attachment of subclavius muscle)

Impression for costoclavicular ligament

Trapezoid line   Conoid tubercle (for trapezoid and conoid parts of coracoclavicular ligament)

Clavicle (inferior view)

Pectoralis major

Deltoid

Subclavius

Trapezius

Muscle attachments (inferior view)

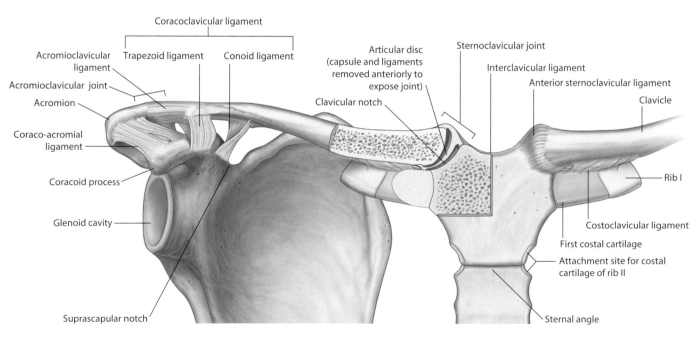

Coracoclavicular ligament

Trapezoid ligament   Conoid ligament

Acromioclavicular ligament

Acromioclavicular joint

Acromion

Coraco-acromial ligament

Coracoid process

Glenoid cavity

Suprascapular notch

Articular disc (capsule and ligaments removed anteriorly to expose joint)

Clavicular notch

Sternoclavicular joint

Interclavicular ligament

Anterior sternoclavicular ligament

Clavicle

Rib I

Costoclavicular ligament

First costal cartilage

Attachment site for costal cartilage of rib II

Sternal angle

Joints and ligaments of the clavicle (anterior view)

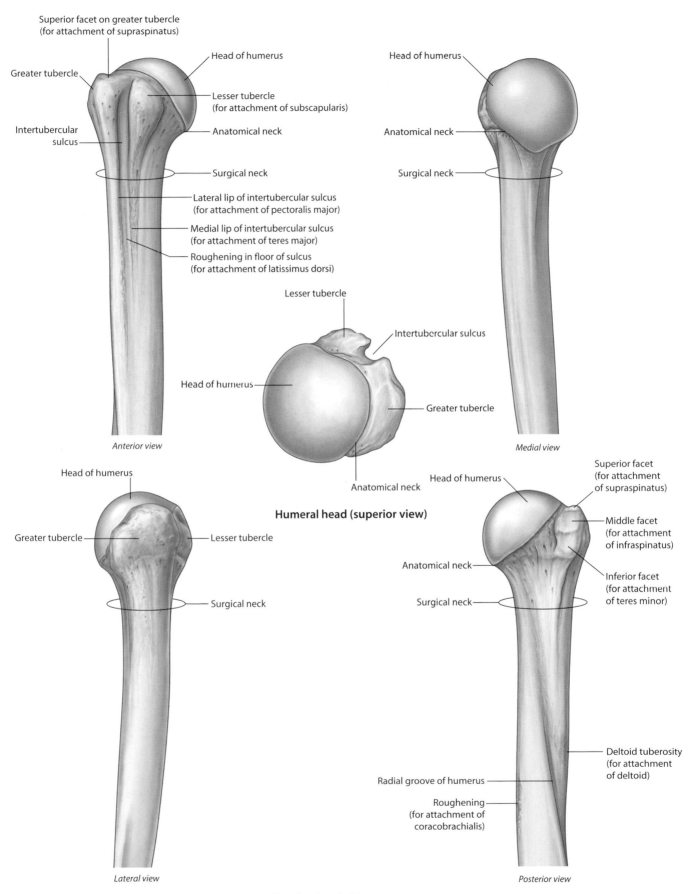

Superior facet on greater tubercle
(for attachment of supraspinatus)

Greater tubercle

Intertubercular
sulcus

Head of humerus

Lesser tubercle
(for attachment of subscapularis)

Anatomical neck

Surgical neck

Lateral lip of intertubercular sulcus
(for attachment of pectoralis major)

Medial lip of intertubercular sulcus
(for attachment of teres major)

Roughening in floor of sulcus
(for attachment of latissimus dorsi)

Anterior view

Head of humerus

Anatomical neck

Surgical neck

Medial view

Lesser tubercle

Intertubercular sulcus

Head of humerus

Greater tubercle

Anatomical neck

Humeral head (superior view)

Head of humerus

Greater tubercle

Lesser tubercle

Surgical neck

Lateral view

Head of humerus

Anatomical neck

Surgical neck

Superior facet
(for attachment
of supraspinatus)

Middle facet
(for attachment
of infraspinatus)

Inferior facet
(for attachment
of teres minor)

Deltoid tuberosity
(for attachment
of deltoid)

Radial groove of humerus

Roughening
(for attachment of
coracobrachialis)

Posterior view

Proximal end of humerus

389

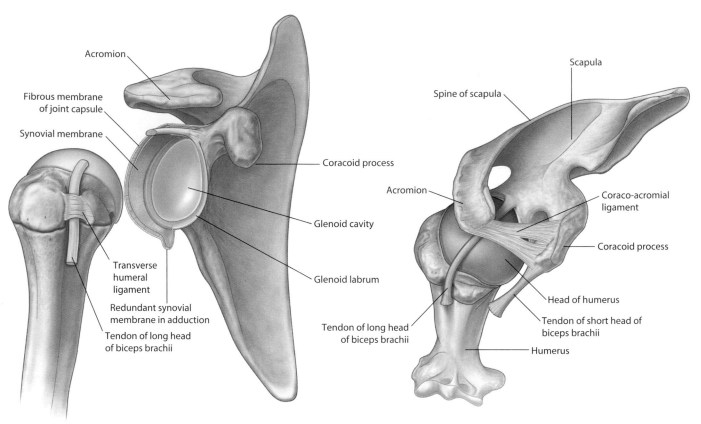

Acromion

Fibrous membrane
of joint capsule

Synovial membrane

Coracoid process

Glenoid cavity

Transverse
humeral
ligament

Glenoid labrum

Redundant synovial
membrane in adduction

Tendon of long head
of biceps brachii

Scapula

Spine of scapula

Acromion

Coraco-acromial
ligament

Coracoid process

Head of humerus

Tendon of long head
of biceps brachii

Tendon of short head of
biceps brachii

Humerus

Origins of biceps brachii tendons (superior view)

Articular surfaces of glenohumeral joint (anterolateral oblique view)

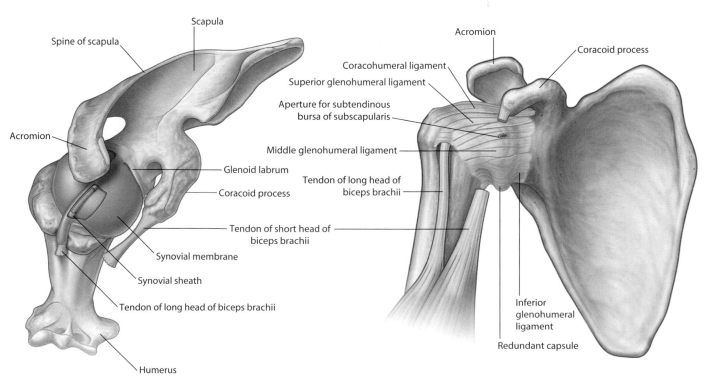

Scapula

Spine of scapula

Acromion

Glenoid labrum

Coracoid process

Synovial membrane

Synovial sheath

Tendon of long head of biceps brachii

Humerus

Acromion

Coracoid process

Coracohumeral ligament

Superior glenohumeral ligament

Aperture for subtendinous
bursa of subscapularis

Middle glenohumeral ligament

Tendon of long head of
biceps brachii

Tendon of short head of
biceps brachii

Inferior
glenohumeral
ligament

Redundant capsule

Synovial membrane (superior view)

Fibrous membrane of joint capsule (anterior view)

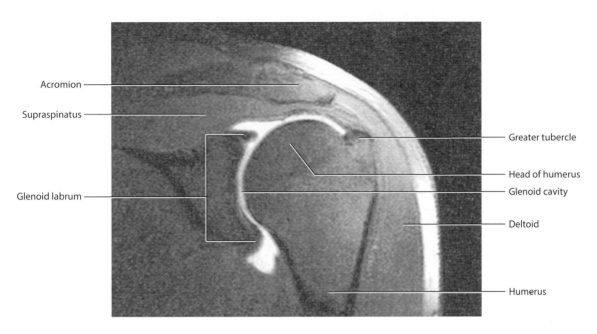

Acromion

Supraspinatus

Glenoid labrum

Greater tubercle

Head of humerus

Glenoid cavity

Deltoid

Humerus

Anterior view of the glenohumeral joint.
T1-weighted MR image in coronal plane

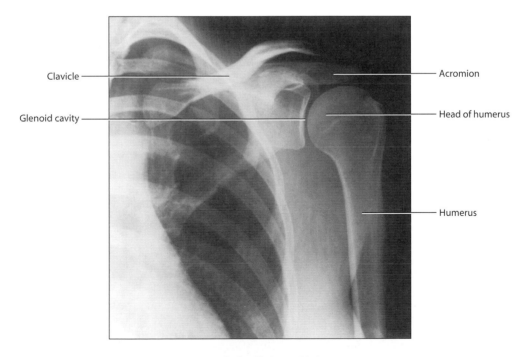

Clavicle

Glenoid cavity

Acromion

Head of humerus

Humerus

Normal glenohumeral joint.
Radiograph, AP view

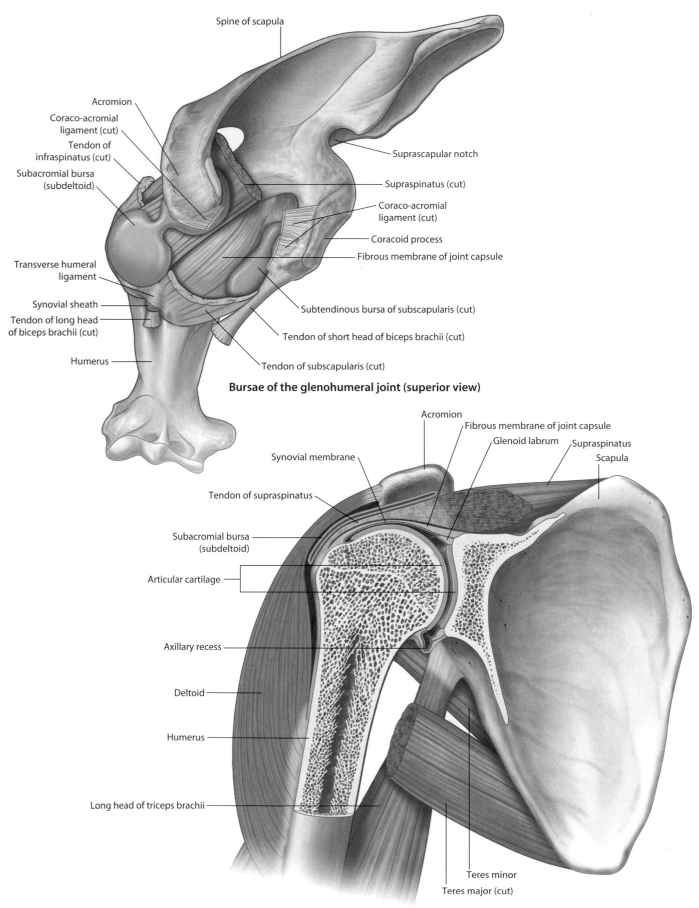

Spine of scapula

Acromion

Coraco-acromial
ligament (cut)

Tendon of
infraspinatus (cut)

Subacromial bursa
(subdeltoid)

Transverse humeral
ligament

Synovial sheath

Tendon of long head
of biceps brachii (cut)

Humerus

Suprascapular notch

Supraspinatus (cut)

Coraco-acromial
ligament (cut)

Coracoid process

Fibrous membrane of joint capsule

Subtendinous bursa of subscapularis (cut)

Tendon of short head of biceps brachii (cut)

Tendon of subscapularis (cut)

Bursae of the glenohumeral joint (superior view)

Acromion

Fibrous membrane of joint capsule

Glenoid labrum

Supraspinatus

Scapula

Synovial membrane

Tendon of supraspinatus

Subacromial bursa
(subdeltoid)

Articular cartilage

Axillary recess

Deltoid

Humerus

Long head of triceps brachii

Teres minor

Teres major (cut)

Glenohumeral joint (anterior view)

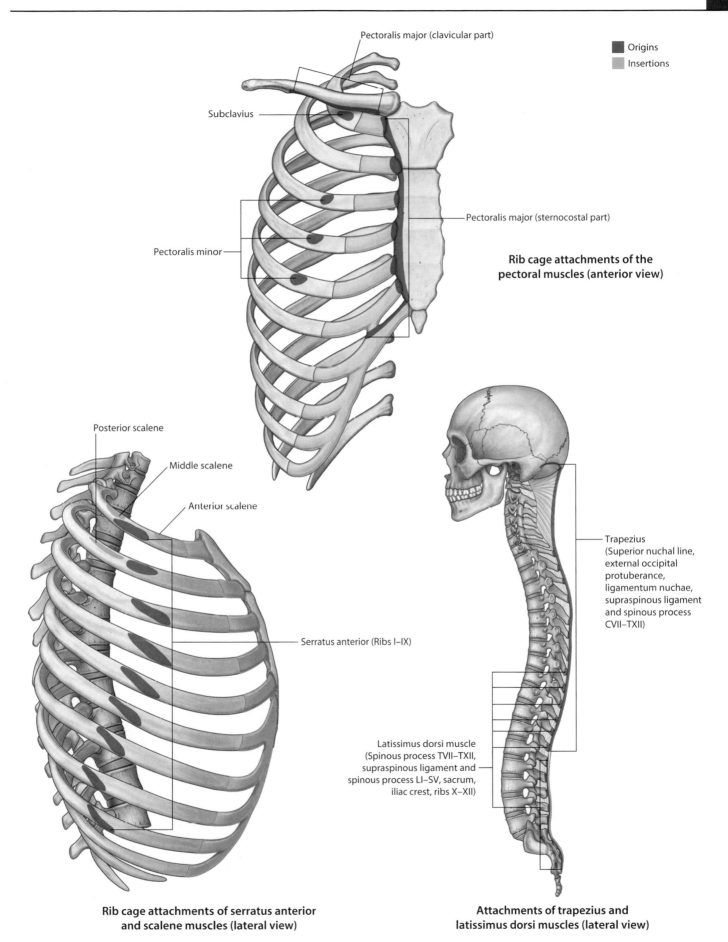

Pectoralis major (clavicular part)

Subclavius

Pectoralis minor

Pectoralis major (sternocostal part)

Origins
Insertions

Rib cage attachments of the pectoral muscles (anterior view)

Posterior scalene

Middle scalene

Anterior scalene

Serratus anterior (Ribs I–IX)

Trapezius
(Superior nuchal line, external occipital protuberance, ligamentum nuchae, supraspinous ligament and spinous process CVII–TXII)

Latissimus dorsi muscle
(Spinous process TVII–TXII, supraspinous ligament and spinous process LI–SV, sacrum, iliac crest, ribs X–XII)

Rib cage attachments of serratus anterior and scalene muscles (lateral view)

Attachments of trapezius and latissimus dorsi muscles (lateral view)

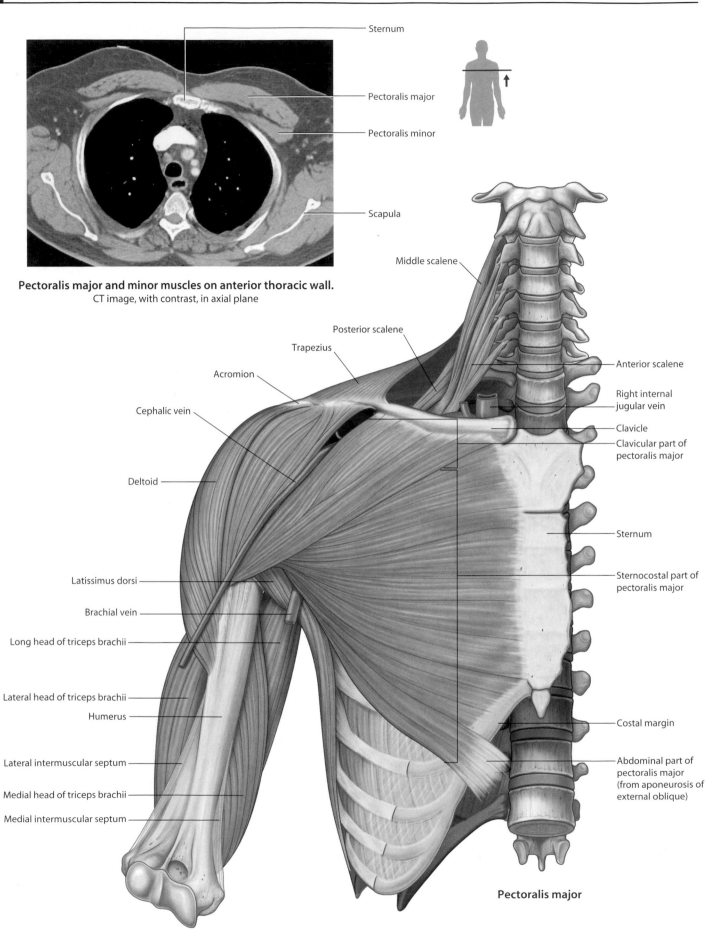

Sternum

Pectoralis major

Pectoralis minor

Scapula

Pectoralis major and minor muscles on anterior thoracic wall.
CT image, with contrast, in axial plane

Middle scalene

Posterior scalene

Trapezius

Acromion

Cephalic vein

Deltoid

Anterior scalene

Right internal
jugular vein

Clavicle

Clavicular part of
pectoralis major

Sternum

Latissimus dorsi

Brachial vein

Long head of triceps brachii

Sternocostal part of
pectoralis major

Lateral head of triceps brachii

Humerus

Lateral intermuscular septum

Medial head of triceps brachii

Medial intermuscular septum

Costal margin

Abdominal part of
pectoralis major
(from aponeurosis of
external oblique)

Pectoralis major

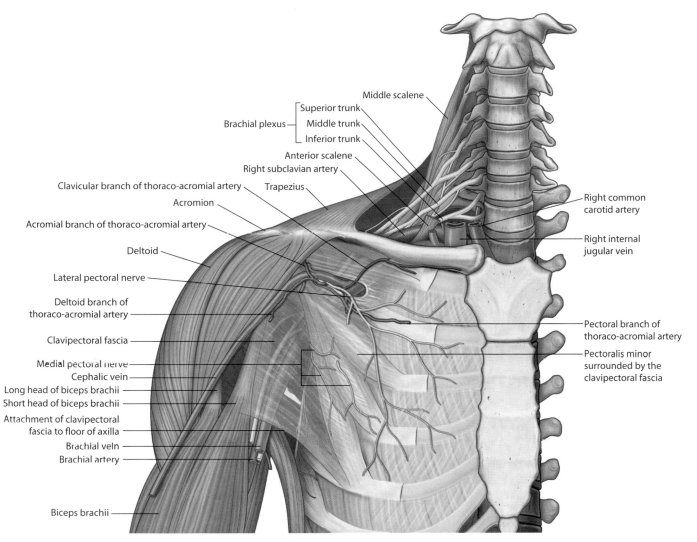

Middle scalene

Brachial plexus —⎡ Superior trunk
                  ⎢ Middle trunk
                  ⎣ Inferior trunk

Anterior scalene

Right subclavian artery

Clavicular branch of thoraco-acromial artery — Trapezius

Acromion

Acromial branch of thoraco-acromial artery

Deltoid

Lateral pectoral nerve

Deltoid branch of thoraco-acromial artery

Clavipectoral fascia

Medial pectoral nerve

Cephalic vein

Long head of biceps brachii

Short head of biceps brachii

Attachment of clavipectoral fascia to floor of axilla

Brachial vein

Brachial artery

Biceps brachii

Right common carotid artery

Right internal jugular vein

Pectoral branch of thoraco-acromial artery

Pectoralis minor surrounded by the clavipectoral fascia

Clavipectoral fascia and related structures

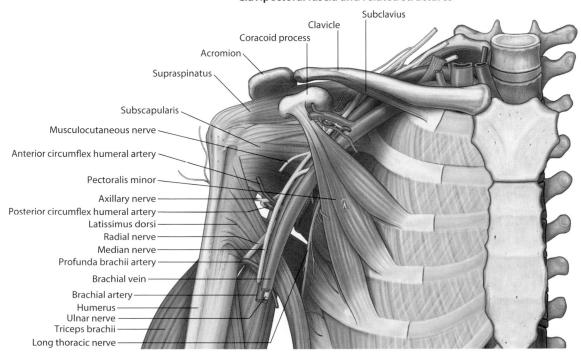

Subclavius

Clavicle

Coracoid process

Acromion

Supraspinatus

Subscapularis

Musculocutaneous nerve

Anterior circumflex humeral artery

Pectoralis minor

Axillary nerve

Posterior circumflex humeral artery

Latissimus dorsi

Radial nerve

Median nerve

Profunda brachii artery

Brachial vein

Brachial artery

Humerus

Ulnar nerve

Triceps brachii

Long thoracic nerve

Pectoralis minor

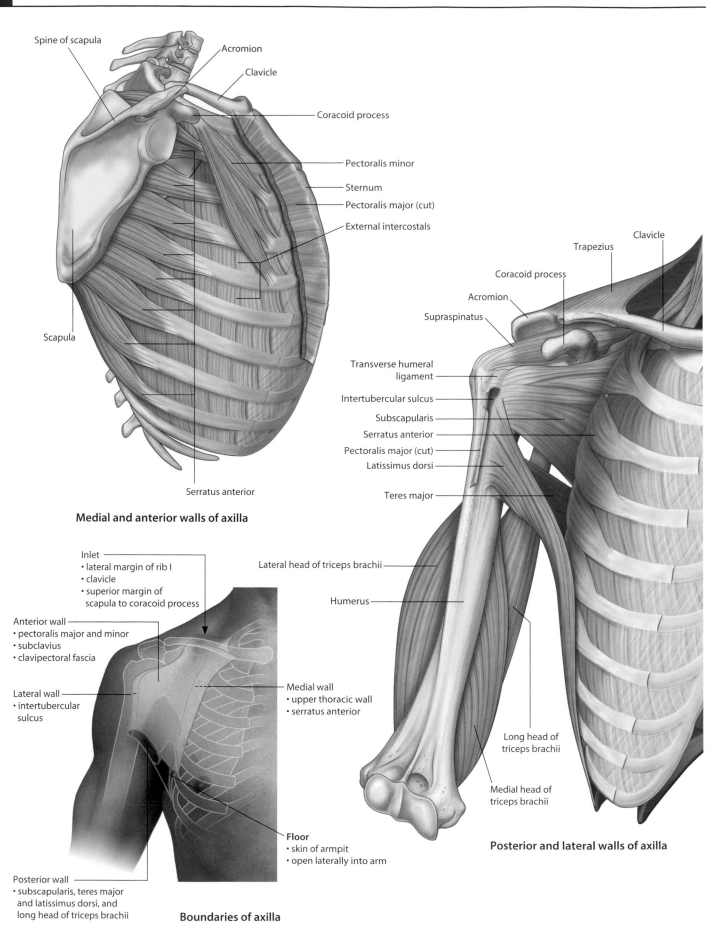

Spine of scapula
Acromion
Clavicle
Coracoid process
Pectoralis minor
Sternum
Pectoralis major (cut)
External intercostals
Scapula
Serratus anterior

Medial and anterior walls of axilla

Clavicle
Trapezius
Coracoid process
Acromion
Supraspinatus
Transverse humeral ligament
Intertubercular sulcus
Subscapularis
Serratus anterior
Pectoralis major (cut)
Latissimus dorsi
Teres major
Lateral head of triceps brachii
Humerus
Long head of triceps brachii
Medial head of triceps brachii

Posterior and lateral walls of axilla

Inlet
• lateral margin of rib I
• clavicle
• superior margin of scapula to coracoid process

Anterior wall
• pectoralis major and minor
• subclavius
• clavipectoral fascia

Lateral wall
• intertubercular sulcus

Medial wall
• upper thoracic wall
• serratus anterior

Floor
• skin of armpit
• open laterally into arm

Posterior wall
• subscapularis, teres major and latissimus dorsi, and long head of triceps brachii

Boundaries of axilla

396

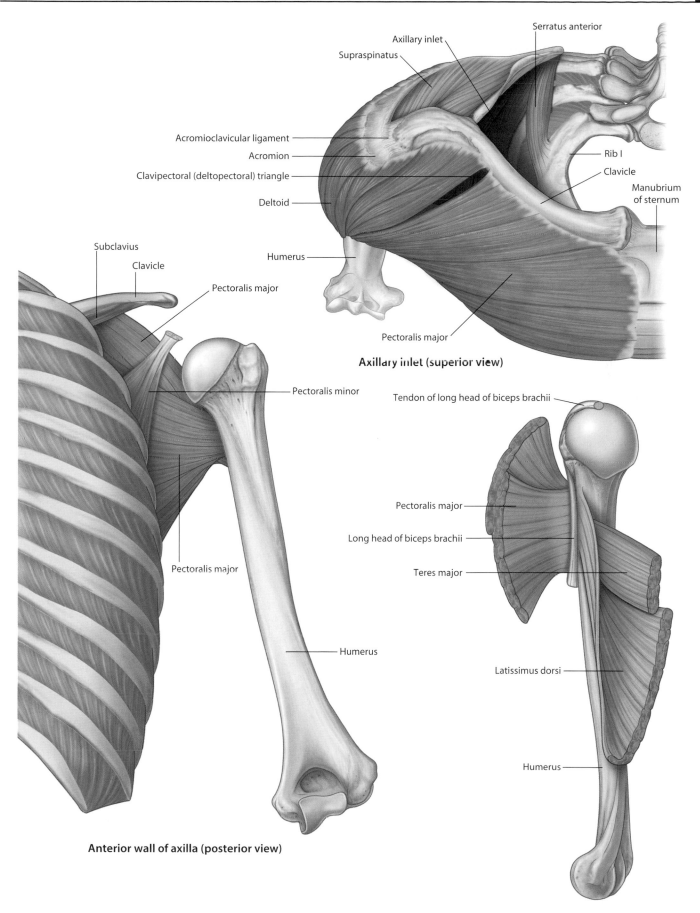

Axillary inlet (superior view)

Anterior wall of axilla (posterior view)

Lateral wall of axilla (medial view)

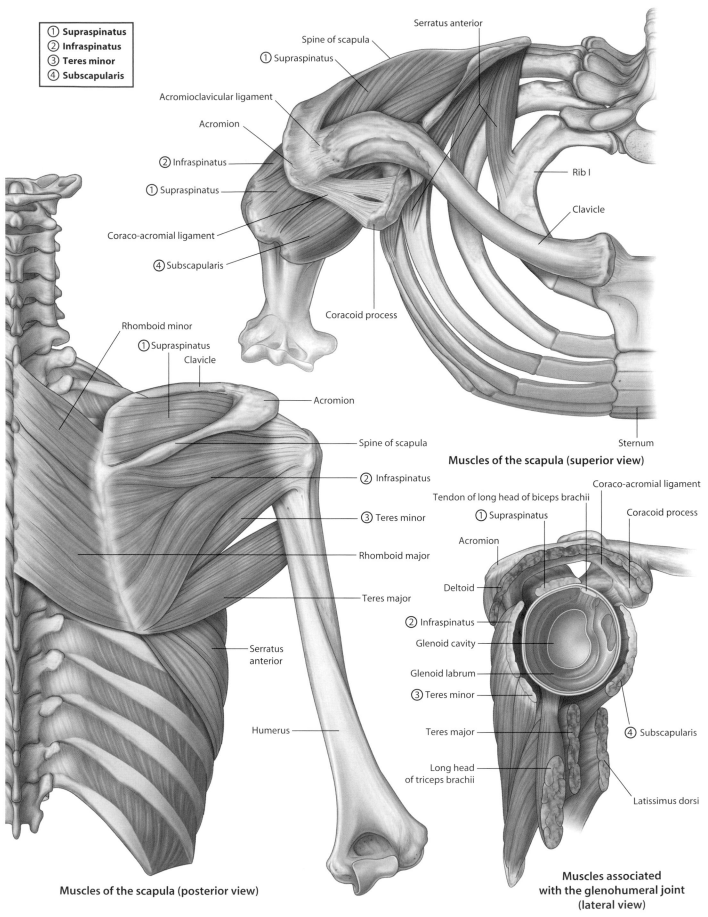

① **Supraspinatus**
② **Infraspinatus**
③ **Teres minor**
④ **Subscapularis**

Spine of scapula
Serratus anterior
① Supraspinatus

Acromioclavicular ligament

Acromion

② Infraspinatus

① Supraspinatus

Coraco-acromial ligament

④ Subscapularis

Coracoid process

Rib I

Clavicle

Sternum

Muscles of the scapula (superior view)

Rhomboid minor
① Supraspinatus
Clavicle

Acromion

Spine of scapula

② Infraspinatus

③ Teres minor

Rhomboid major

Teres major

Serratus anterior

Humerus

Muscles of the scapula (posterior view)

Coraco-acromial ligament
Coracoid process

Tendon of long head of biceps brachii
① Supraspinatus

Acromion

Deltoid

② Infraspinatus

Glenoid cavity

Glenoid labrum

③ Teres minor

Teres major

Long head of triceps brachii

④ Subscapularis

Latissimus dorsi

Muscles associated with the glenohumeral joint (lateral view)

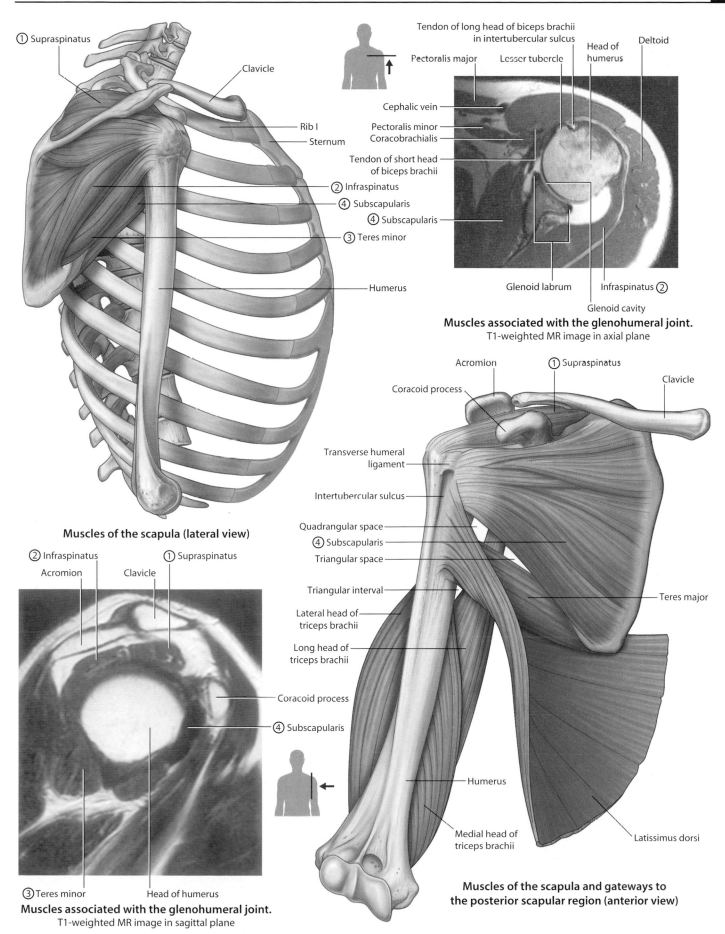

① Supraspinatus

Clavicle

Rib I

Sternum

② Infraspinatus

④ Subscapularis

④ Subscapularis

③ Teres minor

Humerus

Muscles of the scapula (lateral view)

Tendon of long head of biceps brachii
in intertubercular sulcus

Pectoralis major   Lesser tubercle   Head of humerus   Deltoid

Cephalic vein

Pectoralis minor
Coracobrachialis

Tendon of short head
of biceps brachii

④ Subscapularis

Glenoid labrum   Infraspinatus ②

Glenoid cavity

Muscles associated with the glenohumeral joint.
T1-weighted MR image in axial plane

② Infraspinatus   ① Supraspinatus
Acromion   Clavicle

③ Teres minor   Head of humerus

Muscles associated with the glenohumeral joint.
T1-weighted MR image in sagittal plane

Acromion   ① Supraspinatus

Coracoid process   Clavicle

Transverse humeral
ligament

Intertubercular sulcus

Quadrangular space

④ Subscapularis

Triangular space

Triangular interval

Lateral head of
triceps brachii

Long head of
triceps brachii

Coracoid process

④ Subscapularis

Teres major

Humerus

Medial head of
triceps brachii

Latissimus dorsi

**Muscles of the scapula and gateways to
the posterior scapular region (anterior view)**

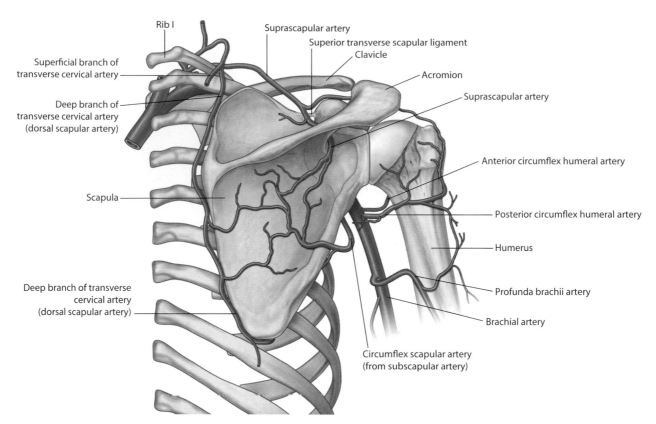

Rib I

Suprascapular artery

Superior transverse scapular ligament

Clavicle

Superficial branch of transverse cervical artery

Acromion

Deep branch of transverse cervical artery (dorsal scapular artery)

Suprascapular artery

Anterior circumflex humeral artery

Scapula

Posterior circumflex humeral artery

Humerus

Deep branch of transverse cervical artery (dorsal scapular artery)

Profunda brachii artery

Brachial artery

Circumflex scapular artery (from subscapular artery)

Arteries of the shoulder (posterior view)

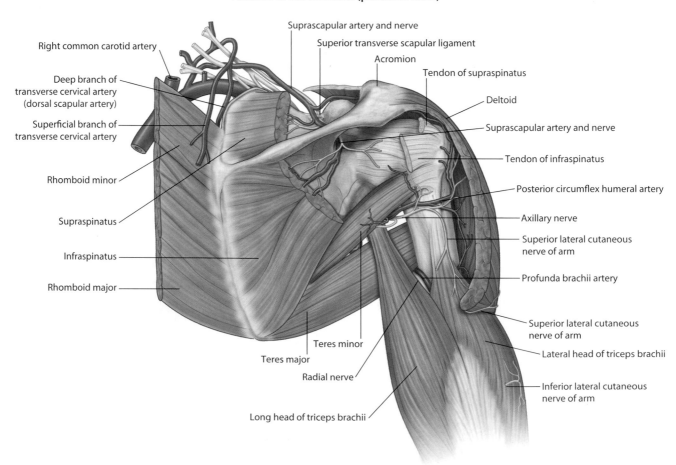

Right common carotid artery

Suprascapular artery and nerve

Superior transverse scapular ligament

Acromion

Deep branch of transverse cervical artery (dorsal scapular artery)

Tendon of supraspinatus

Deltoid

Superficial branch of transverse cervical artery

Suprascapular artery and nerve

Rhomboid minor

Tendon of infraspinatus

Supraspinatus

Posterior circumflex humeral artery

Axillary nerve

Infraspinatus

Superior lateral cutaneous nerve of arm

Rhomboid major

Profunda brachii artery

Superior lateral cutaneous nerve of arm

Teres minor

Lateral head of triceps brachii

Teres major

Radial nerve

Inferior lateral cutaneous nerve of arm

Long head of triceps brachii

Deep arteries and nerves of the shoulder (posterior view)

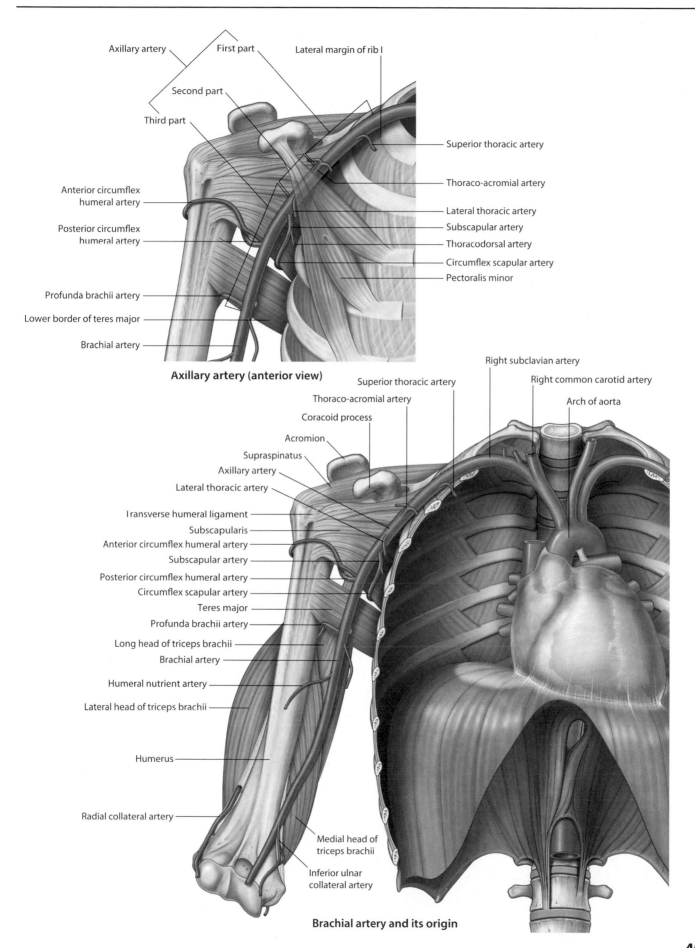

Axillary artery
First part
Second part
Third part
Lateral margin of rib I

Anterior circumflex humeral artery
Posterior circumflex humeral artery

Profunda brachii artery
Lower border of teres major
Brachial artery

Superior thoracic artery
Thoraco-acromial artery
Lateral thoracic artery
Subscapular artery
Thoracodorsal artery
Circumflex scapular artery
Pectoralis minor

Axillary artery (anterior view)

Superior thoracic artery
Thoraco-acromial artery
Coracoid process
Acromion
Supraspinatus
Axillary artery
Lateral thoracic artery
Transverse humeral ligament
Subscapularis
Anterior circumflex humeral artery
Subscapular artery
Posterior circumflex humeral artery
Circumflex scapular artery
Teres major
Profunda brachii artery
Long head of triceps brachii
Brachial artery
Humeral nutrient artery
Lateral head of triceps brachii
Humerus
Radial collateral artery

Right subclavian artery
Right common carotid artery
Arch of aorta

Medial head of triceps brachii
Inferior ulnar collateral artery

Brachial artery and its origin

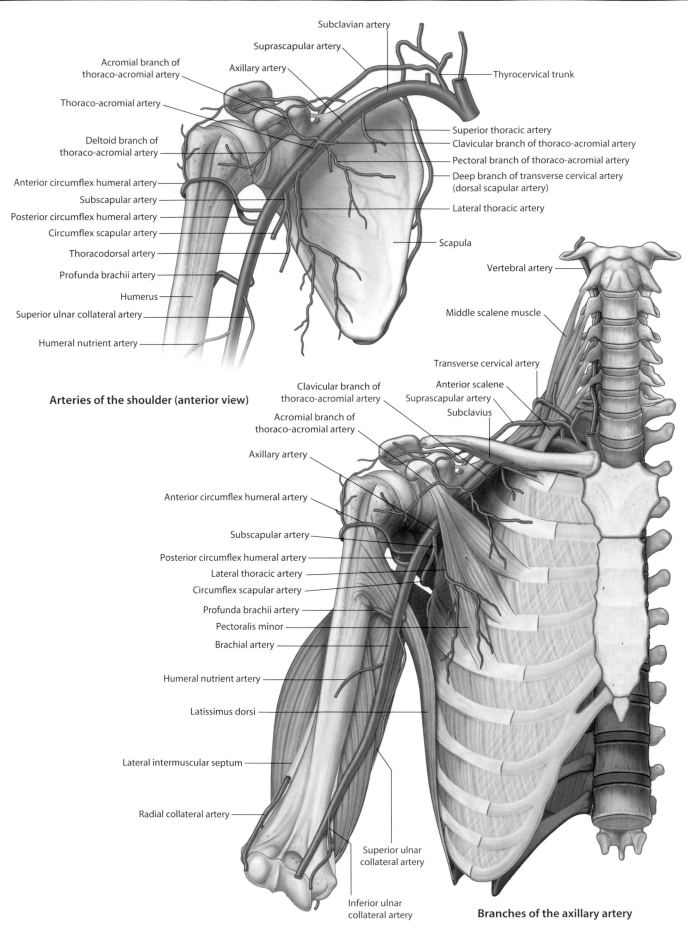

Subclavian artery

Suprascapular artery

Axillary artery

Acromial branch of
thoraco-acromial artery

Thoraco-acromial artery

Deltoid branch of
thoraco-acromial artery

Anterior circumflex humeral artery

Subscapular artery

Posterior circumflex humeral artery

Circumflex scapular artery

Thoracodorsal artery

Profunda brachii artery

Humerus

Superior ulnar collateral artery

Humeral nutrient artery

Thyrocervical trunk

Superior thoracic artery

Clavicular branch of thoraco-acromial artery

Pectoral branch of thoraco-acromial artery

Deep branch of transverse cervical artery
(dorsal scapular artery)

Lateral thoracic artery

Scapula

Arteries of the shoulder (anterior view)

Clavicular branch of
thoraco-acromial artery

Acromial branch of
thoraco-acromial artery

Axillary artery

Anterior circumflex humeral artery

Subscapular artery

Posterior circumflex humeral artery

Lateral thoracic artery

Circumflex scapular artery

Profunda brachii artery

Pectoralis minor

Brachial artery

Humeral nutrient artery

Latissimus dorsi

Lateral intermuscular septum

Radial collateral artery

Vertebral artery

Middle scalene muscle

Transverse cervical artery

Anterior scalene

Suprascapular artery

Subclavius

Inferior ulnar
collateral artery

Superior ulnar
collateral artery

Branches of the axillary artery

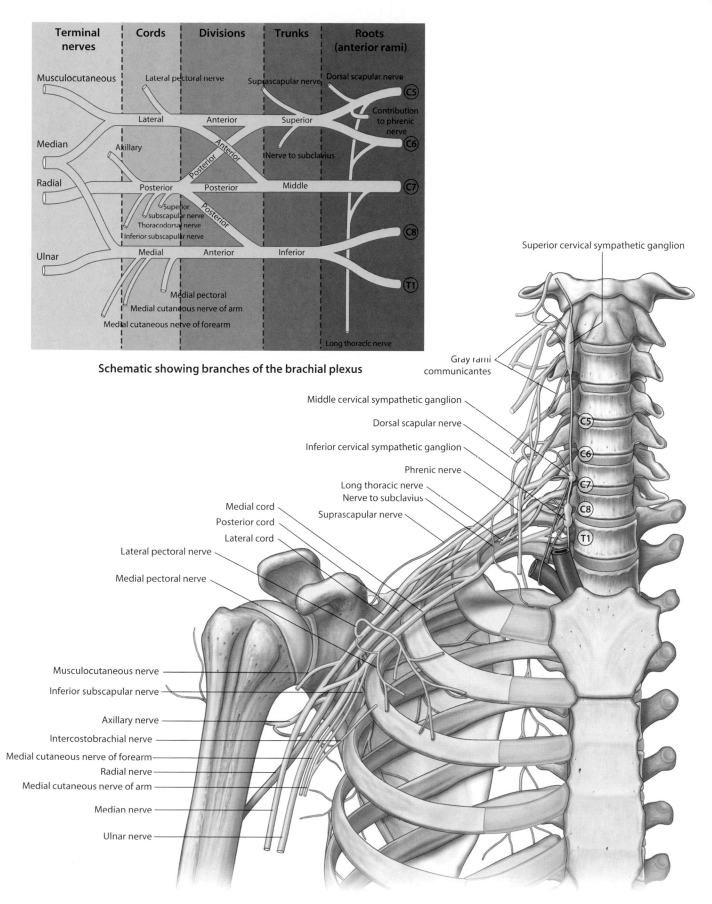

Terminal nerves	Cords	Divisions	Trunks	Roots (anterior rami)

Musculocutaneous — Lateral pectoral nerve — Suprascapular nerve — Dorsal scapular nerve — C5

Lateral — Anterior — Superior

Contribution to phrenic nerve — C6

Median — Axillary

Anterior

Nerve to subclavius

Radial — Posterior — Posterior — Middle — C7

Superior subscapular nerve
Thoracodorsal nerve
Inferior subscapular nerve

Posterior

C8

Ulnar — Medial — Anterior — Inferior

Medial pectoral
Medial cutaneous nerve of arm
Medial cutaneous nerve of forearm

T1

Long thoracic nerve

Schematic showing branches of the brachial plexus

Superior cervical sympathetic ganglion

Gray rami communicantes

Middle cervical sympathetic ganglion

Dorsal scapular nerve

Inferior cervical sympathetic ganglion

Phrenic nerve

Long thoracic nerve
Nerve to subclavius

Suprascapular nerve

C5
C6
C7
C8
T1

Medial cord
Posterior cord
Lateral cord

Lateral pectoral nerve

Medial pectoral nerve

Musculocutaneous nerve

Inferior subscapular nerve

Axillary nerve

Intercostobrachial nerve

Medial cutaneous nerve of forearm

Radial nerve

Medial cutaneous nerve of arm

Median nerve

Ulnar nerve

Brachial plexus

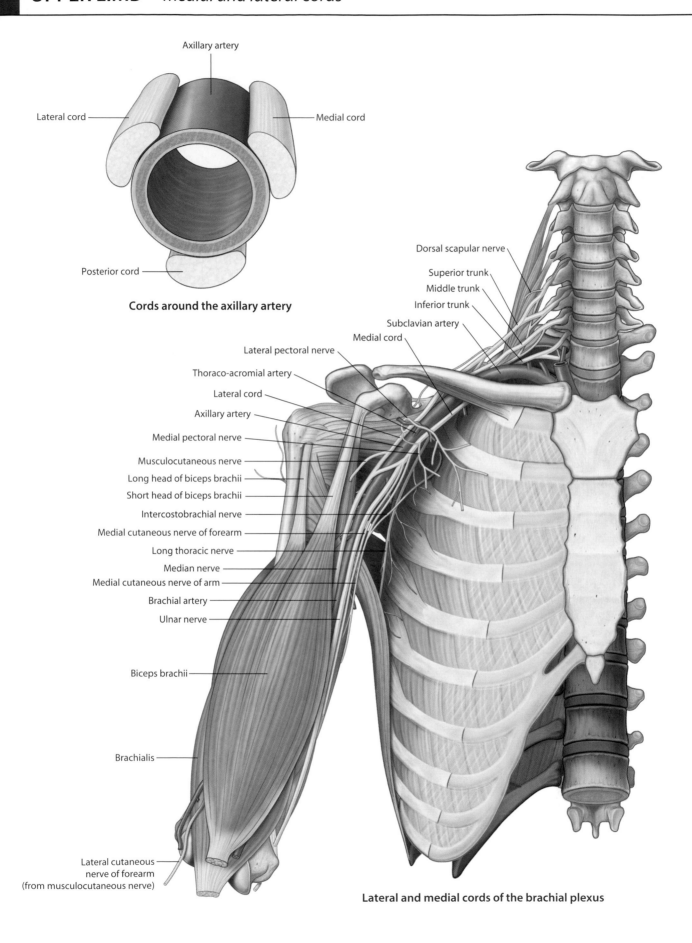

Axillary artery

Lateral cord

Medial cord

Posterior cord

Cords around the axillary artery

Dorsal scapular nerve

Superior trunk

Middle trunk

Inferior trunk

Subclavian artery

Medial cord

Lateral pectoral nerve

Thoraco-acromial artery

Lateral cord

Axillary artery

Medial pectoral nerve

Musculocutaneous nerve

Long head of biceps brachii

Short head of biceps brachii

Intercostobrachial nerve

Medial cutaneous nerve of forearm

Long thoracic nerve

Median nerve

Medial cutaneous nerve of arm

Brachial artery

Ulnar nerve

Biceps brachii

Brachialis

Lateral cutaneous
nerve of forearm
(from musculocutaneous nerve)

Lateral and medial cords of the brachial plexus

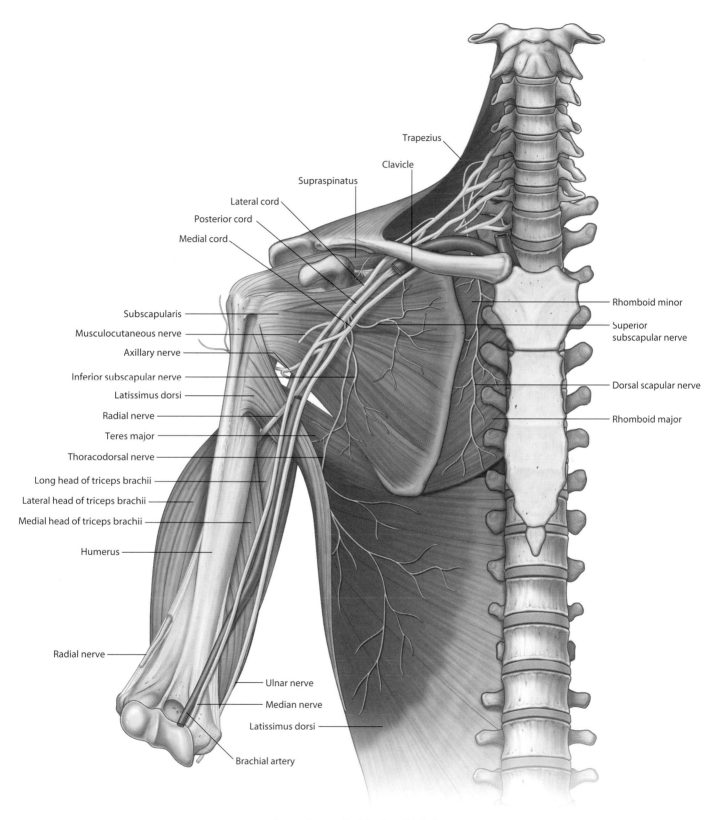

Trapezius

Clavicle

Supraspinatus

Lateral cord

Posterior cord

Medial cord

Subscapularis

Musculocutaneous nerve

Axillary nerve

Inferior subscapular nerve

Latissimus dorsi

Radial nerve

Teres major

Thoracodorsal nerve

Long head of triceps brachii

Lateral head of triceps brachii

Medial head of triceps brachii

Humerus

Radial nerve

Ulnar nerve

Median nerve

Latissimus dorsi

Brachial artery

Rhomboid minor

Superior subscapular nerve

Dorsal scapular nerve

Rhomboid major

**Posterior cord of the brachial plexus
(ribs and associated muscles removed)**

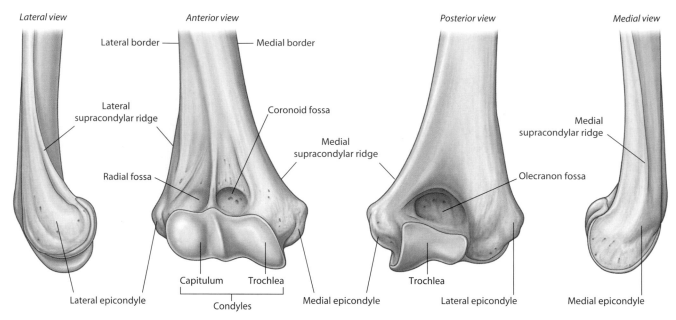

Lateral view

Lateral border — — Medial border

Lateral supracondylar ridge

Coronoid fossa

Medial supracondylar ridge

Radial fossa

Capitulum Trochlea

Condyles

Lateral epicondyle

Medial epicondyle

Anterior view

Posterior view

Medial supracondylar ridge

Olecranon fossa

Trochlea

Lateral epicondyle

Medial view

Medial epicondyle

Distal end of humerus

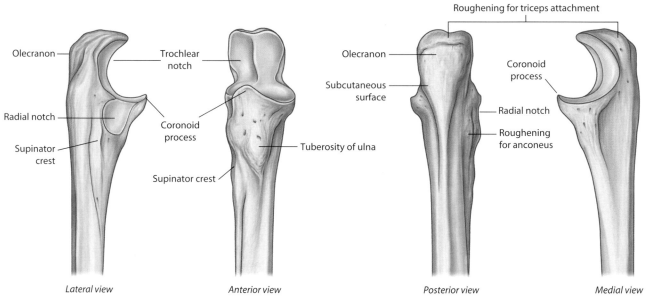

Olecranon

Radial notch

Supinator crest

Trochlear notch

Coronoid process

Supinator crest

Tuberosity of ulna

Lateral view

Anterior view

Roughening for triceps attachment

Olecranon

Subcutaneous surface

Coronoid process

Radial notch

Roughening for anconeus

Posterior view

Medial view

Proximal end of ulna

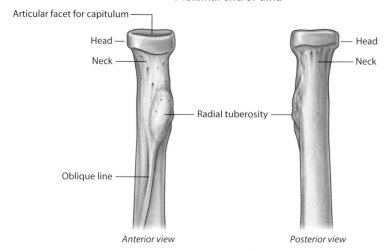

Articular facet for capitulum

Head —

Neck —

Radial tuberosity

Oblique line

Head

Neck

Anterior view

Posterior view

Proximal end of radius

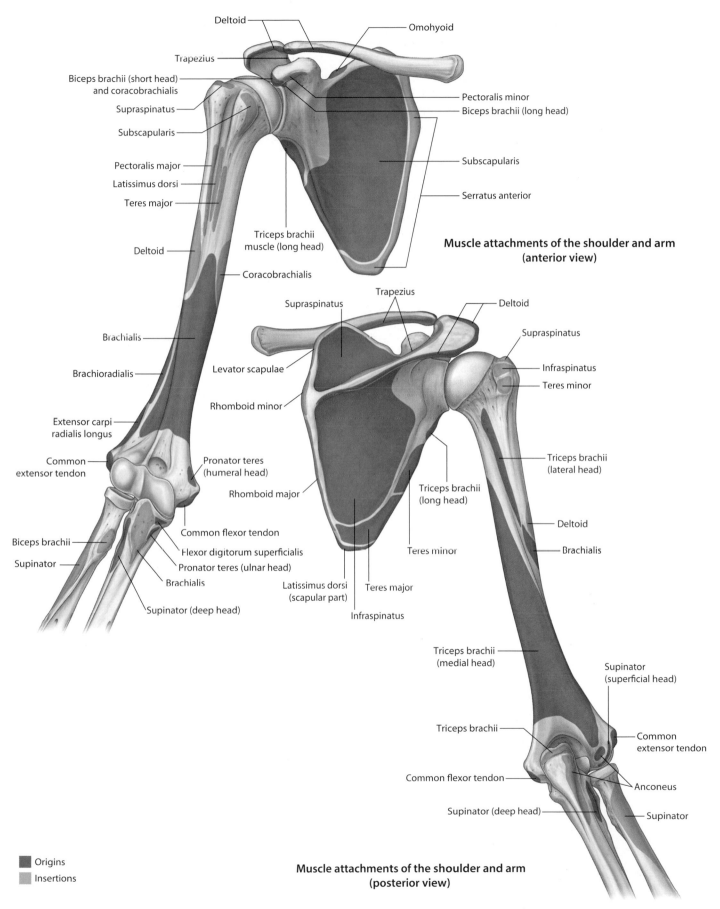

Deltoid
Omohyoid
Trapezius
Biceps brachii (short head) and coracobrachialis
Supraspinatus
Subscapularis
Pectoralis minor
Biceps brachii (long head)
Pectoralis major
Latissimus dorsi
Teres major
Subscapularis
Serratus anterior
Deltoid
Triceps brachii muscle (long head)
Coracobrachialis

Muscle attachments of the shoulder and arm (anterior view)

Brachialis
Brachioradialis
Extensor carpi radialis longus
Common extensor tendon
Biceps brachii
Supinator
Pronator teres (humeral head)
Common flexor tendon
Flexor digitorum superficialis
Pronator teres (ulnar head)
Brachialis
Supinator (deep head)

Supraspinatus
Trapezius
Deltoid
Supraspinatus
Infraspinatus
Teres minor
Levator scapulae
Rhomboid minor
Rhomboid major
Triceps brachii (long head)
Triceps brachii (lateral head)
Deltoid
Brachialis
Latissimus dorsi (scapular part)
Teres major
Infraspinatus
Teres minor

Triceps brachii (medial head)
Triceps brachii
Common flexor tendon
Supinator (deep head)
Supinator (superficial head)
Common extensor tendon
Anconeus
Supinator

■ Origins
■ Insertions

Muscle attachments of the shoulder and arm (posterior view)

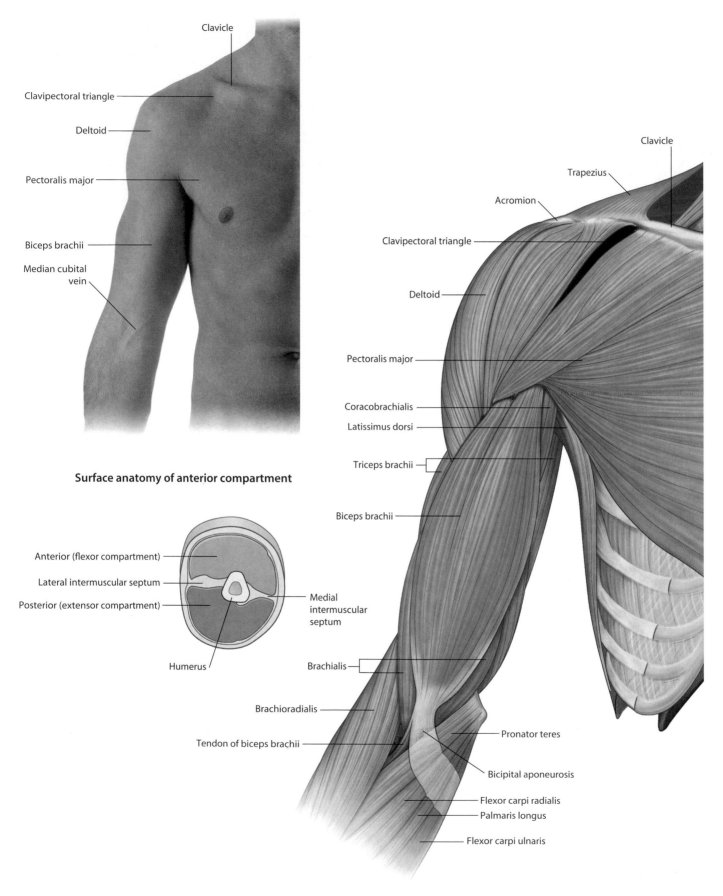

Clavicle

Clavipectoral triangle

Deltoid

Pectoralis major

Biceps brachii

Median cubital vein

Surface anatomy of anterior compartment

Clavicle

Trapezius

Acromion

Clavipectoral triangle

Deltoid

Pectoralis major

Coracobrachialis

Latissimus dorsi

Triceps brachii

Biceps brachii

Anterior (flexor compartment)

Lateral intermuscular septum

Posterior (extensor compartment)

Medial intermuscular septum

Humerus

Brachialis

Brachioradialis

Pronator teres

Tendon of biceps brachii

Bicipital aponeurosis

Flexor carpi radialis

Palmaris longus

Flexor carpi ulnaris

Muscles of anterior compartment of arm

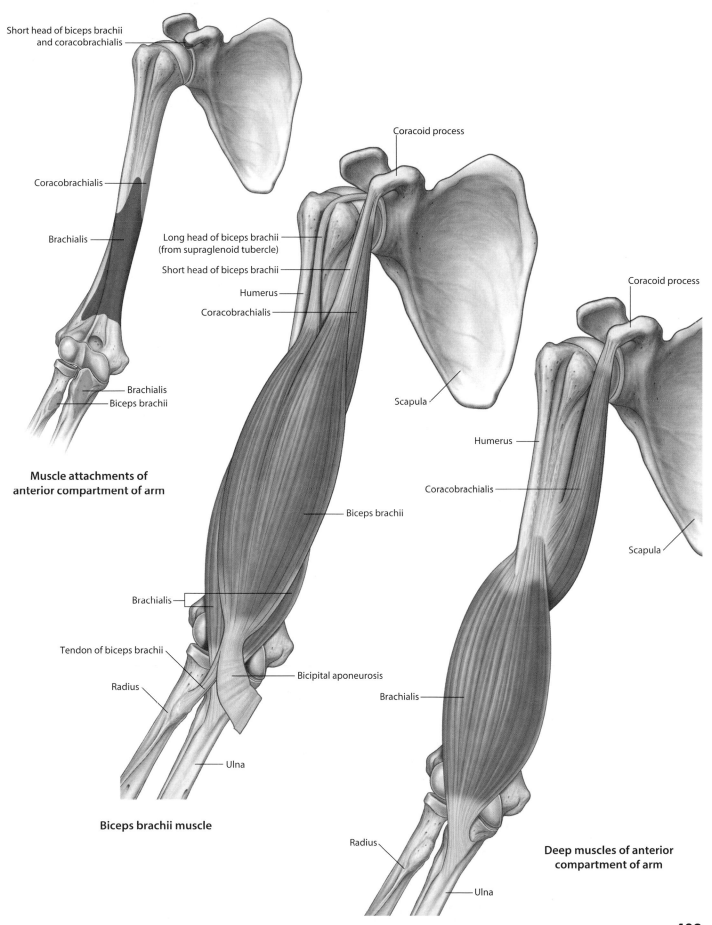

Short head of biceps brachii
and coracobrachialis

Coracobrachialis

Brachialis

Coracoid process

Long head of biceps brachii
(from supraglenoid tubercle)

Short head of biceps brachii

Humerus

Coracobrachialis

Scapula

Coracoid process

Humerus

Coracobrachialis

Scapula

Brachialis
Biceps brachii

**Muscle attachments of
anterior compartment of arm**

Biceps brachii

Brachialis

Tendon of biceps brachii

Radius

Bicipital aponeurosis

Brachialis

Ulna

Biceps brachii muscle

Radius

Ulna

**Deep muscles of anterior
compartment of arm**

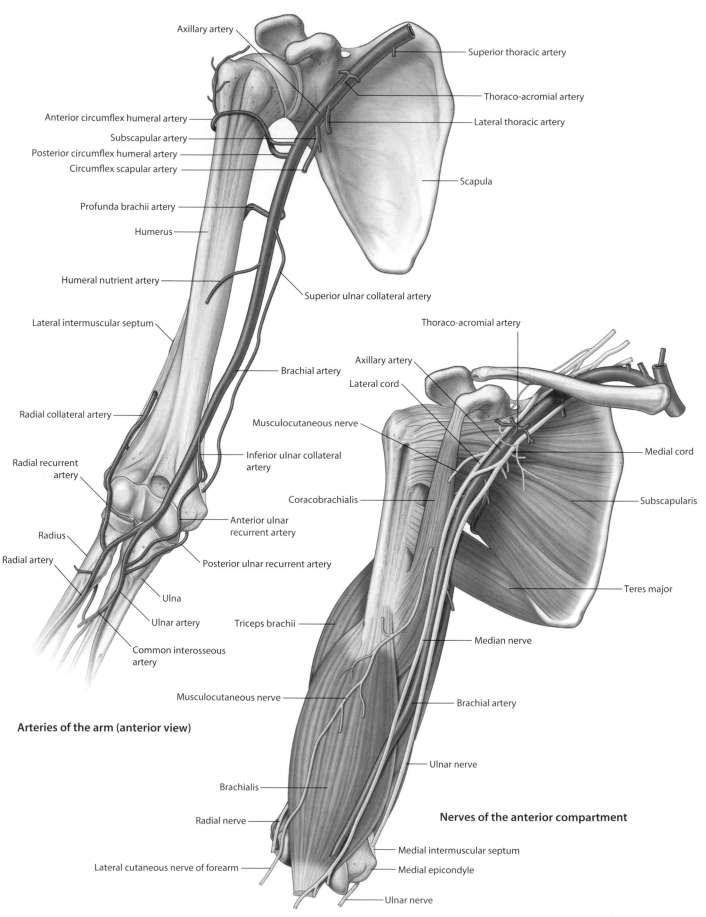

Axillary artery

Superior thoracic artery

Thoraco-acromial artery

Anterior circumflex humeral artery

Subscapular artery

Posterior circumflex humeral artery

Circumflex scapular artery

Lateral thoracic artery

Scapula

Profunda brachii artery

Humerus

Humeral nutrient artery

Superior ulnar collateral artery

Lateral intermuscular septum

Thoraco-acromial artery

Axillary artery

Lateral cord

Brachial artery

Musculocutaneous nerve

Radial collateral artery

Medial cord

Radial recurrent artery

Inferior ulnar collateral artery

Coracobrachialis

Subscapularis

Radius

Anterior ulnar recurrent artery

Radial artery

Posterior ulnar recurrent artery

Teres major

Ulna

Ulnar artery

Triceps brachii

Median nerve

Common interosseous artery

Musculocutaneous nerve

Brachial artery

Arteries of the arm (anterior view)

Ulnar nerve

Brachialis

Radial nerve

Nerves of the anterior compartment

Medial intermuscular septum

Medial epicondyle

Lateral cutaneous nerve of forearm

Ulnar nerve

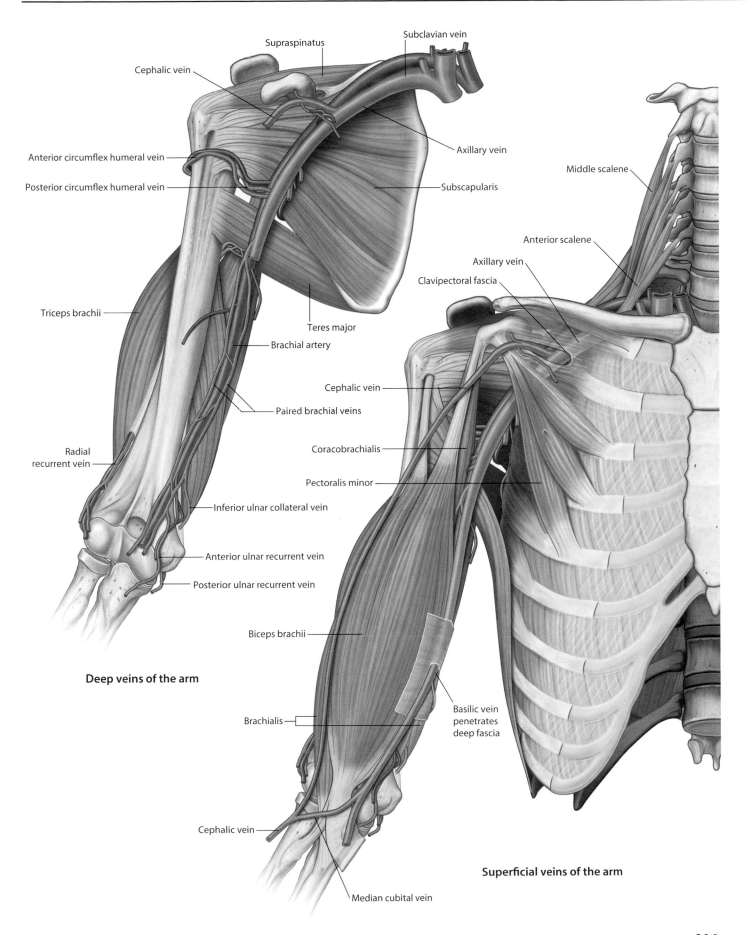

Supraspinatus

Subclavian vein

Cephalic vein

Anterior circumflex humeral vein

Posterior circumflex humeral vein

Axillary vein

Subscapularis

Middle scalene

Anterior scalene

Axillary vein

Clavipectoral fascia

Triceps brachii

Cephalic vein

Teres major

Brachial artery

Paired brachial veins

Coracobrachialis

Radial
recurrent vein

Pectoralis minor

Inferior ulnar collateral vein

Anterior ulnar recurrent vein

Posterior ulnar recurrent vein

Biceps brachii

Deep veins of the arm

Brachialis

Basilic vein
penetrates
deep fascia

Cephalic vein

Superficial veins of the arm

Median cubital vein

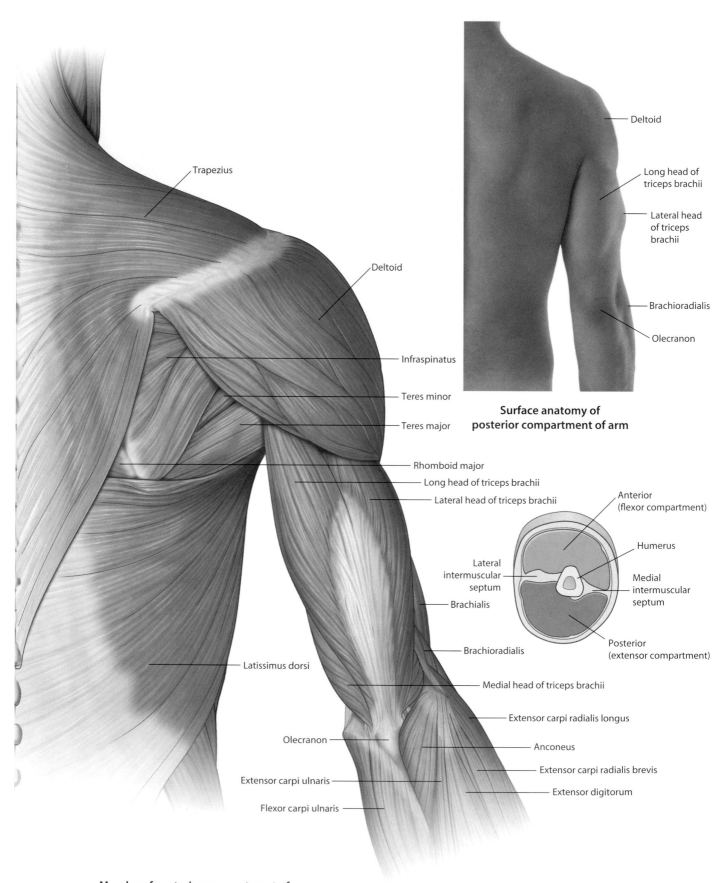

Trapezius

Deltoid

Infraspinatus

Teres minor

Teres major

Rhomboid major

Long head of triceps brachii

Lateral head of triceps brachii

Brachialis

Brachioradialis

Latissimus dorsi

Medial head of triceps brachii

Olecranon

Extensor carpi ulnaris

Flexor carpi ulnaris

Extensor carpi radialis longus

Anconeus

Extensor carpi radialis brevis

Extensor digitorum

Deltoid

Long head of triceps brachii

Lateral head of triceps brachii

Brachioradialis

Olecranon

Surface anatomy of posterior compartment of arm

Anterior (flexor compartment)

Humerus

Lateral intermuscular septum

Medial intermuscular septum

Posterior (extensor compartment)

Muscles of posterior compartment of arm

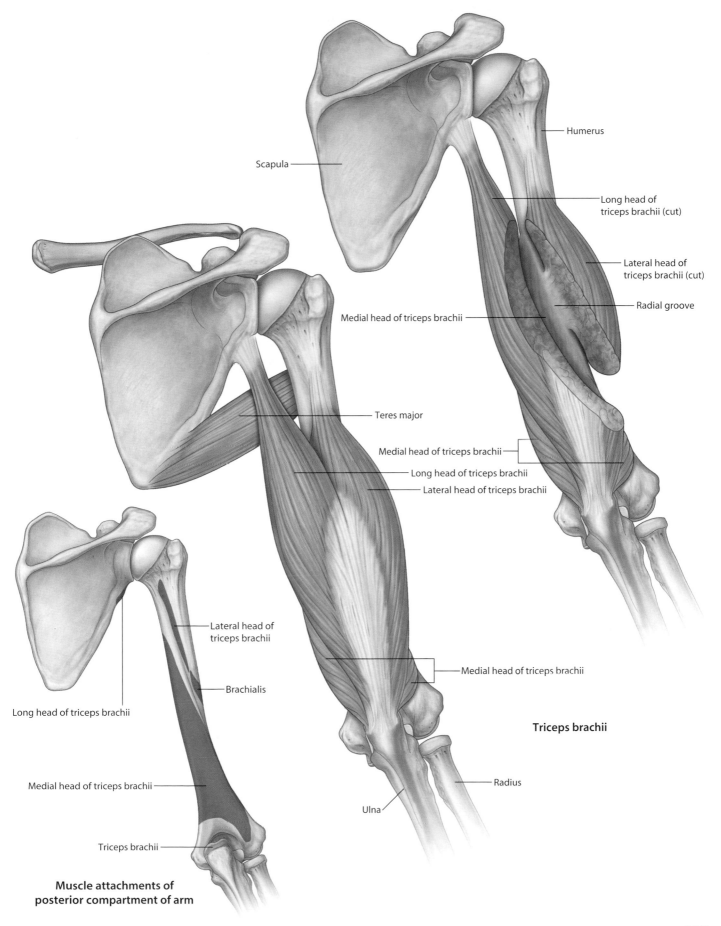

Scapula

Humerus

Long head of triceps brachii (cut)

Lateral head of triceps brachii (cut)

Medial head of triceps brachii

Radial groove

Teres major

Medial head of triceps brachii

Long head of triceps brachii

Lateral head of triceps brachii

Medial head of triceps brachii

Triceps brachii

Radius

Ulna

Lateral head of triceps brachii

Brachialis

Long head of triceps brachii

Medial head of triceps brachii

Triceps brachii

Muscle attachments of posterior compartment of arm

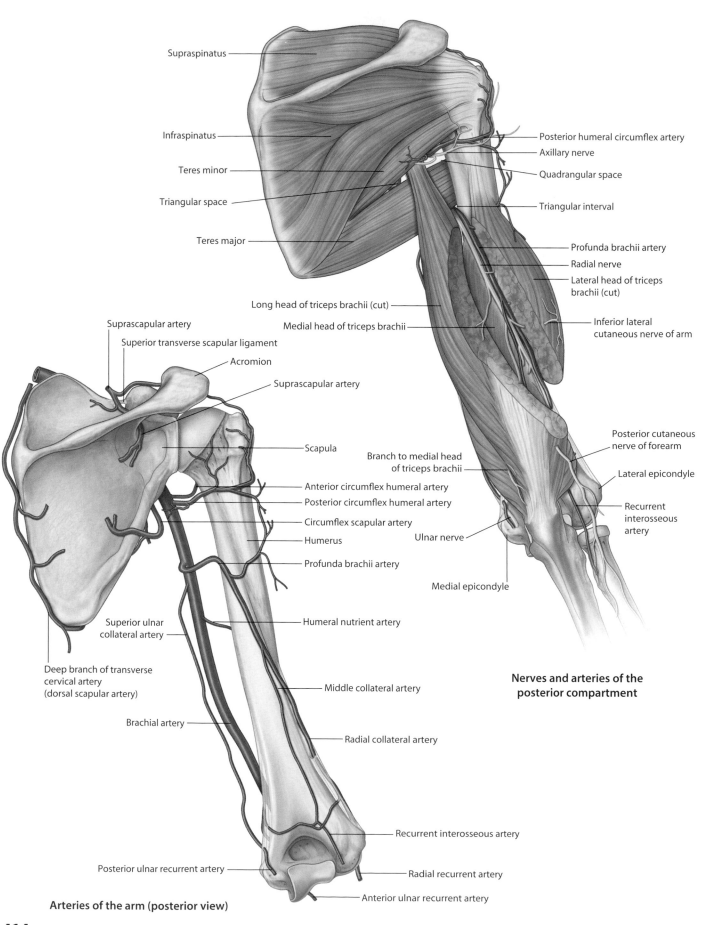

Supraspinatus

Infraspinatus

Teres minor

Triangular space

Teres major

Posterior humeral circumflex artery

Axillary nerve

Quadrangular space

Triangular interval

Profunda brachii artery

Radial nerve

Lateral head of triceps brachii (cut)

Long head of triceps brachii (cut)

Medial head of triceps brachii

Inferior lateral cutaneous nerve of arm

Suprascapular artery

Superior transverse scapular ligament

Acromion

Suprascapular artery

Scapula

Branch to medial head of triceps brachii

Anterior circumflex humeral artery

Posterior circumflex humeral artery

Circumflex scapular artery

Humerus

Profunda brachii artery

Posterior cutaneous nerve of forearm

Lateral epicondyle

Ulnar nerve

Recurrent interosseous artery

Medial epicondyle

Nerves and arteries of the posterior compartment

Superior ulnar collateral artery

Humeral nutrient artery

Deep branch of transverse cervical artery (dorsal scapular artery)

Middle collateral artery

Brachial artery

Radial collateral artery

Recurrent interosseous artery

Posterior ulnar recurrent artery

Radial recurrent artery

Anterior ulnar recurrent artery

Arteries of the arm (posterior view)

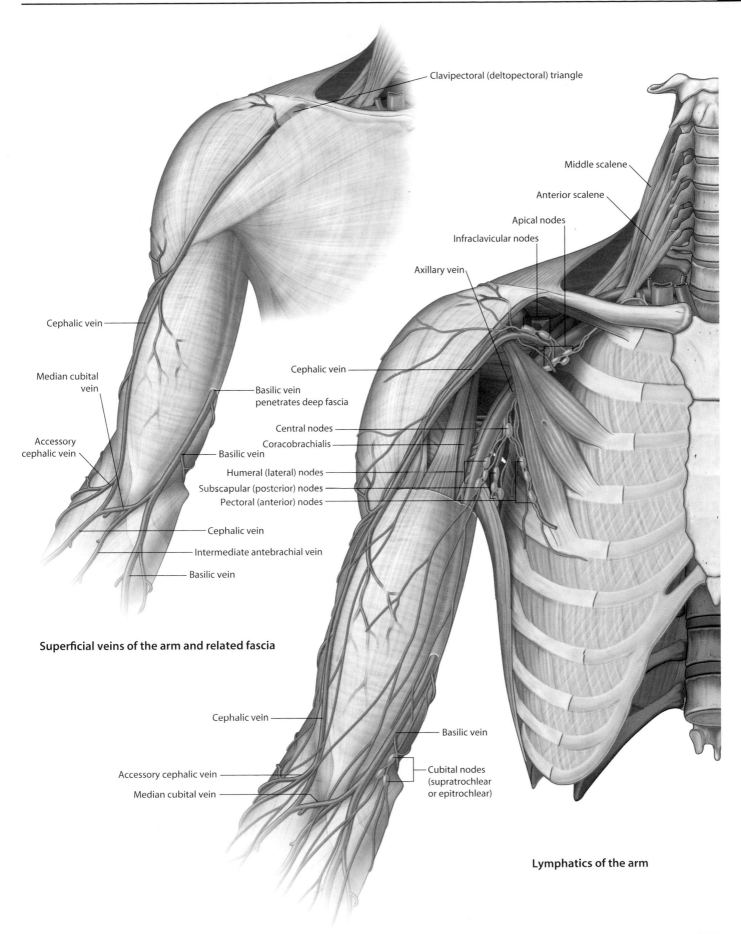

Clavipectoral (deltopectoral) triangle

Middle scalene

Anterior scalene

Apical nodes

Infraclavicular nodes

Axillary vein

Cephalic vein

Cephalic vein

Basilic vein penetrates deep fascia

Central nodes

Coracobrachialis

Basilic vein

Humeral (lateral) nodes

Subscapular (posterior) nodes

Pectoral (anterior) nodes

Cephalic vein

Median cubital vein

Accessory cephalic vein

Cephalic vein

Intermediate antebrachial vein

Basilic vein

Superficial veins of the arm and related fascia

Cephalic vein

Basilic vein

Accessory cephalic vein

Cubital nodes (supratrochlear or epitrochlear)

Median cubital vein

Lymphatics of the arm

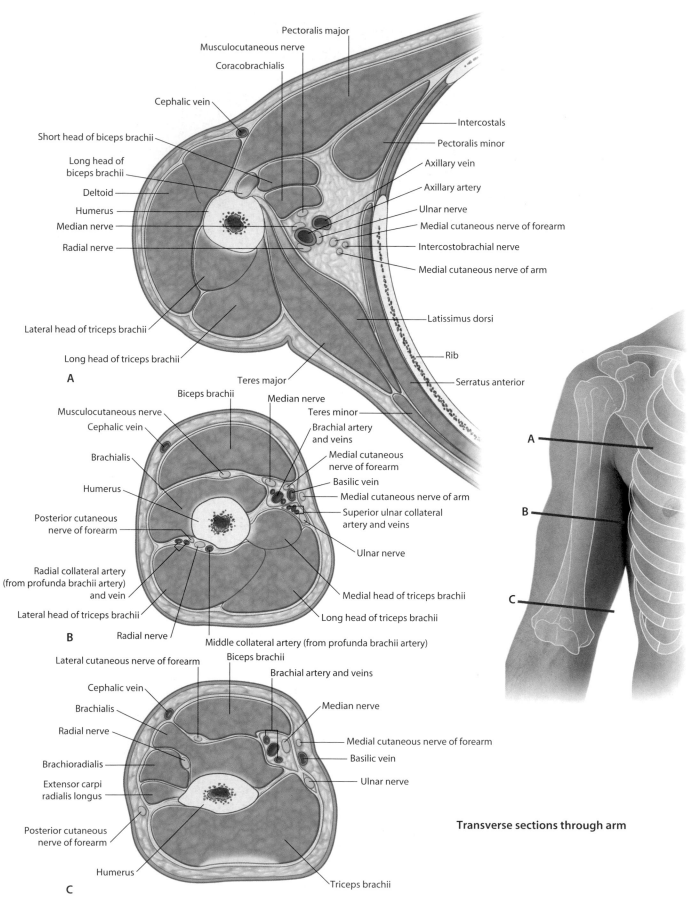

Pectoralis major
Musculocutaneous nerve
Coracobrachialis
Cephalic vein
Short head of biceps brachii
Long head of biceps brachii
Deltoid
Humerus
Median nerve
Radial nerve
Lateral head of triceps brachii
Long head of triceps brachii

Intercostals
Pectoralis minor
Axillary vein
Axillary artery
Ulnar nerve
Medial cutaneous nerve of forearm
Intercostobrachial nerve
Medial cutaneous nerve of arm
Latissimus dorsi
Rib
Serratus anterior

A

Teres major
Biceps brachii
Median nerve
Teres minor

Musculocutaneous nerve
Cephalic vein
Brachialis
Humerus
Posterior cutaneous nerve of forearm
Radial collateral artery (from profunda brachii artery) and vein
Lateral head of triceps brachii
Radial nerve

Brachial artery and veins
Medial cutaneous nerve of forearm
Basilic vein
Medial cutaneous nerve of arm
Superior ulnar collateral artery and veins
Ulnar nerve
Medial head of triceps brachii
Long head of triceps brachii

B

Middle collateral artery (from profunda brachii artery)
Biceps brachii
Brachial artery and veins

Lateral cutaneous nerve of forearm
Cephalic vein
Brachialis
Radial nerve
Brachioradialis
Extensor carpi radialis longus
Posterior cutaneous nerve of forearm
Humerus

Median nerve
Medial cutaneous nerve of forearm
Basilic vein
Ulnar nerve
Triceps brachii

C

Transverse sections through arm

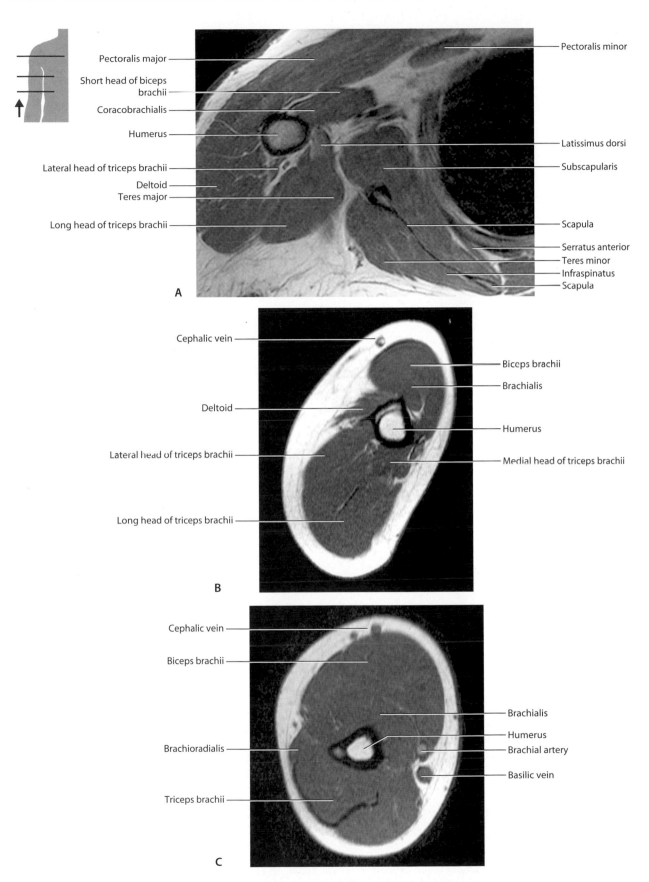

Pectoralis major

Short head of biceps brachii

Coracobrachialis

Humerus

Lateral head of triceps brachii

Deltoid

Teres major

Long head of triceps brachii

A

Pectoralis minor

Latissimus dorsi

Subscapularis

Scapula

Serratus anterior

Teres minor

Infraspinatus

Scapula

Cephalic vein

Deltoid

Lateral head of triceps brachii

Long head of triceps brachii

B

Biceps brachii

Brachialis

Humerus

Medial head of triceps brachii

Cephalic vein

Biceps brachii

Brachioradialis

Triceps brachii

C

Brachialis

Humerus

Brachial artery

Basilic vein

Transverse/axial sections through the arm.
A. Proximal/upper arm. B. Middle arm. C. Distal/lower arm.
T1-weighted MR images in axial plane

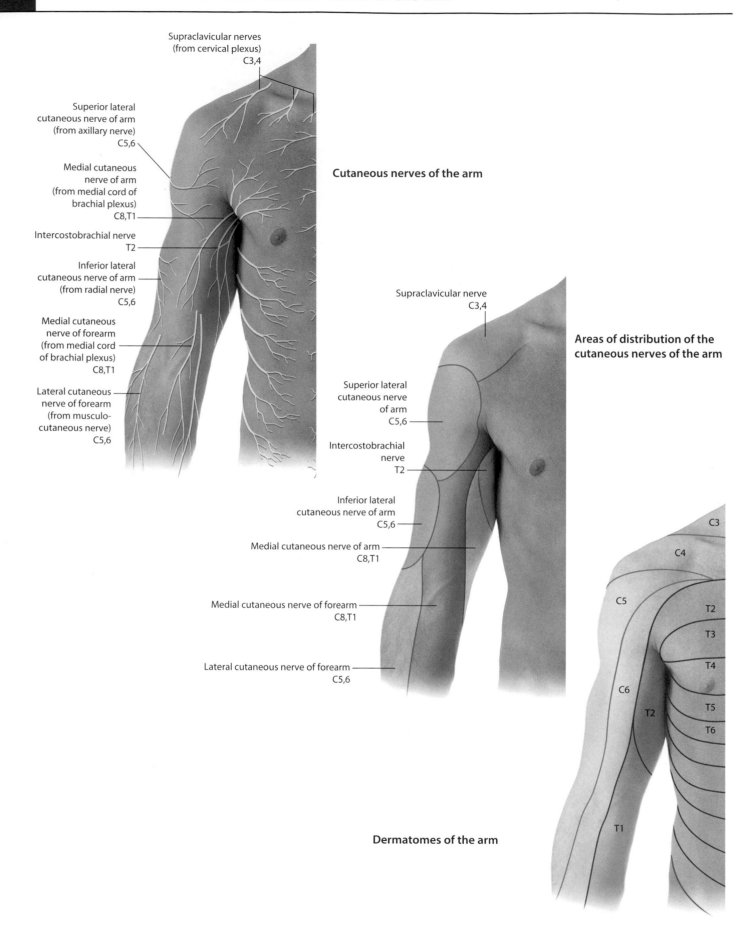

Supraclavicular nerves
(from cervical plexus)
C3,4

Superior lateral
cutaneous nerve of arm
(from axillary nerve)
C5,6

Medial cutaneous
nerve of arm
(from medial cord of
brachial plexus)
C8,T1

Intercostobrachial nerve
T2

Inferior lateral
cutaneous nerve of arm
(from radial nerve)
C5,6

Medial cutaneous
nerve of forearm
(from medial cord
of brachial plexus)
C8,T1

Lateral cutaneous
nerve of forearm
(from musculo-
cutaneous nerve)
C5,6

Cutaneous nerves of the arm

Supraclavicular nerve
C3,4

**Areas of distribution of the
cutaneous nerves of the arm**

Superior lateral
cutaneous nerve
of arm
C5,6

Intercostobrachial
nerve
T2

Inferior lateral
cutaneous nerve of arm
C5,6

Medial cutaneous nerve of arm
C8,T1

Medial cutaneous nerve of forearm
C8,T1

Lateral cutaneous nerve of forearm
C5,6

C3
C4
C5
T2
T3
T4
C6
T5
T2
T6
T1

Dermatomes of the arm

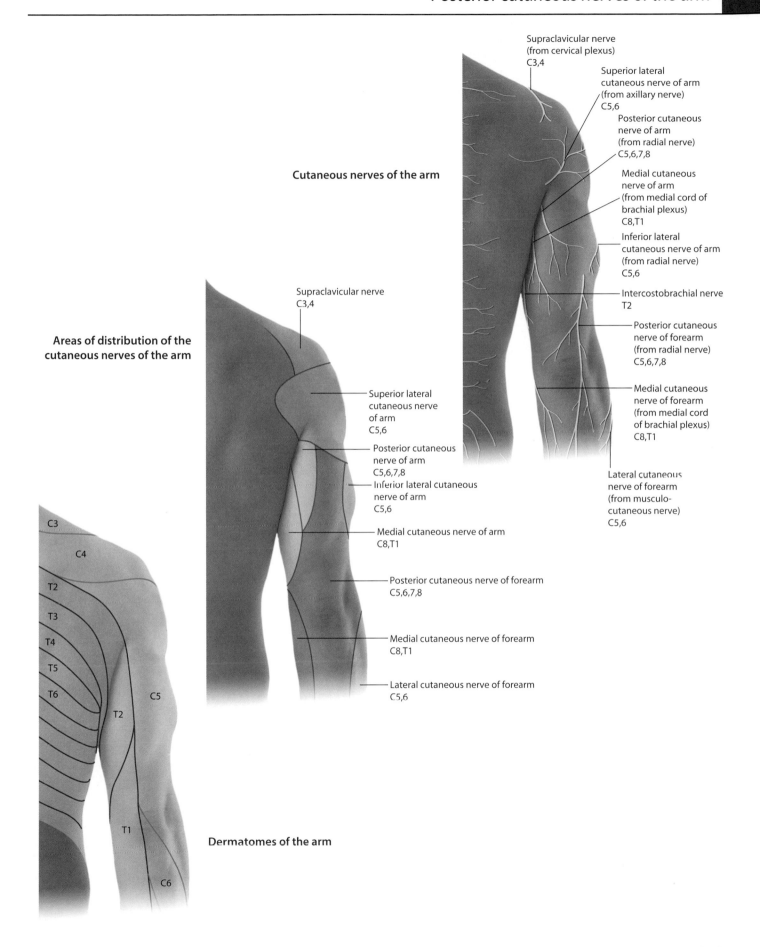

Cutaneous nerves of the arm

Supraclavicular nerve
(from cervical plexus)
C3,4

Superior lateral
cutaneous nerve of arm
(from axillary nerve)
C5,6

Posterior cutaneous
nerve of arm
(from radial nerve)
C5,6,7,8

Medial cutaneous
nerve of arm
(from medial cord of
brachial plexus)
C8,T1

Inferior lateral
cutaneous nerve of arm
(from radial nerve)
C5,6

Intercostobrachial nerve
T2

Posterior cutaneous
nerve of forearm
(from radial nerve)
C5,6,7,8

Medial cutaneous
nerve of forearm
(from medial cord
of brachial plexus)
C8,T1

Lateral cutaneous
nerve of forearm
(from musculo-
cutaneous nerve)
C5,6

Areas of distribution of the
cutaneous nerves of the arm

Supraclavicular nerve
C3,4

Superior lateral
cutaneous nerve
of arm
C5,6

Posterior cutaneous
nerve of arm
C5,6,7,8

Inferior lateral cutaneous
nerve of arm
C5,6

Medial cutaneous nerve of arm
C8,T1

Posterior cutaneous nerve of forearm
C5,6,7,8

Medial cutaneous nerve of forearm
C8,T1

Lateral cutaneous nerve of forearm
C5,6

C3
C4
T2
T3
T4
T5
T6
C5
T2
T1
C6

Dermatomes of the arm

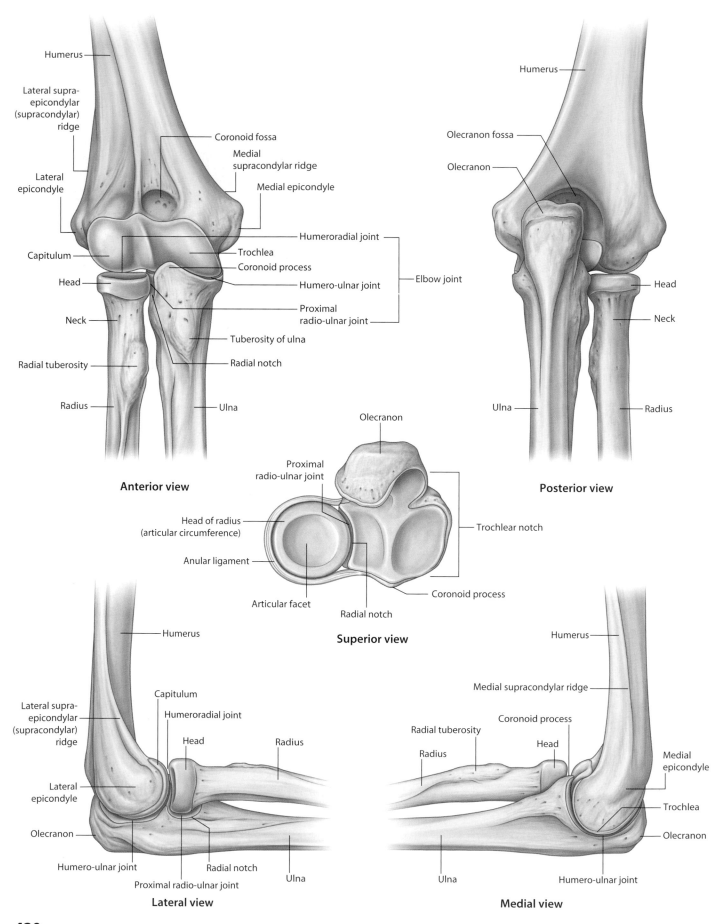

Anterior view

Humerus

Lateral supra-epicondylar (supracondylar) ridge

Lateral epicondyle

Capitulum

Head

Neck

Radial tuberosity

Radius

Coronoid fossa

Medial supracondylar ridge

Medial epicondyle

Humeroradial joint

Trochlea

Coronoid process

Humero-ulnar joint

Proximal radio-ulnar joint

Tuberosity of ulna

Radial notch

Ulna

Elbow joint

Posterior view

Humerus

Olecranon fossa

Olecranon

Head

Neck

Ulna

Radius

Superior view

Olecranon

Proximal radio-ulnar joint

Head of radius (articular circumference)

Anular ligament

Articular facet

Radial notch

Trochlear notch

Coronoid process

Lateral view

Humerus

Lateral supra-epicondylar (supracondylar) ridge

Lateral epicondyle

Olecranon

Humero-ulnar joint

Proximal radio-ulnar joint

Capitulum

Humeroradial joint

Head

Radius

Radial notch

Ulna

Medial view

Humerus

Medial supracondylar ridge

Coronoid process

Radial tuberosity

Radius

Head

Medial epicondyle

Trochlea

Olecranon

Humero-ulnar joint

Ulna

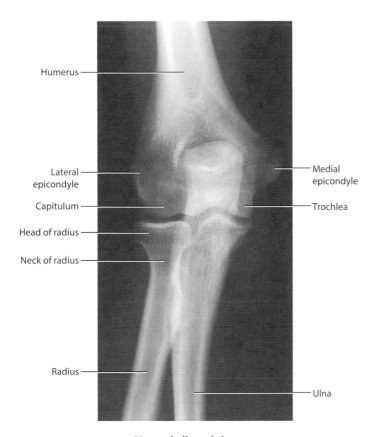

Humerus

Lateral epicondyle

Capitulum

Head of radius

Neck of radius

Radius

Medial epicondyle

Trochlea

Ulna

Normal elbow joint.
Radiograph, AP view

Radial tuberosity   Capitulum   Humerus

Coronoid process   Trochlear notch   Olecranon

Normal elbow joint.
Radiograph, lateral view

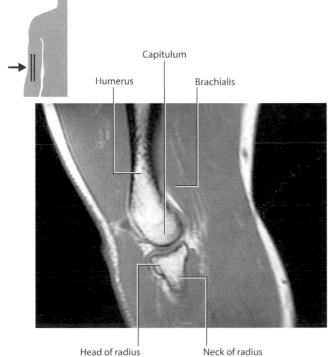

Humerus

Capitulum

Brachialis

Head of radius   Neck of radius

Articulation of the capitulum of the humerus and the head of the radius at the elbow joint.
T2-weighted MR image in sagittal plane

Triceps brachii   Humerus   Brachialis

Olecranon   Ulna   Trochlea

Articulation of the trochlea of the humerus and the trochlear notch of the ulna.
T2-weighted MR image in sagittal plane

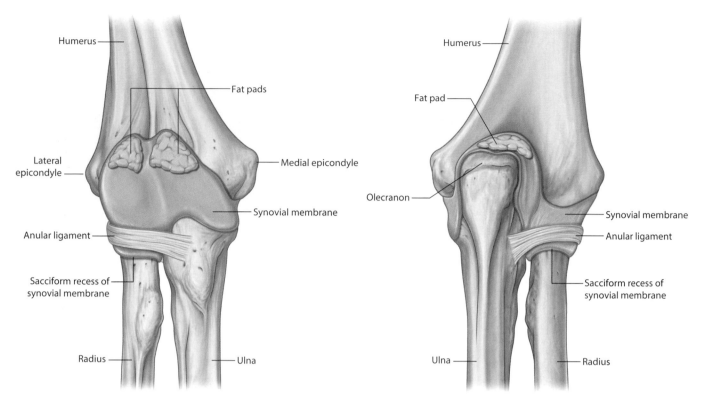

**Synovial membrane of the elbow joint
(anterior view)**

**Synovial membrane of the elbow joint
(posterior view)**

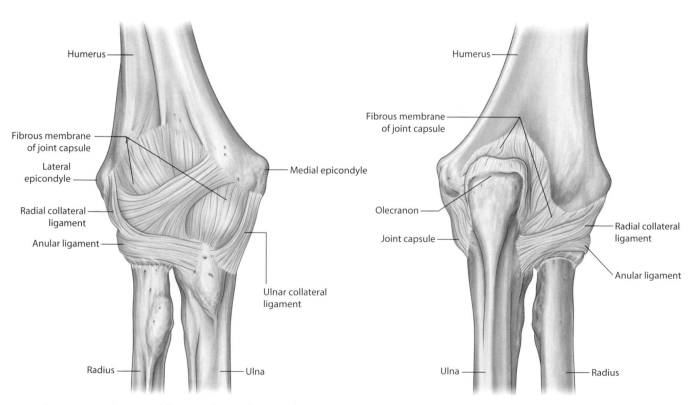

**Fibrous membrane of joint capsule and ligaments
of the elbow joint (anterior view)**

**Fibrous membrane of joint capsule and ligaments
of the elbow joint (posterior view)**

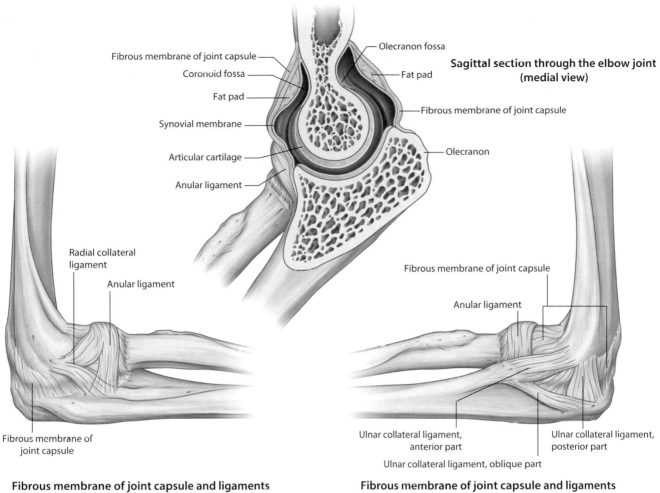

Fibrous membrane of joint capsule

Coronoid fossa

Fat pad

Synovial membrane

Articular cartilage

Anular ligament

Olecranon fossa

Fat pad

Sagittal section through the elbow joint (medial view)

Fibrous membrane of joint capsule

Olecranon

Radial collateral ligament

Anular ligament

Fibrous membrane of joint capsule

Fibrous membrane of joint capsule

Anular ligament

Ulnar collateral ligament, anterior part

Ulnar collateral ligament, oblique part

Ulnar collateral ligament, posterior part

Fibrous membrane of joint capsule and ligaments of the elbow joint (lateral view)

Fibrous membrane of joint capsule and ligaments of the elbow joint (medial view)

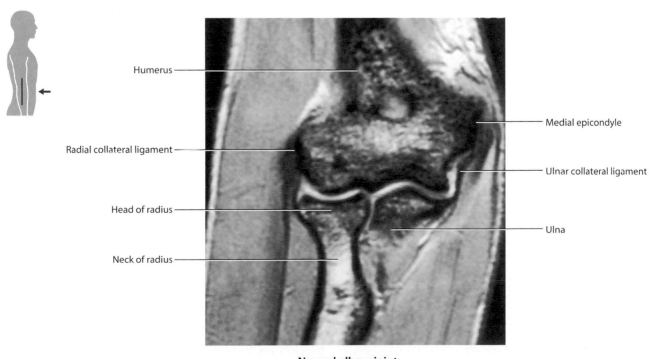

Humerus

Radial collateral ligament

Head of radius

Neck of radius

Medial epicondyle

Ulnar collateral ligament

Ulna

Normal elbow joint.
T2-weighted MR image in coronal plane

423

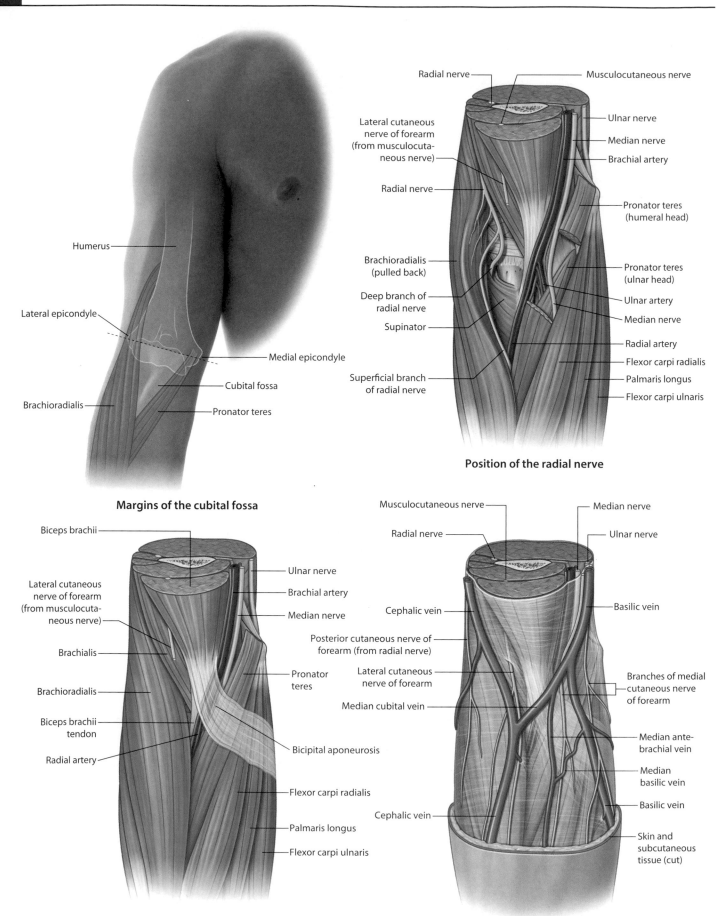

Radial nerve

Musculocutaneous nerve

Lateral cutaneous
nerve of forearm
(from musculocuta-
neous nerve)

Ulnar nerve

Median nerve

Brachial artery

Radial nerve

Pronator teres
(humeral head)

Brachioradialis
(pulled back)

Deep branch of
radial nerve

Pronator teres
(ulnar head)

Ulnar artery

Supinator

Median nerve

Radial artery

Superficial branch
of radial nerve

Flexor carpi radialis

Palmaris longus

Flexor carpi ulnaris

Position of the radial nerve

Humerus

Lateral epicondyle

Medial epicondyle

Cubital fossa

Brachioradialis

Pronator teres

Margins of the cubital fossa

Biceps brachii

Lateral cutaneous
nerve of forearm
(from musculocuta-
neous nerve)

Brachialis

Brachioradialis

Biceps brachii
tendon

Radial artery

Ulnar nerve

Brachial artery

Median nerve

Pronator
teres

Bicipital aponeurosis

Flexor carpi radialis

Palmaris longus

Flexor carpi ulnaris

Contents of the cubital fossa

Musculocutaneous nerve

Median nerve

Radial nerve

Ulnar nerve

Cephalic vein

Basilic vein

Posterior cutaneous nerve of
forearm (from radial nerve)

Lateral cutaneous
nerve of forearm

Median cubital vein

Branches of medial
cutaneous nerve
of forearm

Median ante-
brachial vein

Median
basilic vein

Cephalic vein

Basilic vein

Skin and
subcutaneous
tissue (cut)

Superficial structures

424

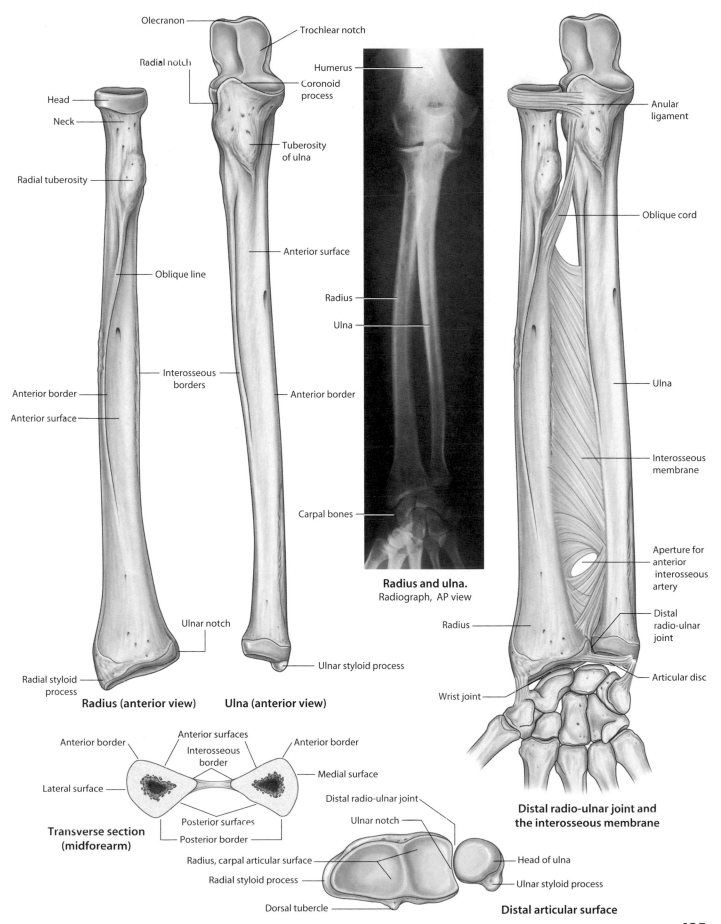

Olecranon

Trochlear notch

Radial notch

Humerus

Head

Coronoid process

Neck

Radial tuberosity

Tuberosity of ulna

Oblique line

Anterior surface

Radius

Ulna

Interosseous borders

Anterior border

Anterior border

Anterior surface

Carpal bones

Ulnar notch

Radial styloid process

Ulnar styloid process

Radius (anterior view)

Ulna (anterior view)

Radius and ulna.
Radiograph, AP view

Anular ligament

Oblique cord

Ulna

Interosseous membrane

Aperture for anterior interosseous artery

Distal radio-ulnar joint

Articular disc

Radius

Wrist joint

Distal radio-ulnar joint and the interosseous membrane

Anterior border

Anterior surfaces

Anterior border

Interosseous border

Lateral surface

Medial surface

Posterior surfaces

Posterior border

Transverse section (midforearm)

Distal radio-ulnar joint

Ulnar notch

Radius, carpal articular surface

Head of ulna

Radial styloid process

Ulnar styloid process

Dorsal tubercle

Distal articular surface

425

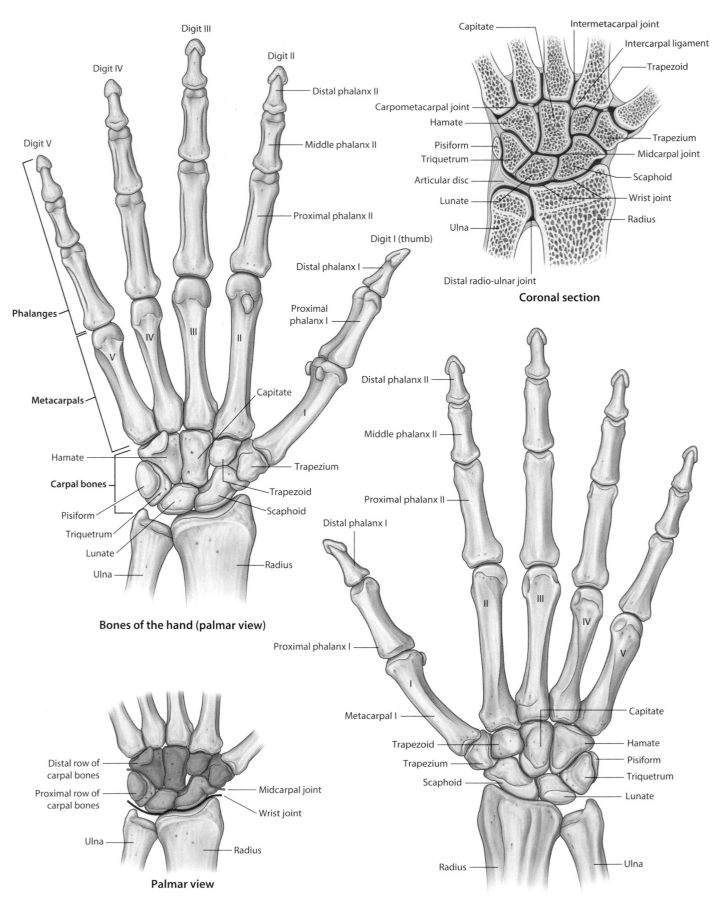

Digit III

Digit IV

Digit II

Distal phalanx II

Middle phalanx II

Digit V

Proximal phalanx II

Phalanges

Digit I (thumb)

Distal phalanx I

Proximal phalanx I

Metacarpals

Capitate

Hamate

Trapezium

Carpal bones

Trapezoid

Pisiform

Scaphoid

Triquetrum

Lunate

Ulna

Radius

Bones of the hand (palmar view)

Capitate

Intermetacarpal joint

Intercarpal ligament

Trapezoid

Carpometacarpal joint

Hamate

Pisiform

Trapezium

Triquetrum

Midcarpal joint

Articular disc

Scaphoid

Lunate

Wrist joint

Ulna

Radius

Distal radio-ulnar joint

Coronal section

Distal phalanx II

Middle phalanx II

Proximal phalanx II

Distal phalanx I

Proximal phalanx I

Metacarpal I

Capitate

Trapezoid

Hamate

Trapezium

Pisiform

Scaphoid

Triquetrum

Lunate

Distal row of carpal bones

Proximal row of carpal bones

Midcarpal joint

Wrist joint

Ulna

Radius

Palmar view

Radius

Ulna

Bones of the hand (dorsal view)

426

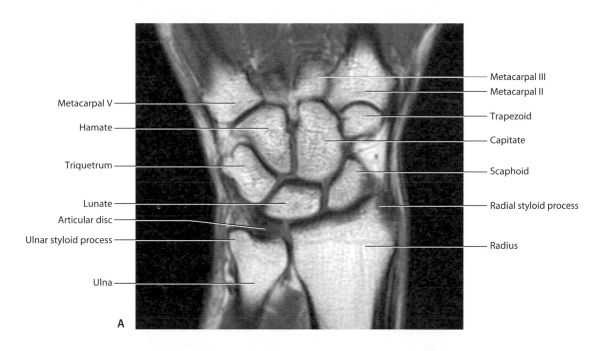

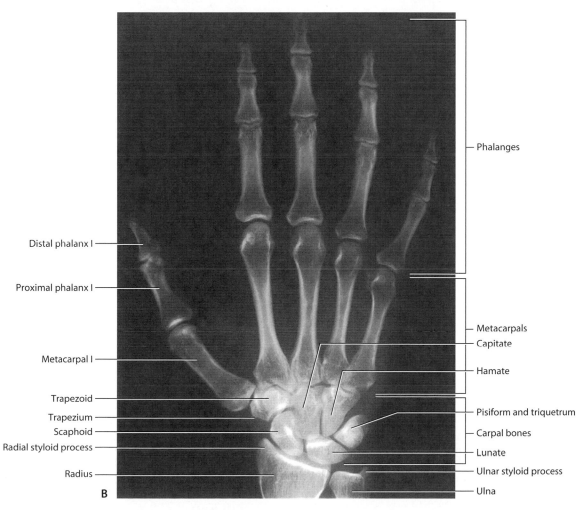

Imaging of the wrist joint, the carpal bones, and the hand.
A. T1-weighted MR image in coronal plane
B. Radiograph, AP view

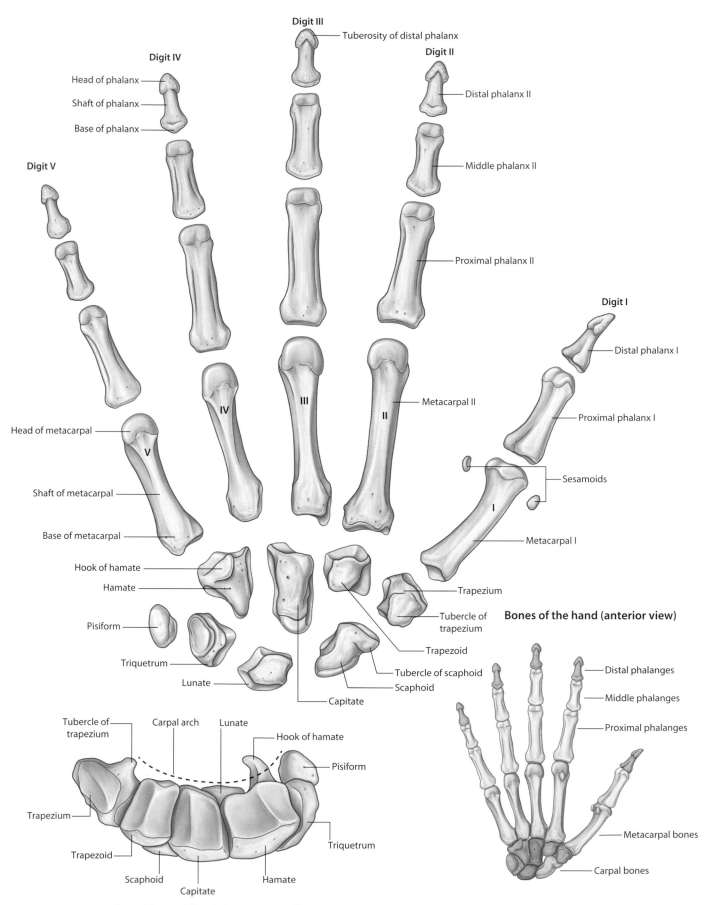

Digit III

Tuberosity of distal phalanx

Digit IV

Head of phalanx

Shaft of phalanx

Base of phalanx

Digit II

Distal phalanx II

Middle phalanx II

Digit V

Proximal phalanx II

Digit I

Distal phalanx I

Metacarpal II

Proximal phalanx I

Sesamoids

Head of metacarpal

Shaft of metacarpal

Base of metacarpal

Metacarpal I

Hook of hamate

Hamate

Trapezium

Tubercle of trapezium

Bones of the hand (anterior view)

Pisiform

Trapezoid

Triquetrum

Tubercle of scaphoid

Lunate

Scaphoid

Capitate

Tubercle of
trapezium

Carpal arch

Lunate

Hook of hamate

Pisiform

Trapezium

Triquetrum

Trapezoid

Scaphoid

Capitate

Hamate

Distal phalanges

Middle phalanges

Proximal phalanges

Metacarpal bones

Carpal bones

Carpal bones (distal view; pronated)

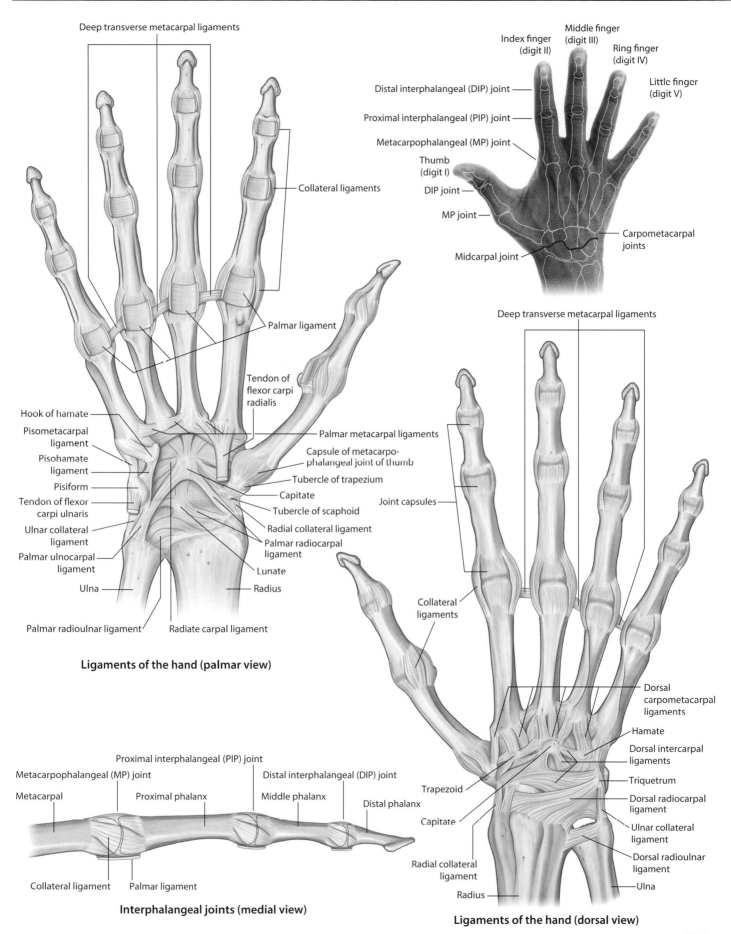

Deep transverse metacarpal ligaments

Collateral ligaments

Palmar ligament

Index finger (digit II)

Middle finger (digit III)

Ring finger (digit IV)

Little finger (digit V)

Distal interphalangeal (DIP) joint

Proximal interphalangeal (PIP) joint

Metacarpophalangeal (MP) joint

Thumb (digit I)

DIP joint

MP joint

Carpometacarpal joints

Midcarpal joint

Tendon of flexor carpi radialis

Deep transverse metacarpal ligaments

Hook of hamate

Pisometacarpal ligament

Pisohamate ligament

Pisiform

Tendon of flexor carpi ulnaris

Ulnar collateral ligament

Palmar ulnocarpal ligament

Ulna

Palmar radioulnar ligament

Radiate carpal ligament

Palmar metacarpal ligaments

Capsule of metacarpo-phalangeal joint of thumb

Tubercle of trapezium

Capitate

Tubercle of scaphoid

Radial collateral ligament

Palmar radiocarpal ligament

Lunate

Radius

Ligaments of the hand (palmar view)

Joint capsules

Collateral ligaments

Dorsal carpometacarpal ligaments

Hamate

Dorsal intercarpal ligaments

Triquetrum

Dorsal radiocarpal ligament

Ulnar collateral ligament

Dorsal radioulnar ligament

Ulna

Trapezoid

Capitate

Radial collateral ligament

Radius

Ligaments of the hand (dorsal view)

Proximal interphalangeal (PIP) joint

Metacarpophalangeal (MP) joint

Distal interphalangeal (DIP) joint

Metacarpal

Proximal phalanx

Middle phalanx

Distal phalanx

Collateral ligament

Palmar ligament

Interphalangeal joints (medial view)

429

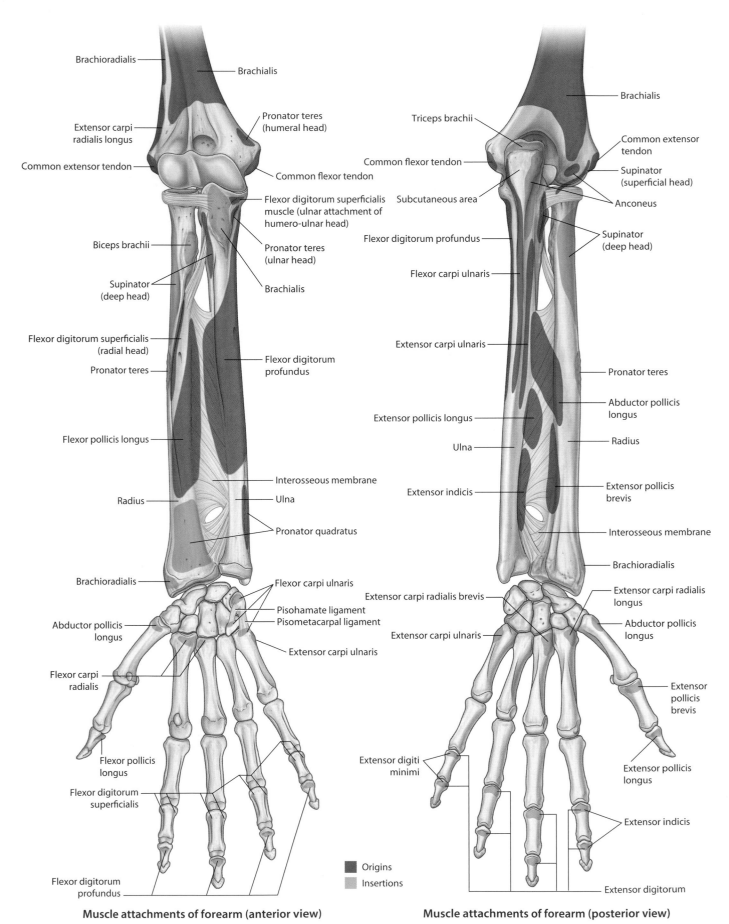

Brachioradialis

Brachialis

Extensor carpi radialis longus

Pronator teres (humeral head)

Common extensor tendon

Common flexor tendon

Flexor digitorum superficialis muscle (ulnar attachment of humero-ulnar head)

Biceps brachii

Pronator teres (ulnar head)

Supinator (deep head)

Brachialis

Flexor digitorum superficialis (radial head)

Pronator teres

Flexor digitorum profundus

Flexor pollicis longus

Interosseous membrane

Radius

Ulna

Pronator quadratus

Brachioradialis

Flexor carpi ulnaris

Pisohamate ligament

Pisometacarpal ligament

Abductor pollicis longus

Extensor carpi ulnaris

Flexor carpi radialis

Flexor pollicis longus

Flexor digitorum superficialis

Flexor digitorum profundus

Triceps brachii

Brachialis

Common flexor tendon

Common extensor tendon

Supinator (superficial head)

Subcutaneous area

Anconeus

Flexor digitorum profundus

Supinator (deep head)

Flexor carpi ulnaris

Extensor carpi ulnaris

Pronator teres

Abductor pollicis longus

Extensor pollicis longus

Radius

Ulna

Extensor indicis

Extensor pollicis brevis

Interosseous membrane

Brachioradialis

Extensor carpi radialis brevis

Extensor carpi radialis longus

Extensor carpi ulnaris

Abductor pollicis longus

Extensor pollicis brevis

Extensor digiti minimi

Extensor indicis

Extensor pollicis longus

Extensor digitorum

Origins

Insertions

Muscle attachments of forearm (anterior view)

Muscle attachments of forearm (posterior view)

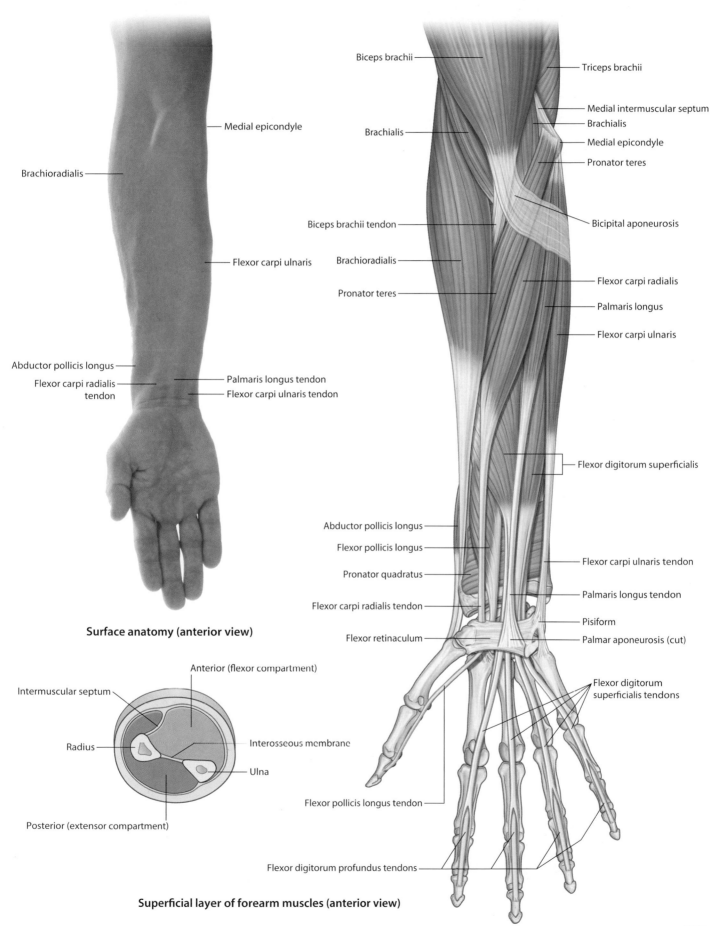

Medial epicondyle

Brachioradialis

Flexor carpi ulnaris

Abductor pollicis longus

Flexor carpi radialis tendon

Palmaris longus tendon

Flexor carpi ulnaris tendon

Surface anatomy (anterior view)

Biceps brachii

Brachialis

Biceps brachii tendon

Brachioradialis

Pronator teres

Abductor pollicis longus

Flexor pollicis longus

Pronator quadratus

Flexor carpi radialis tendon

Flexor retinaculum

Flexor pollicis longus tendon

Triceps brachii

Medial intermuscular septum

Brachialis

Medial epicondyle

Pronator teres

Bicipital aponeurosis

Flexor carpi radialis

Palmaris longus

Flexor carpi ulnaris

Flexor digitorum superficialis

Flexor carpi ulnaris tendon

Palmaris longus tendon

Pisiform

Palmar aponeurosis (cut)

Flexor digitorum superficialis tendons

Flexor digitorum profundus tendons

Superficial layer of forearm muscles (anterior view)

Anterior (flexor compartment)

Intermuscular septum

Radius

Interosseous membrane

Ulna

Posterior (extensor compartment)

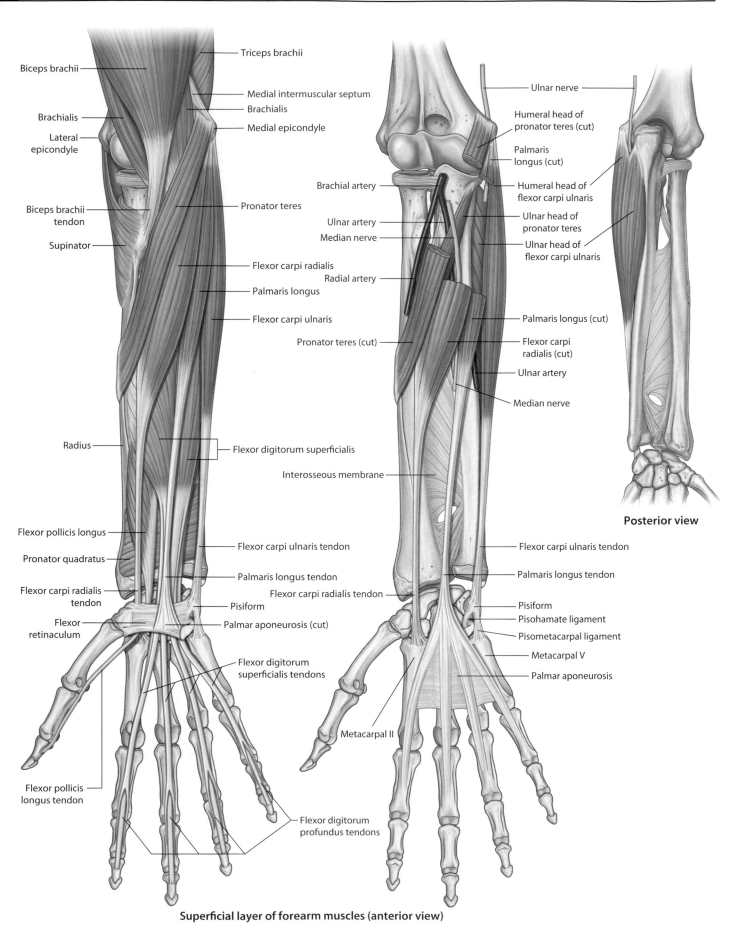

Triceps brachii

Biceps brachii

Medial intermuscular septum

Brachialis

Brachialis

Medial epicondyle

Lateral epicondyle

Biceps brachii tendon

Pronator teres

Supinator

Flexor carpi radialis

Palmaris longus

Flexor carpi ulnaris

Radius

Flexor digitorum superficialis

Flexor pollicis longus

Flexor carpi ulnaris tendon

Pronator quadratus

Palmaris longus tendon

Flexor carpi radialis tendon

Flexor carpi radialis tendon

Pisiform

Flexor retinaculum

Palmar aponeurosis (cut)

Flexor digitorum superficialis tendons

Flexor pollicis longus tendon

Flexor digitorum profundus tendons

Ulnar nerve

Humeral head of pronator teres (cut)

Palmaris longus (cut)

Brachial artery

Humeral head of flexor carpi ulnaris

Ulnar artery

Ulnar head of pronator teres

Median nerve

Ulnar head of flexor carpi ulnaris

Radial artery

Pronator teres (cut)

Palmaris longus (cut)

Flexor carpi radialis (cut)

Ulnar artery

Median nerve

Interosseous membrane

Flexor carpi ulnaris tendon

Palmaris longus tendon

Flexor carpi radialis tendon

Pisiform

Pisohamate ligament

Pisometacarpal ligament

Metacarpal V

Palmar aponeurosis

Metacarpal II

Posterior view

Flexor carpi ulnaris tendon

Superficial layer of forearm muscles (anterior view)

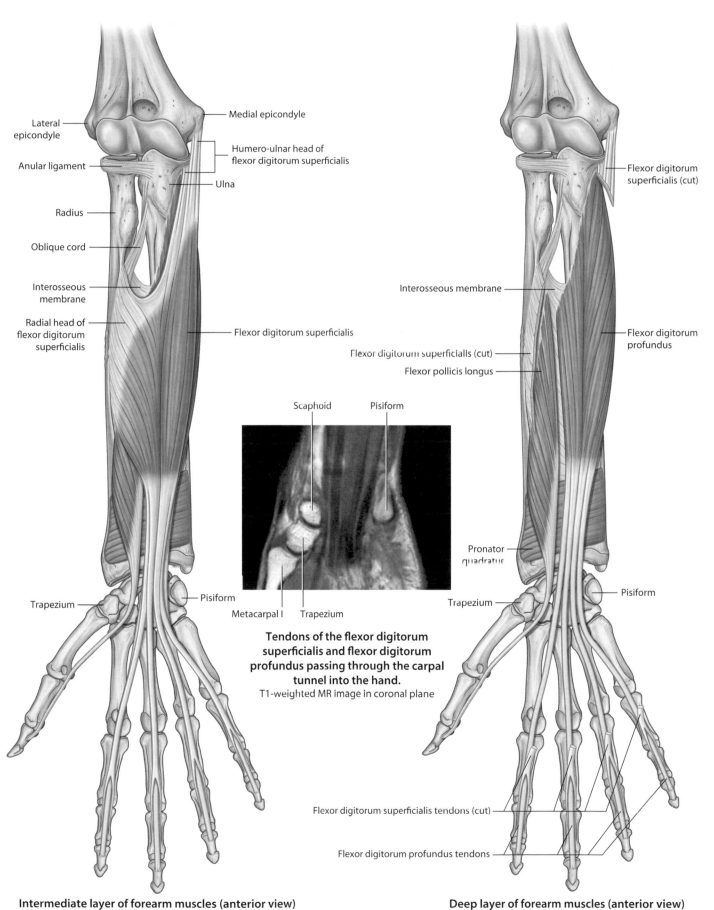

Lateral epicondyle

Anular ligament

Radius

Oblique cord

Interosseous membrane

Radial head of flexor digitorum superficialis

Trapezium

Medial epicondyle

Humero-ulnar head of flexor digitorum superficialis

Ulna

Flexor digitorum superficialis

Pisiform

Flexor digitorum superficialis (cut)

Interosseous membrane

Flexor digitorum superficialis (cut)

Flexor pollicis longus

Flexor digitorum profundus

Pronator quadratus

Trapezium

Pisiform

Scaphoid

Pisiform

Metacarpal I

Trapezium

Tendons of the flexor digitorum superficialis and flexor digitorum profundus passing through the carpal tunnel into the hand.
T1-weighted MR image in coronal plane

Flexor digitorum superficialis tendons (cut)

Flexor digitorum profundus tendons

Intermediate layer of forearm muscles (anterior view)

Deep layer of forearm muscles (anterior view)

433

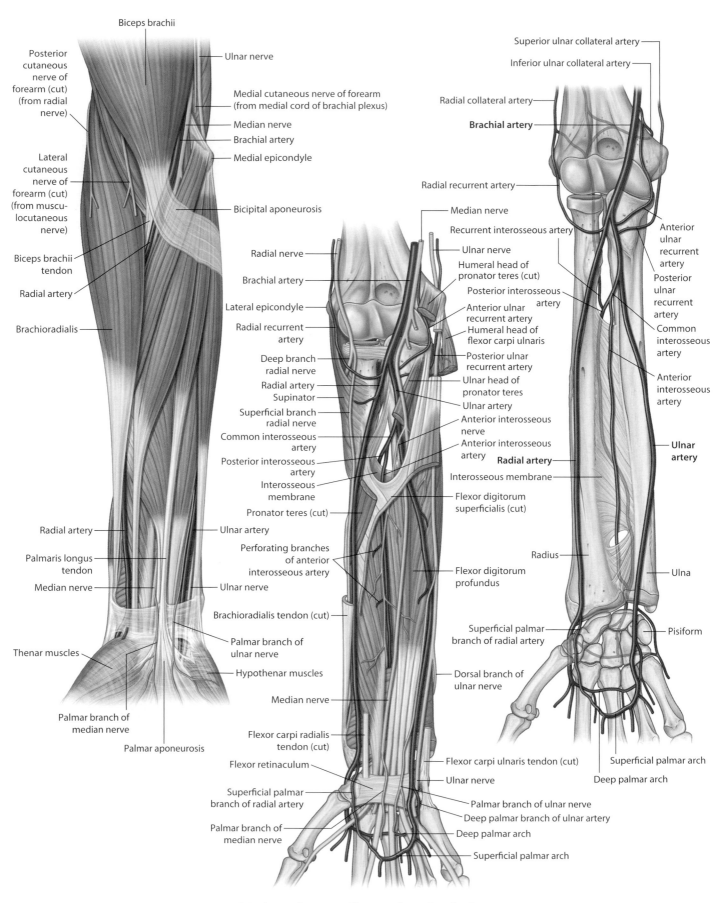

Biceps brachii

Posterior cutaneous nerve of forearm (cut) (from radial nerve)

Lateral cutaneous nerve of forearm (cut) (from musculocutaneous nerve)

Biceps brachii tendon

Radial artery

Brachioradialis

Radial artery

Palmaris longus tendon

Median nerve

Thenar muscles

Palmar branch of median nerve

Palmar aponeurosis

Ulnar nerve

Medial cutaneous nerve of forearm (from medial cord of brachial plexus)

Median nerve

Brachial artery

Medial epicondyle

Bicipital aponeurosis

Radial nerve

Brachial artery

Lateral epicondyle

Radial recurrent artery

Deep branch radial nerve

Radial artery

Supinator

Superficial branch radial nerve

Common interosseous artery

Posterior interosseous artery

Interosseous membrane

Pronator teres (cut)

Ulnar artery

Perforating branches of anterior interosseous artery

Brachioradialis tendon (cut)

Palmar branch of ulnar nerve

Hypothenar muscles

Median nerve

Flexor carpi radialis tendon (cut)

Flexor retinaculum

Superficial palmar branch of radial artery

Palmar branch of median nerve

Median nerve

Recurrent interosseous artery

Ulnar nerve

Humeral head of pronator teres (cut)

Posterior interosseous artery

Anterior ulnar recurrent artery

Humeral head of flexor carpi ulnaris

Posterior ulnar recurrent artery

Ulnar head of pronator teres

Ulnar artery

Anterior interosseous nerve

Anterior interosseous artery

Flexor digitorum superficialis (cut)

Flexor digitorum profundus

Dorsal branch of ulnar nerve

Flexor carpi ulnaris tendon (cut)

Ulnar nerve

Palmar branch of ulnar nerve

Deep palmar branch of ulnar artery

Deep palmar arch

Superficial palmar arch

Superior ulnar collateral artery

Inferior ulnar collateral artery

Radial collateral artery

Brachial artery

Radial recurrent artery

Anterior ulnar recurrent artery

Posterior ulnar recurrent artery

Common interosseous artery

Anterior interosseous artery

Ulnar artery

Radial artery

Interosseous membrane

Radius

Ulna

Superficial palmar branch of radial artery

Pisiform

Superficial palmar arch

Deep palmar arch

Arteries and nerves of forearm (anterior view)

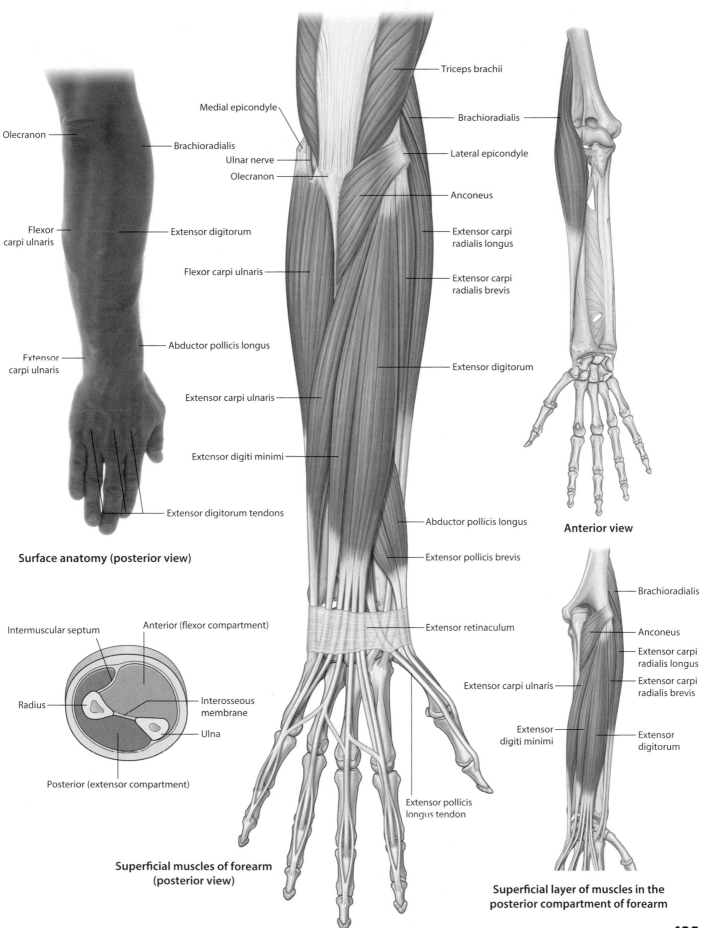

Olecranon

Brachioradialis

Flexor carpi ulnaris

Extensor carpi ulnaris

Surface anatomy (posterior view)

Medial epicondyle

Ulnar nerve

Olecranon

Extensor digitorum

Flexor carpi ulnaris

Abductor pollicis longus

Extensor carpi ulnaris

Extensor digiti minimi

Extensor digitorum tendons

Triceps brachii

Brachioradialis

Lateral epicondyle

Anconeus

Extensor carpi radialis longus

Extensor carpi radialis brevis

Extensor digitorum

Abductor pollicis longus

Extensor pollicis brevis

Extensor retinaculum

Extensor pollicis longus tendon

Anterior view

Intermuscular septum

Anterior (flexor compartment)

Radius

Interosseous membrane

Ulna

Posterior (extensor compartment)

Superficial muscles of forearm (posterior view)

Brachioradialis

Anconeus

Extensor carpi radialis longus

Extensor carpi radialis brevis

Extensor carpi ulnaris

Extensor digiti minimi

Extensor digitorum

Superficial layer of muscles in the posterior compartment of forearm

435

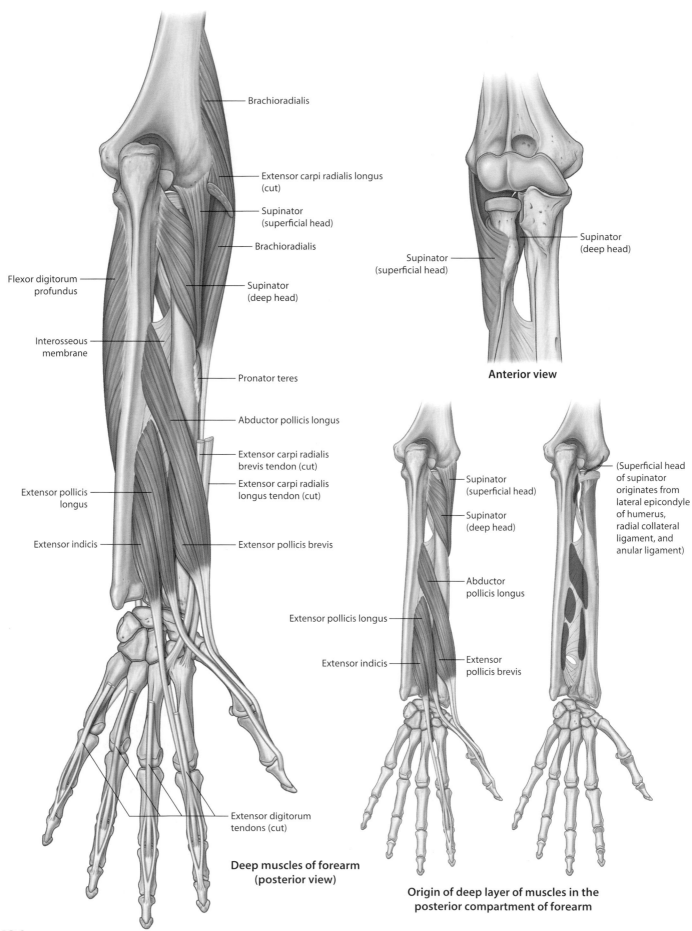

Brachioradialis

Extensor carpi radialis longus (cut)

Supinator (superficial head)

Brachioradialis

Supinator (deep head)

Flexor digitorum profundus

Interosseous membrane

Pronator teres

Abductor pollicis longus

Extensor carpi radialis brevis tendon (cut)

Extensor carpi radialis longus tendon (cut)

Extensor pollicis longus

Extensor indicis

Extensor pollicis brevis

Extensor digitorum tendons (cut)

Deep muscles of forearm (posterior view)

Supinator (deep head)

Supinator (superficial head)

Anterior view

Supinator (superficial head)

Supinator (deep head)

Abductor pollicis longus

Extensor pollicis longus

Extensor indicis

Extensor pollicis brevis

(Superficial head of supinator originates from lateral epicondyle of humerus, radial collateral ligament, and anular ligament)

Origin of deep layer of muscles in the posterior compartment of forearm

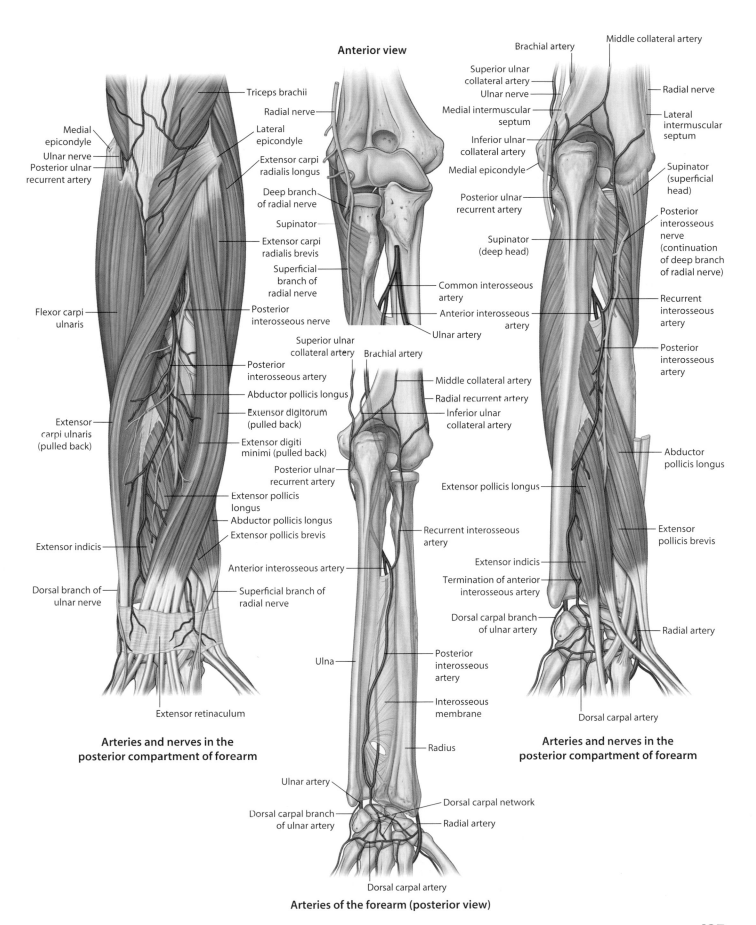

Anterior view

Triceps brachii

Radial nerve

Lateral epicondyle

Extensor carpi radialis longus

Deep branch of radial nerve

Supinator

Extensor carpi radialis brevis

Superficial branch of radial nerve

Posterior interosseous nerve

Medial epicondyle

Ulnar nerve

Posterior ulnar recurrent artery

Flexor carpi ulnaris

Extensor carpi ulnaris (pulled back)

Extensor indicis

Dorsal branch of ulnar nerve

Posterior interosseous artery

Abductor pollicis longus

Extensor digitorum (pulled back)

Extensor digiti minimi (pulled back)

Posterior ulnar recurrent artery

Extensor pollicis longus

Abductor pollicis longus

Extensor pollicis brevis

Anterior interosseous artery

Superficial branch of radial nerve

Extensor retinaculum

Arteries and nerves in the posterior compartment of forearm

Brachial artery

Middle collateral artery

Superior ulnar collateral artery

Ulnar nerve

Medial intermuscular septum

Inferior ulnar collateral artery

Medial epicondyle

Posterior ulnar recurrent artery

Supinator (deep head)

Common interosseous artery

Anterior interosseous artery

Ulnar artery

Radial nerve

Lateral intermuscular septum

Supinator (superficial head)

Posterior interosseous nerve (continuation of deep branch of radial nerve)

Recurrent interosseous artery

Posterior interosseous artery

Abductor pollicis longus

Extensor pollicis brevis

Dorsal carpal artery

Arteries and nerves in the posterior compartment of forearm

Superior ulnar collateral artery

Brachial artery

Middle collateral artery

Radial recurrent artery

Inferior ulnar collateral artery

Posterior ulnar recurrent artery

Recurrent interosseous artery

Extensor pollicis longus

Extensor indicis

Termination of anterior interosseous artery

Dorsal carpal branch of ulnar artery

Radial artery

Ulna

Posterior interosseous artery

Interosseous membrane

Radius

Ulnar artery

Dorsal carpal branch of ulnar artery

Dorsal carpal network

Radial artery

Dorsal carpal artery

Arteries of the forearm (posterior view)

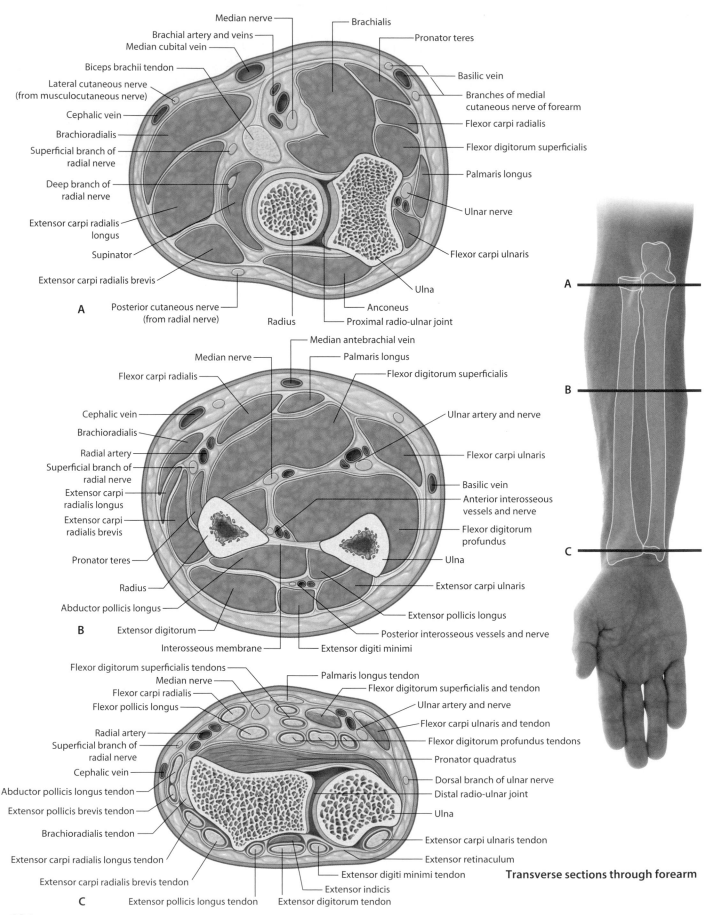

Median nerve
Brachial artery and veins
Median cubital vein
Biceps brachii tendon
Lateral cutaneous nerve
(from musculocutaneous nerve)
Cephalic vein
Brachioradialis
Superficial branch of
radial nerve
Deep branch of
radial nerve
Extensor carpi radialis
longus
Supinator
Extensor carpi radialis brevis

Brachialis
Pronator teres
Basilic vein
Branches of medial
cutaneous nerve of forearm
Flexor carpi radialis
Flexor digitorum superficialis
Palmaris longus
Ulnar nerve
Flexor carpi ulnaris
Ulna
Anconeus
Proximal radio-ulnar joint

A
Posterior cutaneous nerve
(from radial nerve)
Radius

Median antebrachial vein
Median nerve
Flexor carpi radialis
Cephalic vein
Brachioradialis
Radial artery
Superficial branch of
radial nerve
Extensor carpi
radialis longus
Extensor carpi
radialis brevis
Pronator teres
Radius
Abductor pollicis longus

Palmaris longus
Flexor digitorum superficialis
Ulnar artery and nerve
Flexor carpi ulnaris
Basilic vein
Anterior interosseous
vessels and nerve
Flexor digitorum
profundus
Ulna
Extensor carpi ulnaris
Extensor pollicis longus
Posterior interosseous vessels and nerve

B
Extensor digitorum
Interosseous membrane
Extensor digiti minimi

Flexor digitorum superficialis tendons
Median nerve
Flexor carpi radialis
Flexor pollicis longus
Radial artery
Superficial branch of
radial nerve
Cephalic vein
Abductor pollicis longus tendon
Extensor pollicis brevis tendon
Brachioradialis tendon
Extensor carpi radialis longus tendon
Extensor carpi radialis brevis tendon

Palmaris longus tendon
Flexor digitorum superficialis and tendon
Ulnar artery and nerve
Flexor carpi ulnaris and tendon
Flexor digitorum profundus tendons
Pronator quadratus
Dorsal branch of ulnar nerve
Distal radio-ulnar joint
Ulna
Extensor carpi ulnaris tendon
Extensor retinaculum
Extensor digiti minimi tendon

C
Extensor pollicis longus tendon
Extensor indicis
Extensor digitorum tendon

A
B
C

Transverse sections through forearm

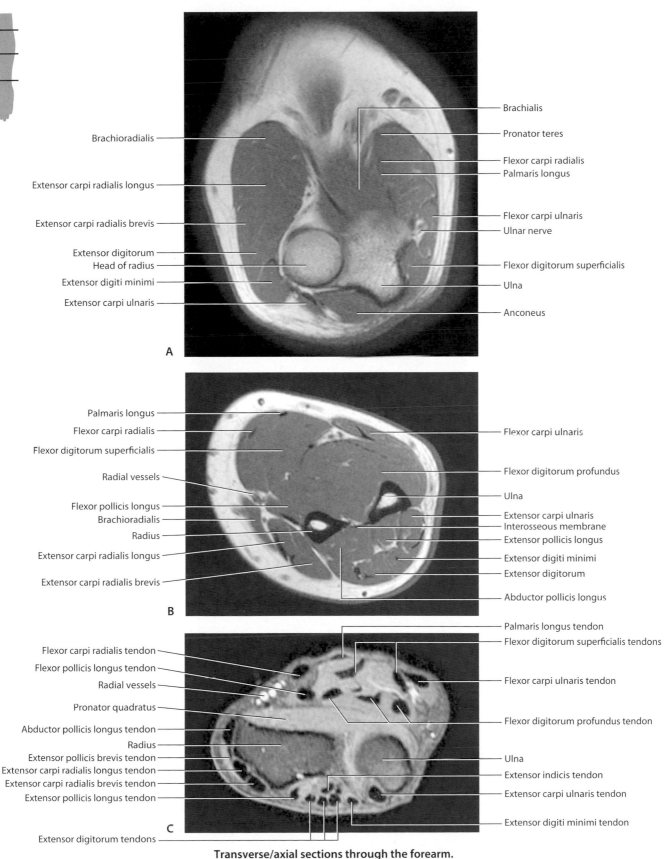

Brachioradialis

Extensor carpi radialis longus

Extensor carpi radialis brevis

Extensor digitorum
Head of radius
Extensor digiti minimi

Extensor carpi ulnaris

Brachialis
Pronator teres
Flexor carpi radialis
Palmaris longus

Flexor carpi ulnaris
Ulnar nerve

Flexor digitorum superficialis
Ulna

Anconeus

A

Palmaris longus
Flexor carpi radialis
Flexor digitorum superficialis

Radial vessels

Flexor pollicis longus
Brachioradialis
Radius

Extensor carpi radialis longus

Extensor carpi radialis brevis

Flexor carpi ulnaris

Flexor digitorum profundus

Ulna

Extensor carpi ulnaris
Interosseous membrane
Extensor pollicis longus
Extensor digiti minimi
Extensor digitorum

Abductor pollicis longus

B

Palmaris longus tendon
Flexor digitorum superficialis tendons

Flexor carpi radialis tendon
Flexor pollicis longus tendon
Radial vessels
Pronator quadratus
Abductor pollicis longus tendon
Radius
Extensor pollicis brevis tendon
Extensor carpi radialis longus tendon
Extensor carpi radialis brevis tendon
Extensor pollicis longus tendon

Extensor digitorum tendons

Flexor carpi ulnaris tendon

Flexor digitorum profundus tendon

Ulna
Extensor indicis tendon
Extensor carpi ulnaris tendon

Extensor digiti minimi tendon

C

Transverse/axial sections through the forearm.
A. Proximal/upper forearm. T1-weighted MR image in axial plane
B. Middle forearm. T1-weighted MR image in axial plane
C. Distal/lower forearm. Fat-saturated proton density MR image in axial plane

439

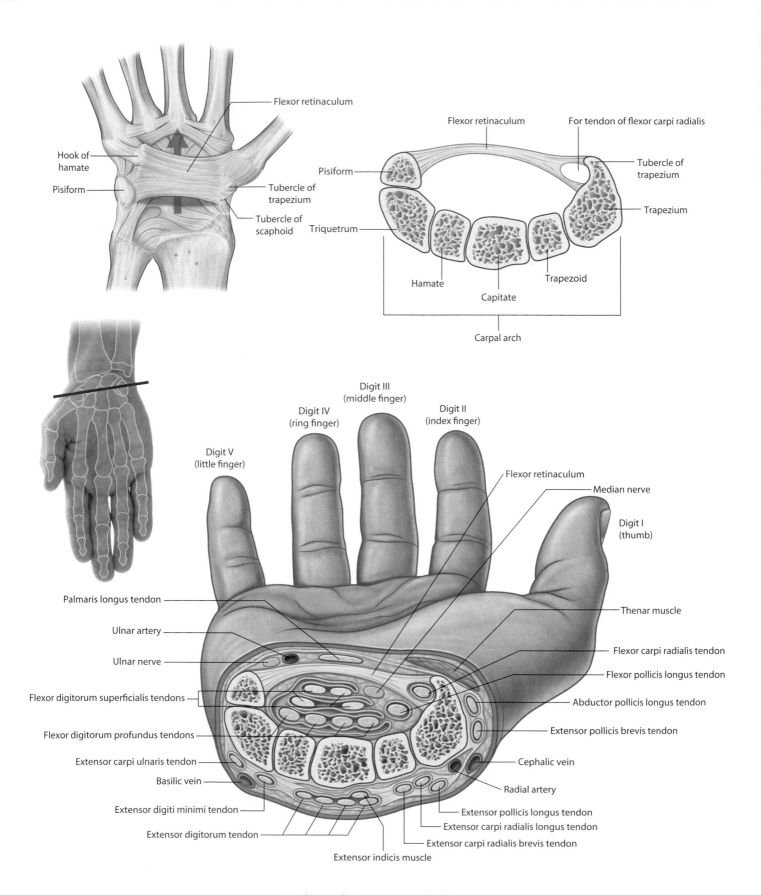

Carpal tunnel, structures and relations

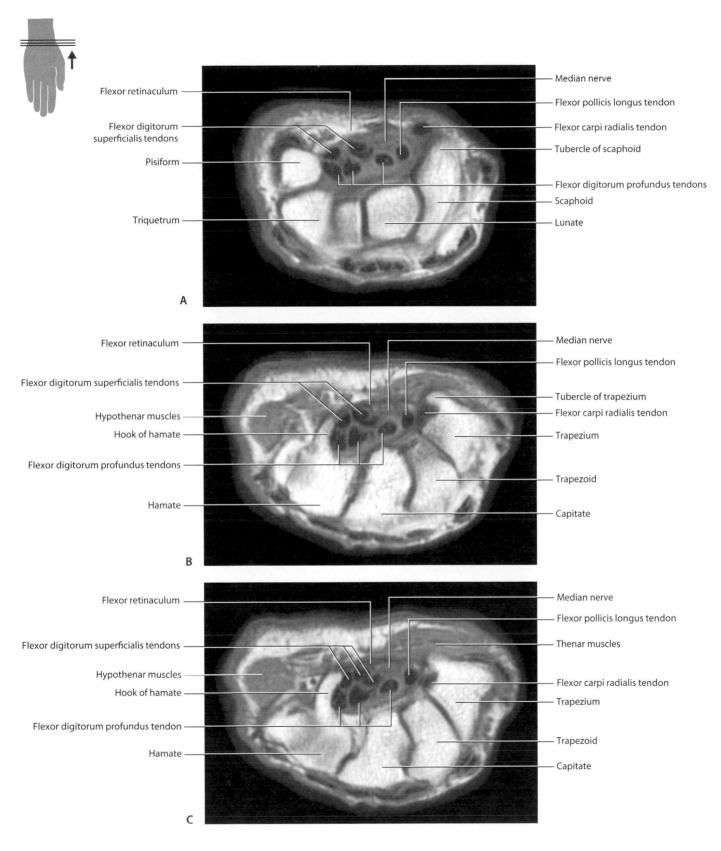

Flexor retinaculum

Flexor digitorum superficialis tendons

Pisiform

Triquetrum

Median nerve

Flexor pollicis longus tendon

Flexor carpi radialis tendon

Tubercle of scaphoid

Flexor digitorum profundus tendons

Scaphoid

Lunate

A

Flexor retinaculum

Flexor digitorum superficialis tendons

Hypothenar muscles

Hook of hamate

Flexor digitorum profundus tendons

Hamate

Median nerve

Flexor pollicis longus tendon

Tubercle of trapezium

Flexor carpi radialis tendon

Trapezium

Trapezoid

Capitate

B

Flexor retinaculum

Flexor digitorum superficialis tendons

Hypothenar muscles

Hook of hamate

Flexor digitorum profundus tendon

Hamate

Median nerve

Flexor pollicis longus tendon

Thenar muscles

Flexor carpi radialis tendon

Trapezium

Trapezoid

Capitate

C

Transverse/axial sections through the carpal tunnel.
A. Proximal end of carpal tunnel.
B. Middle portion of carpal tunnel.
C. Distal portion of carpal tunnel.
T1-weighted MR images in axial plane

441

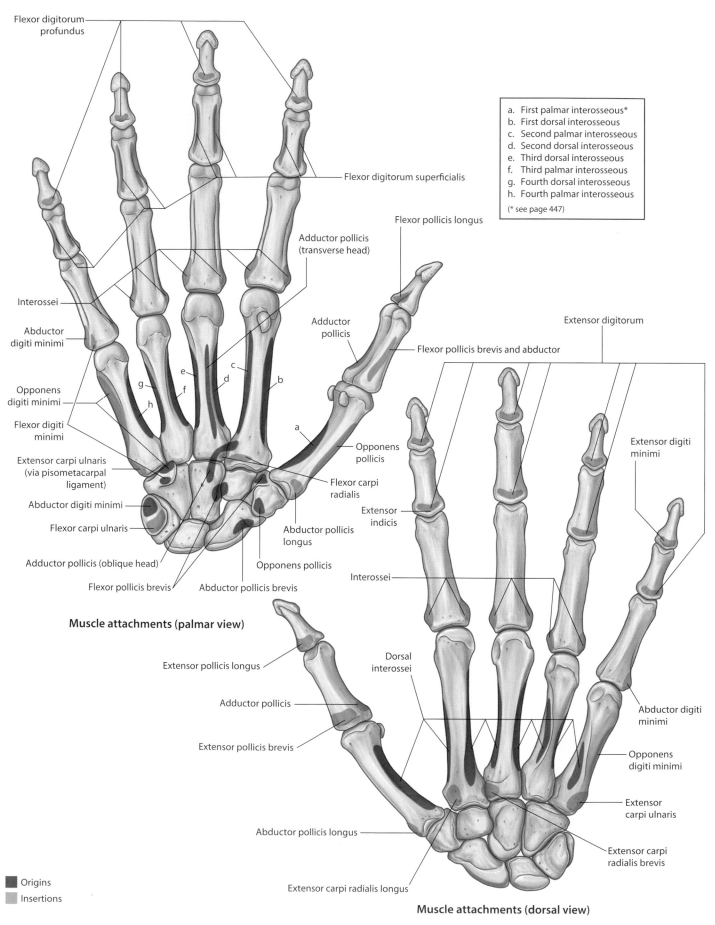

Flexor digitorum profundus

Flexor digitorum superficialis

a. First palmar interosseous*
b. First dorsal interosseous
c. Second palmar interosseous
d. Second dorsal interosseous
e. Third dorsal interosseous
f. Third palmar interosseous
g. Fourth dorsal interosseous
h. Fourth palmar interosseous

(* see page 447)

Flexor pollicis longus

Adductor pollicis (transverse head)

Adductor pollicis

Flexor pollicis brevis and abductor

Extensor digitorum

Interossei

Abductor digiti minimi

Extensor digiti minimi

Opponens digiti minimi

Flexor digiti minimi

Opponens pollicis

Extensor carpi ulnaris (via pisometacarpal ligament)

Flexor carpi radialis

Extensor indicis

Abductor digiti minimi

Flexor carpi ulnaris

Abductor pollicis longus

Interossei

Adductor pollicis (oblique head)

Opponens pollicis

Flexor pollicis brevis

Abductor pollicis brevis

Muscle attachments (palmar view)

Extensor pollicis longus

Dorsal interossei

Adductor pollicis

Abductor digiti minimi

Extensor pollicis brevis

Opponens digiti minimi

Extensor carpi ulnaris

Abductor pollicis longus

Extensor carpi radialis brevis

Extensor carpi radialis longus

Muscle attachments (dorsal view)

■ Origins
■ Insertions

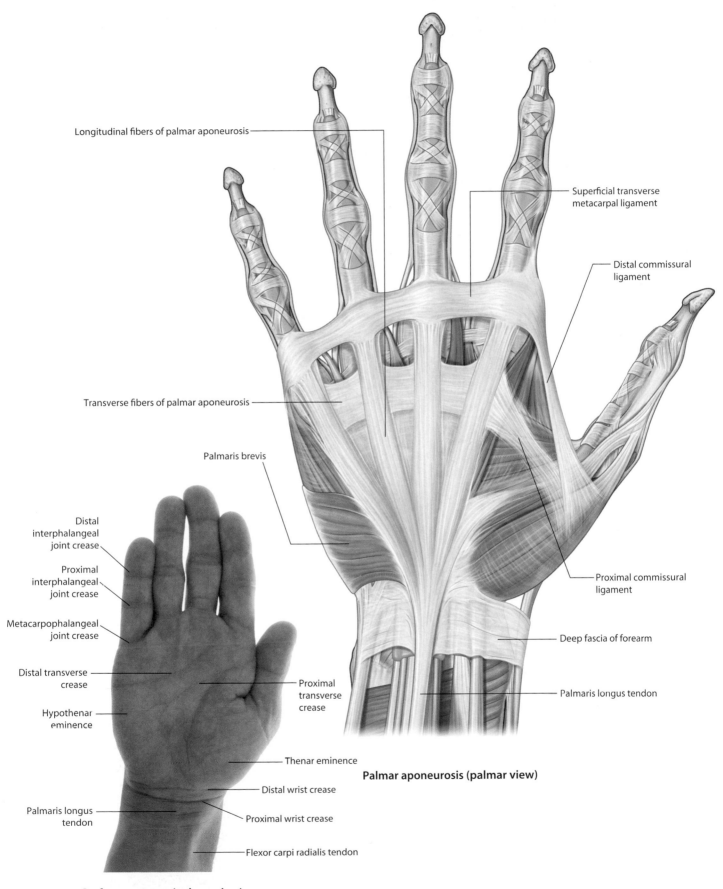

Longitudinal fibers of palmar aponeurosis

Superficial transverse metacarpal ligament

Distal commissural ligament

Transverse fibers of palmar aponeurosis

Palmaris brevis

Distal interphalangeal joint crease

Proximal interphalangeal joint crease

Metacarpophalangeal joint crease

Distal transverse crease

Hypothenar eminence

Palmaris longus tendon

Proximal transverse crease

Thenar eminence

Distal wrist crease

Proximal wrist crease

Flexor carpi radialis tendon

Proximal commissural ligament

Deep fascia of forearm

Palmaris longus tendon

Palmar aponeurosis (palmar view)

Surface anatomy (palmar view)

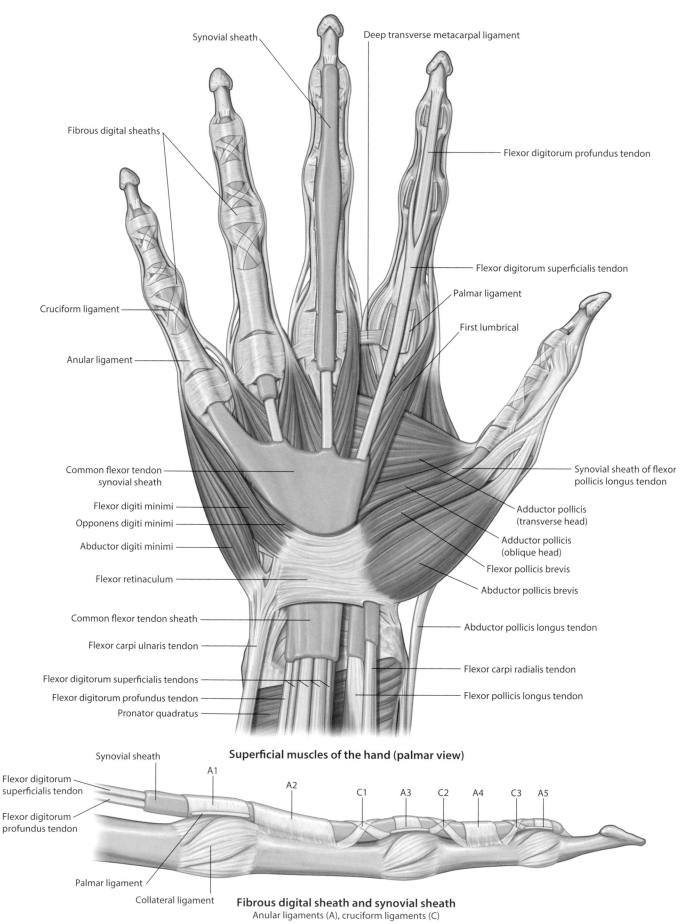

Synovial sheath

Deep transverse metacarpal ligament

Fibrous digital sheaths

Flexor digitorum profundus tendon

Cruciform ligament

Flexor digitorum superficialis tendon

Palmar ligament

First lumbrical

Anular ligament

Common flexor tendon synovial sheath

Synovial sheath of flexor pollicis longus tendon

Flexor digiti minimi

Adductor pollicis (transverse head)

Opponens digiti minimi

Adductor pollicis (oblique head)

Abductor digiti minimi

Flexor pollicis brevis

Flexor retinaculum

Abductor pollicis brevis

Common flexor tendon sheath

Abductor pollicis longus tendon

Flexor carpi ulnaris tendon

Flexor carpi radialis tendon

Flexor digitorum superficialis tendons

Flexor digitorum profundus tendon

Flexor pollicis longus tendon

Pronator quadratus

Superficial muscles of the hand (palmar view)

Synovial sheath

A1   A2   C1   A3   C2   A4   C3   A5

Flexor digitorum superficialis tendon

Flexor digitorum profundus tendon

Palmar ligament

Collateral ligament

Fibrous digital sheath and synovial sheath
Anular ligaments (A), cruciform ligaments (C)

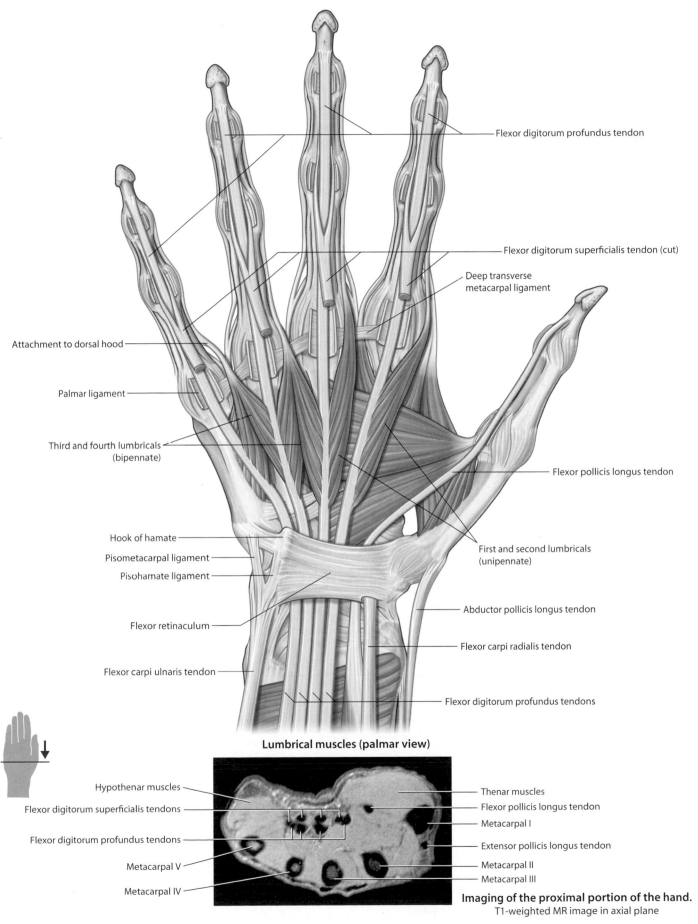

Flexor digitorum profundus tendon

Flexor digitorum superficialis tendon (cut)

Deep transverse metacarpal ligament

Attachment to dorsal hood

Palmar ligament

Third and fourth lumbricals (bipennate)

Flexor pollicis longus tendon

Hook of hamate

Pisometacarpal ligament

Pisohamate ligament

First and second lumbricals (unipennate)

Abductor pollicis longus tendon

Flexor retinaculum

Flexor carpi radialis tendon

Flexor carpi ulnaris tendon

Flexor digitorum profundus tendons

Lumbrical muscles (palmar view)

Hypothenar muscles

Thenar muscles

Flexor digitorum superficialis tendons

Flexor pollicis longus tendon

Metacarpal I

Flexor digitorum profundus tendons

Extensor pollicis longus tendon

Metacarpal V

Metacarpal II

Metacarpal III

Metacarpal IV

Imaging of the proximal portion of the hand.
T1-weighted MR image in axial plane

445

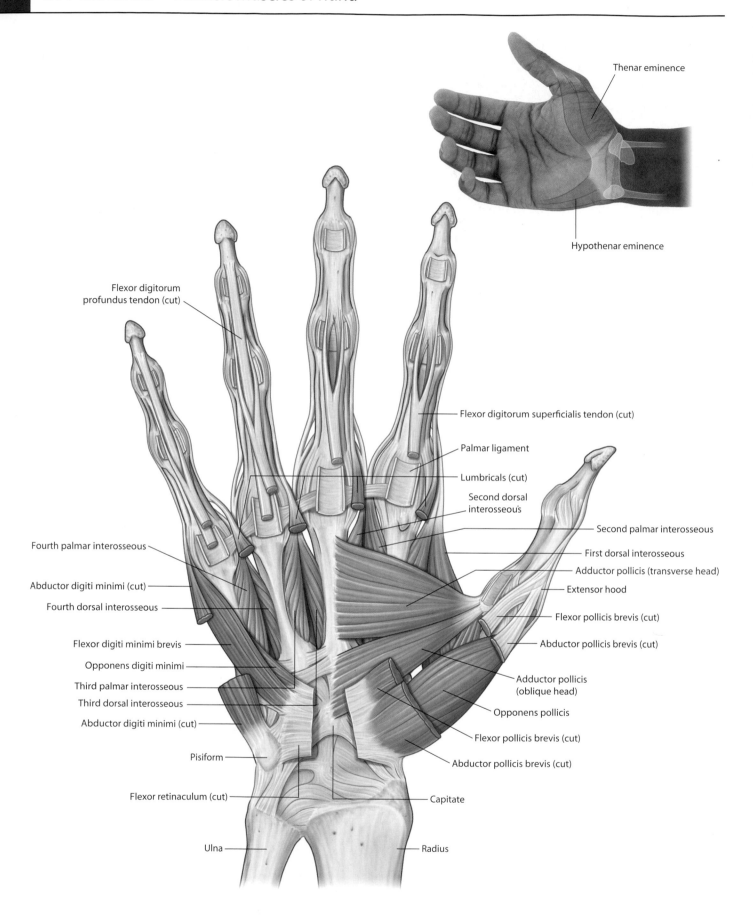

Thenar eminence

Hypothenar eminence

Flexor digitorum profundus tendon (cut)

Flexor digitorum superficialis tendon (cut)

Palmar ligament

Lumbricals (cut)

Second dorsal interosseous

Second palmar interosseous

First dorsal interosseous

Adductor pollicis (transverse head)

Extensor hood

Flexor pollicis brevis (cut)

Abductor pollicis brevis (cut)

Adductor pollicis (oblique head)

Opponens pollicis

Flexor pollicis brevis (cut)

Abductor pollicis brevis (cut)

Capitate

Radius

Fourth palmar interosseous

Abductor digiti minimi (cut)

Fourth dorsal interosseous

Flexor digiti minimi brevis

Opponens digiti minimi

Third palmar interosseous

Third dorsal interosseous

Abductor digiti minimi (cut)

Pisiform

Flexor retinaculum (cut)

Ulna

Deep muscles of the hand (palmar view)

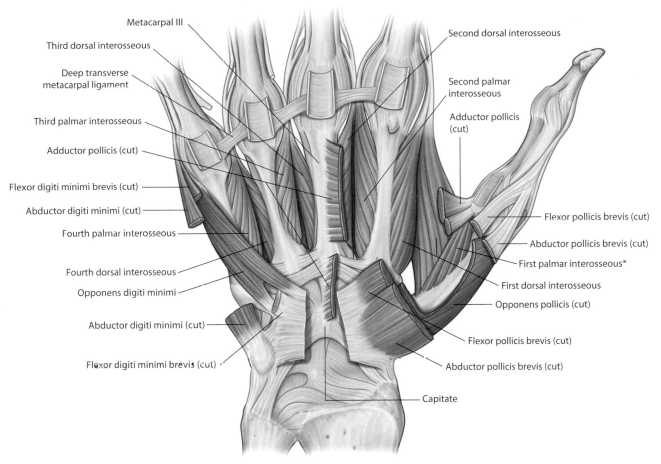

Metacarpal III

Third dorsal interosseous

Deep transverse metacarpal ligament

Third palmar interosseous

Adductor pollicis (cut)

Flexor digiti minimi brevis (cut)

Abductor digiti minimi (cut)

Fourth palmar interosseous

Fourth dorsal interosseous

Opponens digiti minimi

Abductor digiti minimi (cut)

Flexor digiti minimi brevis (cut)

Second dorsal interosseous

Second palmar interosseous

Adductor pollicis (cut)

Flexor pollicis brevis (cut)

Abductor pollicis brevis (cut)

First palmar interosseous*

First dorsal interosseous

Opponens pollicis (cut)

Flexor pollicis brevis (cut)

Abductor pollicis brevis (cut)

Capitate

Deep muscles of the hand (palmar view)

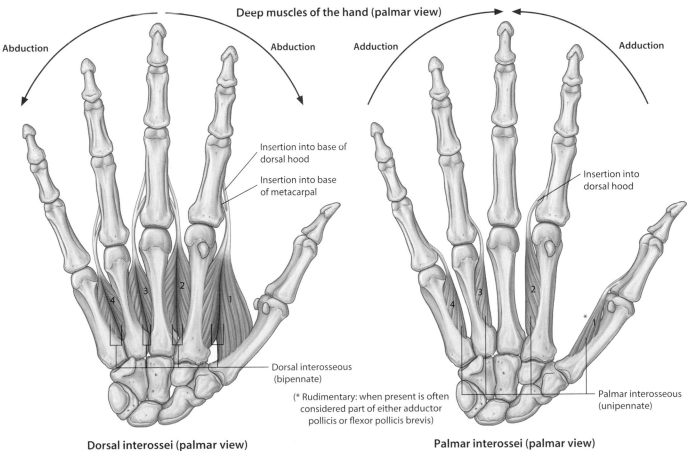

Abduction

Abduction

Adduction

Adduction

Insertion into base of dorsal hood

Insertion into base of metacarpal

Insertion into dorsal hood

4 3 2 1

4 3 2 *1

Dorsal interosseous (bipennate)

(* Rudimentary: when present is often considered part of either adductor pollicis or flexor pollicis brevis)

Palmar interosseous (unipennate)

Dorsal interossei (palmar view)

Palmar interossei (palmar view)

447

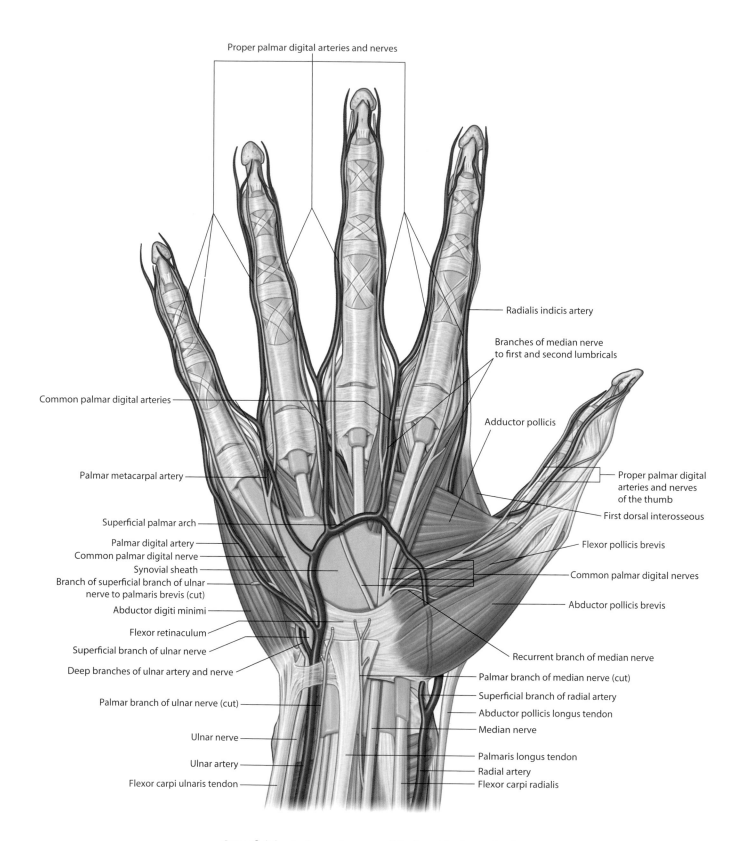

Proper palmar digital arteries and nerves

Radialis indicis artery

Branches of median nerve to first and second lumbricals

Common palmar digital arteries

Adductor pollicis

Palmar metacarpal artery

Proper palmar digital arteries and nerves of the thumb

First dorsal interosseous

Superficial palmar arch

Palmar digital artery

Flexor pollicis brevis

Common palmar digital nerve

Synovial sheath

Common palmar digital nerves

Branch of superficial branch of ulnar nerve to palmaris brevis (cut)

Abductor pollicis brevis

Abductor digiti minimi

Flexor retinaculum

Recurrent branch of median nerve

Superficial branch of ulnar nerve

Palmar branch of median nerve (cut)

Deep branches of ulnar artery and nerve

Superficial branch of radial artery

Palmar branch of ulnar nerve (cut)

Abductor pollicis longus tendon

Median nerve

Ulnar nerve

Palmaris longus tendon

Ulnar artery

Radial artery

Flexor carpi ulnaris tendon

Flexor carpi radialis

Superficial arteries and nerves of the hand (palmar view)

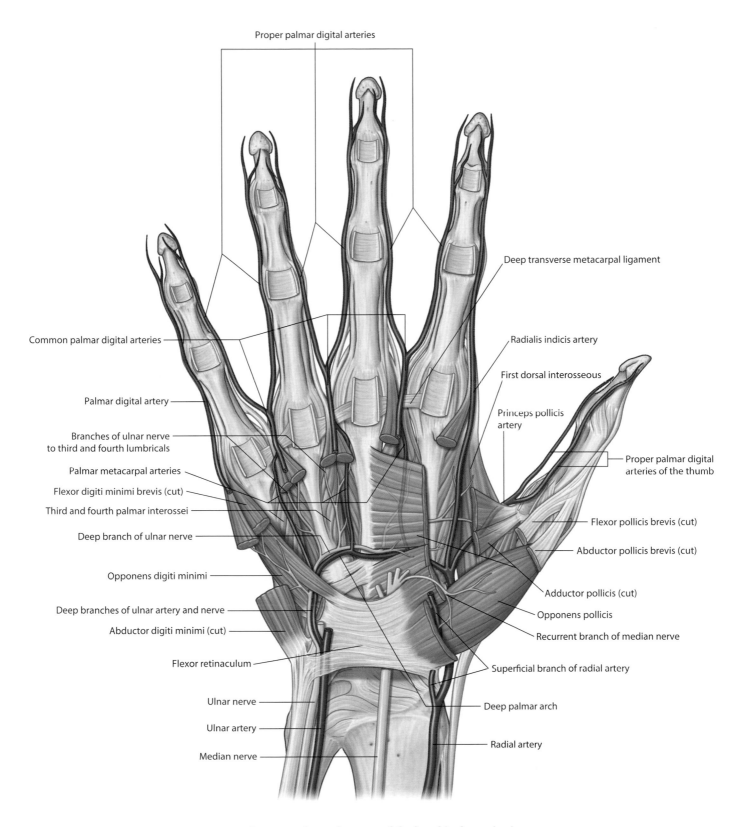

Proper palmar digital arteries

Deep transverse metacarpal ligament

Common palmar digital arteries

Radialis indicis artery

First dorsal interosseous

Palmar digital artery

Princeps pollicis artery

Branches of ulnar nerve to third and fourth lumbricals

Proper palmar digital arteries of the thumb

Palmar metacarpal arteries

Flexor digiti minimi brevis (cut)

Flexor pollicis brevis (cut)

Third and fourth palmar interossei

Abductor pollicis brevis (cut)

Deep branch of ulnar nerve

Opponens digiti minimi

Adductor pollicis (cut)

Deep branches of ulnar artery and nerve

Opponens pollicis

Abductor digiti minimi (cut)

Recurrent branch of median nerve

Flexor retinaculum

Superficial branch of radial artery

Ulnar nerve

Deep palmar arch

Ulnar artery

Median nerve

Radial artery

Deep arteries and nerves of the hand (palmar view)

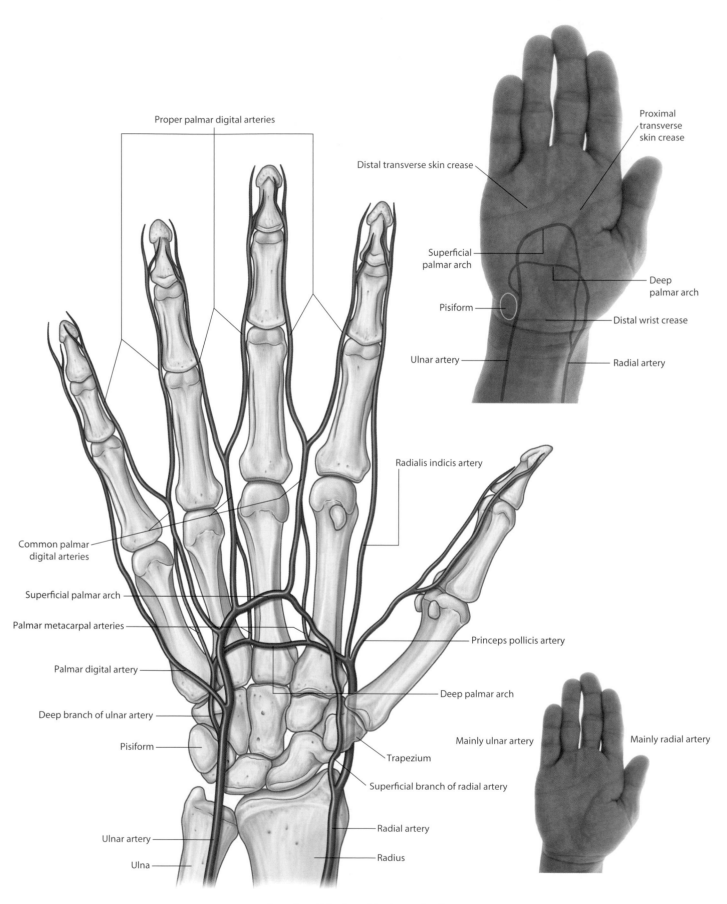

Proper palmar digital arteries

Proximal transverse skin crease

Distal transverse skin crease

Superficial palmar arch

Deep palmar arch

Pisiform

Distal wrist crease

Ulnar artery

Radial artery

Radialis indicis artery

Common palmar digital arteries

Superficial palmar arch

Palmar metacarpal arteries

Princeps pollicis artery

Palmar digital artery

Deep palmar arch

Deep branch of ulnar artery

Mainly ulnar artery

Mainly radial artery

Pisiform

Trapezium

Superficial branch of radial artery

Ulnar artery

Radial artery

Ulna

Radius

Arteries of the hand (palmar view)

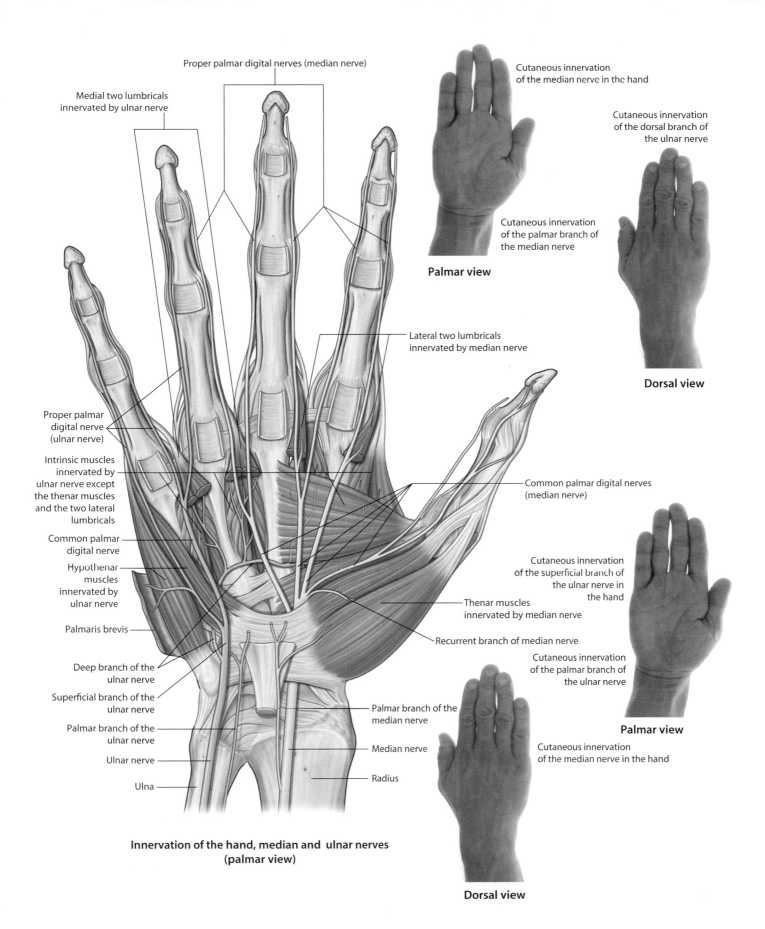

Proper palmar digital nerves (median nerve)

Medial two lumbricals innervated by ulnar nerve

Cutaneous innervation of the median nerve in the hand

Cutaneous innervation of the dorsal branch of the ulnar nerve

Cutaneous innervation of the palmar branch of the median nerve

Palmar view

Dorsal view

Lateral two lumbricals innervated by median nerve

Proper palmar digital nerve (ulnar nerve)

Intrinsic muscles innervated by ulnar nerve except the thenar muscles and the two lateral lumbricals

Common palmar digital nerve

Hypothenar muscles innervated by ulnar nerve

Palmaris brevis

Deep branch of the ulnar nerve

Superficial branch of the ulnar nerve

Palmar branch of the ulnar nerve

Ulnar nerve

Ulna

Common palmar digital nerves (median nerve)

Cutaneous innervation of the superficial branch of the ulnar nerve in the hand

Thenar muscles innervated by median nerve

Recurrent branch of median nerve

Cutaneous innervation of the palmar branch of the ulnar nerve

Palmar view

Palmar branch of the median nerve

Median nerve

Radius

Cutaneous innervation of the median nerve in the hand

Innervation of the hand, median and ulnar nerves (palmar view)

Dorsal view

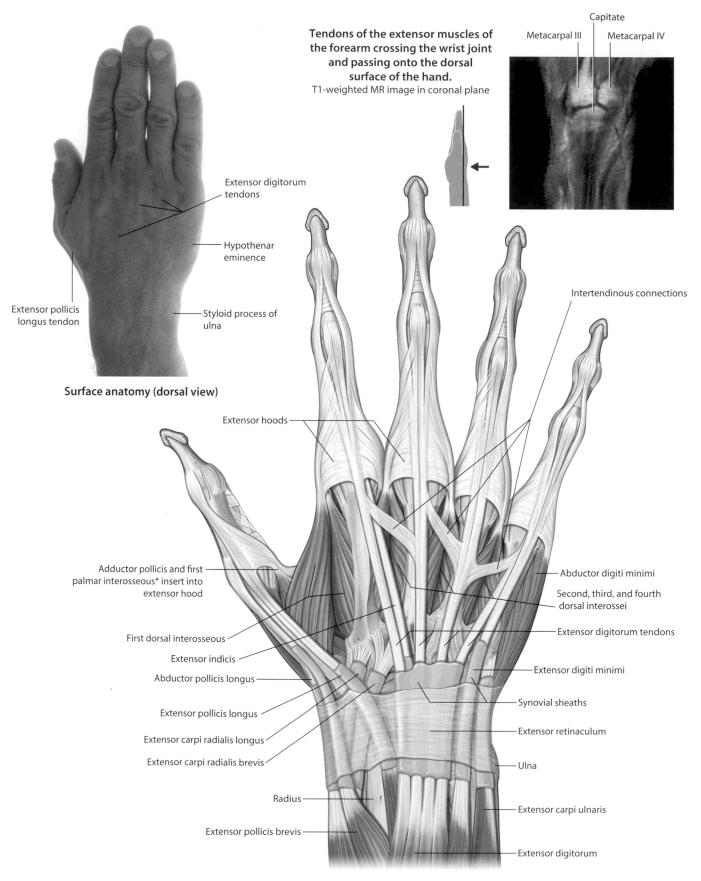

Surface anatomy (dorsal view)

Tendons of the extensor muscles of the forearm crossing the wrist joint and passing onto the dorsal surface of the hand.
T1-weighted MR image in coronal plane

Capitate

Metacarpal III

Metacarpal IV

Extensor digitorum tendons

Hypothenar eminence

Extensor pollicis longus tendon

Styloid process of ulna

Intertendinous connections

Extensor hoods

Adductor pollicis and first palmar interosseous* insert into extensor hood

First dorsal interosseous

Extensor indicis

Abductor pollicis longus

Extensor pollicis longus

Extensor carpi radialis longus

Extensor carpi radialis brevis

Radius

Extensor pollicis brevis

Abductor digiti minimi

Second, third, and fourth dorsal interossei

Extensor digitorum tendons

Extensor digiti minimi

Synovial sheaths

Extensor retinaculum

Ulna

Extensor carpi ulnaris

Extensor digitorum

Superficial structures of the hand (dorsal view)
(* see page 447)

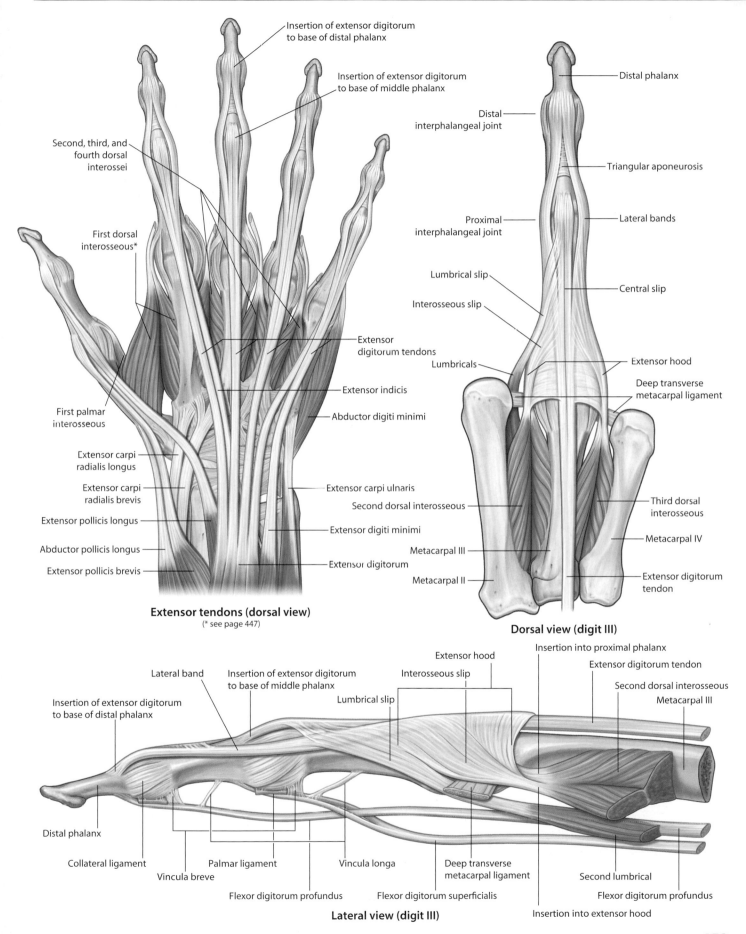

Insertion of extensor digitorum to base of distal phalanx

Insertion of extensor digitorum to base of middle phalanx

Second, third, and fourth dorsal interossei

First dorsal interosseous*

First palmar interosseous

Extensor carpi radialis longus

Extensor carpi radialis brevis

Extensor pollicis longus

Abductor pollicis longus

Extensor pollicis brevis

Extensor digitorum tendons

Extensor indicis

Abductor digiti minimi

Extensor carpi ulnaris

Extensor digiti minimi

Extensor digitorum

Extensor tendons (dorsal view)
(* see page 447)

Distal phalanx

Distal interphalangeal joint

Proximal interphalangeal joint

Lumbrical slip

Interosseous slip

Lumbricals

Triangular aponeurosis

Lateral bands

Central slip

Extensor hood

Deep transverse metacarpal ligament

Second dorsal interosseous

Metacarpal III

Metacarpal II

Third dorsal interosseous

Metacarpal IV

Extensor digitorum tendon

Dorsal view (digit III)

Insertion of extensor digitorum to base of distal phalanx

Lateral band

Insertion of extensor digitorum to base of middle phalanx

Lumbrical slip

Extensor hood

Interosseous slip

Insertion into proximal phalanx

Extensor digitorum tendon

Second dorsal interosseous

Metacarpal III

Distal phalanx

Collateral ligament

Vincula breve

Palmar ligament

Flexor digitorum profundus

Vincula longa

Flexor digitorum superficialis

Deep transverse metacarpal ligament

Insertion into extensor hood

Second lumbrical

Flexor digitorum profundus

Lateral view (digit III)

453

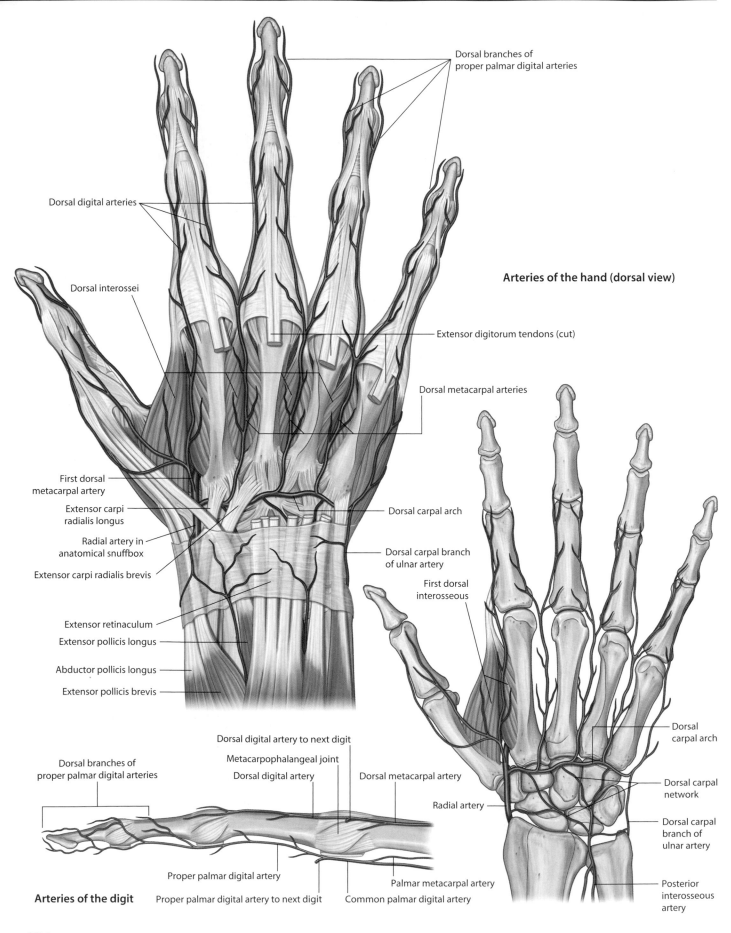

Dorsal branches of
proper palmar digital arteries

Dorsal digital arteries

Dorsal interossei

Arteries of the hand (dorsal view)

Extensor digitorum tendons (cut)

Dorsal metacarpal arteries

First dorsal
metacarpal artery

Extensor carpi
radialis longus

Radial artery in
anatomical snuffbox

Extensor carpi radialis brevis

Extensor retinaculum

Extensor pollicis longus

Abductor pollicis longus

Extensor pollicis brevis

Dorsal carpal arch

Dorsal carpal branch
of ulnar artery

First dorsal
interosseous

Dorsal branches of
proper palmar digital arteries

Dorsal digital artery to next digit

Metacarpophalangeal joint

Dorsal digital artery

Dorsal metacarpal artery

Radial artery

Proper palmar digital artery

Proper palmar digital artery to next digit

Arteries of the digit

Palmar metacarpal artery

Common palmar digital artery

Dorsal
carpal arch

Dorsal carpal
network

Dorsal carpal
branch of
ulnar artery

Posterior
interosseous
artery

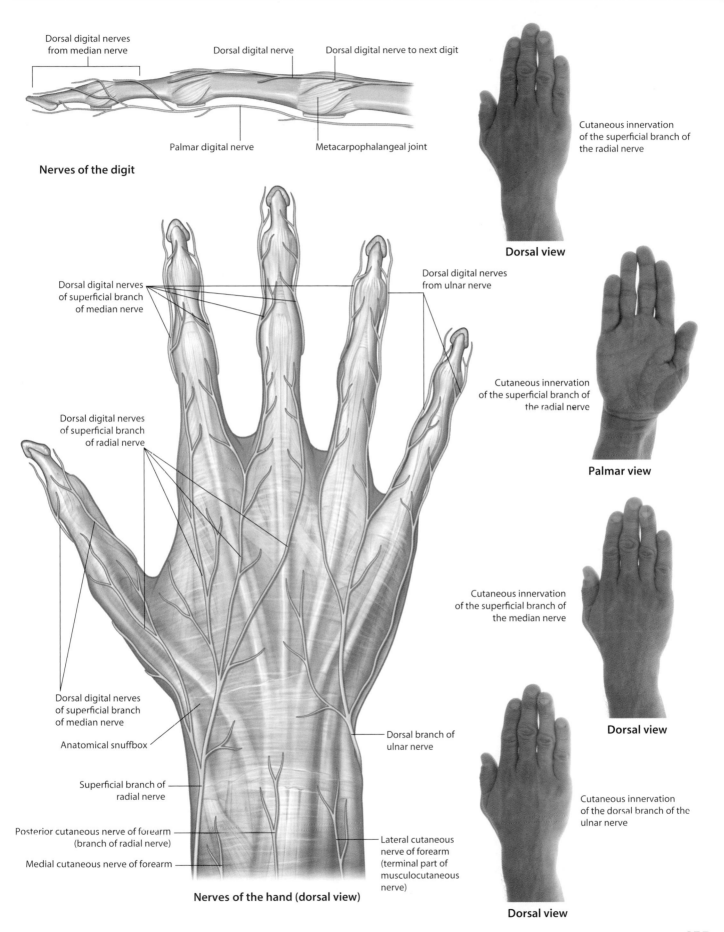

Dorsal digital nerves from median nerve

Dorsal digital nerve

Dorsal digital nerve to next digit

Palmar digital nerve

Metacarpophalangeal joint

Nerves of the digit

Dorsal digital nerves of superficial branch of median nerve

Dorsal digital nerves from ulnar nerve

Dorsal digital nerves of superficial branch of radial nerve

Dorsal digital nerves of superficial branch of median nerve

Anatomical snuffbox

Superficial branch of radial nerve

Posterior cutaneous nerve of forearm (branch of radial nerve)

Medial cutaneous nerve of forearm

Dorsal branch of ulnar nerve

Lateral cutaneous nerve of forearm (terminal part of musculocutaneous nerve)

Nerves of the hand (dorsal view)

Cutaneous innervation of the superficial branch of the radial nerve

Dorsal view

Cutaneous innervation of the superficial branch of the radial nerve

Palmar view

Cutaneous innervation of the superficial branch of the median nerve

Dorsal view

Cutaneous innervation of the dorsal branch of the ulnar nerve

Dorsal view

455

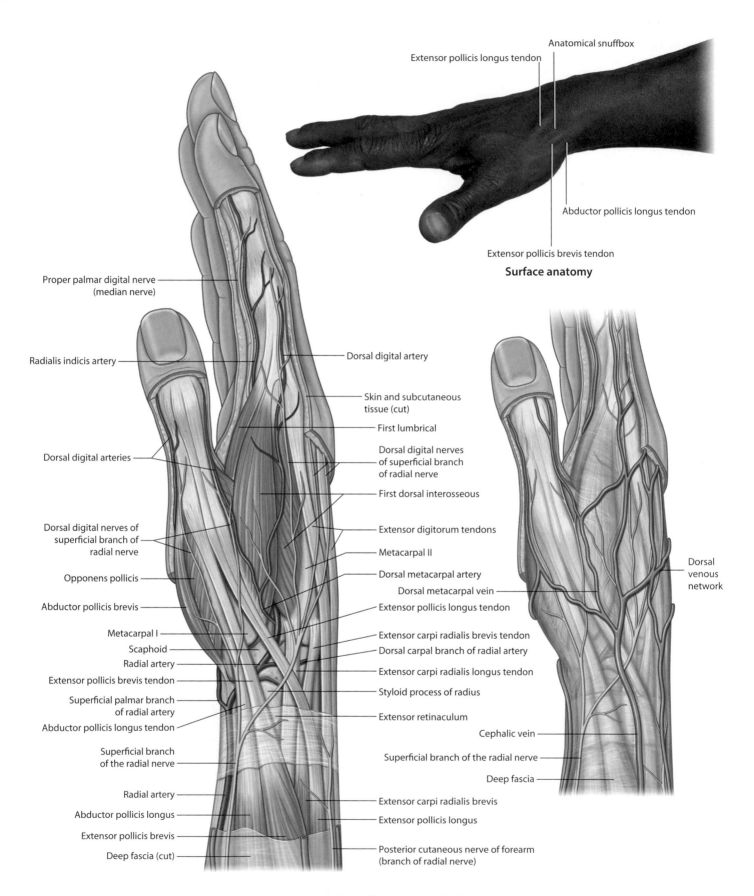

Extensor pollicis longus tendon

Anatomical snuffbox

Abductor pollicis longus tendon

Extensor pollicis brevis tendon

Surface anatomy

Proper palmar digital nerve (median nerve)

Radialis indicis artery

Dorsal digital arteries

Dorsal digital nerves of superficial branch of radial nerve

Opponens pollicis

Abductor pollicis brevis

Metacarpal I

Scaphoid

Radial artery

Extensor pollicis brevis tendon

Superficial palmar branch of radial artery

Abductor pollicis longus tendon

Superficial branch of the radial nerve

Radial artery

Abductor pollicis longus

Extensor pollicis brevis

Deep fascia (cut)

Dorsal digital artery

Skin and subcutaneous tissue (cut)

First lumbrical

Dorsal digital nerves of superficial branch of radial nerve

First dorsal interosseous

Extensor digitorum tendons

Metacarpal II

Dorsal metacarpal artery

Extensor pollicis longus tendon

Extensor carpi radialis brevis tendon

Dorsal carpal branch of radial artery

Extensor carpi radialis longus tendon

Styloid process of radius

Extensor retinaculum

Extensor carpi radialis brevis

Extensor pollicis longus

Posterior cutaneous nerve of forearm (branch of radial nerve)

Dorsal venous network

Dorsal metacarpal vein

Cephalic vein

Superficial branch of the radial nerve

Deep fascia

Anatomical snuffbox (lateral view)

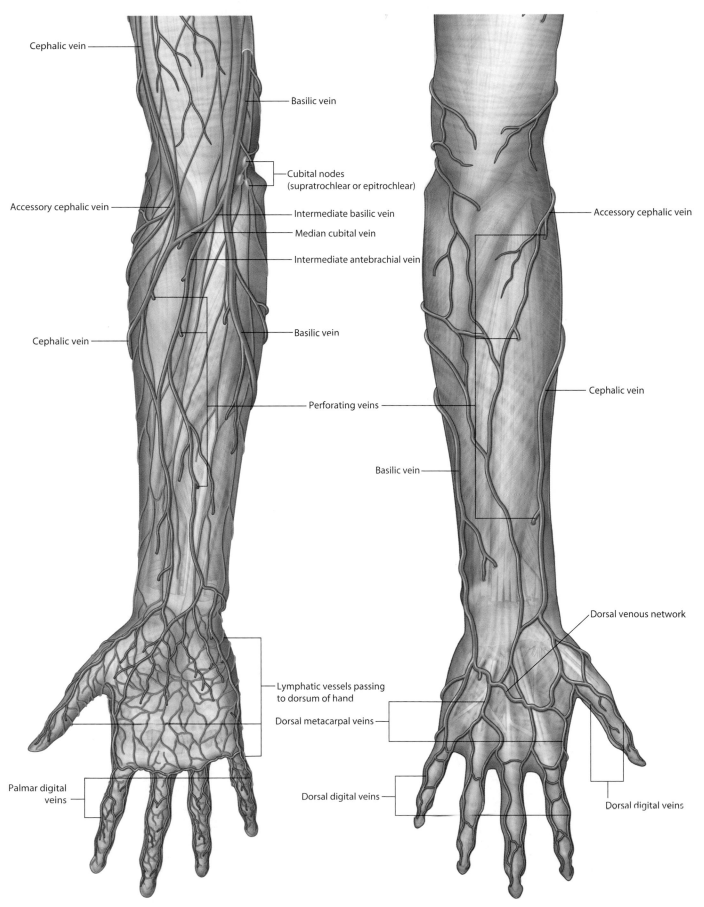

Cephalic vein

Basilic vein

Cubital nodes
(supratrochlear or epitrochlear)

Accessory cephalic vein

Intermediate basilic vein

Median cubital vein

Intermediate antebrachial vein

Cephalic vein

Basilic vein

Accessory cephalic vein

Perforating veins

Cephalic vein

Basilic vein

Dorsal venous network

Lymphatic vessels passing
to dorsum of hand

Dorsal metacarpal veins

Palmar digital
veins

Dorsal digital veins

Dorsal digital veins

Superficial veins and lymphatics of the forearm (palmar view)

Superficial veins of the forearm (dorsal view)

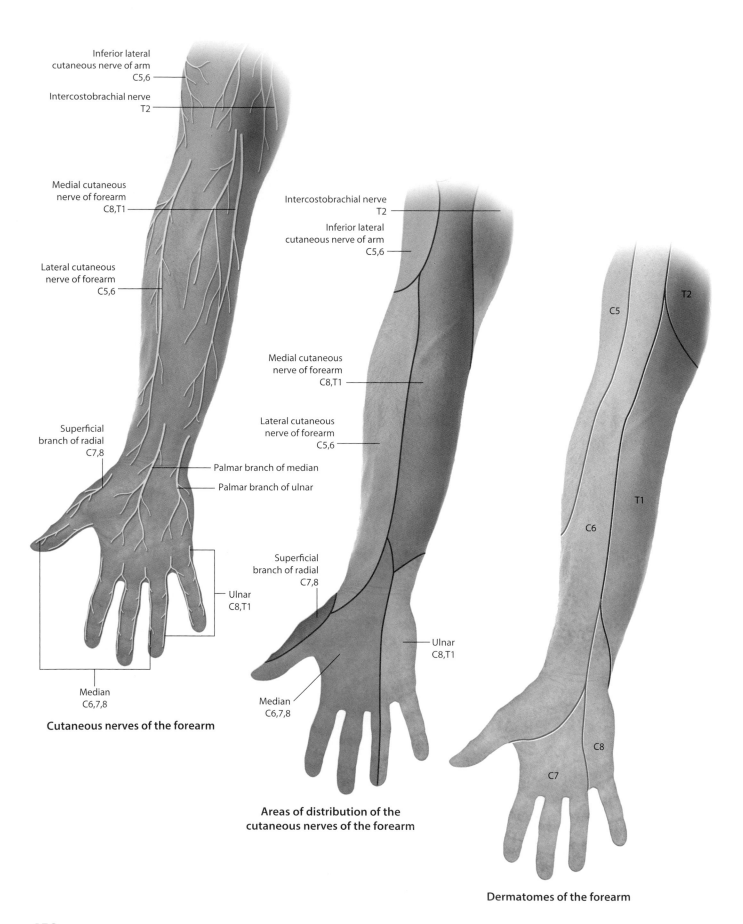

Inferior lateral
cutaneous nerve of arm
C5,6

Intercostobrachial nerve
T2

Medial cutaneous
nerve of forearm
C8,T1

Lateral cutaneous
nerve of forearm
C5,6

Superficial
branch of radial
C7,8

Palmar branch of median

Palmar branch of ulnar

Ulnar
C8,T1

Median
C6,7,8

Cutaneous nerves of the forearm

Intercostobrachial nerve
T2

Inferior lateral
cutaneous nerve of arm
C5,6

Medial cutaneous
nerve of forearm
C8,T1

Lateral cutaneous
nerve of forearm
C5,6

Superficial
branch of radial
C7,8

Ulnar
C8,T1

Median
C6,7,8

**Areas of distribution of the
cutaneous nerves of the forearm**

C5

T2

T1

C6

C8

C7

Dermatomes of the forearm

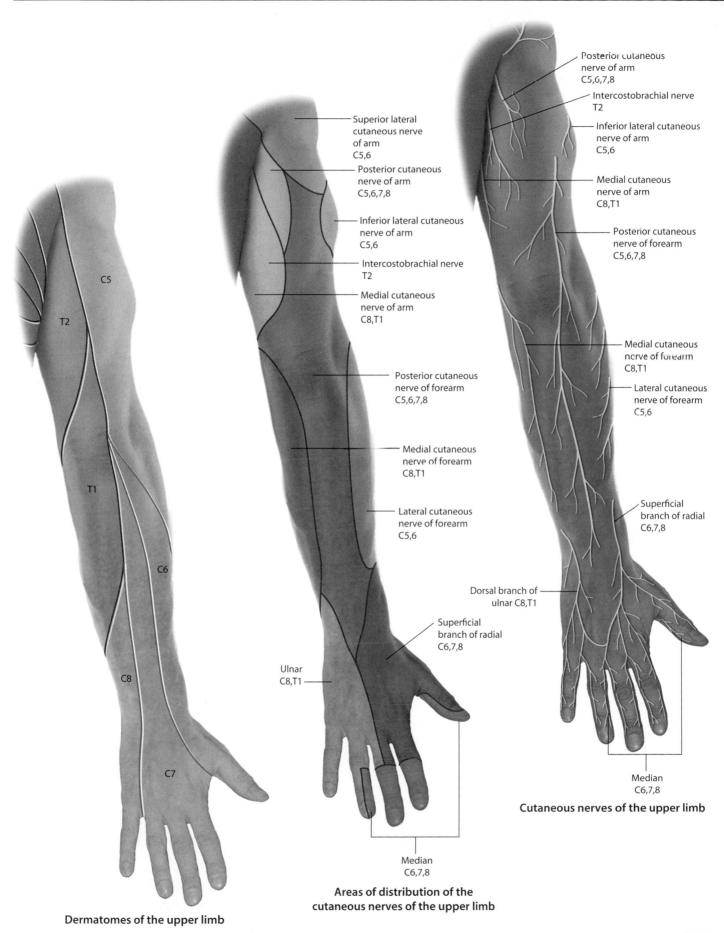

Superior lateral
cutaneous nerve
of arm
C5,6

Posterior cutaneous
nerve of arm
C5,6,7,8

Inferior lateral cutaneous
nerve of arm
C5,6

Intercostobrachial nerve
T2

Medial cutaneous
nerve of arm
C8,T1

Posterior cutaneous
nerve of forearm
C5,6,7,8

Medial cutaneous
nerve of forearm
C8,T1

Lateral cutaneous
nerve of forearm
C5,6

Medial cutaneous
nerve of forearm
C8,T1

Superficial
branch of radial
C6,7,8

Ulnar
C8,T1

Median
C6,7,8

**Areas of distribution of the
cutaneous nerves of the upper limb**

Posterior cutaneous
nerve of arm
C5,6,7,8

Intercostobrachial nerve
T2

Inferior lateral cutaneous
nerve of arm
C5,6

Medial cutaneous
nerve of arm
C8,T1

Posterior cutaneous
nerve of forearm
C5,6,7,8

Medial cutaneous
nerve of forearm
C8,T1

Lateral cutaneous
nerve of forearm
C5,6

Superficial
branch of radial
C6,7,8

Dorsal branch of
ulnar C8,T1

Median
C6,7,8

Cutaneous nerves of the upper limb

C5

T2

T1

C6

C8

C7

Dermatomes of the upper limb

Branches of the brachial plexus

Branch		Origin	Spinal segments	Function: motor	Function: sensory
Dorsal scapular	1	C5 root	C5	Rhomboid major, rhomboid minor	
Long thoracic	2	C5 to C7 roots	C5 to C7	Serratus anterior	
Suprascapular	3	Superior trunk	C5, C6	Supraspinatus, infraspinatus	
Nerve to subclavius	4	Superior trunk	C5, C6	Subclavius	
Lateral pectoral	5	Lateral cord	C5 to C7	Pectoralis major	
Musculocutaneous	6	Lateral cord	C5 to C7	All muscles in the anterior compartment of the arm	Skin on lateral side of forearm
Medial pectoral	7	Medial cord	C8, T1 (also receives contributions from spinal segments C5 to C7 through a communication with the lateral pectoral nerve)	Pectoralis major, pectoralis minor	
Medial cutaneous of arm	8	Medial cord	Spinal segments: C8, T1		Skin on medial side of distal one third of arm
Medial cutaneous of forearm	9	Medial cord	C8, T1		Skin on medial side of forearm
Median	10	Medial and lateral cords	(C5), C6 to T1	All muscles in the anterior compartment of the forearm (except flexor carpi ulnaris and medial half of flexor digitorum profundus), three thenar muscles of the thumb, and two lateral lumbrical muscles	Skin over the palmar surface of the lateral three and one half digits and over the lateral side of the palm and middle of the wrist
Ulnar	11	Medial cord	(C7), C8, T1	All intrinsic muscles of the hand (except three thenar muscles and two lateral lumbricals); also flexor carpi ulnaris and the medial half of flexor digitorum profundus in the forearm	Skin over the palmar surface of the medial one and one half digits and associated palm and wrist, and skin over the dorsal surface of the medial one and one half digits
Superior subscapular	12	Posterior cord	C5, C6	Subscapularis	
Thoracodorsal	13	Posterior cord	C6 to C8	Latissimus dorsi	

Branches of the brachial plexus

Branch		Origin	Spinal segments	Function: motor	Function: sensory
Inferior subscapular	14	Posterior cord	C5, C6	Subscapularis, teres major	
Axillary	15	Posterior cord	C5, C6	Deltoid, teres minor	Skin over upper lateral part of arm
Radial	16	Posterior cord	C5 to C8, (T1)	All muscles in the posterior compartments of arm and forearm	Skin on the posterior aspects of the arm and forearm, the lower lateral surface of the arm, and the dorsal lateral surface of the hand

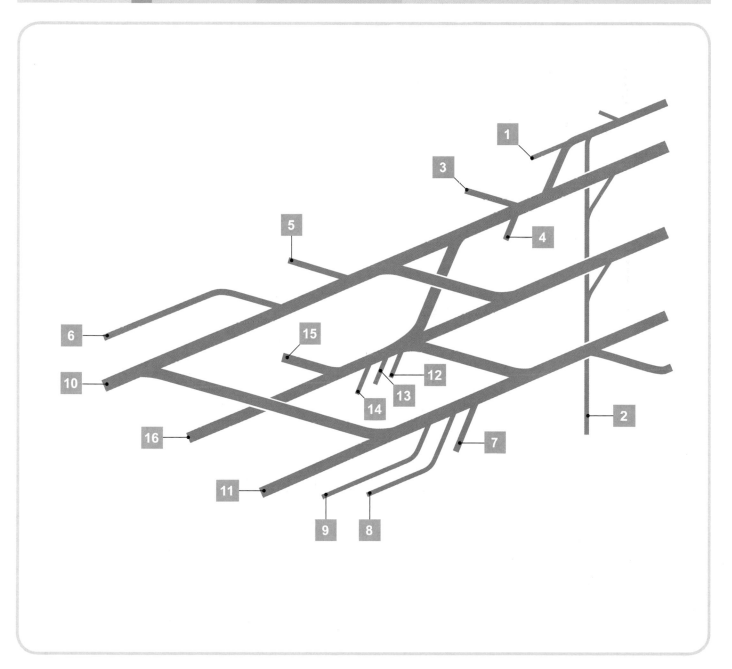

Muscles of the shoulder

(muscles of the shoulder spinal segments indicated in bold are the major segments innervating the muscle)

Muscle		Origin	Insertion	Innervation	Function
Trapezius	1	Superior nuchal line, external occipital protuberance, medial margin of the ligamentum nuchae, spinous processes of CVII to TXII and the related supraspinous ligaments	Superior edge of the crest of the spine of the scapula, acromion, posterior border of lateral one third of clavicle	Motor spinal part of accessory nerve [XI]. Sensory (proprioception) anterior rami of C3 and C4	Powerful elevator of the scapula; rotates the scapula during abduction of humerus above horizontal; middle fibers retract scapula; lower fibers depress scapula
Deltoid	2	Inferior edge of the crest of the spine of the scapula, lateral margin of the acromion, anterior border of lateral one third of clavicle	Deltoid tuberosity of humerus	Axillary nerve [**C5**, **C6**]	Major abductor of arm (abducts arm beyond initial 15° done by supraspinatus); clavicular fibers assist in flexing the arm; posterior fibers assist in extending the arm
Levator scapulae	3	Transverse processes of CI and CII vertebrae and posterior tubercles of transverse processes of CIII and CIV vertebrae	Posterior surface of medial border of scapula from superior angle to root of spine of the scapula	Branches directly from anterior rami of **C3** and **C4** spinal nerves and by branches [**C5**] from the dorsal scapular nerve	Elevates the scapula
Rhomboid minor	4	Lower end of ligamentum nuchae and spinous processes of CVII and TI vertebrae	Posterior surface of medial border of scapula at the root of the spine of the scapula	Dorsal scapular nerve [C4, **C5**]	Elevates and retracts the scapula
Rhomboid major	5	Spinous processes of TII–TV vertebrae and intervening supraspinous ligaments	Posterior surface of medial border of scapula from the root of the spine of the scapula to the inferior angle	Dorsal scapular nerve [**C4**, **C5**]	Elevates and retracts the scapula

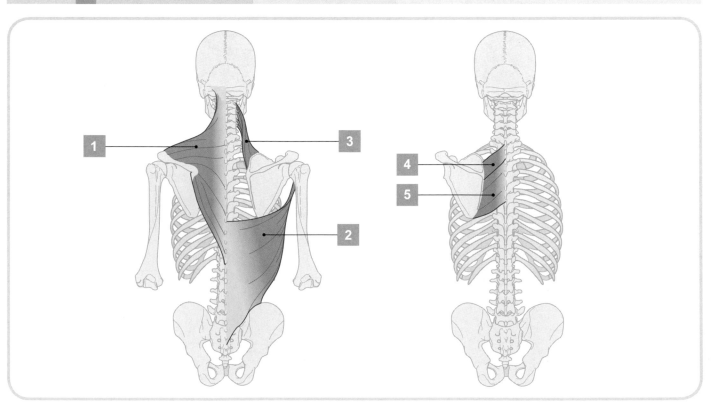

Muscles of the posterior scapular region

(spinal segments in bold are the major segments innervating the muscle)

Muscle		Origin	Insertion	Innervation	Function
Supraspinatus	1	Medial two thirds of the supraspinous fossa of the scapula and the deep fascia that covers the muscle	Most superior facet on the greater tubercle of the humerus	Suprascapular nerve [**C5**, C6]	Rotator cuff muscle; initiation of abduction of arm to 15° at glenohumeral joint
Infraspinatus	2	Medial two thirds of the infraspinous fossa of the scapula and the deep fascia that covers the muscle	Middle facet on posterior surface of the greater tubercle of the humerus	Suprascapular nerve [**C5**, C6]	Rotator cuff muscle; lateral rotation of arm at the glenohumeral joint
Teres minor	3	Upper two thirds of a flattened strip of bone on the posterior surface of the scapula immediately adjacent to the lateral border of the scapula	Inferior facet on the posterior surface of the greater tubercle of the humerus	Axillary nerve [**C5**, C6]	Rotator cuff muscle; lateral rotation of arm at the glenohumeral joint
Teres major	4	Elongate oval area on the posterior surface of the inferior angle of the scapula	Medial lip of the intertubercular sulcus on the anterior surface of the humerus	Inferior subscapular nerve [**C5**, **C6**, **C7**]	Medial rotation and extension of the arm at the glenohumeral joint
Long head of triceps brachii	5	Infraglenoid tubercle on scapula	Common tendon of insertion with medial and lateral heads on the olecranon process of ulna	Radial nerve [C6, **C7**, C8]	Extension of the forearm at the elbow joint; accessory adductor and extensor of the arm at the glenohumeral joint

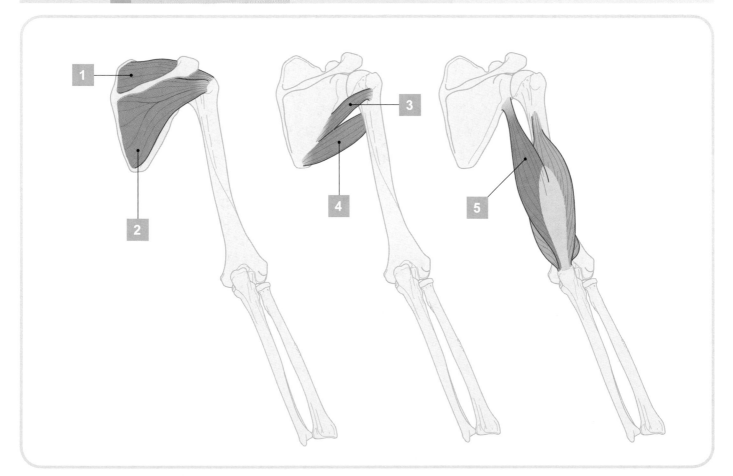

Muscles of the anterior wall of the axilla

(spinal segments in bold are the major segments innervating the muscle)

Muscle		Origin	Insertion	Innervation	Function
Pectoralis major	1	Clavicular head—anterior surface of medial half of clavicle; sternocostal head—anterior surface of sternum; first seven costal cartilages; sternal end of sixth rib; aponeurosis of external oblique	Lateral lip of intertubercular sulcus of humerus	Medial and lateral pectoral nerves; clavicular head [**C5**, C6]; sternocostal head [C6, C7, C8, T1]	Flexion, adduction, and medial rotation of arm at glenohumeral joint; clavicular head—flexion of extended arm; sternocostal head—extension of flexed arm
Subclavius	2	First rib at junction between rib and costal cartilage	Groove on inferior surface of middle one third of clavicle	Nerve to subclavius [**C5**, **C6**]	Pulls tip of shoulder down; pulls clavicle medially to stabilize sternoclavicular joint
Pectoralis minor	3	Anterior surfaces and superior borders of ribs III to V; and from deep fascia overlying the related intercostal spaces	Coracoid process of scapula (medial border and upper surface)	Medial pectoral nerve [C5, C6, **C7**, **C8**, T1]	Pulls tip of shoulder down; protracts scapula

Muscles of the medial wall of the axilla

Serratus anterior	4	Lateral surfaces of upper 8–9 ribs and deep fascia overlying the related intercostal spaces	Costal surface of medial border of scapula	Long thoracic nerve [**C5**, C6, C7]	Protraction and rotation of the scapula; keeps medial border and inferior angle of scapula opposed to thoracic wall

Muscles of the lateral and posterior wall of the axilla

(spinal segments enclosed in parentheses do not consistently innervate the muscle)

Subscapularis	5	Medial two thirds of subscapular fossa	Lesser tubercle of humerus	Upper and lower subscapular nerves [C5, **C6**, (C7)]	Rotator cuff muscle; medial rotation of the arm at the glenohumeral joint
Teres major	6	Elongate oval area on the posterior surface of the inferior angle of the scapula	Medial lip of the intertubercular sulcus on the anterior surface of the humerus	Lower subscapular nerve [**C5**, **C6**, **C7**]	Medial rotation and extension of the arm at the glenohumeral joint
Latissimus dorsi	7	Spinous processes of lower six thoracic vertebrae and related interspinous ligaments; via the thoracolumbar fascia to the spinous processes of the lumbar vertebrae, related interspinous ligaments, and iliac crest; lower 3–4 ribs	Floor of intertubercular sulcus	Thoracodorsal nerve [C6, **C7**, C8]	Adduction, medial rotation, and extension of the arm at the glenohumeral joint
Long head of triceps brachii	8	Infraglenoid tubercle on scapula	Common tendon of insertion with medial and lateral heads on the olecranon process of ulna	Radial nerve [C6, **C7**, C8]	Extension of the forearm at the elbow joint; accessory adductor and extensor of the arm at the glenohumeral joint

Muscles having parts that pass through the axilla

(spinal segments in bold are the major segments innervating the muscle)

Muscle		Origin	Insertion	Innervation	Function
Biceps brachii	1	Long head—supraglenoid tubercle of scapula; short head—apex of coracoid process	Tuberosity of radius	Musculocutaneous nerve [**C5**, **C6**]	Powerful flexor of the forearm at the elbow joint and supinator of the forearm; accessory flexor of the arm at the glenohumeral joint
Coracobrachialis	2	Apex of coracoid process	Linear roughening on midshaft of humerus on medial side	Musculocutaneous nerve [**C5**, **C6**, **C7**]	Flexor of the arm at the glenohumeral joint; adducts arm

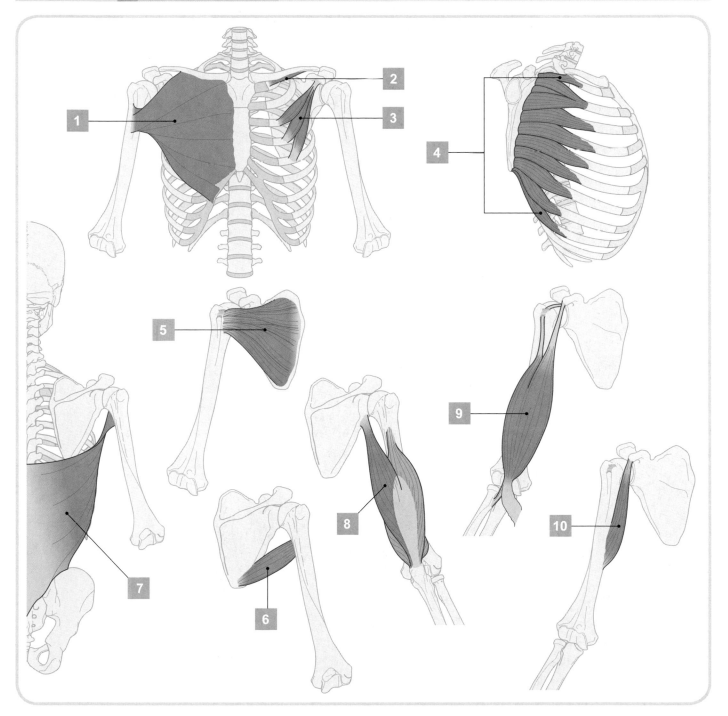

Muscles of the anterior compartment of the arm
(spinal segments in bold are the major segments innervating the muscle)

Muscle		Origin	Insertion	Innervation	Function
Coracobrachialis	1	Apex of coracoid process	Linear roughening on midshaft of humerus on medial side	Musculocutaneous nerve [**C5**, **C6**, **C7**]	Flexor of the arm at the glenohumeral joint
Biceps brachii	2	Long head— supraglenoid tubercle of scapula; short head— apex of coracoid process	Radial tuberosity	Musculocutaneous nerve [**C5**, **C6**]	Powerful flexor of the forearm at the elbow joint and supinator of the forearm; accessory flexor of the arm at the glenohumeral joint
Brachialis	3	Anterior aspect of humerus (medial and lateral surfaces) and adjacent intermuscular septae	Tuberosity of the ulna	Musculocutaneous nerve [C5, **C6**]; (small contribution by the radial nerve [C7] to lateral part of muscle)	Powerful flexor of the forearm at the elbow joint

Muscle of the posterior compartment of the arm

Muscle		Origin	Insertion	Innervation	Function
Triceps brachii	4	Long head—infraglenoid tubercle of scapula; medial head—posterior surface of humerus; lateral head— posterior surface of humerus	Olecranon	Radial nerve [C6, **C7**, C8]	Extension of the forearm at the elbow joint. Long head can also extend and adduct the arm at the shoulder joint

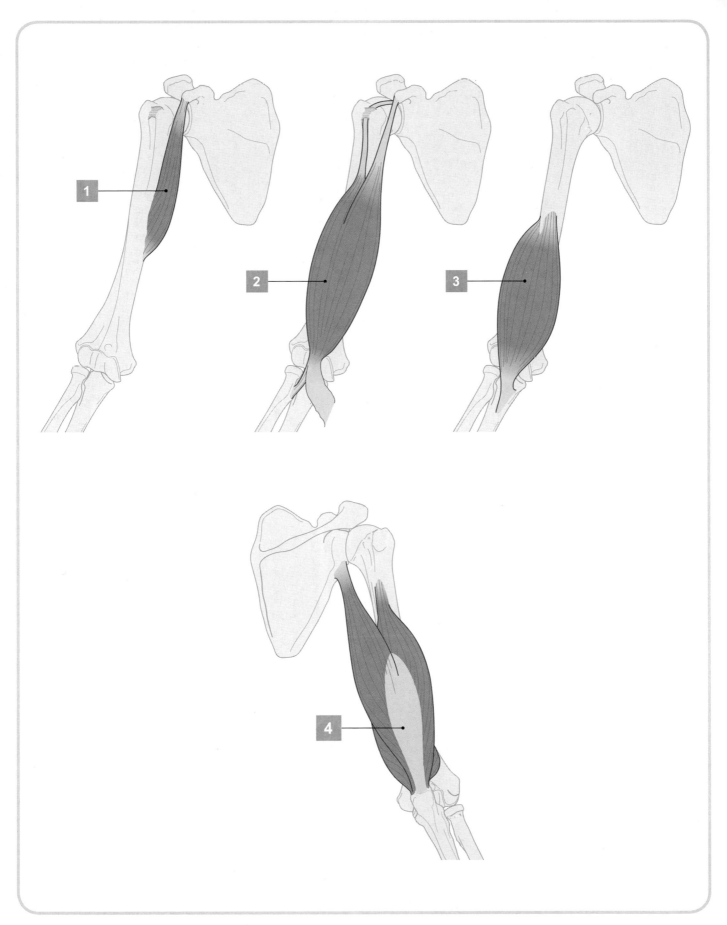

Superficial layer of muscles in the anterior compartment of the forearm

(spinal segments indicated in bold are the major segments innervating the muscle)

Muscle		Origin	Insertion	Innervation	Function
Flexor carpi ulnaris	1	Humeral head—medial epicondyle of humerus; ulnar head—olecranon and posterior border of ulna	Pisiform bone, and then via pisohamate and pisometacarpal ligaments into the hamate and base of metacarpal V	Ulnar nerve [C7, **C8**, T1]	Flexes and adducts the wrist joint
Palmaris longus	2	Medial epicondyle of humerus	Palmar aponeurosis of hand	Median nerve [**C7**, **C8**]	Flexes wrist joint; because the palmar aponeurosis anchors skin of the hand, contraction of the muscle resists shearing forces when gripping
Flexor carpi radialis	3	Medial epicondyle of humerus	Base of metacarpals II and III	Median nerve [**C6**, **C7**]	Flexes and abducts the wrist
Pronator teres	4	Humeral head—medial epicondyle and adjacent supracondylar ridge; ulnar head—medial side of coronoid process	Roughening on lateral surface, midshaft, of radius	Median nerve [**C6**, **C7**]	Pronation

Intermediate layer of muscles in the anterior compartment of the forearm

Muscle		Origin	Insertion	Innervation	Function
Flexor digitorum superficialis	5	Humero-ulnar head—medial epicondyle of humerus and adjacent margin of coronoid process; radial head—oblique line of radius	Four tendons, which attach to the palmar surfaces of the middle phalanges of the index, middle, ring, and little fingers	Median nerve [**C8**, T1]	Flexes proximal interphalangeal joints of the index, middle, ring, and little fingers; can also flex metacarpophalangeal joints of the same fingers and the wrist joint

Deep layer of muscles in the anterior compartment of the forearm

Muscle		Origin	Insertion	Innervation	Function
Flexor digitorum profundus	6	Anterior and medial surfaces of ulna and anterior medial half of interosseous membrane	Four tendons, which attach to the palmar surfaces of the distal phalanges of the index, middle, ring, and little fingers	Lateral half by median nerve (anterior interosseous nerve); medial half by ulnar nerve [**C8**, T1]	Flexes distal interphalangeal joints of the index, middle, ring, and little fingers; can also flex metacarpophalangeal joints of the same fingers and the wrist joint
Flexor pollicis longus	7	Anterior surface of radius and radial half of interosseous membrane	Palmar surface of base of distal phalanx of thumb	Median nerve (anterior interosseous nerve) [C7, **C8**]	Flexes interphalangeal joint of the thumb; can also flex metacarpophalangeal joint of the thumb
Pronator quadratus	8	Linear ridge on distal anterior surface of ulna	Distal anterior surface of radius	Median nerve (anterior interosseous nerve) [C7, **C8**]	Pronation

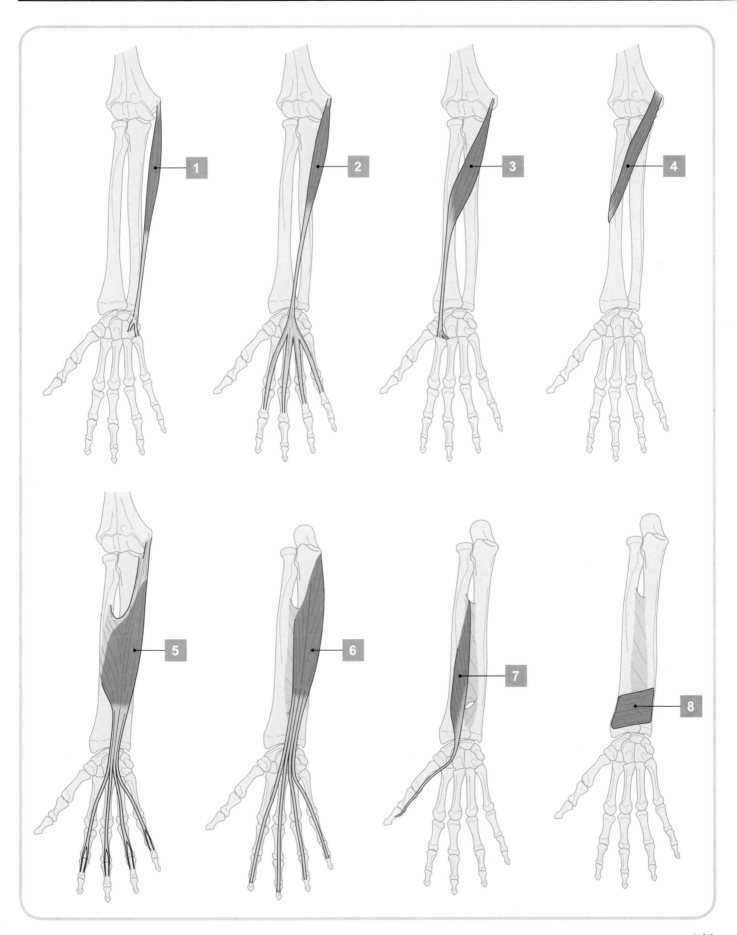

Superficial layer of muscles in the posterior compartment of the forearm

(spinal segments indicated in bold are the major segments innervating the muscle)

Muscle		Origin	Insertion	Innervation	Function
Brachioradialis	1	Proximal part of lateral supracondylar ridge of humerus and adjacent intermuscular septum	Lateral surface of distal end of radius	Radial nerve [C5, **C6**] before division into superficial and deep branches	Accessory flexor of elbow joint when forearm is midpronated
Extensor carpi radialis longus	2	Distal part of lateral supracondylar ridge of humerus and adjacent intermuscular septum	Dorsal surface of base of metacarpal II	Radial nerve [**C6**, C7] before division into superficial and deep branches	Extends and abducts the wrist
Extensor carpi radialis brevis	3	Lateral epicondyle of humerus and adjacent intermuscular septum	Dorsal surface of base of metacarpals II and III	Deep branch of radial nerve [**C7**, C8] before penetrating supinator muscle	Extends and abducts the wrist
Extensor digitorum	4	Lateral epicondyle of humerus and adjacent intermuscular septum and deep fascia	Four tendons, which insert via extensor hoods into the dorsal aspects of the bases of the middle and distal phalanges of the index, middle, ring, and little fingers	Posterior interosseous nerve [**C7**, C8]	Extends the index, middle, ring, and little fingers; can also extend the wrist
Extensor digiti minimi	5	Lateral epicondyle of humerus and adjacent intermuscular septum together with extensor digitorum	Extensor hood of the little finger	Posterior interosseous nerve [**C7**, C8]	Extends the little finger
Extensor carpi ulnaris	6	Lateral epicondyle of humerus and posterior border of ulna	Tubercle on the base of the medial side of metacarpal V	Posterior interosseous nerve [**C7**, C8]	Extends and adducts the wrist
Anconeus	7	Lateral epicondyle of humerus	Olecranon and proximal posterior surface of ulna	Radial nerve [**C6, C7, C8**] (via branch to medial head of triceps brachii)	Abduction of the ulna in pronation; accessory extensor of the elbow joint

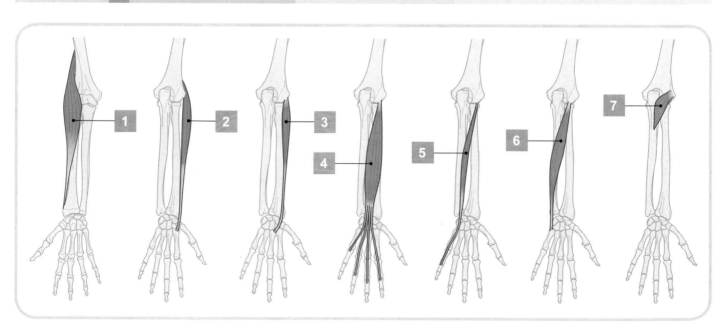

Deep layer of muscles in the posterior compartment of the forearm

(spinal segments indicated in bold are the major segments innervating the muscle)

Muscle		Origin	Insertion	Innervation	Function
Supinator	1	Superficial part—lateral epicondyle of humerus, radial collateral and anular ligaments; deep part—supinator crest of the ulna	Lateral surface of radius superior to the anterior oblique line	Posterior interosseous nerve [**C6**, C7]	Supination
Abductor pollicis longus	2	Posterior surfaces of ulna and radius (distal to the attachments of supinator and anconeus) and intervening interosseous membrane	Lateral side of base of metacarpal I	Posterior interosseous nerve [**C7**, C8]	Abducts carpometacarpal joint of thumb; accessory extensor of the thumb
Extensor pollicis brevis	3	Posterior surface of radius (distal to abductor pollicis longus) and the adjacent interosseous membrane	Dorsal surface of base of proximal phalanx of the thumb	Posterior interosseous nerve [**C7**, C8]	Extends metacarpophalangeal joint of the thumb; can also extend the carpometacarpal joint of the thumb
Extensor pollicis longus	4	Posterior surface of ulna (distal to the abductor pollicis longus) and the adjacent interosseous membrane	Dorsal surface of base of distal phalanx of thumb	Posterior interosseous nerve [**C7**, C8]	Extends interphalangeal joint of the thumb; can also extend carpometacarpal and metacarpophalangeal joints of the thumb
Extensor indicis	5	Posterior surface of ulna (distal to extensor pollicis longus) and adjacent interosseous membrane	Extensor hood of index finger	Posterior interosseous nerve [**C7**, C8]	Extends index finger

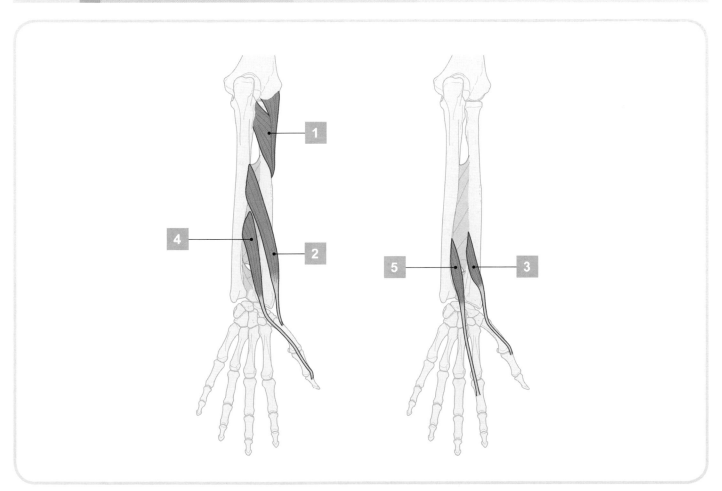

Intrinsic muscles of the hand

(spinal segments indicated in bold are the major segments innervating the muscle)

Muscle		Origin	Insertion	Innervation	Function
Palmaris brevis	1	Palmar aponeurosis and flexor retinaculum	Dermis of skin on the medial margin of the hand	Superficial branch of the ulnar nerve [C8, **T1**]	Improves grip
Dorsal interossei (four muscles)	2	Adjacent sides of metacarpals	Extensor hood and base of proximal phalanges of index, middle, and ring fingers	Deep branch of ulnar nerve [C8, **T1**]	Abduction of index, middle, and ring fingers at the metacarpophalangeal joints
Palmar interossei (four muscles)	3	Sides of metacarpals	Extensor hoods of the thumb, index, ring, and little fingers and the proximal phalanx of thumb	Deep branch of ulnar nerve [C8, **T1**]	Adduction of the thumb, index, ring, and little fingers at the metacarpophalangeal joints
Adductor pollicis	4	Transverse head—metacarpal III; oblique head—capitate and bases of metacarpals II and III	Base of proximal phalanx and extensor hood of thumb	Deep branch of ulnar nerve [C8, **T1**]	Adducts thumb
Lumbricals (four muscles)	5	Tendons of flexor digitorum profundus	Extensor hoods of index, ring, middle, and little fingers	Medial two by the deep branch of the ulnar nerve; lateral two by digital branches of the median nerve	Flex metacarpophalangeal joints while extending interphalangeal joints
Thenar muscles					
Opponens pollicis	6	Tubercle of trapezium and flexor retinaculum	Lateral margin and adjacent palmar surface of metacarpal I	Recurrent branch of median nerve [C8, **T1**]	Medially rotates thumb
Abductor pollicis brevis	7	Tubercles of scaphoid and trapezium and adjacent flexor retinaculum	Proximal phalanx and extensor hood of thumb	Recurrent branch of median nerve [C8, **T1**]	Abducts thumb at metacarpophalangeal joint
Flexor pollicis brevis	8	Tubercle of the trapezium and flexor retinaculum	Proximal phalanx of the thumb	Recurrent branch of median nerve [C8, **T1**]	Flexes thumb at metacarpophalangeal joint
Hypothenar muscles					
Opponens digiti minimi	9	Hook of hamate and flexor retinaculum	Medial aspect of metacarpal V	Deep branch of ulnar nerve [C8, **T1**]	Laterally rotates metacarpal V
Abductor digiti minimi	10	Pisiform, the pisohamate ligament, and tendon of flexor carpi ulnaris	Proximal phalanx of little finger	Deep branch of ulnar nerve [C8, **T1**]	Abducts little finger at metacarpophalangeal joint
Flexor digiti minimi brevis	11	Hook of the hamate and flexor retinaculum	Proximal phalanx of little finger	Deep branch of ulnar nerve [C8, **T1**]	Flexes little finger at metacarpophalangeal joint

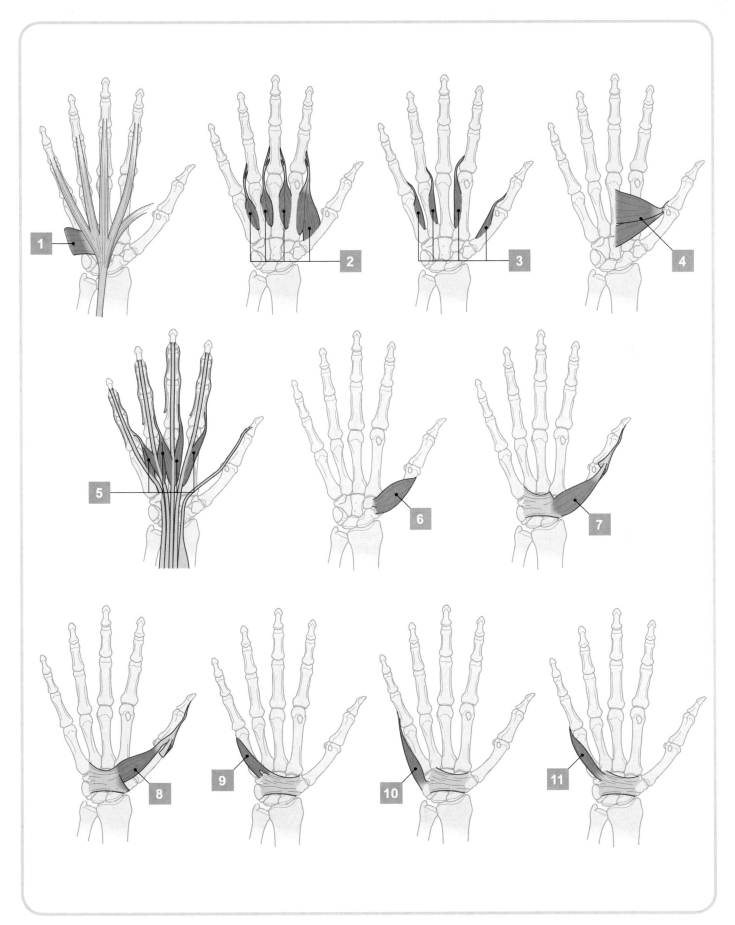

8

HEAD AND NECK

CONTENTS

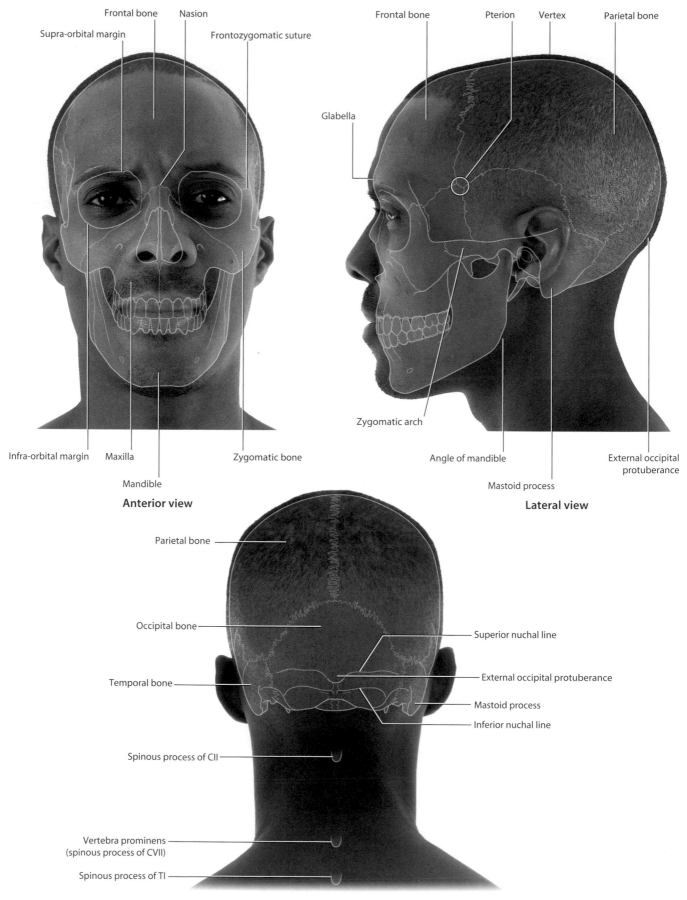

Frontal bone
Nasion
Supra-orbital margin
Frontozygomatic suture

Frontal bone
Pterion
Vertex
Parietal bone

Glabella

Infra-orbital margin
Maxilla
Mandible
Zygomatic bone

Anterior view

Zygomatic arch

Angle of mandible
Mastoid process
External occipital protuberance

Lateral view

Parietal bone

Occipital bone
Superior nuchal line

Temporal bone
External occipital protuberance
Mastoid process
Inferior nuchal line

Spinous process of CII

Vertebra prominens (spinous process of CVII)
Spinous process of TI

Posterior view

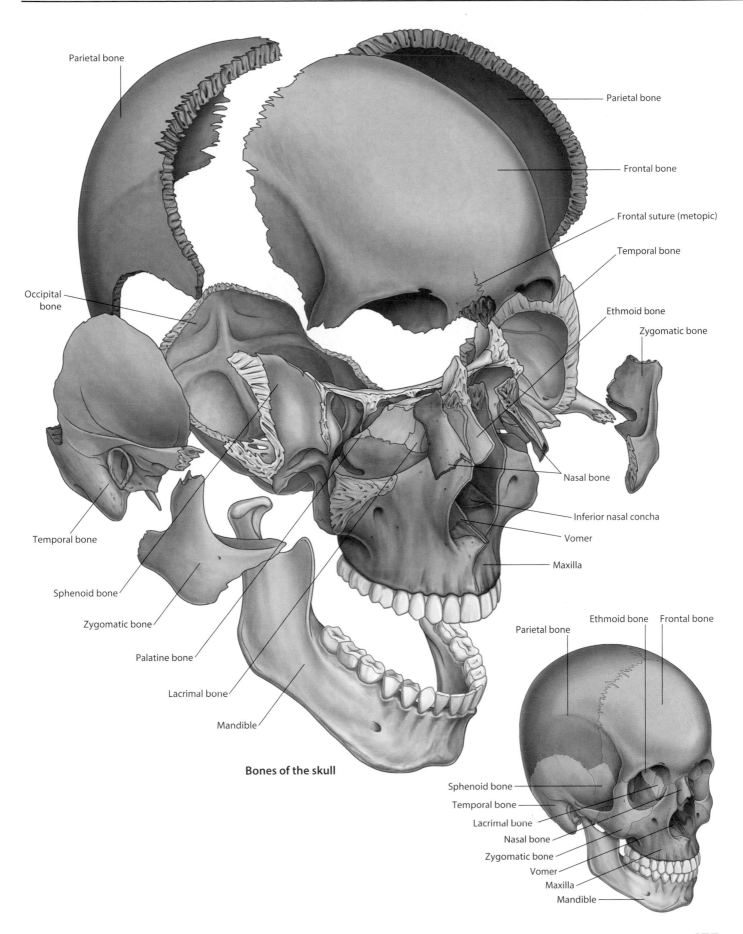

Parietal bone

Parietal bone

Frontal bone

Frontal suture (metopic)

Temporal bone

Occipital bone

Ethmoid bone

Zygomatic bone

Nasal bone

Inferior nasal concha

Temporal bone

Vomer

Sphenoid bone

Maxilla

Zygomatic bone

Palatine bone

Ethmoid bone   Frontal bone

Parietal bone

Lacrimal bone

Mandible

Sphenoid bone

Temporal bone

Lacrimal bone

Nasal bone

Zygomatic bone

Vomer

Maxilla

Mandible

Bones of the skull

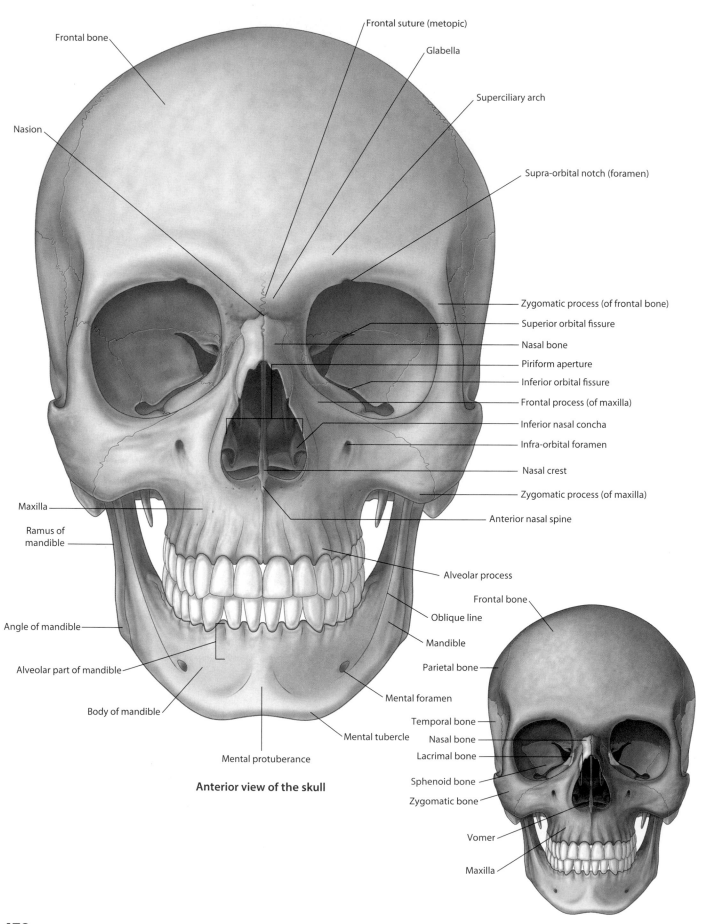

Frontal suture (metopic)

Glabella

Superciliary arch

Supra-orbital notch (foramen)

Frontal bone

Nasion

Zygomatic process (of frontal bone)

Superior orbital fissure

Nasal bone

Piriform aperture

Inferior orbital fissure

Frontal process (of maxilla)

Inferior nasal concha

Infra-orbital foramen

Nasal crest

Zygomatic process (of maxilla)

Anterior nasal spine

Maxilla

Ramus of mandible

Alveolar process

Frontal bone

Oblique line

Mandible

Parietal bone

Angle of mandible

Mental foramen

Alveolar part of mandible

Temporal bone

Nasal bone

Lacrimal bone

Body of mandible

Sphenoid bone

Zygomatic bone

Mental tubercle

Mental protuberance

Vomer

Anterior view of the skull

Maxilla

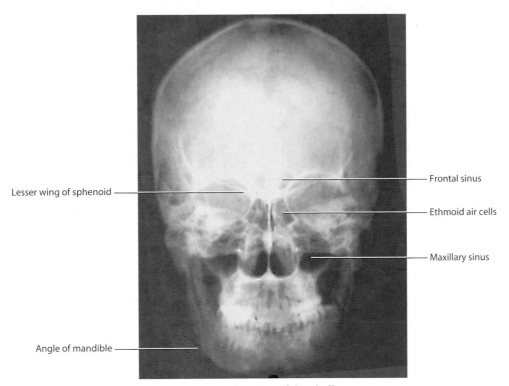

Lesser wing of sphenoid

Angle of mandible

Frontal sinus

Ethmoid air cells

Maxillary sinus

Anterior view of the skull.
Radiograph, AP view

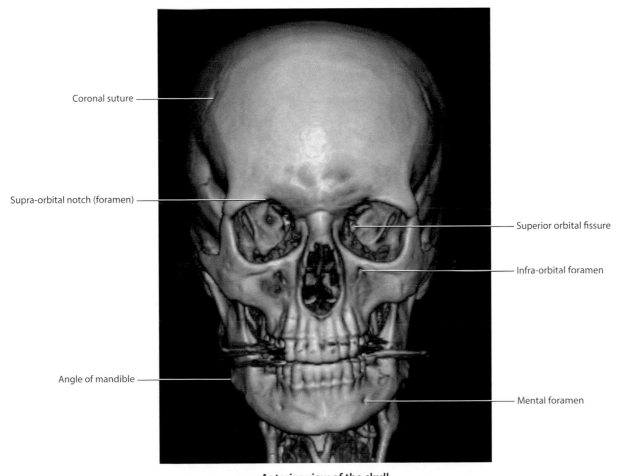

Coronal suture

Supra-orbital notch (foramen)

Angle of mandible

Superior orbital fissure

Infra-orbital foramen

Mental foramen

Anterior view of the skull.
Volume-rendered anterior view using multidetector computed tomography

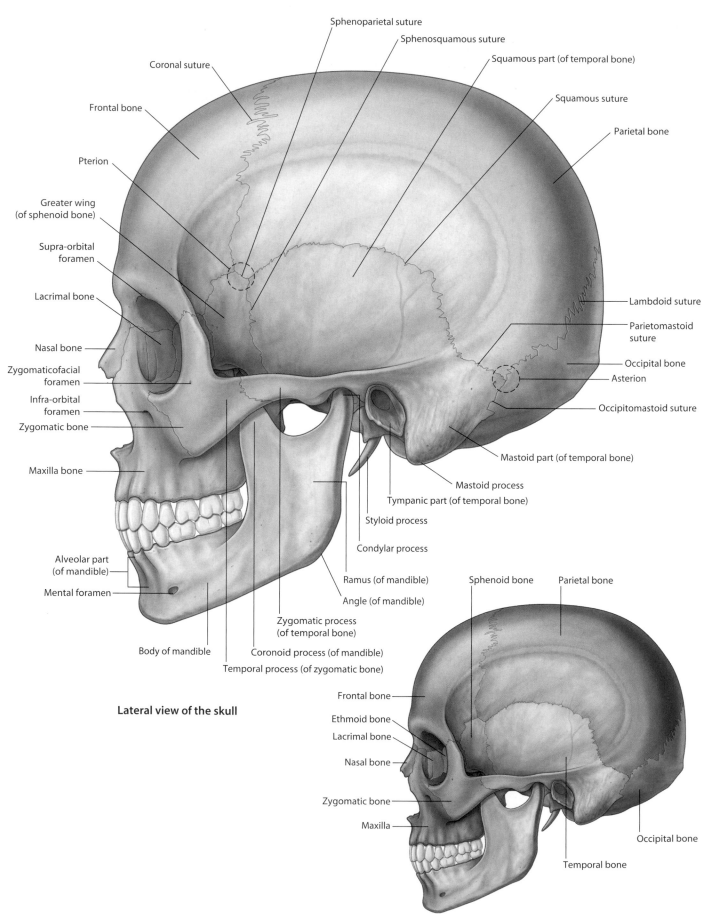

Sphenoparietal suture

Sphenosquamous suture

Squamous part (of temporal bone)

Coronal suture

Squamous suture

Frontal bone

Parietal bone

Pterion

Greater wing
(of sphenoid bone)

Supra-orbital
foramen

Lacrimal bone

Lambdoid suture

Parietomastoid
suture

Nasal bone

Occipital bone

Zygomaticofacial
foramen

Asterion

Infra-orbital
foramen

Occipitomastoid suture

Zygomatic bone

Maxilla bone

Mastoid part (of temporal bone)

Mastoid process

Tympanic part (of temporal bone)

Styloid process

Condylar process

Alveolar part
(of mandible)

Ramus (of mandible)

Mental foramen

Angle (of mandible)

Zygomatic process
(of temporal bone)

Body of mandible

Coronoid process (of mandible)

Temporal process (of zygomatic bone)

Lateral view of the skull

Sphenoid bone

Parietal bone

Frontal bone

Ethmoid bone

Lacrimal bone

Nasal bone

Zygomatic bone

Maxilla

Occipital bone

Temporal bone

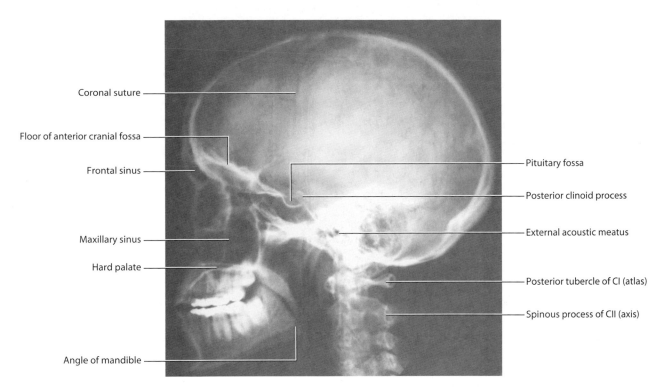

Coronal suture

Floor of anterior cranial fossa

Frontal sinus

Maxillary sinus

Hard palate

Angle of mandible

Pituitary fossa

Posterior clinoid process

External acoustic meatus

Posterior tubercle of CI (atlas)

Spinous process of CII (axis)

Lateral view of the skull.
Radiograph, lateral view

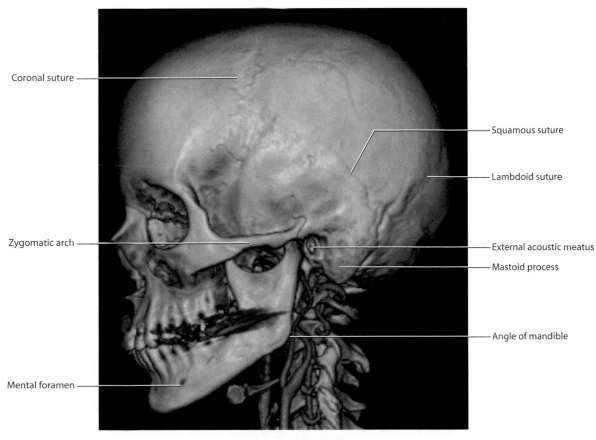

Coronal suture

Zygomatic arch

Mental foramen

Squamous suture

Lambdoid suture

External acoustic meatus

Mastoid process

Angle of mandible

Lateral view of the skull.
Volume-rendered lateral view using multidetector computed tomography

481

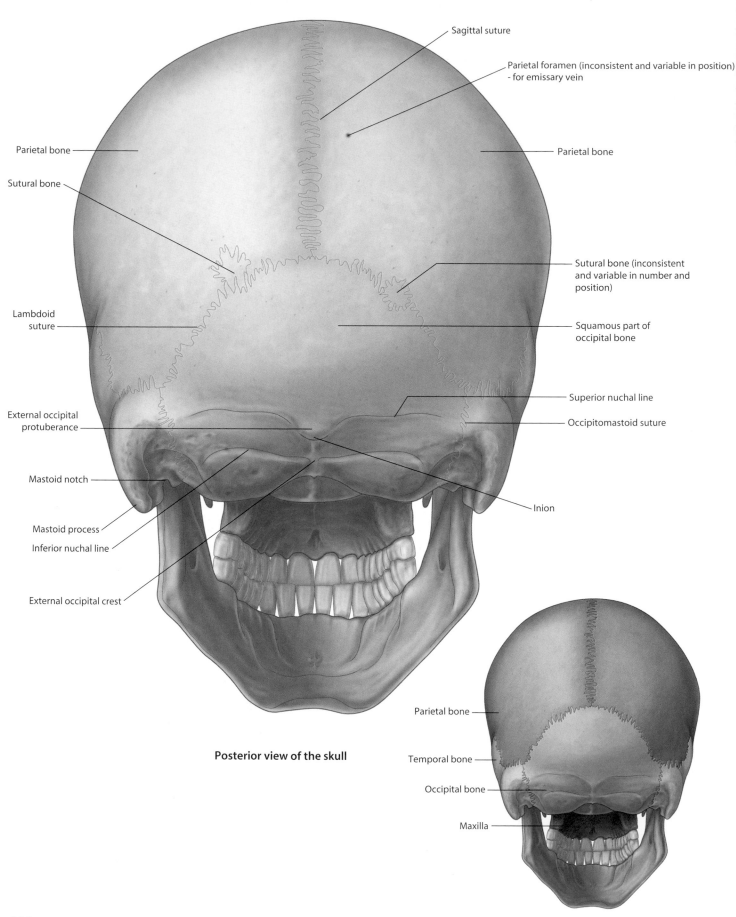

Sagittal suture

Parietal foramen (inconsistent and variable in position) - for emissary vein

Parietal bone

Sutural bone

Parietal bone

Sutural bone (inconsistent and variable in number and position)

Lambdoid suture

Squamous part of occipital bone

External occipital protuberance

Superior nuchal line

Occipitomastoid suture

Mastoid notch

Mastoid process

Inferior nuchal line

Inion

External occipital crest

Posterior view of the skull

Parietal bone

Temporal bone

Occipital bone

Maxilla

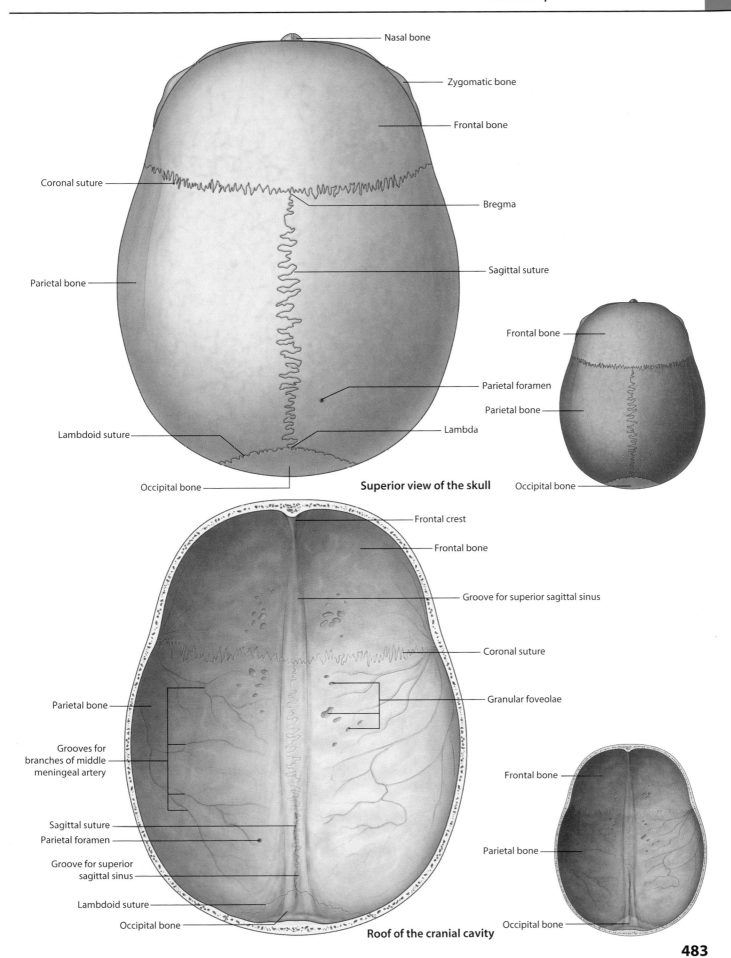

Nasal bone

Zygomatic bone

Frontal bone

Coronal suture

Bregma

Sagittal suture

Frontal bone

Parietal bone

Parietal foramen

Parietal bone

Lambdoid suture

Lambda

Occipital bone

Superior view of the skull

Occipital bone

Frontal crest

Frontal bone

Groove for superior sagittal sinus

Coronal suture

Parietal bone

Granular foveolae

Grooves for branches of middle meningeal artery

Frontal bone

Sagittal suture

Parietal foramen

Parietal bone

Groove for superior sagittal sinus

Lambdoid suture

Occipital bone

Occipital bone

Roof of the cranial cavity

483

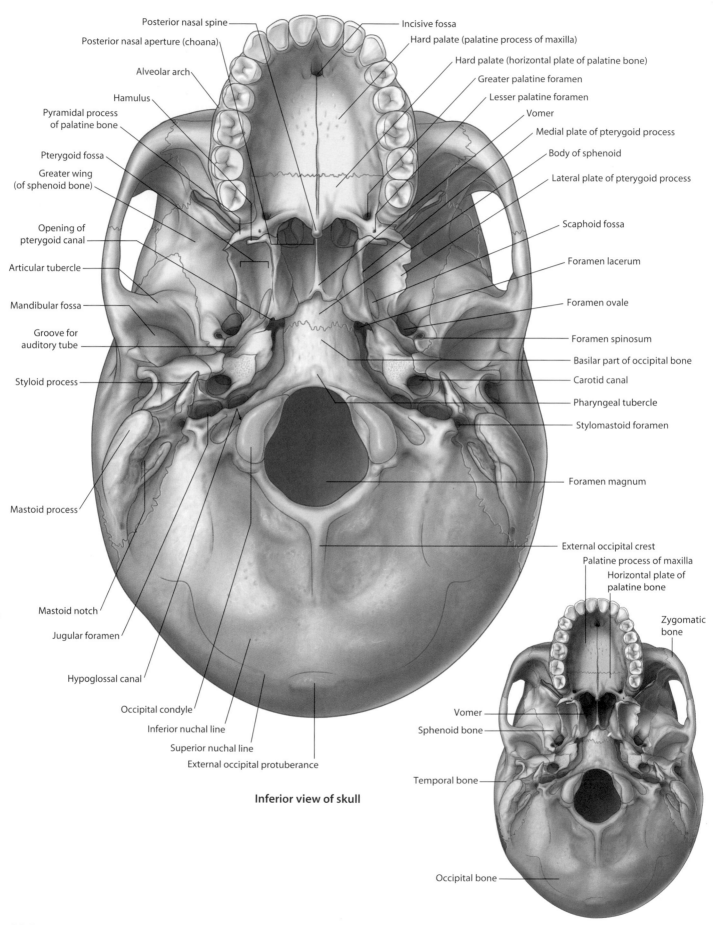

Posterior nasal spine

Posterior nasal aperture (choana)

Alveolar arch

Hamulus

Pyramidal process of palatine bone

Pterygoid fossa

Greater wing (of sphenoid bone)

Opening of pterygoid canal

Articular tubercle

Mandibular fossa

Groove for auditory tube

Styloid process

Mastoid process

Mastoid notch

Jugular foramen

Hypoglossal canal

Occipital condyle

Inferior nuchal line

Superior nuchal line

External occipital protuberance

Incisive fossa

Hard palate (palatine process of maxilla)

Hard palate (horizontal plate of palatine bone)

Greater palatine foramen

Lesser palatine foramen

Vomer

Medial plate of pterygoid process

Body of sphenoid

Lateral plate of pterygoid process

Scaphoid fossa

Foramen lacerum

Foramen ovale

Foramen spinosum

Basilar part of occipital bone

Carotid canal

Pharyngeal tubercle

Stylomastoid foramen

Foramen magnum

External occipital crest

Palatine process of maxilla

Horizontal plate of palatine bone

Zygomatic bone

Vomer

Sphenoid bone

Temporal bone

Occipital bone

Inferior view of skull

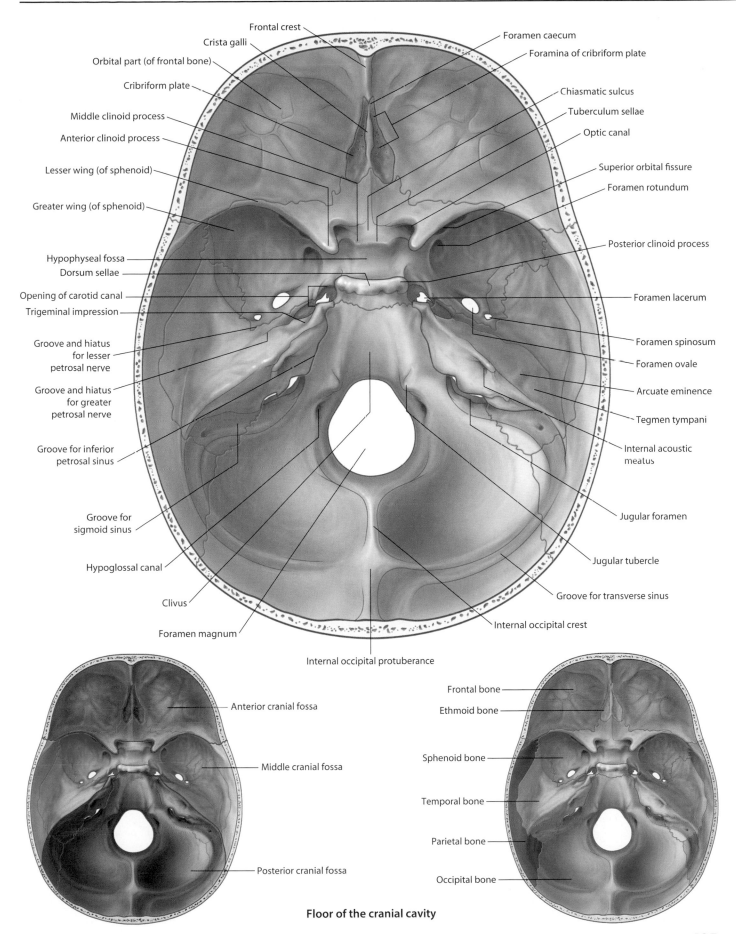

Frontal crest
Crista galli
Orbital part (of frontal bone)
Cribriform plate
Middle clinoid process
Anterior clinoid process
Lesser wing (of sphenoid)
Greater wing (of sphenoid)
Hypophyseal fossa
Dorsum sellae
Opening of carotid canal
Trigeminal impression
Groove and hiatus for lesser petrosal nerve
Groove and hiatus for greater petrosal nerve
Groove for inferior petrosal sinus
Groove for sigmoid sinus
Hypoglossal canal
Clivus
Foramen magnum

Foramen caecum
Foramina of cribriform plate
Chiasmatic sulcus
Tuberculum sellae
Optic canal
Superior orbital fissure
Foramen rotundum
Posterior clinoid process
Foramen lacerum
Foramen spinosum
Foramen ovale
Arcuate eminence
Tegmen tympani
Internal acoustic meatus
Jugular foramen
Jugular tubercle
Groove for transverse sinus
Internal occipital crest

Internal occipital protuberance

Anterior cranial fossa
Middle cranial fossa
Posterior cranial fossa

Frontal bone
Ethmoid bone
Sphenoid bone
Temporal bone
Parietal bone
Occipital bone

Floor of the cranial cavity

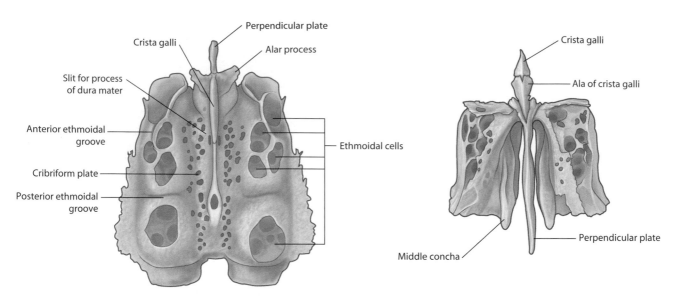

Crista galli

Perpendicular plate

Alar process

Slit for process
of dura mater

Anterior ethmoidal
groove

Cribriform plate

Posterior ethmoidal
groove

Ethmoidal cells

Ethmoid bone (superior view)

Crista galli

Ala of crista galli

Perpendicular plate

Middle concha

Ethmoid bone (posterior view)

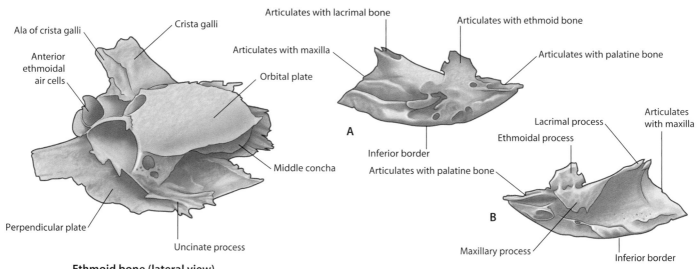

Ala of crista galli

Crista galli

Anterior
ethmoidal
air cells

Orbital plate

Middle concha

Perpendicular plate

Uncinate process

Ethmoid bone (lateral view)

Articulates with lacrimal bone

Articulates with maxilla

Articulates with ethmoid bone

Articulates with palatine bone

A

Inferior border

Lacrimal process

Ethmoidal process

Articulates
with maxilla

Articulates with palatine bone

B

Maxillary process

Inferior border

**Right inferior concha
A. Medial view   B. Lateral view**

Articulates with frontal bone

Orbital surface

Lacrimal groove (for lacrimal sac)

Articulates
with ethmoid
bone

Articulates
with
maxilla

Nasal surface

Posterior
lacrimal crest

Lacrimal
hamulus

A

B

Descending process
for inferior nasal
concha

**Right lacrimal bone
A. Lateral view   B. Medial view**

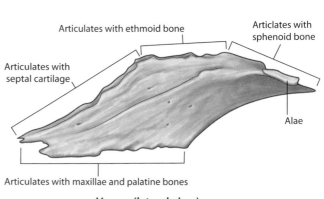

Articulates with ethmoid bone

Articlates with
sphenoid bone

Articulates with
septal cartilage

Alae

Articulates with maxillae and palatine bones

Vomer (lateral view)

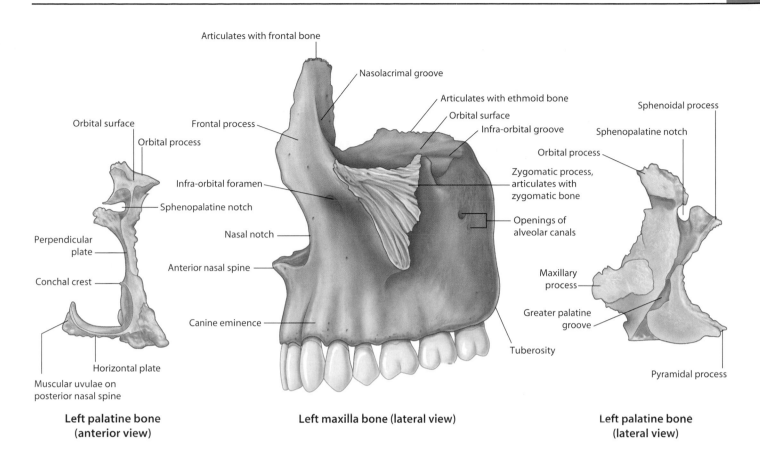

Left palatine bone (anterior view)

Orbital surface
Orbital process
Infra-orbital foramen
Sphenopalatine notch
Perpendicular plate
Conchal crest
Horizontal plate
Muscular uvulae on posterior nasal spine

Left maxilla bone (lateral view)

Articulates with frontal bone
Nasolacrimal groove
Frontal process
Articulates with ethmoid bone
Orbital surface
Infra-orbital groove
Zygomatic process, articulates with zygomatic bone
Openings of alveolar canals
Nasal notch
Anterior nasal spine
Canine eminence
Tuberosity

Left palatine bone (lateral view)

Sphenoidal process
Sphenopalatine notch
Orbital process
Maxillary process
Greater palatine groove
Pyramidal process

Left palatine bone (medial view)

Sphenoidal process
Sphenopalatine notch
Orbital process
Ethmoidal crest
Greater palatine canal
Maxillary process
Conchal crest
Horizontal plate
Pyramidal process
Articulates with perpendicular plate of palatine bone

Left maxilla bone (medial view)

Articulates with frontal bone
Maxillary hiatus
Nasolacrimal groove
Articulates with perpendicular plate of palatine bone
Ethmoidal crest
Middle meatus
Conchal crest
Inferior meatus
Anterior nasal spine
Articulates with lateral pterygoid plate
Palatine process

Left palatine bone (posterior view)

Orbital process
Orbital surface
Completes wall of sphenoidal sinus
Sphenopalatine notch
Articular surface
Sphenoidal process
Perpendicular plate
Conchal crest
Horizontal plate
Articulates with medial pterygoid plate
Pyramidal process

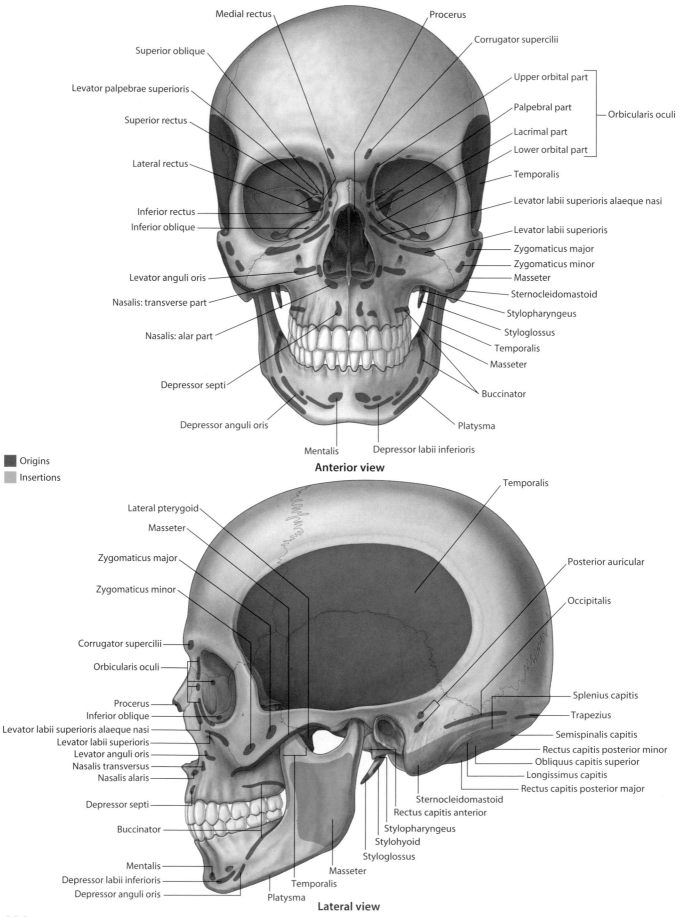

Medial rectus

Procerus

Superior oblique

Corrugator supercilii

Levator palpebrae superioris

Upper orbital part

Palpebral part

Superior rectus

Lacrimal part

Orbicularis oculi

Lower orbital part

Lateral rectus

Temporalis

Levator labii superioris alaeque nasi

Inferior rectus

Levator labii superioris

Inferior oblique

Zygomaticus major

Zygomaticus minor

Masseter

Levator anguli oris

Sternocleidomastoid

Nasalis: transverse part

Stylopharyngeus

Styloglossus

Temporalis

Nasalis: alar part

Masseter

Buccinator

Depressor septi

Platysma

Depressor anguli oris

Mentalis

Depressor labii inferioris

Anterior view

Origins

Insertions

Temporalis

Lateral pterygoid

Masseter

Posterior auricular

Zygomaticus major

Occipitalis

Zygomaticus minor

Corrugator supercilii

Orbicularis oculi

Splenius capitis

Procerus

Trapezius

Inferior oblique

Levator labii superioris alaeque nasi

Semispinalis capitis

Levator labii superioris

Rectus capitis posterior minor

Levator anguli oris

Obliquus capitis superior

Nasalis transversus

Longissimus capitis

Nasalis alaris

Rectus capitis posterior major

Depressor septi

Sternocleidomastoid

Buccinator

Rectus capitis anterior

Stylopharyngeus

Mentalis

Stylohyoid

Depressor labii inferioris

Styloglossus

Depressor anguli oris

Masseter

Temporalis

Platysma

Lateral view

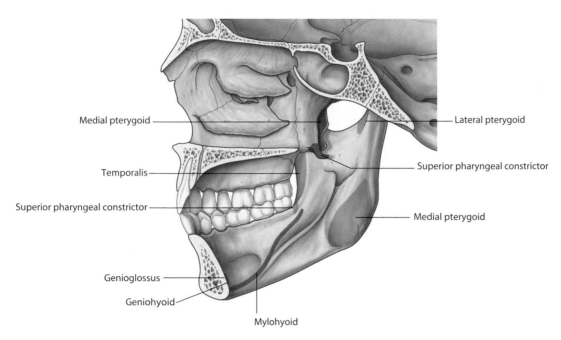

Medial pterygoid

Lateral pterygoid

Temporalis

Superior pharyngeal constrictor

Superior pharyngeal constrictor

Medial pterygoid

Genioglossus

Geniohyoid

Mylohyoid

Medial view

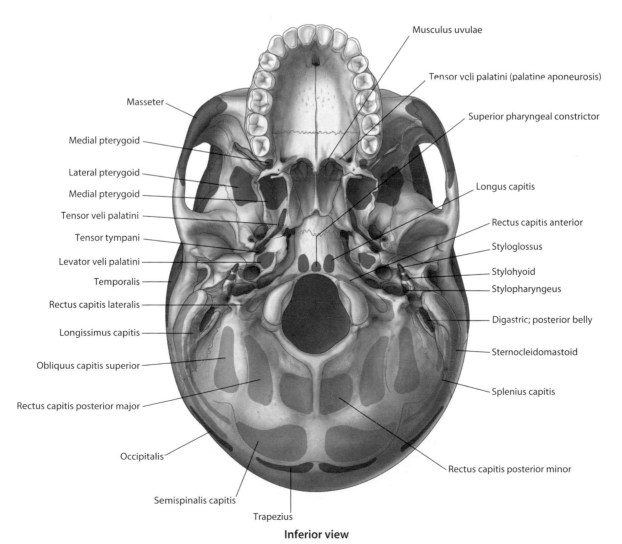

Musculus uvulae

Tensor veli palatini (palatine aponeurosis)

Masseter

Superior pharyngeal constrictor

Medial pterygoid

Lateral pterygoid

Longus capitis

Medial pterygoid

Rectus capitis anterior

Tensor veli palatini

Tensor tympani

Styloglossus

Levator veli palatini

Stylohyoid

Temporalis

Stylopharyngeus

Rectus capitis lateralis

Digastric; posterior belly

Longissimus capitis

Sternocleidomastoid

Obliquus capitis superior

Rectus capitis posterior major

Splenius capitis

Occipitalis

Rectus capitis posterior minor

Semispinalis capitis

Trapezius

Inferior view

489

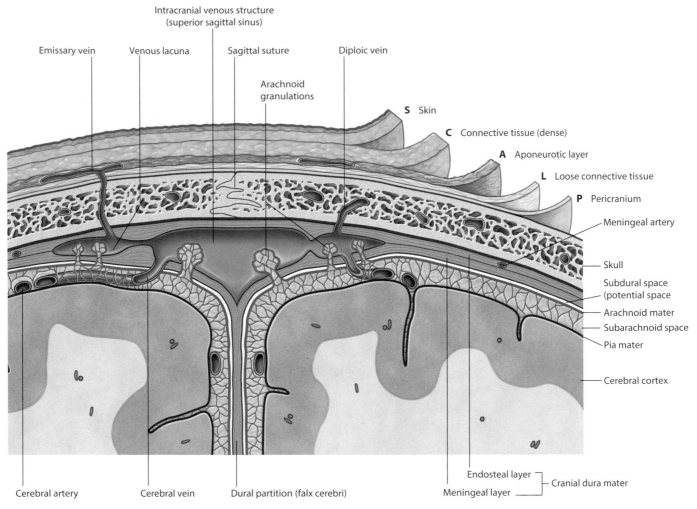

Intracranial venous structure
(superior sagittal sinus)

Emissary vein Venous lacuna Sagittal suture Diploic vein

Arachnoid
granulations

S Skin

C Connective tissue (dense)

A Aponeurotic layer

L Loose connective tissue

P Pericranium

Meningeal artery

Skull

Subdural space
(potential space)

Arachnoid mater

Subarachnoid space

Pia mater

Cerebral cortex

Cerebral artery Cerebral vein Dural partition (falx cerebri)

Endosteal layer
Meningeal layer } Cranial dura mater

Scalp and cranial meninges

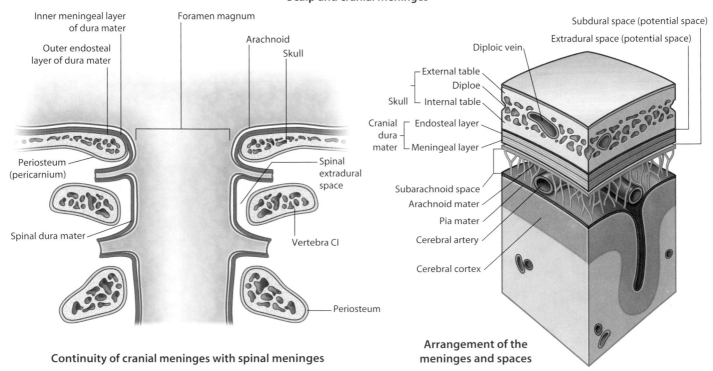

Inner meningeal layer
of dura mater

Outer endosteal
layer of dura mater

Foramen magnum

Arachnoid

Skull

Periosteum
(pericarnium)

Spinal dura mater

Spinal
extradural
space

Vertebra CI

Periosteum

Continuity of cranial meninges with spinal meninges

Subdural space (potential space)

Extradural space (potential space)

Diploic vein

External table

Diploe

Skull Internal table

Cranial
dura
mater

Endosteal layer

Meningeal layer

Subarachnoid space

Arachnoid mater

Pia mater

Cerebral artery

Cerebral cortex

**Arrangement of the
meninges and spaces**

490

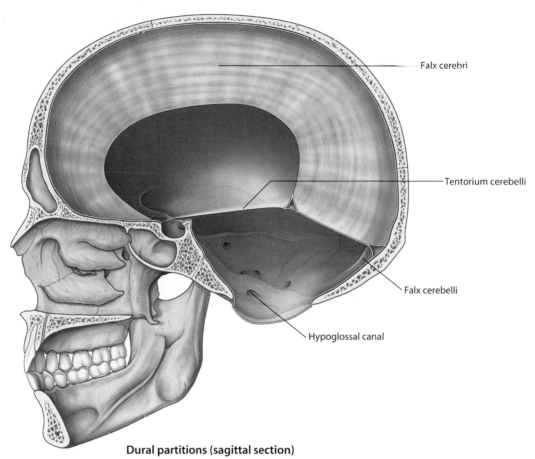

Dural partitions (sagittal section)

Falx cerebri

Tentorium cerebelli

Falx cerebelli

Hypoglossal canal

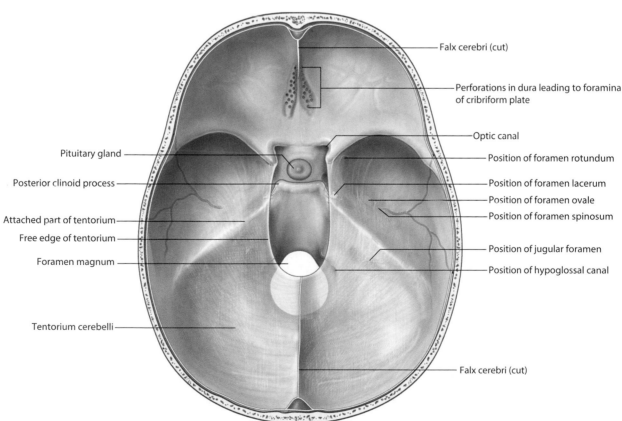

Falx cerebri (cut)

Perforations in dura leading to foramina of cribriform plate

Optic canal

Position of foramen rotundum

Position of foramen lacerum

Position of foramen ovale

Position of foramen spinosum

Position of jugular foramen

Position of hypoglossal canal

Pituitary gland

Posterior clinoid process

Attached part of tentorium

Free edge of tentorium

Foramen magnum

Tentorium cerebelli

Falx cerebri (cut)

Cranial cavity (superior view)

491

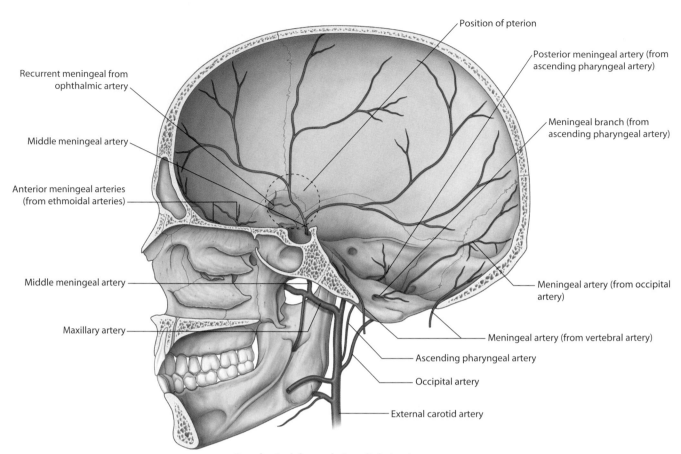

Position of pterion

Posterior meningeal artery (from ascending pharyngeal artery)

Recurrent meningeal from ophthalmic artery

Middle meningeal artery

Meningeal branch (from ascending pharyngeal artery)

Anterior meningeal arteries (from ethmoidal arteries)

Middle meningeal artery

Maxillary artery

Meningeal artery (from occipital artery)

Meningeal artery (from vertebral artery)

Ascending pharyngeal artery

Occipital artery

External carotid artery

Dural arterial supply (medial view)

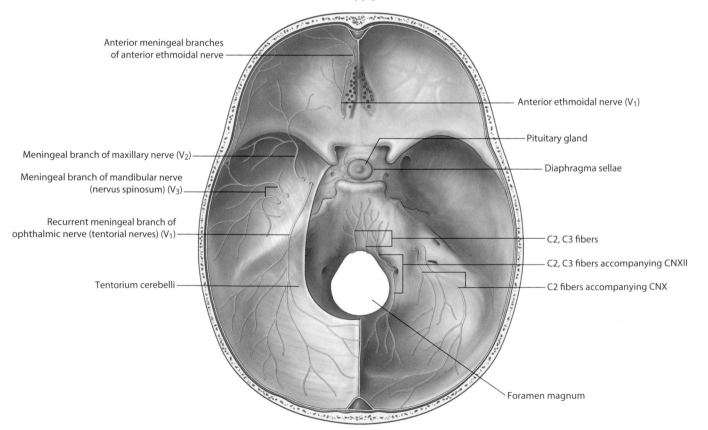

Anterior meningeal branches of anterior ethmoidal nerve

Anterior ethmoidal nerve (V$_1$)

Pituitary gland

Diaphragma sellae

Meningeal branch of maxillary nerve (V$_2$)

Meningeal branch of mandibular nerve (nervus spinosum) (V$_3$)

Recurrent meningeal branch of ophthalmic nerve (tentorial nerves) (V$_1$)

C2, C3 fibers

C2, C3 fibers accompanying CNXII

C2 fibers accompanying CNX

Tentorium cerebelli

Foramen magnum

Dural innervation (superior view)

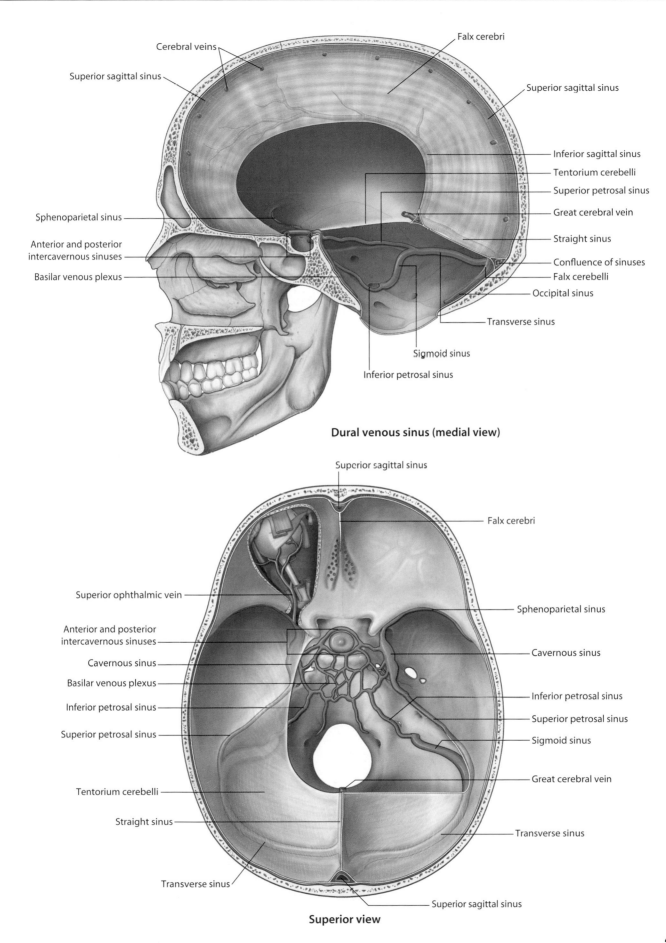

Cerebral veins

Superior sagittal sinus

Falx cerebri

Superior sagittal sinus

Inferior sagittal sinus

Tentorium cerebelli

Superior petrosal sinus

Sphenoparietal sinus

Great cerebral vein

Anterior and posterior intercavernous sinuses

Straight sinus

Basilar venous plexus

Confluence of sinuses

Falx cerebelli

Occipital sinus

Transverse sinus

Sigmoid sinus

Inferior petrosal sinus

Dural venous sinus (medial view)

Superior sagittal sinus

Falx cerebri

Superior ophthalmic vein

Sphenoparietal sinus

Anterior and posterior intercavernous sinuses

Cavernous sinus

Cavernous sinus

Basilar venous plexus

Inferior petrosal sinus

Inferior petrosal sinus

Superior petrosal sinus

Superior petrosal sinus

Sigmoid sinus

Tentorium cerebelli

Great cerebral vein

Straight sinus

Transverse sinus

Transverse sinus

Superior sagittal sinus

Superior view

493

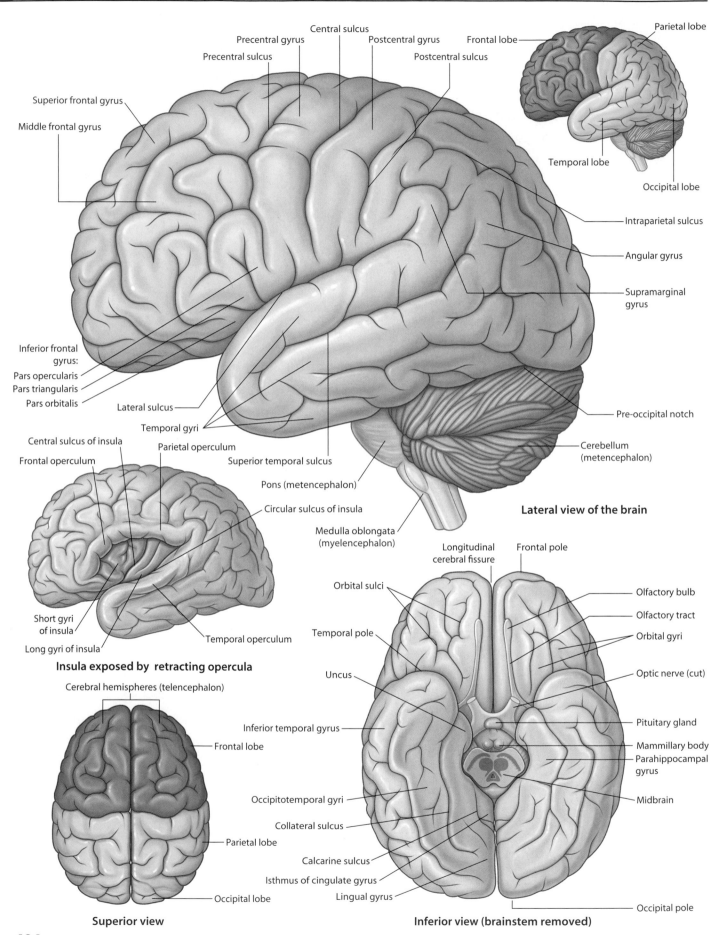

Precentral gyrus
Central sulcus
Precentral sulcus
Postcentral gyrus
Postcentral sulcus
Frontal lobe
Parietal lobe
Superior frontal gyrus
Middle frontal gyrus
Temporal lobe
Occipital lobe
Intraparietal sulcus
Angular gyrus
Supramarginal gyrus
Inferior frontal gyrus:
Pars opercularis
Pars triangularis
Pars orbitalis
Lateral sulcus
Temporal gyri
Pre-occipital notch
Cerebellum (metencephalon)
Central sulcus of insula
Frontal operculum
Parietal operculum
Superior temporal sulcus
Pons (metencephalon)
Circular sulcus of insula
Short gyri of insula
Long gyri of insula
Temporal operculum
Medulla oblongata (myelencephalon)

Lateral view of the brain

Insula exposed by retracting opercula

Longitudinal cerebral fissure
Frontal pole
Orbital sulci
Olfactory bulb
Olfactory tract
Temporal pole
Orbital gyri
Uncus
Optic nerve (cut)
Cerebral hemispheres (telencephalon)
Frontal lobe
Pituitary gland
Mammillary body
Parahippocampal gyrus
Inferior temporal gyrus
Midbrain
Occipitotemporal gyri
Collateral sulcus
Parietal lobe
Calcarine sulcus
Isthmus of cingulate gyrus
Lingual gyrus
Occipital lobe
Occipital pole

Superior view

Inferior view (brainstem removed)

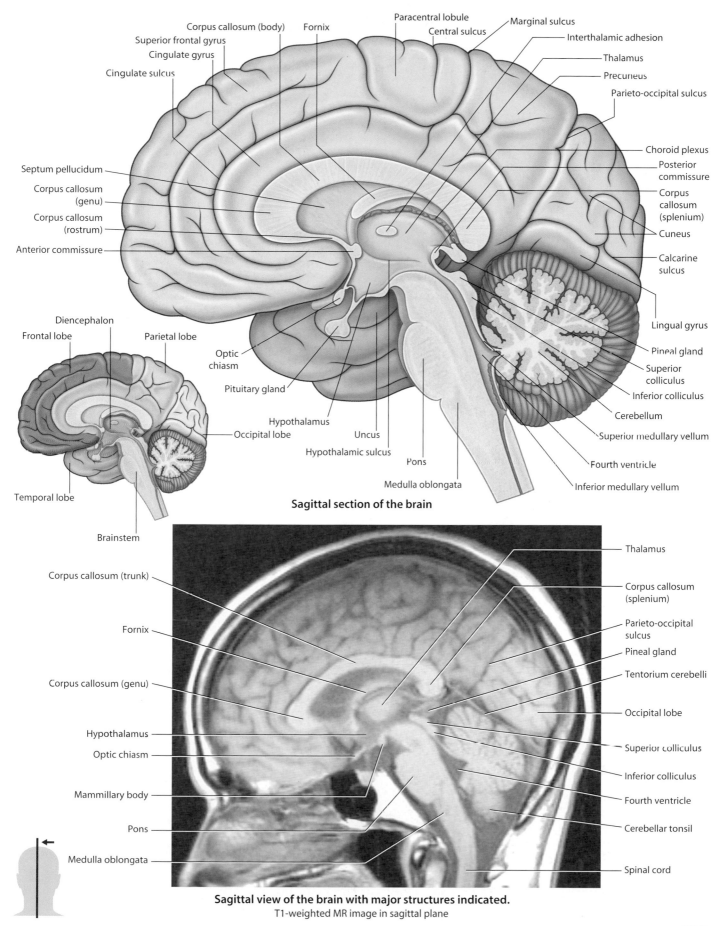

Sagittal section of the brain

Sagittal view of the brain with major structures indicated.
T1-weighted MR image in sagittal plane

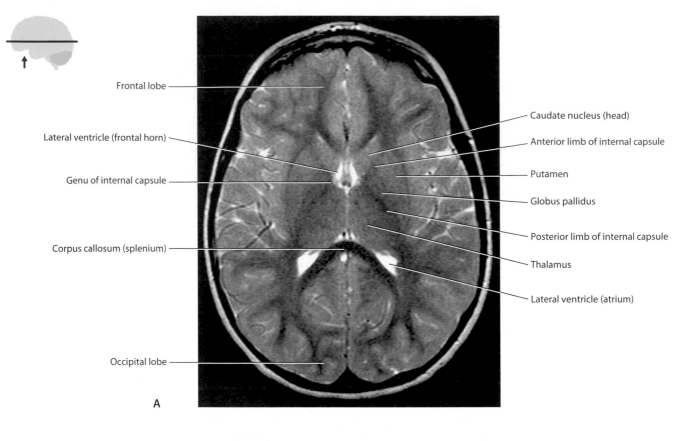

Frontal lobe

Lateral ventricle (frontal horn)

Genu of internal capsule

Corpus callosum (splenium)

Occipital lobe

Caudate nucleus (head)

Anterior limb of internal capsule

Putamen

Globus pallidus

Posterior limb of internal capsule

Thalamus

Lateral ventricle (atrium)

A

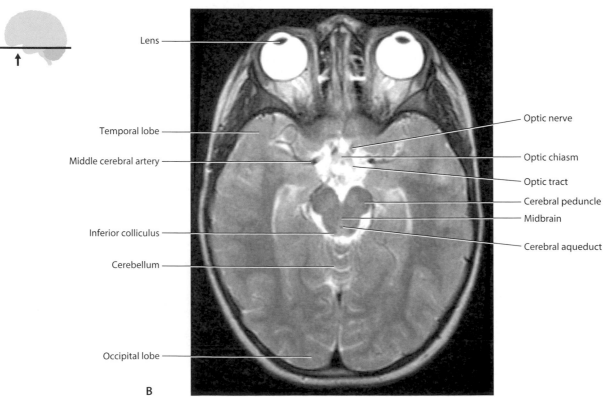

Lens

Temporal lobe

Middle cerebral artery

Inferior colliculus

Cerebellum

Occipital lobe

Optic nerve

Optic chiasm

Optic tract

Cerebral peduncle

Midbrain

Cerebral aqueduct

B

Axial or horizontal sections through the brain with major structures indicated.
A. Section showing structures related to the internal capsule.
B. Section showing structures related to the midbrain.
T1-weighted MR images in axial plane

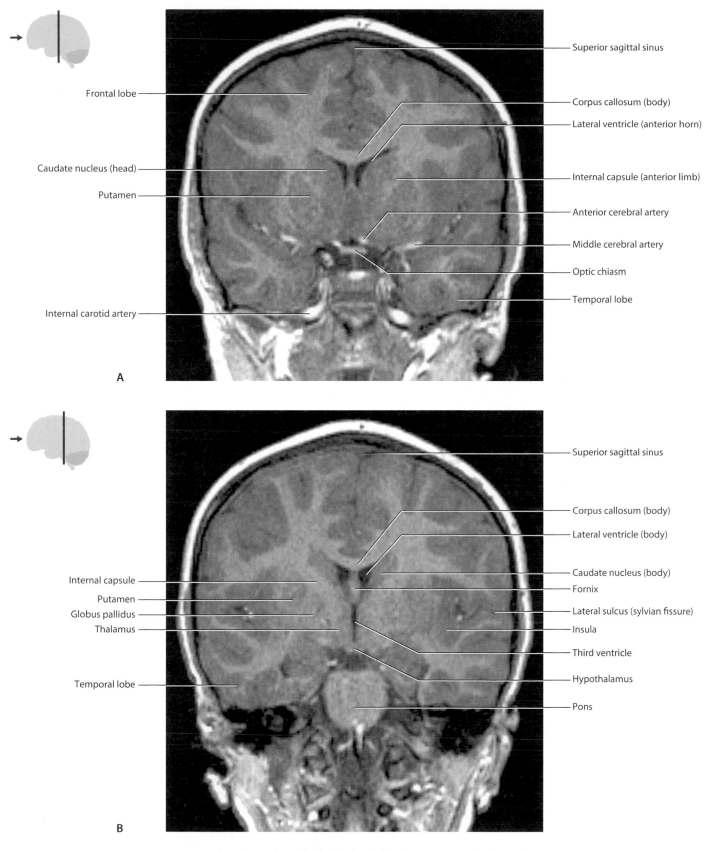

Frontal lobe

Caudate nucleus (head)

Putamen

Internal carotid artery

A

Superior sagittal sinus

Corpus callosum (body)

Lateral ventricle (anterior horn)

Internal capsule (anterior limb)

Anterior cerebral artery

Middle cerebral artery

Optic chiasm

Temporal lobe

Internal capsule

Putamen

Globus pallidus

Thalamus

Temporal lobe

B

Superior sagittal sinus

Corpus callosum (body)

Lateral ventricle (body)

Caudate nucleus (body)

Fornix

Lateral sulcus (sylvian fissure)

Insula

Third ventricle

Hypothalamus

Pons

Coronal sections through the brain with major structures indicated.
A. Section showing structures related to the optic chiasm.
B. Section showing structures related to the third ventricle.
T1-weighted MR images in coronal plane

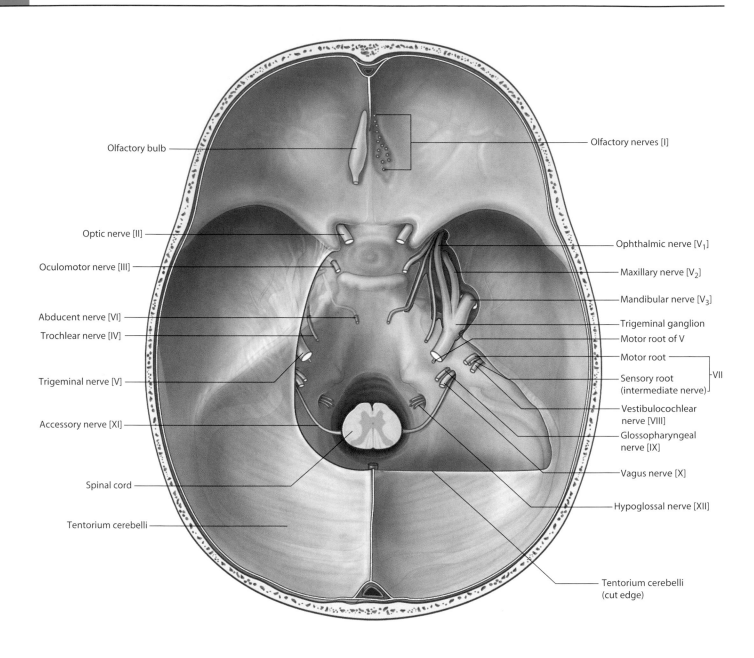

Olfactory bulb

Olfactory nerves [I]

Optic nerve [II]

Ophthalmic nerve [V₁]

Oculomotor nerve [III]

Maxillary nerve [V₂]

Mandibular nerve [V₃]

Abducent nerve [VI]

Trigeminal ganglion

Trochlear nerve [IV]

Motor root of V

Motor root

Sensory root (intermediate nerve)

⎱VII

Trigeminal nerve [V]

Vestibulocochlear nerve [VIII]

Accessory nerve [XI]

Glossopharyngeal nerve [IX]

Vagus nerve [X]

Spinal cord

Hypoglossal nerve [XII]

Tentorium cerebelli

Tentorium cerebelli (cut edge)

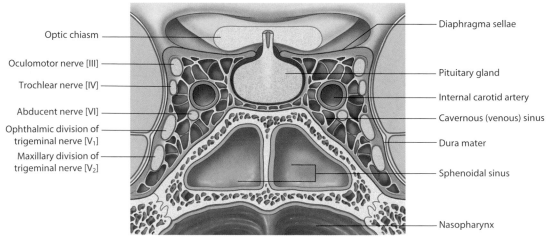

Optic chiasm

Diaphragma sellae

Oculomotor nerve [III]

Pituitary gland

Trochlear nerve [IV]

Internal carotid artery

Abducent nerve [VI]

Cavernous (venous) sinus

Ophthalmic division of trigeminal nerve [V₁]

Dura mater

Maxillary division of trigeminal nerve [V₂]

Sphenoidal sinus

Nasopharynx

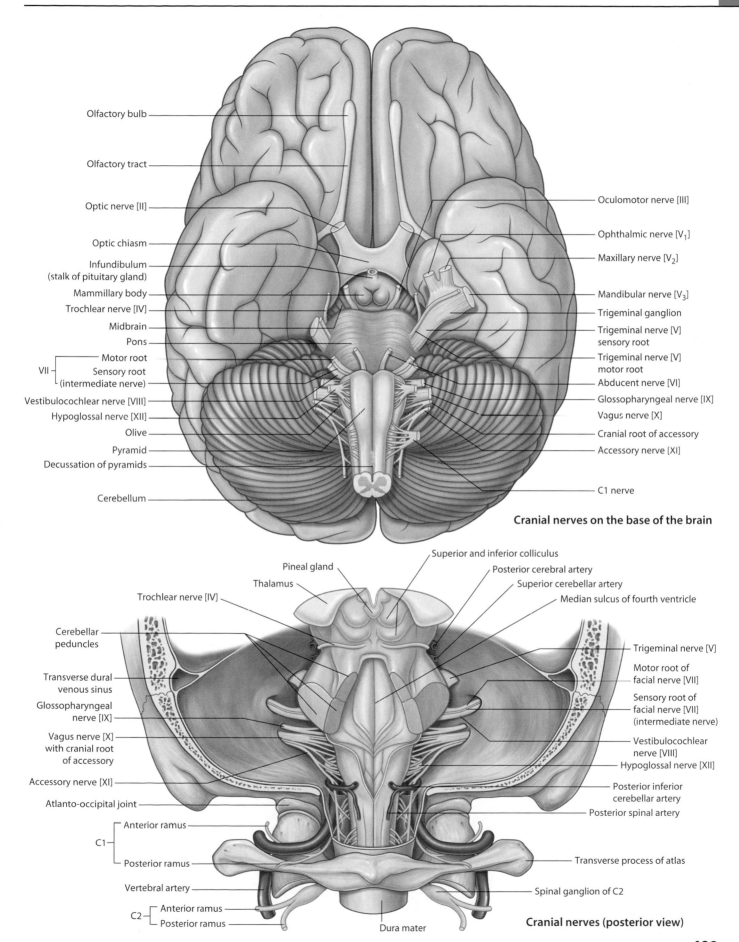

Olfactory bulb

Olfactory tract

Optic nerve [II]

Optic chiasm

Infundibulum
(stalk of pituitary gland)

Mammillary body

Trochlear nerve [IV]

Midbrain

Pons

VII {
Motor root
Sensory root
(intermediate nerve)
}

Vestibulocochlear nerve [VIII]

Hypoglossal nerve [XII]

Olive

Pyramid

Decussation of pyramids

Cerebellum

Oculomotor nerve [III]

Ophthalmic nerve [V₁]

Maxillary nerve [V₂]

Mandibular nerve [V₃]

Trigeminal ganglion

Trigeminal nerve [V]
sensory root

Trigeminal nerve [V]
motor root

Abducent nerve [VI]

Glossopharyngeal nerve [IX]

Vagus nerve [X]

Cranial root of accessory

Accessory nerve [XI]

C1 nerve

Cranial nerves on the base of the brain

Pineal gland

Thalamus

Trochlear nerve [IV]

Cerebellar
peduncles

Transverse dural
venous sinus

Glossopharyngeal
nerve [IX]

Vagus nerve [X]
with cranial root
of accessory

Accessory nerve [XI]

Atlanto-occipital joint

C1 {
Anterior ramus
Posterior ramus
}

Vertebral artery

C2 {
Anterior ramus
Posterior ramus
}

Superior and inferior colliculus

Posterior cerebral artery

Superior cerebellar artery

Median sulcus of fourth ventricle

Trigeminal nerve [V]

Motor root of
facial nerve [VII]

Sensory root of
facial nerve [VII]
(intermediate nerve)

Vestibulocochlear
nerve [VIII]

Hypoglossal nerve [XII]

Posterior inferior
cerebellar artery

Posterior spinal artery

Transverse process of atlas

Spinal ganglion of C2

Dura mater

Cranial nerves (posterior view)

499

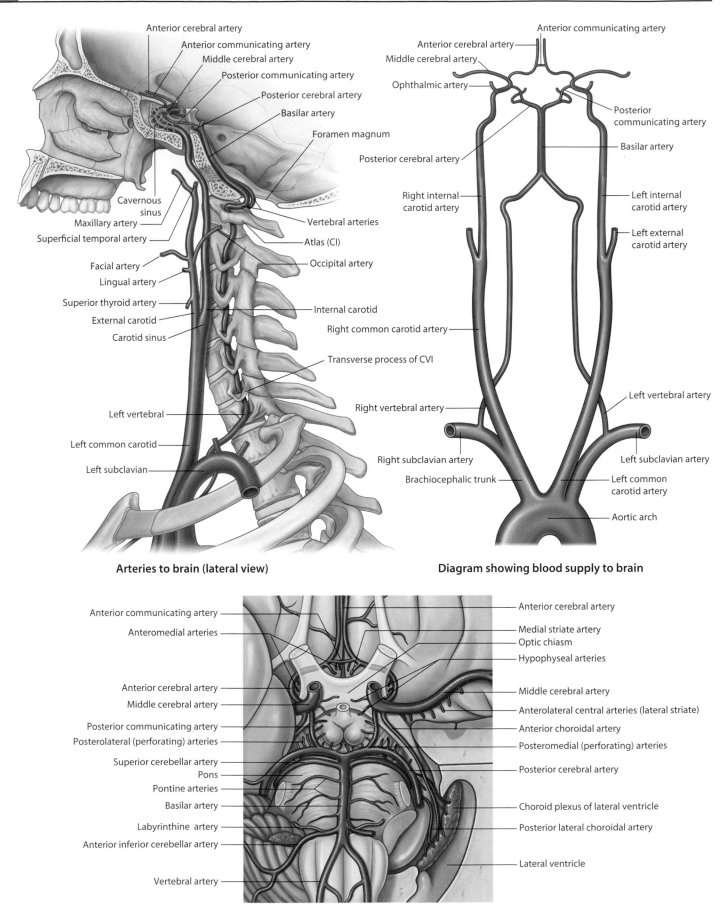

Arteries to brain (lateral view)

Anterior cerebral artery
Anterior communicating artery
Middle cerebral artery
Posterior communicating artery
Posterior cerebral artery
Basilar artery
Foramen magnum
Cavernous sinus
Maxillary artery
Superficial temporal artery
Facial artery
Lingual artery
Superior thyroid artery
External carotid
Carotid sinus
Vertebral arteries
Atlas (CI)
Occipital artery
Internal carotid
Right common carotid artery
Transverse process of CVI
Left vertebral
Left common carotid
Left subclavian

Diagram showing blood supply to brain

Anterior communicating artery
Anterior cerebral artery
Middle cerebral artery
Ophthalmic artery
Posterior communicating artery
Posterior cerebral artery
Basilar artery
Right internal carotid artery
Left internal carotid artery
Left external carotid artery
Right vertebral artery
Left vertebral artery
Right subclavian artery
Left subclavian artery
Brachiocephalic trunk
Left common carotid artery
Aortic arch

Cerebral arterial circle (of Willis)

Anterior communicating artery
Anteromedial arteries
Anterior cerebral artery
Middle cerebral artery
Posterior communicating artery
Posterolateral (perforating) arteries
Superior cerebellar artery
Pons
Pontine arteries
Basilar artery
Labyrinthine artery
Anterior inferior cerebellar artery
Vertebral artery
Anterior cerebral artery
Medial striate artery
Optic chiasm
Hypophyseal arteries
Middle cerebral artery
Anterolateral central arteries (lateral striate)
Anterior choroidal artery
Posteromedial (perforating) arteries
Posterior cerebral artery
Choroid plexus of lateral ventricle
Posterior lateral choroidal artery
Lateral ventricle

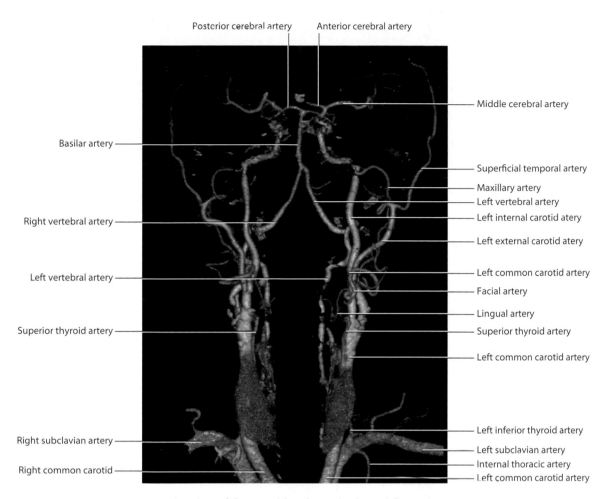

Posterior cerebral artery

Anterior cerebral artery

Middle cerebral artery

Basilar artery

Superficial temporal artery

Maxillary artery

Left vertebral artery

Left internal carotid atery

Left external carotid atery

Right vertebral artery

Left common carotid artery

Facial artery

Left vertebral artery

Lingual artery

Superior thyroid artery

Superior thyroid artery

Left common carotid artery

Left inferior thyroid artery

Right subclavian artery

Left subclavian artery

Internal thoracic artery

Right common carotid

Left common carotid artery

Anterior view of the carotid and vertebral arterial systems.
Volume-rendered anterior view using multidetector computed tomography

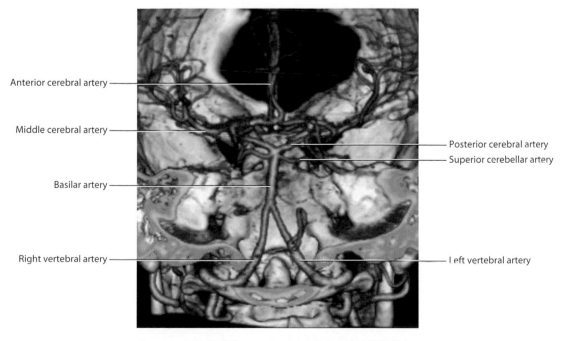

Anterior cerebral artery

Middle cerebral artery

Posterior cerebral artery

Superior cerebellar artery

Basilar artery

Right vertebral artery

Left vertebral artery

Posterior view of the cerebral arterial circle (of Willis).
Volume-rendered posterior view using multidetector computed tomography

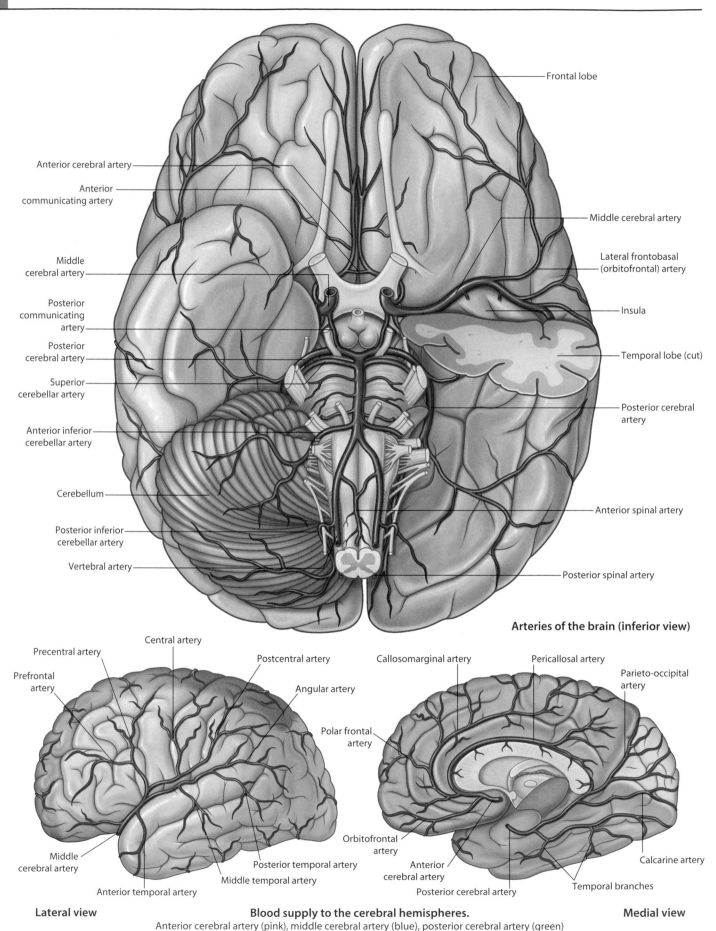

Anterior cerebral artery

Anterior communicating artery

Middle cerebral artery

Posterior communicating artery

Posterior cerebral artery

Superior cerebellar artery

Anterior inferior cerebellar artery

Cerebellum

Posterior inferior cerebellar artery

Vertebral artery

Frontal lobe

Middle cerebral artery

Lateral frontobasal (orbitofrontal) artery

Insula

Temporal lobe (cut)

Posterior cerebral artery

Anterior spinal artery

Posterior spinal artery

Arteries of the brain (inferior view)

Precentral artery

Central artery

Postcentral artery

Prefrontal artery

Angular artery

Prefrontal artery

Callosomarginal artery

Pericallosal artery

Parieto-occipital artery

Polar frontal artery

Middle cerebral artery

Posterior temporal artery

Middle temporal artery

Anterior temporal artery

Orbitofrontal artery

Anterior cerebral artery

Posterior cerebral artery

Temporal branches

Calcarine artery

Lateral view

Blood supply to the cerebral hemispheres.
Anterior cerebral artery (pink), middle cerebral artery (blue), posterior cerebral artery (green)

Medial view

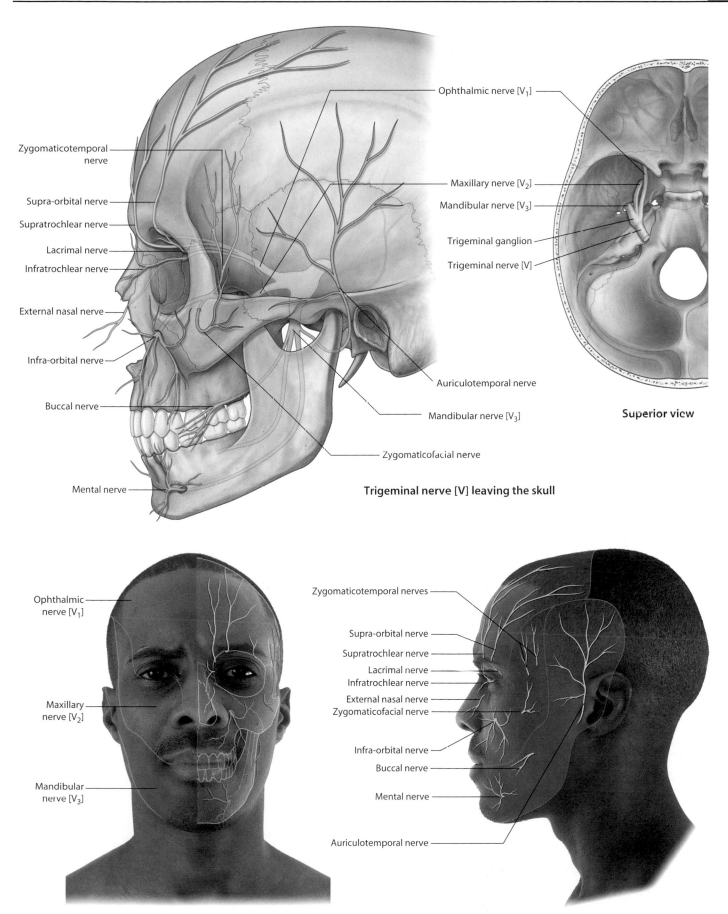

Zygomaticotemporal nerve
Supra-orbital nerve
Supratrochlear nerve
Lacrimal nerve
Infratrochlear nerve
External nasal nerve
Infra-orbital nerve
Buccal nerve
Mental nerve

Ophthalmic nerve [V₁]

Auriculotemporal nerve
Mandibular nerve [V₃]
Zygomaticofacial nerve

Trigeminal nerve [V] leaving the skull

Ophthalmic nerve [V₁]
Maxillary nerve [V₂]
Mandibular nerve [V₃]
Trigeminal ganglion
Trigeminal nerve [V]

Superior view

Ophthalmic nerve [V₁]
Maxillary nerve [V₂]
Mandibular nerve [V₃]

Zygomaticotemporal nerves
Supra-orbital nerve
Supratrochlear nerve
Lacrimal nerve
Infratrochlear nerve
External nasal nerve
Zygomaticofacial nerve
Infra-orbital nerve
Buccal nerve
Mental nerve
Auriculotemporal nerve

Cutaneous distribution of the trigeminal nerve [V]

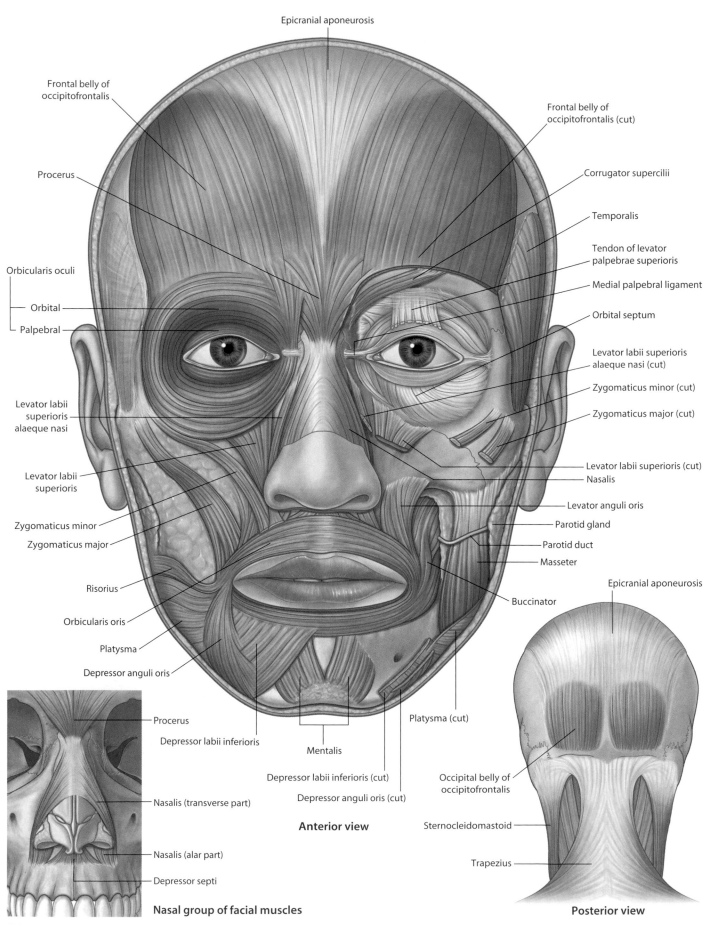

Epicranial aponeurosis

Frontal belly of occipitofrontalis

Procerus

Orbicularis oculi

Orbital

Palpebral

Levator labii superioris alaeque nasi

Levator labii superioris

Zygomaticus minor

Zygomaticus major

Risorius

Orbicularis oris

Platysma

Depressor anguli oris

Frontal belly of occipitofrontalis (cut)

Corrugator supercilii

Temporalis

Tendon of levator palpebrae superioris

Medial palpebral ligament

Orbital septum

Levator labii superioris alaeque nasi (cut)

Zygomaticus minor (cut)

Zygomaticus major (cut)

Levator labii superioris (cut)

Nasalis

Levator anguli oris

Parotid gland

Parotid duct

Masseter

Buccinator

Platysma (cut)

Depressor labii inferioris (cut)

Depressor anguli oris (cut)

Mentalis

Depressor labii inferioris

Anterior view

Procerus

Nasalis (transverse part)

Nasalis (alar part)

Depressor septi

Nasal group of facial muscles

Epicranial aponeurosis

Occipital belly of occipitofrontalis

Sternocleidomastoid

Trapezius

Posterior view

504

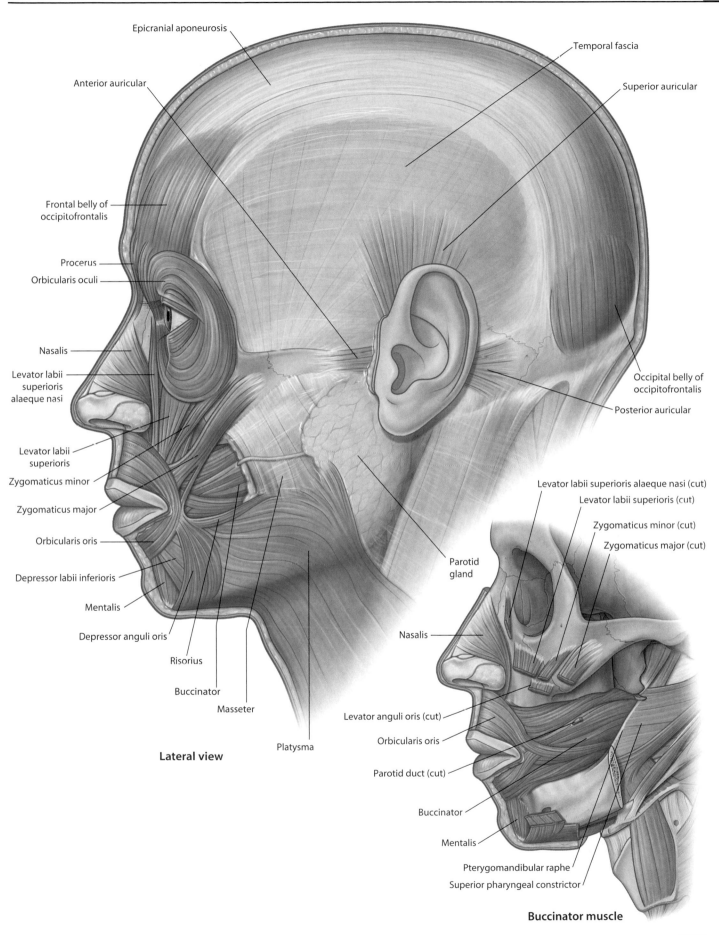

Epicranial aponeurosis

Anterior auricular

Temporal fascia

Superior auricular

Frontal belly of occipitofrontalis

Procerus

Orbicularis oculi

Nasalis

Levator labii superioris alaeque nasi

Levator labii superioris

Zygomaticus minor

Zygomaticus major

Orbicularis oris

Depressor labii inferioris

Mentalis

Depressor anguli oris

Risorius

Buccinator

Masseter

Platysma

Occipital belly of occipitofrontalis

Posterior auricular

Parotid gland

Lateral view

Levator labii superioris alaeque nasi (cut)

Levator labii superioris (cut)

Zygomaticus minor (cut)

Zygomaticus major (cut)

Nasalis

Levator anguli oris (cut)

Orbicularis oris

Parotid duct (cut)

Buccinator

Mentalis

Pterygomandibular raphe

Superior pharyngeal constrictor

Buccinator muscle

505

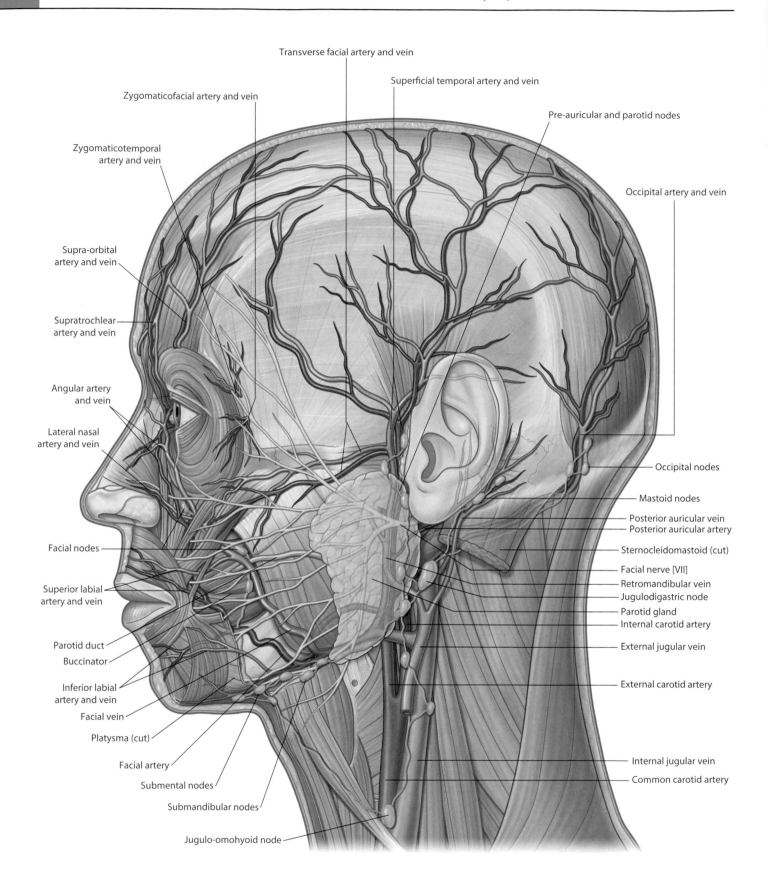

Transverse facial artery and vein

Superficial temporal artery and vein

Zygomaticofacial artery and vein

Zygomaticotemporal artery and vein

Pre-auricular and parotid nodes

Occipital artery and vein

Supra-orbital artery and vein

Supratrochlear artery and vein

Angular artery and vein

Lateral nasal artery and vein

Occipital nodes

Mastoid nodes

Posterior auricular vein
Posterior auricular artery

Facial nodes

Sternocleidomastoid (cut)

Facial nerve [VII]
Retromandibular vein
Jugulodigastric node
Parotid gland
Internal carotid artery

Superior labial artery and vein

External jugular vein

Parotid duct

Buccinator

External carotid artery

Inferior labial artery and vein

Facial vein

Platysma (cut)

Facial artery

Internal jugular vein

Common carotid artery

Submental nodes

Submandibular nodes

Jugulo-omohyoid node

Vasculature, facial nerve [VII], and lymphatics of the face

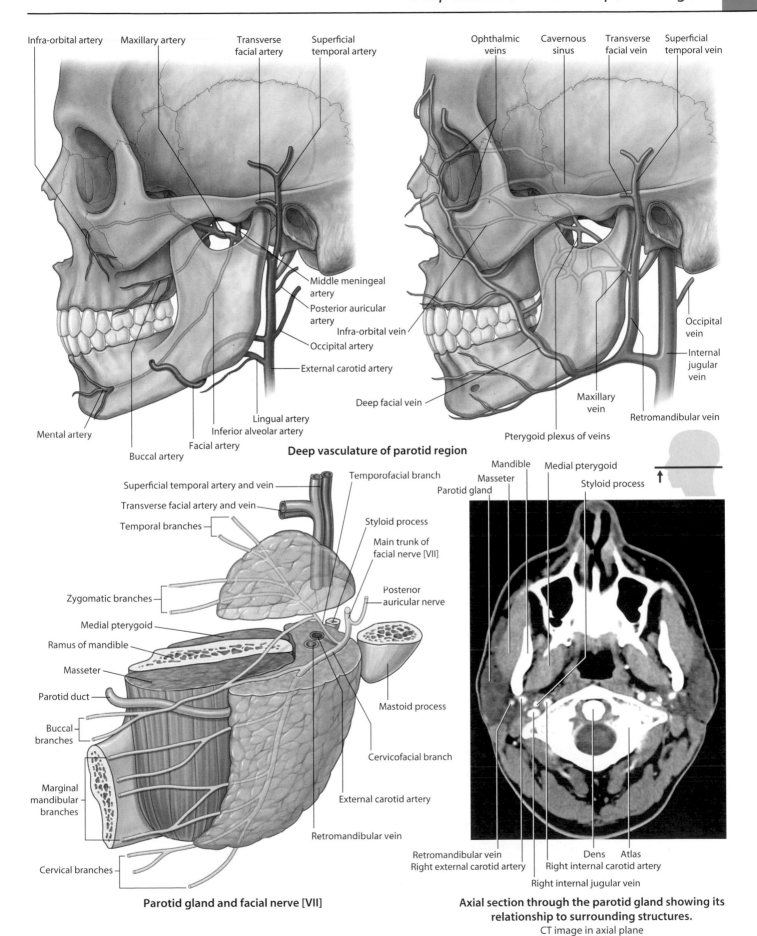

Infra-orbital artery | Maxillary artery | Transverse facial artery | Superficial temporal artery

Ophthalmic veins | Cavernous sinus | Transverse facial vein | Superficial temporal vein

Middle meningeal artery
Posterior auricular artery
Infra-orbital vein
Occipital artery
External carotid artery

Mental artery
Buccal artery
Facial artery
Inferior alveolar artery
Lingual artery

Occipital vein
Internal jugular vein

Deep facial vein
Maxillary vein
Retromandibular vein
Pterygoid plexus of veins

Deep vasculature of parotid region

Superficial temporal artery and vein
Transverse facial artery and vein
Temporal branches
Zygomatic branches
Medial pterygoid
Ramus of mandible
Masseter
Parotid duct
Buccal branches
Marginal mandibular branches
Cervical branches

Temporofacial branch
Styloid process
Main trunk of facial nerve [VII]
Posterior auricular nerve
Mastoid process
Cervicofacial branch
External carotid artery
Retromandibular vein

Parotid gland and facial nerve [VII]

Mandible | Medial pterygoid
Masseter | Styloid process
Parotid gland

Retromandibular vein
Right external carotid artery
Right internal jugular vein
Dens | Atlas
Right internal carotid artery

Axial section through the parotid gland showing its relationship to surrounding structures.
CT image in axial plane

507

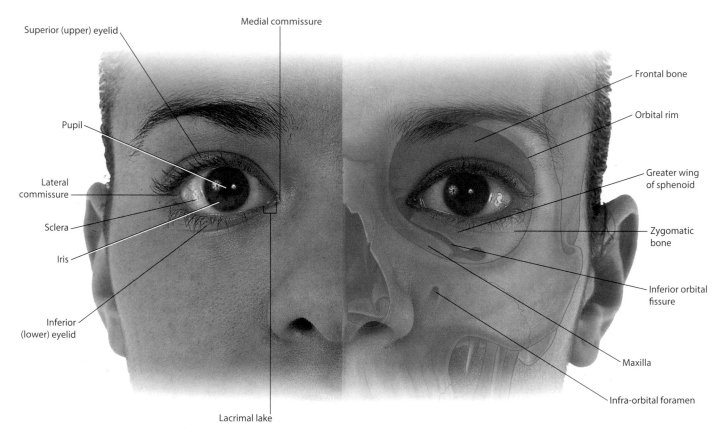

Superior (upper) eyelid

Medial commissure

Frontal bone

Orbital rim

Pupil

Greater wing
of sphenoid

Lateral
commissure

Zygomatic
bone

Sclera

Iris

Inferior orbital
fissure

Inferior
(lower) eyelid

Maxilla

Lacrimal lake

Infra-orbital foramen

Surface anatomy

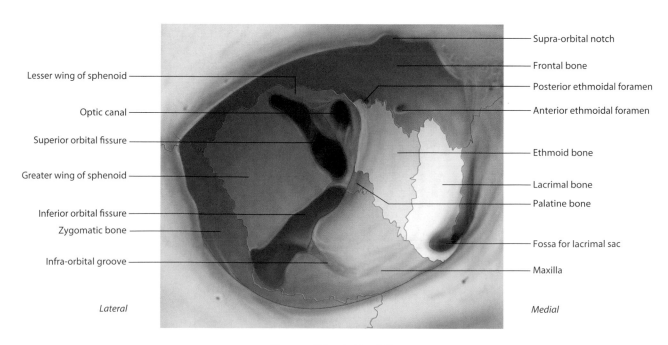

Lesser wing of sphenoid

Supra-orbital notch

Frontal bone

Optic canal

Posterior ethmoidal foramen

Anterior ethmoidal foramen

Superior orbital fissure

Greater wing of sphenoid

Ethmoid bone

Lacrimal bone

Inferior orbital fissure

Palatine bone

Zygomatic bone

Fossa for lacrimal sac

Infra-orbital groove

Maxilla

Lateral

Medial

Bones of the right orbit

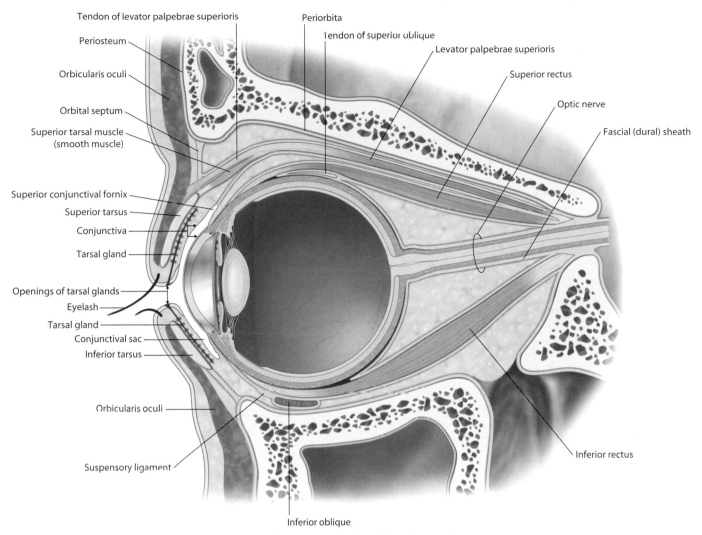

Tendon of levator palpebrae superioris
Periosteum
Orbicularis oculi
Orbital septum
Superior tarsal muscle (smooth muscle)
Superior conjunctival fornix
Superior tarsus
Conjunctiva
Tarsal gland
Openings of tarsal glands
Eyelash
Tarsal gland
Conjunctival sac
Inferior tarsus
Orbicularis oculi
Suspensory ligament
Periorbita
Tendon of superior oblique
Levator palpebrae superioris
Superior rectus
Optic nerve
Fascial (dural) sheath
Inferior rectus
Inferior oblique

Sagittal section through orbit and eyeball

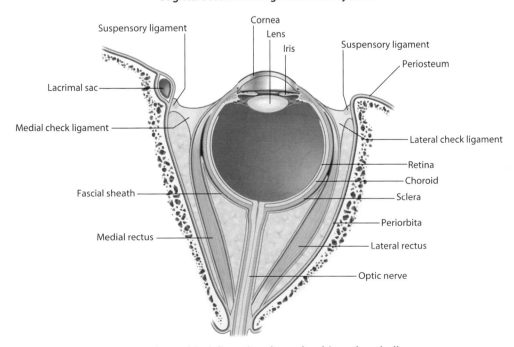

Suspensory ligament
Lacrimal sac
Medial check ligament
Fascial sheath
Medial rectus
Cornea
Lens
Iris
Suspensory ligament
Periosteum
Lateral check ligament
Retina
Choroid
Sclera
Periorbita
Lateral rectus
Optic nerve

Horizontal (axial) section through orbit and eyeball

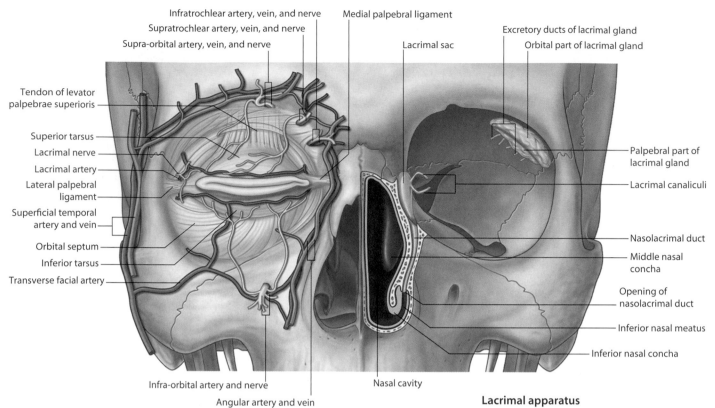

Infratrochlear artery, vein, and nerve
Supratrochlear artery, vein, and nerve
Supra-orbital artery, vein, and nerve

Tendon of levator palpebrae superioris

Superior tarsus
Lacrimal nerve
Lacrimal artery
Lateral palpebral ligament
Superficial temporal artery and vein
Orbital septum
Inferior tarsus
Transverse facial artery

Medial palpebral ligament
Lacrimal sac

Excretory ducts of lacrimal gland
Orbital part of lacrimal gland

Palpebral part of lacrimal gland
Lacrimal canaliculi

Nasolacrimal duct
Middle nasal concha
Opening of nasolacrimal duct
Inferior nasal meatus
Inferior nasal concha

Infra-orbital artery and nerve
Angular artery and vein
Nasal cavity

Lacrimal apparatus

Vasculature and nerves of the eyelids

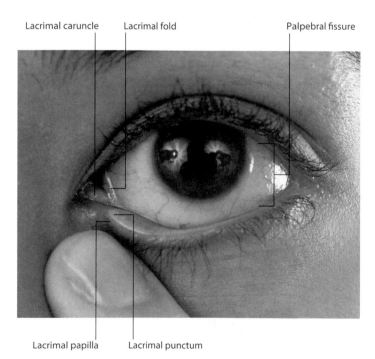

Lacrimal caruncle
Lacrimal fold
Palpebral fissure

Lacrimal papilla
Lacrimal punctum

Lacrimal papilla and punctum of left eye

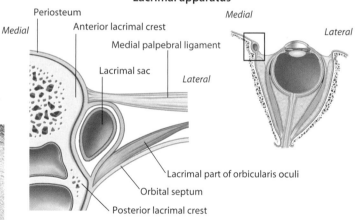

Periosteum
Anterior lacrimal crest
Medial palpebral ligament
Lacrimal sac
Medial
Lateral
Medial
Lateral

Lacrimal part of orbicularis oculi
Orbital septum
Posterior lacrimal crest

Lacrimal sac (horizontal section)

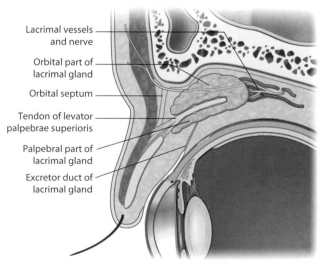

Lacrimal vessels and nerve
Orbital part of lacrimal gland
Orbital septum
Tendon of levator palpebrae superioris
Palpebral part of lacrimal gland
Excretor duct of lacrimal gland

Lacrimal gland and levator palpebrae superioris (parasagittal section)

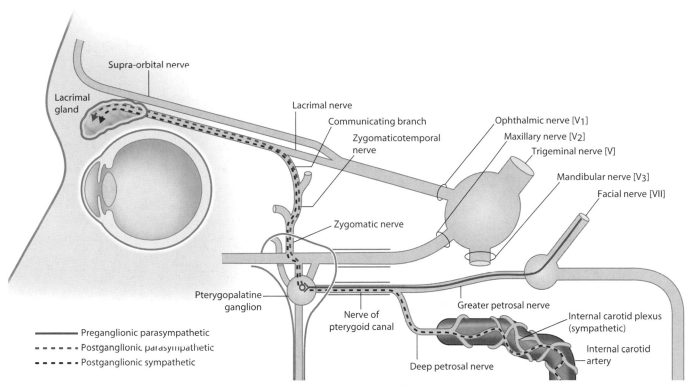

Visceral efferent (motor) innervation of the lacrimal gland

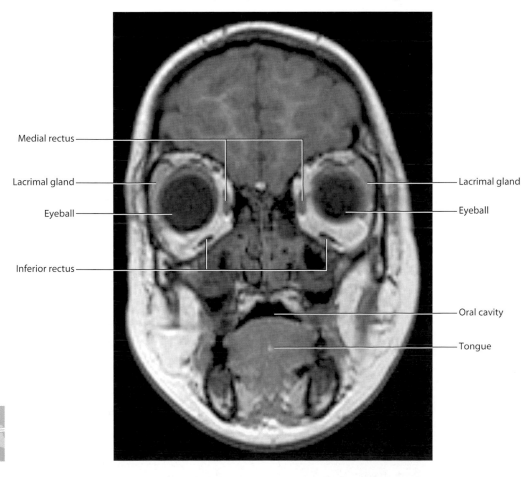

**Coronal section through the orbit showing the lacrimal gland
and its relationship to surrounding structures.**
T1-weighted MR image in coronal plane

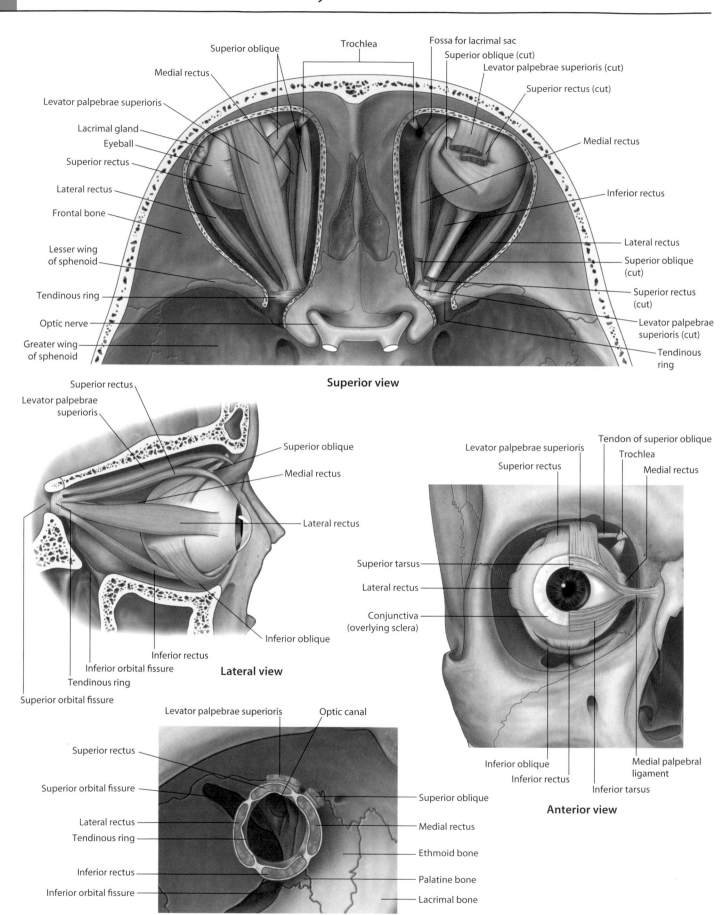

Superior view

Trochlea

Superior oblique

Medial rectus

Levator palpebrae superioris

Lacrimal gland

Eyeball

Superior rectus

Lateral rectus

Frontal bone

Lesser wing of sphenoid

Tendinous ring

Optic nerve

Greater wing of sphenoid

Fossa for lacrimal sac

Superior oblique (cut)

Levator palpebrae superioris (cut)

Superior rectus (cut)

Medial rectus

Inferior rectus

Lateral rectus

Superior oblique (cut)

Superior rectus (cut)

Levator palpebrae superioris (cut)

Tendinous ring

Lateral view

Superior rectus

Levator palpebrae superioris

Superior oblique

Medial rectus

Lateral rectus

Inferior oblique

Inferior rectus

Inferior orbital fissure

Tendinous ring

Superior orbital fissure

Anterior view

Levator palpebrae superioris

Superior rectus

Tendon of superior oblique

Trochlea

Medial rectus

Superior tarsus

Lateral rectus

Conjunctiva (overlying sclera)

Inferior oblique

Inferior rectus

Inferior tarsus

Medial palpebral ligament

Origins of muscles of the eyeball

Levator palpebrae superioris

Optic canal

Superior rectus

Superior orbital fissure

Lateral rectus

Tendinous ring

Inferior rectus

Inferior orbital fissure

Superior oblique

Medial rectus

Ethmoid bone

Palatine bone

Lacrimal bone

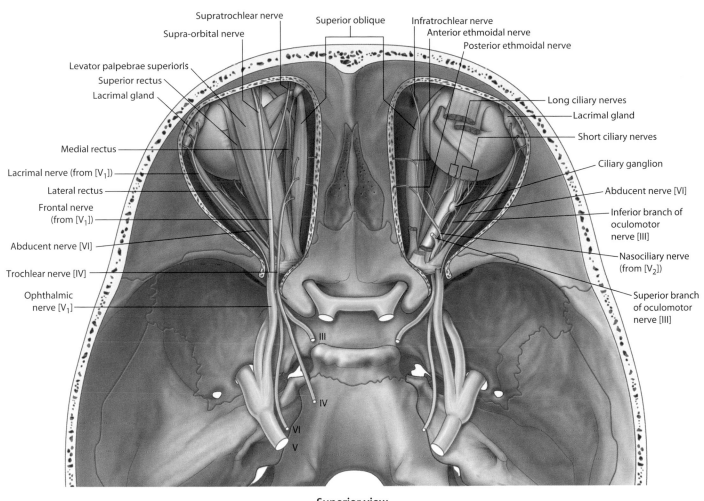

Supratrochlear nerve

Supra-orbital nerve

Levator palpebrae superioris

Superior rectus

Lacrimal gland

Medial rectus

Lacrimal nerve (from [V₁])

Lateral rectus

Frontal nerve (from [V₁])

Abducent nerve [VI]

Trochlear nerve [IV]

Ophthalmic nerve [V₁]

Superior oblique

Infratrochlear nerve

Anterior ethmoidal nerve

Posterior ethmoidal nerve

Long ciliary nerves

Lacrimal gland

Short ciliary nerves

Ciliary ganglion

Abducent nerve [VI]

Inferior branch of oculomotor nerve [III]

Nasociliary nerve (from [V₂])

Superior branch of oculomotor nerve [III]

III

IV

VI

V

Superior view

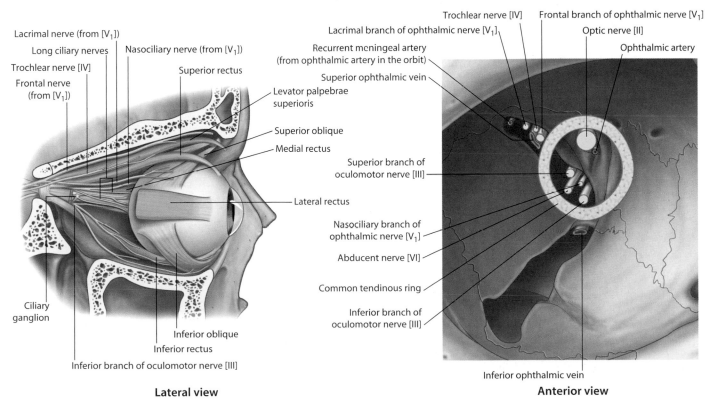

Lacrimal nerve (from [V₁])

Long ciliary nerves

Trochlear nerve [IV]

Frontal nerve (from [V₁])

Nasociliary nerve (from [V₁])

Superior rectus

Levator palpebrae superioris

Superior oblique

Medial rectus

Lateral rectus

Ciliary ganglion

Inferior oblique

Inferior rectus

Inferior branch of oculomotor nerve [III]

Lateral view

Trochlear nerve [IV]

Lacrimal branch of ophthalmic nerve [V₁]

Recurrent meningeal artery (from ophthalmic artery in the orbit)

Superior ophthalmic vein

Frontal branch of ophthalmic nerve [V₁]

Optic nerve [II]

Ophthalmic artery

Superior branch of oculomotor nerve [III]

Nasociliary branch of ophthalmic nerve [V₁]

Abducent nerve [VI]

Common tendinous ring

Inferior branch of oculomotor nerve [III]

Inferior ophthalmic vein

Anterior view

513

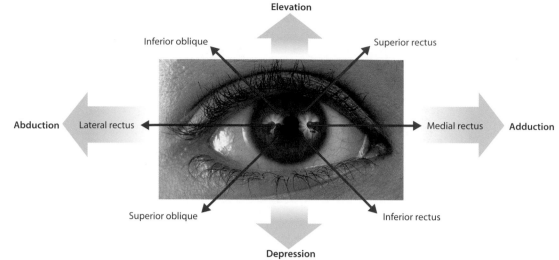

Elevation

Inferior oblique

Superior rectus

Abduction — Lateral rectus

Medial rectus — Adduction

Superior oblique

Inferior rectus

Depression

Actions of individual muscles (anatomical action)

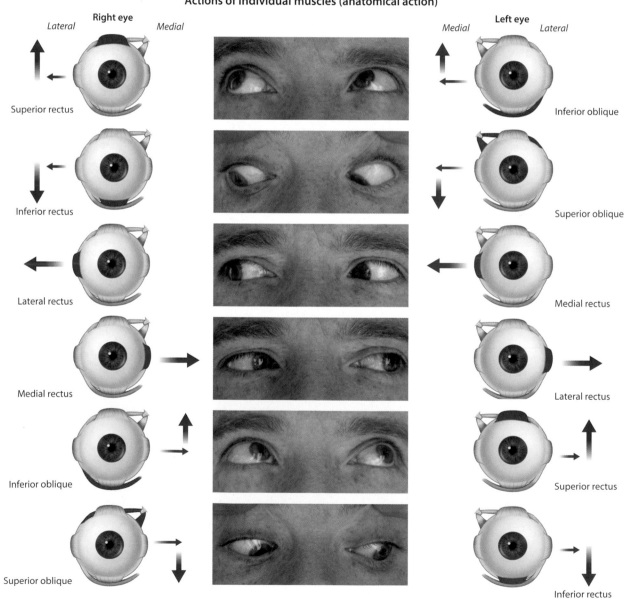

Right eye

Lateral / *Medial*

Superior rectus

Inferior rectus

Lateral rectus

Medial rectus

Inferior oblique

Superior oblique

Left eye

Medial / *Lateral*

Inferior oblique

Superior oblique

Medial rectus

Lateral rectus

Superior rectus

Inferior rectus

Movement of eyes when testing specific muscle (clinical testing).

For testing some muscles, a patient is "asked" first to move the eye into a position (small arrow) where the indicated muscle can best be tested. The large arrow indicates the direction the patient is then "asked" to move the eye to test the muscle

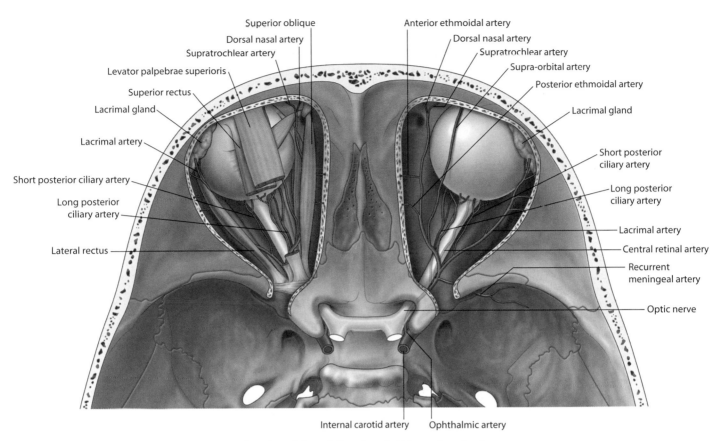

Superior oblique
Dorsal nasal artery
Supratrochlear artery
Levator palpebrae superioris
Superior rectus
Lacrimal gland
Lacrimal artery
Short posterior ciliary artery
Long posterior ciliary artery
Lateral rectus

Anterior ethmoidal artery
Dorsal nasal artery
Supratrochlear artery
Supra-orbital artery
Posterior ethmoidal artery
Lacrimal gland
Short posterior ciliary artery
Long posterior ciliary artery
Lacrimal artery
Central retinal artery
Recurrent meningeal artery
Optic nerve

Internal carotid artery   Ophthalmic artery

Arteries of the orbit and eyeball (superior view)

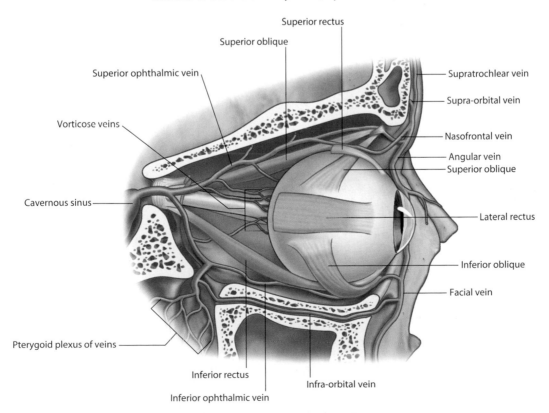

Superior rectus
Superior oblique
Superior ophthalmic vein
Vorticose veins
Cavernous sinus
Pterygoid plexus of veins

Supratrochlear vein
Supra-orbital vein
Nasofrontal vein
Angular vein
Superior oblique
Lateral rectus
Inferior oblique
Facial vein

Inferior rectus
Inferior ophthalmic vein
Infra-orbital vein

Veins of the orbit and eyeball (lateral view)

515

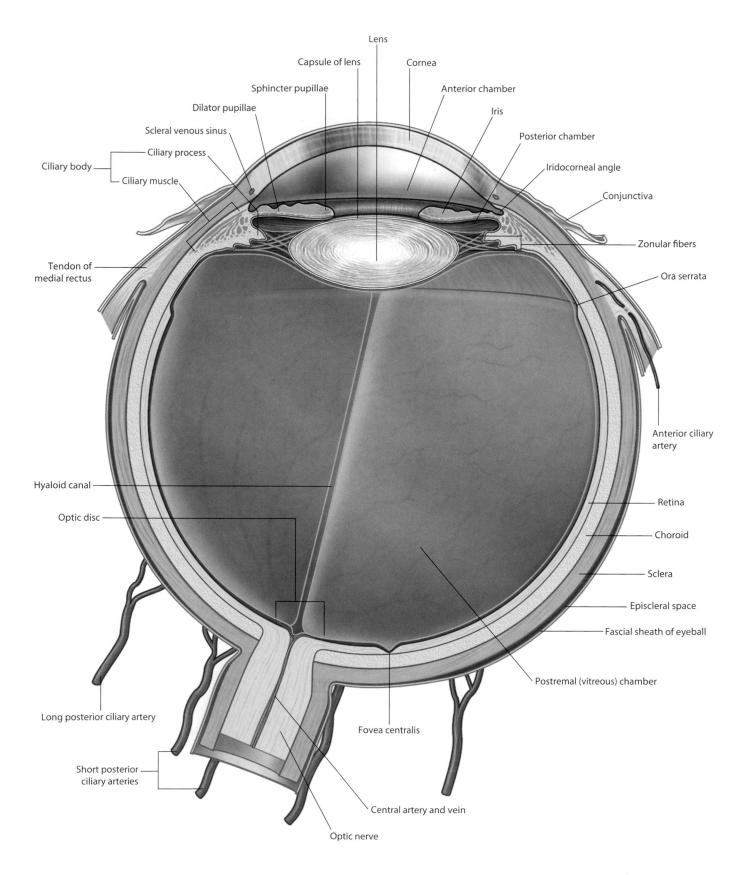

Lens

Capsule of lens

Cornea

Sphincter pupillae

Anterior chamber

Dilator pupillae

Iris

Scleral venous sinus

Posterior chamber

Ciliary process

Iridocorneal angle

Ciliary body

Ciliary muscle

Conjunctiva

Tendon of
medial rectus

Zonular fibers

Ora serrata

Anterior ciliary
artery

Hyaloid canal

Retina

Optic disc

Choroid

Sclera

Episcleral space

Fascial sheath of eyeball

Postremal (vitreous) chamber

Long posterior ciliary artery

Short posterior
ciliary arteries

Fovea centralis

Central artery and vein

Optic nerve

Eyeball (horizontal section)

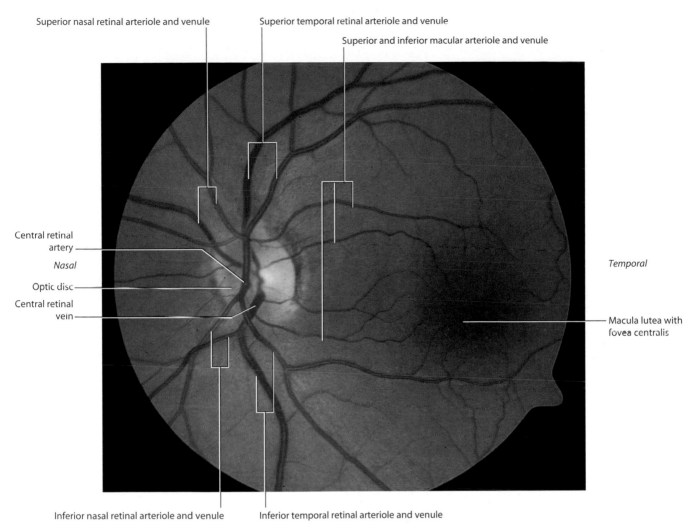

Superior nasal retinal arteriole and venule

Superior temporal retinal arteriole and venule

Superior and inferior macular arteriole and venule

Central retinal artery

Nasal

Optic disc

Central retinal vein

Temporal

Macula lutea with fovea centralis

Inferior nasal retinal arteriole and venule

Inferior temporal retinal arteriole and venule

Ophthalmoscopic view of the left retina showing the optic disc, the macula lutea, and the retinal vasculature

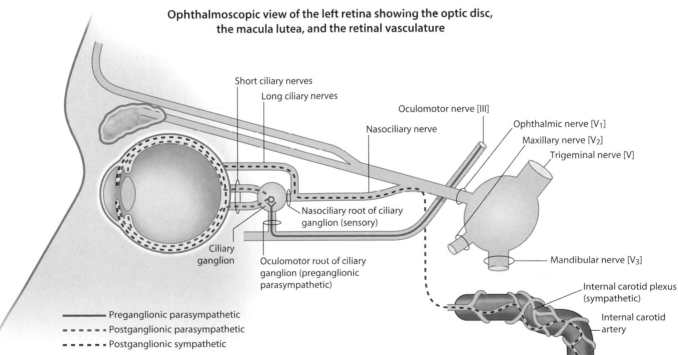

Short ciliary nerves

Long ciliary nerves

Oculomotor nerve [III]

Nasociliary nerve

Ophthalmic nerve [V₁]

Maxillary nerve [V₂]

Trigeminal nerve [V]

Nasociliary root of ciliary ganglion (sensory)

Ciliary ganglion

Oculomotor root of ciliary ganglion (preganglionic parasympathetic)

Mandibular nerve [V₃]

Internal carotid plexus (sympathetic)

Internal carotid artery

——— Preganglionic parasympathetic
- - - - Postganglionic parasympathetic
- - - - Postganglionic sympathetic

Visceral efferent (motor) innervation of eyeball (iris and ciliary body)

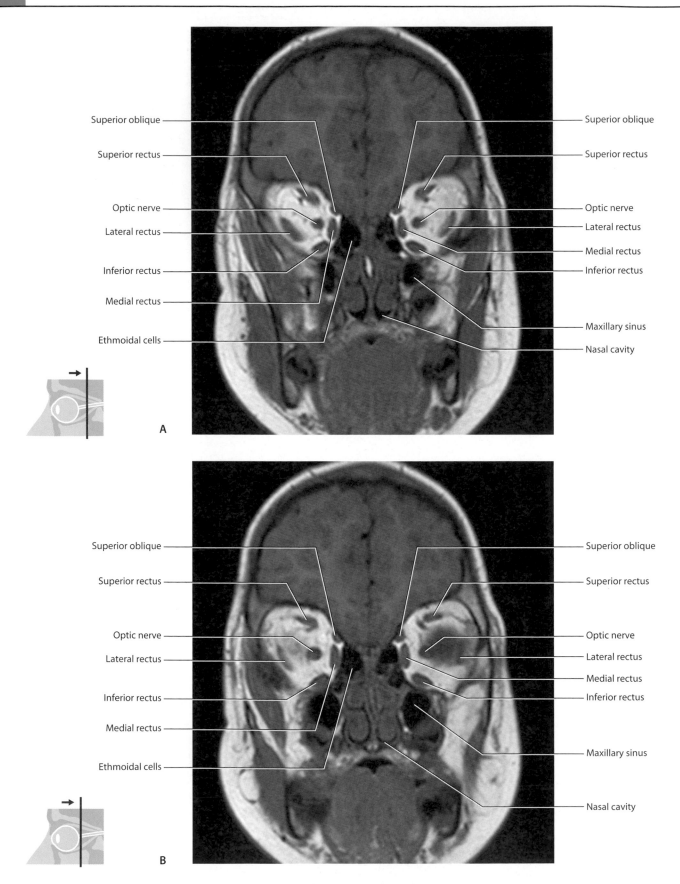

Superior oblique

Superior rectus

Optic nerve

Lateral rectus

Inferior rectus

Medial rectus

Ethmoidal cells

Superior oblique

Superior rectus

Optic nerve

Lateral rectus

Medial rectus

Inferior rectus

Maxillary sinus

Nasal cavity

A

Superior oblique

Superior rectus

Optic nerve

Lateral rectus

Inferior rectus

Medial rectus

Ethmoidal cells

Superior oblique

Superior rectus

Optic nerve

Lateral rectus

Medial rectus

Inferior rectus

Maxillary sinus

Nasal cavity

B

A through D – Coronal sections that pass through the orbit from posterior to anterior showing the extrinsic (extra-ocular) muscles and their relationships with each other and with other structures.

T1-weighted MR images in coronal plane

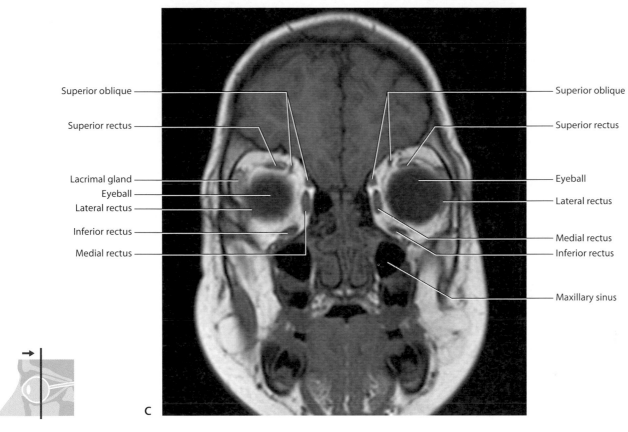

Superior oblique

Superior rectus

Lacrimal gland
Eyeball
Lateral rectus
Inferior rectus
Medial rectus

Superior oblique

Superior rectus

Eyeball

Lateral rectus

Medial rectus
Inferior rectus

Maxillary sinus

C

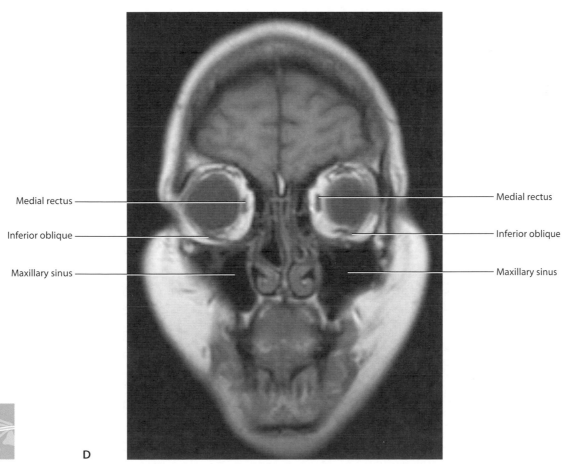

Medial rectus

Inferior oblique

Maxillary sinus

Medial rectus

Inferior oblique

Maxillary sinus

D

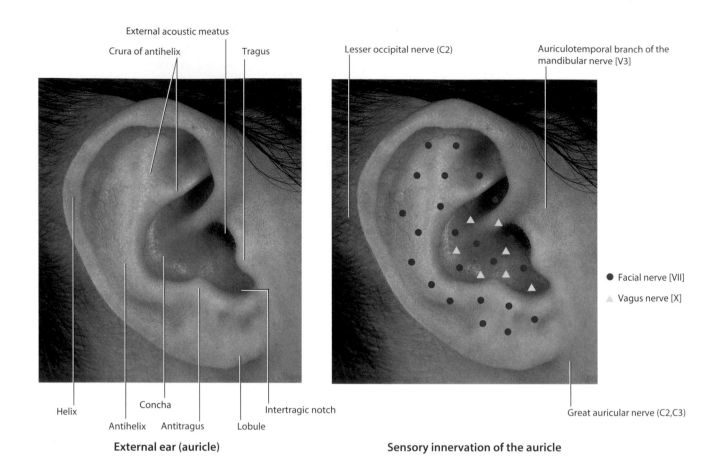

External acoustic meatus
Crura of antihelix
Tragus

Helix
Antihelix
Concha
Antitragus
Lobule
Intertragic notch

External ear (auricle)

Lesser occipital nerve (C2)
Auriculotemporal branch of the mandibular nerve [V3]

● Facial nerve [VII]
▲ Vagus nerve [X]

Great auricular nerve (C2,C3)

Sensory innervation of the auricle

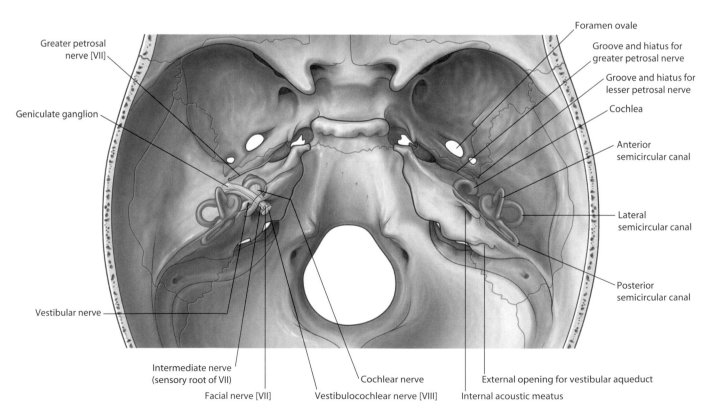

Greater petrosal nerve [VII]
Geniculate ganglion
Vestibular nerve
Intermediate nerve (sensory root of VII)
Facial nerve [VII]
Vestibulocochlear nerve [VIII]
Cochlear nerve

Foramen ovale
Groove and hiatus for greater petrosal nerve
Groove and hiatus for lesser petrosal nerve
Cochlea
Anterior semicircular canal
Lateral semicircular canal
Posterior semicircular canal
External opening for vestibular aqueduct
Internal acoustic meatus

Superior projection of internal ear in the temporal bone

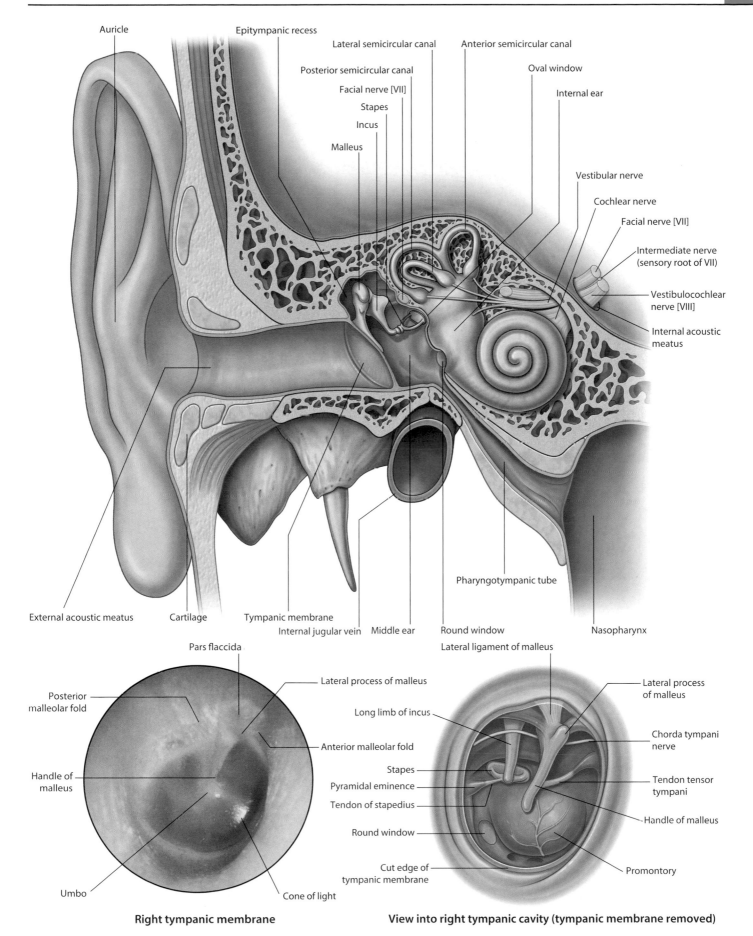

Auricle

Epitympanic recess

Lateral semicircular canal

Posterior semicircular canal

Anterior semicircular canal

Facial nerve [VII]

Oval window

Stapes

Internal ear

Incus

Malleus

Vestibular nerve

Cochlear nerve

Facial nerve [VII]

Intermediate nerve (sensory root of VII)

Vestibulocochlear nerve [VIII]

Internal acoustic meatus

External acoustic meatus

Cartilage

Tympanic membrane

Internal jugular vein

Middle ear

Round window

Pharyngotympanic tube

Nasopharynx

Pars flaccida

Lateral ligament of malleus

Posterior malleolar fold

Lateral process of malleus

Lateral process of malleus

Long limb of incus

Chorda tympani nerve

Handle of malleus

Anterior malleolar fold

Stapes

Pyramidal eminence

Tendon of stapedius

Tendon tensor tympani

Handle of malleus

Round window

Umbo

Cut edge of tympanic membrane

Promontory

Cone of light

Right tympanic membrane

View into right tympanic cavity (tympanic membrane removed)

521

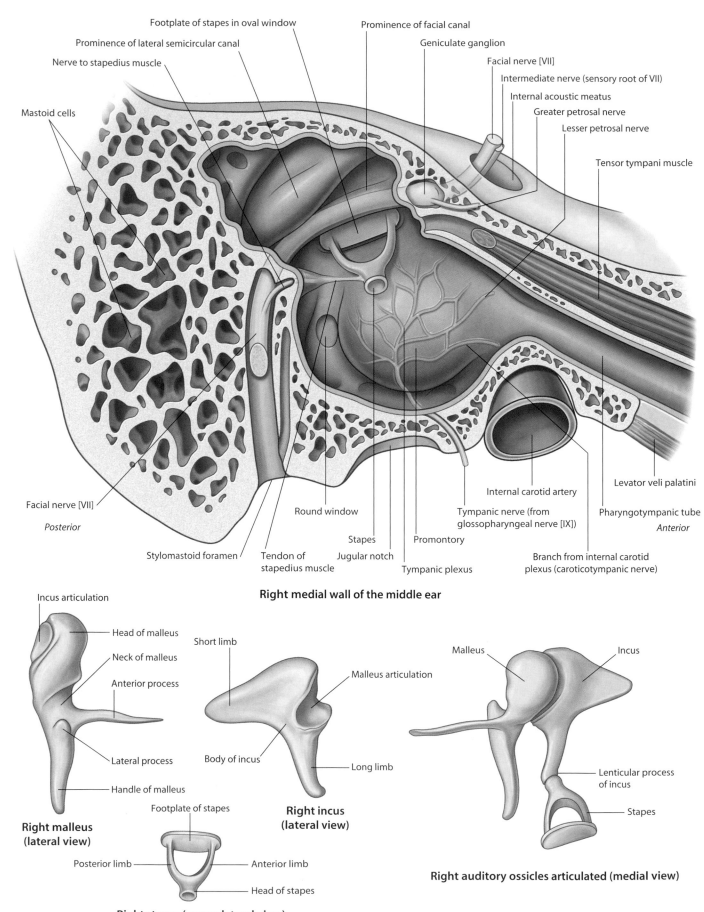

Footplate of stapes in oval window

Prominence of lateral semicircular canal

Nerve to stapedius muscle

Prominence of facial canal

Geniculate ganglion

Facial nerve [VII]

Intermediate nerve (sensory root of VII)

Internal acoustic meatus

Greater petrosal nerve

Lesser petrosal nerve

Tensor tympani muscle

Mastoid cells

Facial nerve [VII]

Posterior

Stylomastoid foramen

Tendon of stapedius muscle

Round window

Stapes

Jugular notch

Promontory

Tympanic plexus

Tympanic nerve (from glossopharyngeal nerve [IX])

Internal carotid artery

Branch from internal carotid plexus (caroticotympanic nerve)

Levator veli palatini

Pharyngotympanic tube

Anterior

Right medial wall of the middle ear

Incus articulation

Head of malleus

Neck of malleus

Anterior process

Lateral process

Handle of malleus

Right malleus (lateral view)

Short limb

Malleus articulation

Body of incus

Long limb

Right incus (lateral view)

Footplate of stapes

Posterior limb

Anterior limb

Head of stapes

Right stapes (superolateral view)

Malleus

Incus

Lenticular process of incus

Stapes

Right auditory ossicles articulated (medial view)

522

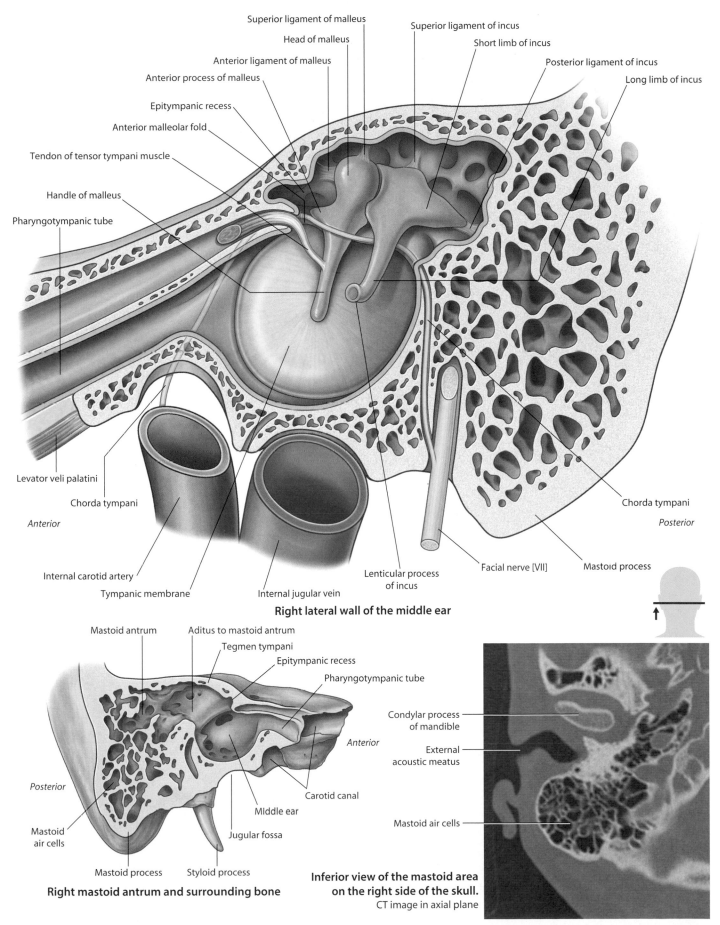

Superior ligament of malleus
Head of malleus
Anterior ligament of malleus
Anterior process of malleus
Epitympanic recess
Anterior malleolar fold
Tendon of tensor tympani muscle
Handle of malleus
Pharyngotympanic tube

Superior ligament of incus
Short limb of incus
Posterior ligament of incus
Long limb of incus

Chorda tympani
Posterior

Levator veli palatini
Chorda tympani
Anterior

Internal carotid artery
Tympanic membrane
Lenticular process of incus
Internal jugular vein
Facial nerve [VII]
Mastoid process

Right lateral wall of the middle ear

Mastoid antrum
Aditus to mastoid antrum
Tegmen tympani
Epitympanic recess
Pharyngotympanic tube
Anterior

Posterior

Mastoid air cells
Mastoid process
Styloid process
Carotid canal
Middle ear
Jugular fossa

Right mastoid antrum and surrounding bone

Condylar process of mandible
External acoustic meatus
Mastoid air cells

Inferior view of the mastoid area on the right side of the skull.
CT image in axial plane

523

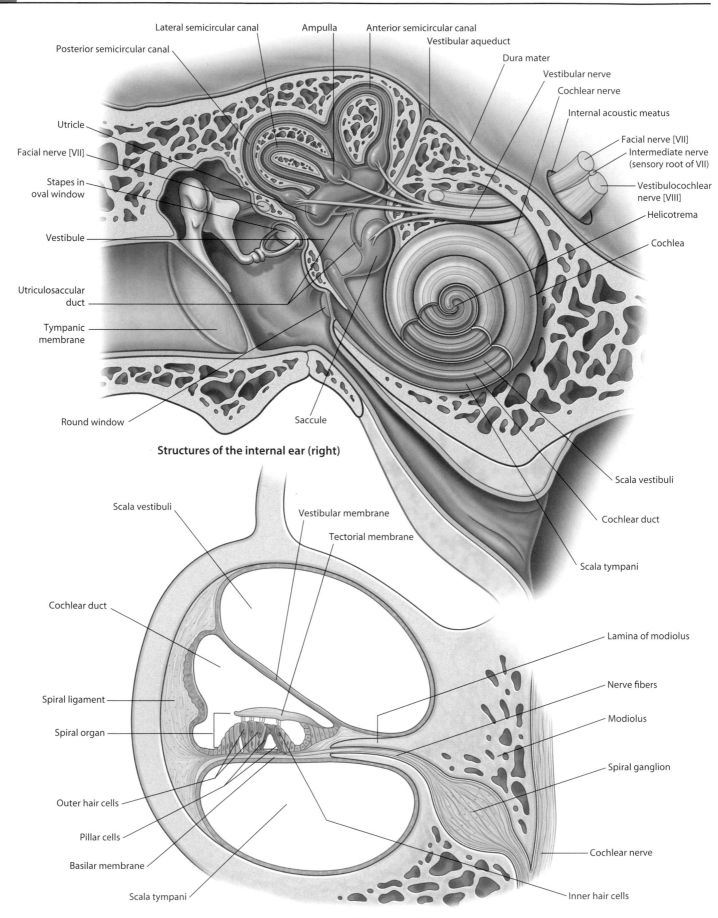

Lateral semicircular canal

Posterior semicircular canal

Ampulla

Anterior semicircular canal

Vestibular aqueduct

Dura mater

Vestibular nerve

Cochlear nerve

Internal acoustic meatus

Utricle

Facial nerve [VII]

Stapes in oval window

Vestibule

Utriculosaccular duct

Tympanic membrane

Round window

Saccule

Facial nerve [VII]

Intermediate nerve (sensory root of VII)

Vestibulocochlear nerve [VIII]

Helicotrema

Cochlea

Scala vestibuli

Cochlear duct

Scala tympani

Structures of the internal ear (right)

Scala vestibuli

Vestibular membrane

Tectorial membrane

Cochlear duct

Lamina of modiolus

Spiral ligament

Nerve fibers

Spiral organ

Modiolus

Outer hair cells

Spiral ganglion

Pillar cells

Basilar membrane

Cochlear nerve

Scala tympani

Inner hair cells

Cross section through cochlea

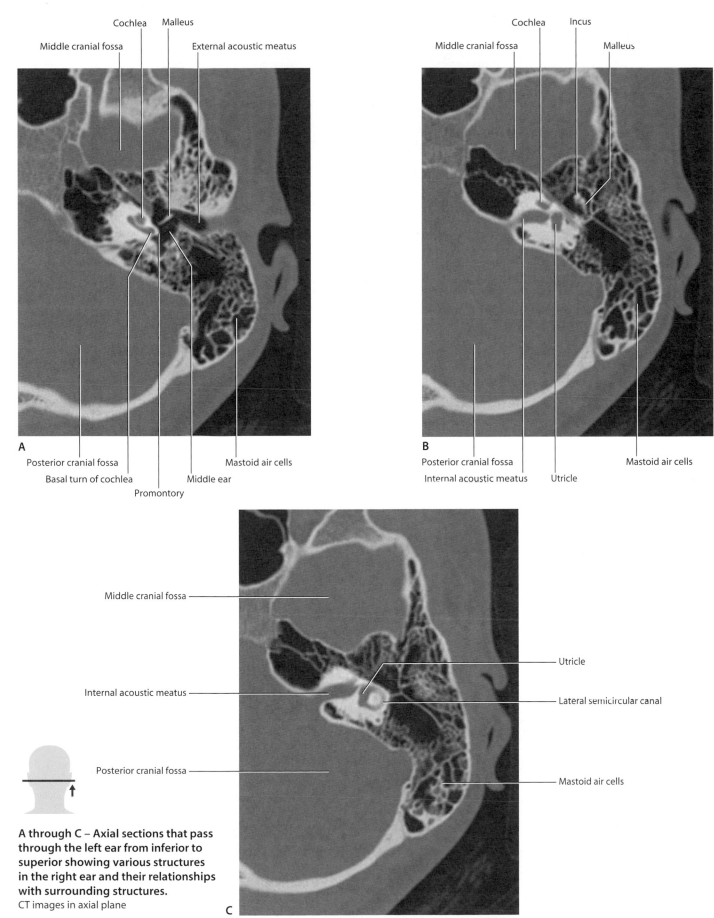

A

Middle cranial fossa
Cochlea
Malleus
External acoustic meatus

Posterior cranial fossa
Basal turn of cochlea
Promontory
Middle ear
Mastoid air cells

B

Middle cranial fossa
Cochlea
Incus
Malleus

Posterior cranial fossa
Internal acoustic meatus
Utricle
Mastoid air cells

C

Middle cranial fossa
Internal acoustic meatus
Posterior cranial fossa

Utricle
Lateral semicircular canal
Mastoid air cells

A through C – Axial sections that pass through the left ear from inferior to superior showing various structures in the right ear and their relationships with surrounding structures.
CT images in axial plane

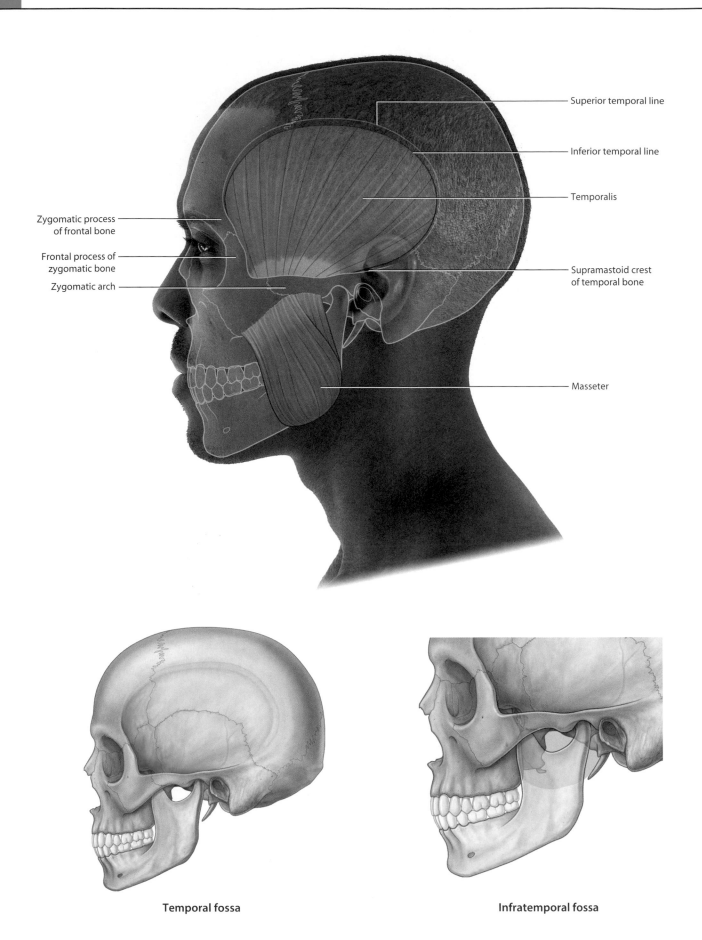

Superior temporal line

Inferior temporal line

Temporalis

Zygomatic process
of frontal bone

Frontal process of
zygomatic bone

Zygomatic arch

Supramastoid crest
of temporal bone

Masseter

Temporal fossa

Infratemporal fossa

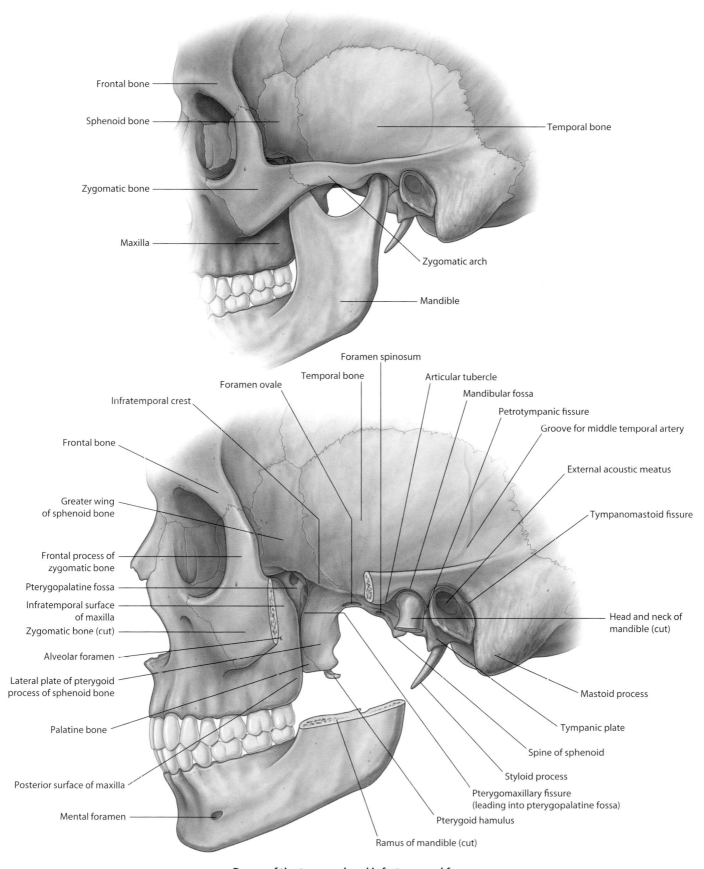

Frontal bone

Sphenoid bone

Temporal bone

Zygomatic bone

Maxilla

Zygomatic arch

Mandible

Foramen spinosum

Temporal bone

Articular tubercle

Mandibular fossa

Foramen ovale

Petrotympanic fissure

Infratemporal crest

Groove for middle temporal artery

Frontal bone

External acoustic meatus

Greater wing
of sphenoid bone

Tympanomastoid fissure

Frontal process of
zygomatic bone

Pterygopalatine fossa

Infratemporal surface
of maxilla

Zygomatic bone (cut)

Head and neck of
mandible (cut)

Alveolar foramen

Lateral plate of pterygoid
process of sphenoid bone

Palatine bone

Mastoid process

Tympanic plate

Spine of sphenoid

Posterior surface of maxilla

Styloid process

Mental foramen

Pterygomaxillary fissure
(leading into pterygopalatine fossa)

Pterygoid hamulus

Ramus of mandible (cut)

Bones of the temporal band infratemporal fossae

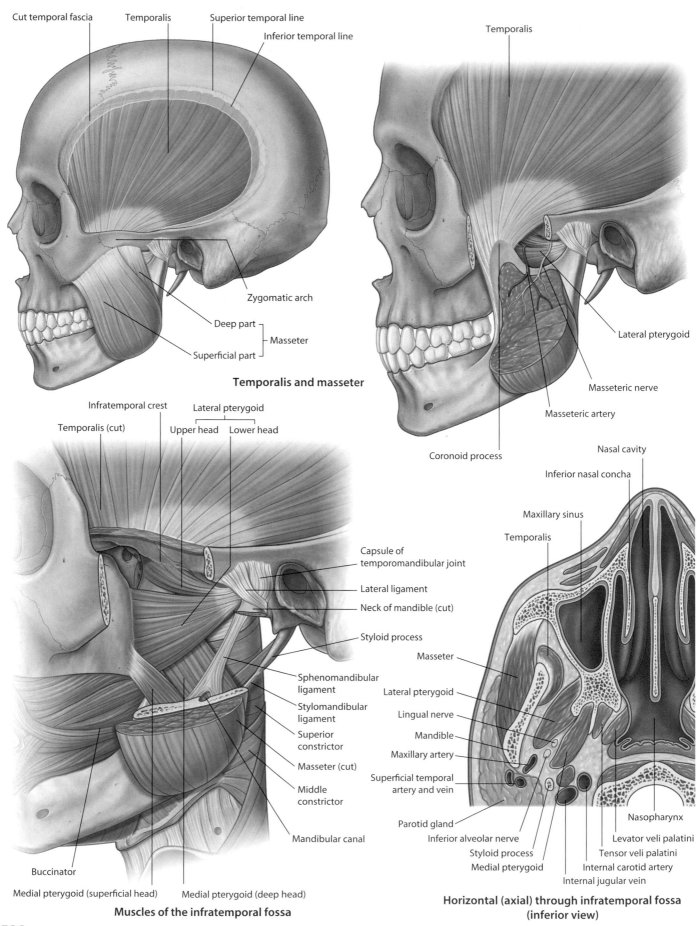

Cut temporal fascia
Temporalis
Superior temporal line
Inferior temporal line
Temporalis

Zygomatic arch

Deep part ⎤
⎥ Masseter
Superficial part ⎦

Temporalis and masseter

Lateral pterygoid

Masseteric nerve

Masseteric artery

Coronoid process

Infratemporal crest
Lateral pterygoid
Temporalis (cut)
Upper head   Lower head

Capsule of temporomandibular joint

Lateral ligament

Neck of mandible (cut)

Styloid process

Sphenomandibular ligament

Stylomandibular ligament

Superior constrictor

Masseter (cut)

Middle constrictor

Mandibular canal

Buccinator

Medial pterygoid (superficial head)

Medial pterygoid (deep head)

Muscles of the infratemporal fossa

Nasal cavity

Inferior nasal concha

Maxillary sinus

Temporalis

Masseter

Lateral pterygoid

Lingual nerve

Mandible

Maxillary artery

Superficial temporal artery and vein

Parotid gland

Inferior alveolar nerve

Styloid process

Medial pterygoid

Nasopharynx

Levator veli palatini

Tensor veli palatini

Internal carotid artery

Internal jugular vein

Horizontal (axial) through infratemporal fossa (inferior view)

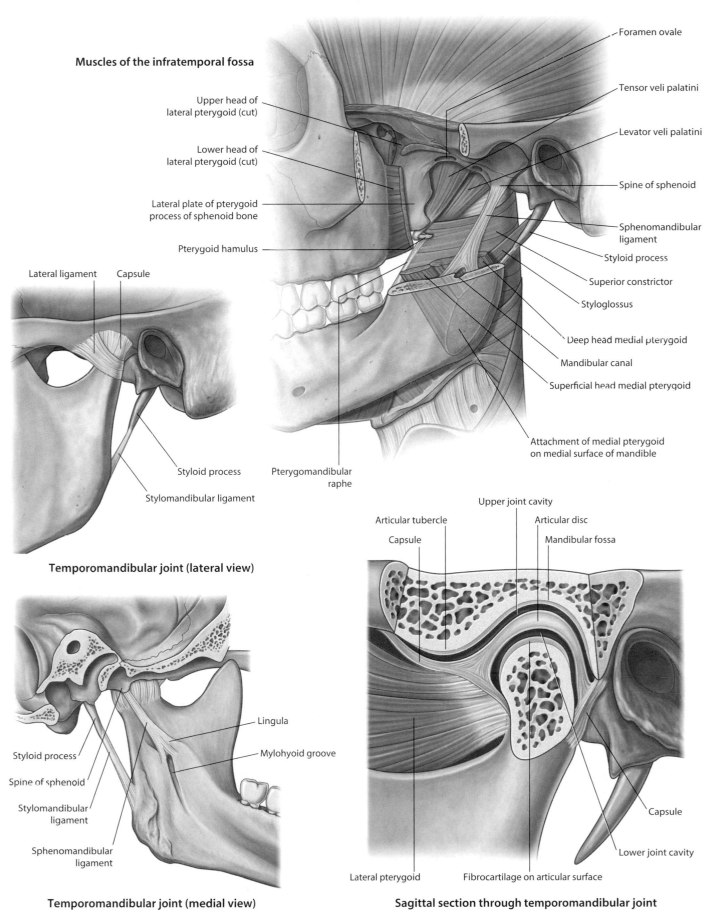

Muscles of the infratemporal fossa

Foramen ovale

Upper head of lateral pterygoid (cut)

Lower head of lateral pterygoid (cut)

Lateral plate of pterygoid process of sphenoid bone

Pterygoid hamulus

Tensor veli palatini

Levator veli palatini

Spine of sphenoid

Sphenomandibular ligament

Styloid process

Superior constrictor

Styloglossus

Deep head medial pterygoid

Mandibular canal

Superficial head medial pterygoid

Attachment of medial pterygoid on medial surface of mandible

Pterygomandibular raphe

Lateral ligament

Capsule

Styloid process

Stylomandibular ligament

Temporomandibular joint (lateral view)

Styloid process

Spine of sphenoid

Stylomandibular ligament

Sphenomandibular ligament

Lingula

Mylohyoid groove

Temporomandibular joint (medial view)

Upper joint cavity

Articular tubercle

Articular disc

Capsule

Mandibular fossa

Capsule

Lower joint cavity

Lateral pterygoid

Fibrocartilage on articular surface

Sagittal section through temporomandibular joint

529

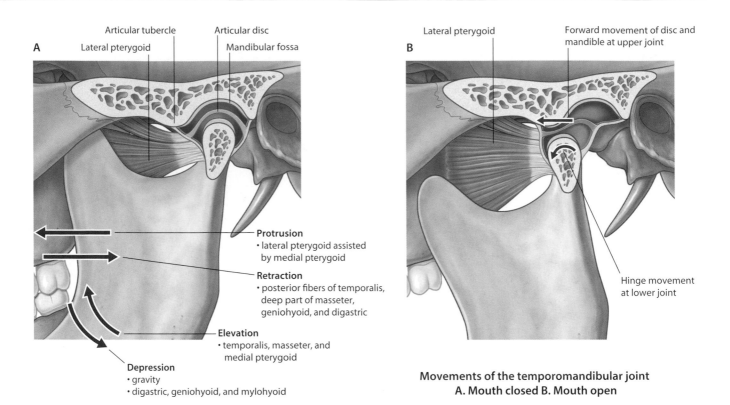

A

Articular tubercle
Lateral pterygoid
Articular disc
Mandibular fossa

Protrusion
• lateral pterygoid assisted by medial pterygoid

Retraction
• posterior fibers of temporalis, deep part of masseter, geniohyoid, and digastric

Elevation
• temporalis, masseter, and medial pterygoid

Depression
• gravity
• digastric, geniohyoid, and mylohyoid

B

Lateral pterygoid
Forward movement of disc and mandible at upper joint

Hinge movement at lower joint

**Movements of the temporomandibular joint
A. Mouth closed B. Mouth open**

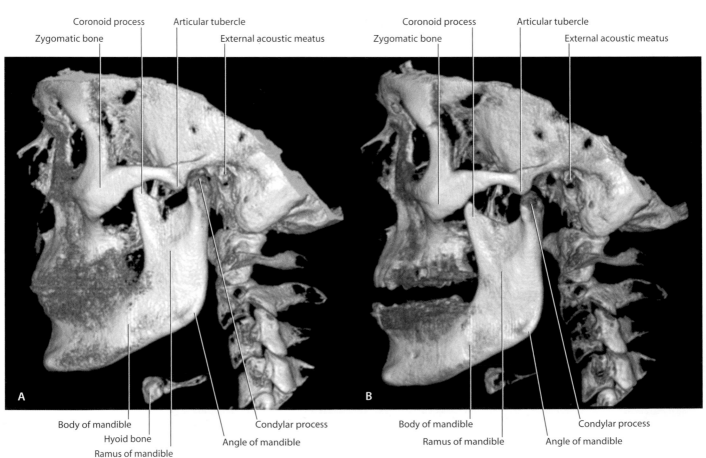

Coronoid process
Zygomatic bone
Articular tubercle
External acoustic meatus

Coronoid process
Zygomatic bone
Articular tubercle
External acoustic meatus

A

B

Body of mandible
Hyoid bone
Ramus of mandible
Angle of mandible
Condylar process

Body of mandible
Ramus of mandible
Angle of mandible
Condylar process

**Lateral view of the right temporomandibular joint
A. Mouth closed B. Mouth open.**
Image taken with Cone Beam Computerized Tomography (CBCT)
technology viewed in the radiographic mode

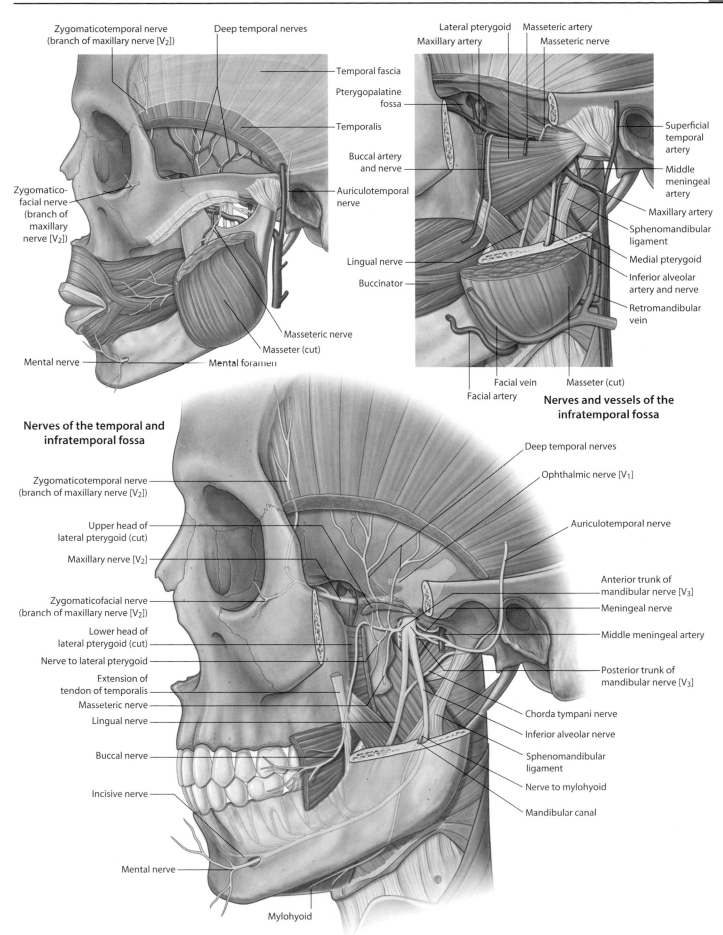

Zygomaticotemporal nerve
(branch of maxillary nerve [V₂])

Deep temporal nerves

Temporal fascia

Pterygopalatine
fossa

Temporalis

Buccal artery
and nerve

Auriculotemporal
nerve

Zygomatico-
facial nerve
(branch of
maxillary
nerve [V₂])

Lingual nerve

Buccinator

Masseteric nerve

Masseter (cut)

Mental nerve

Mental foramen

Lateral pterygoid   Masseteric artery
Maxillary artery   Masseteric nerve

Superficial
temporal
artery

Middle
meningeal
artery

Maxillary artery

Sphenomandibular
ligament

Medial pterygoid

Inferior alveolar
artery and nerve

Retromandibular
vein

Facial vein   Masseter (cut)
Facial artery

**Nerves and vessels of the
infratemporal fossa**

**Nerves of the temporal and
infratemporal fossa**

Zygomaticotemporal nerve
(branch of maxillary nerve [V₂])

Upper head of
lateral pterygoid (cut)

Maxillary nerve [V₂]

Zygomaticofacial nerve
(branch of maxillary nerve [V₂])

Lower head of
lateral pterygoid (cut)

Nerve to lateral pterygoid

Extension of
tendon of temporalis

Masseteric nerve

Lingual nerve

Buccal nerve

Incisive nerve

Mental nerve

Mylohyoid

Deep temporal nerves

Ophthalmic nerve [V₁]

Auriculotemporal nerve

Anterior trunk of
mandibular nerve [V₃]

Meningeal nerve

Middle meningeal artery

Posterior trunk of
mandibular nerve [V₃]

Chorda tympani nerve

Inferior alveolar nerve

Sphenomandibular
ligament

Nerve to mylohyoid

Mandibular canal

531

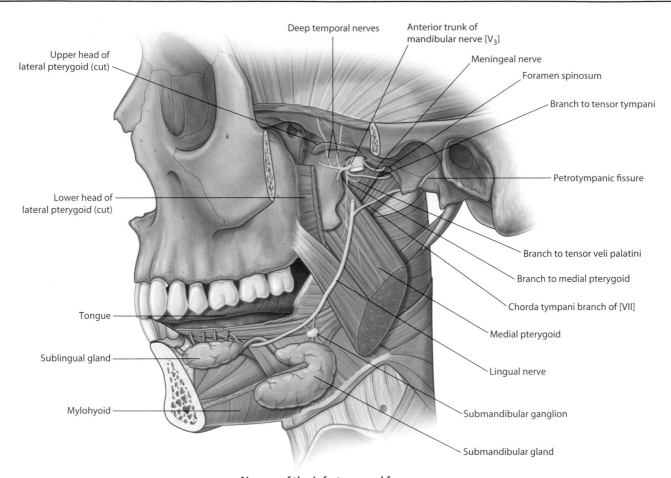

Nerves of the infratemporal fossa

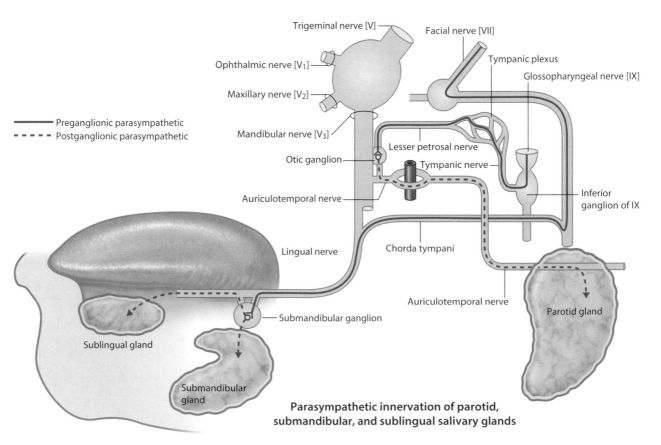

Parasympathetic innervation of parotid, submandibular, and sublingual salivary glands

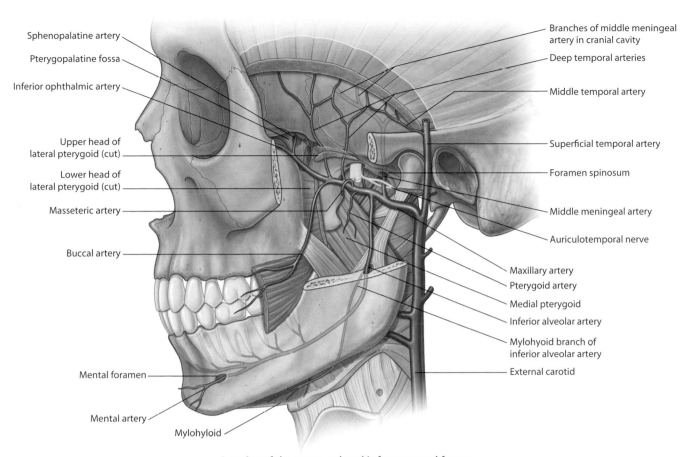

Sphenopalatine artery
Pterygopalatine fossa
Inferior ophthalmic artery
Upper head of lateral pterygoid (cut)
Lower head of lateral pterygoid (cut)
Masseteric artery
Buccal artery
Mental foramen
Mental artery
Mylohyoid

Branches of middle meningeal artery in cranial cavity
Deep temporal arteries
Middle temporal artery
Superficial temporal artery
Foramen spinosum
Middle meningeal artery
Auriculotemporal nerve
Maxillary artery
Pterygoid artery
Medial pterygoid
Inferior alveolar artery
Mylohyoid branch of inferior alveolar artery
External carotid

Arteries of the temporal and infratemporal fossae

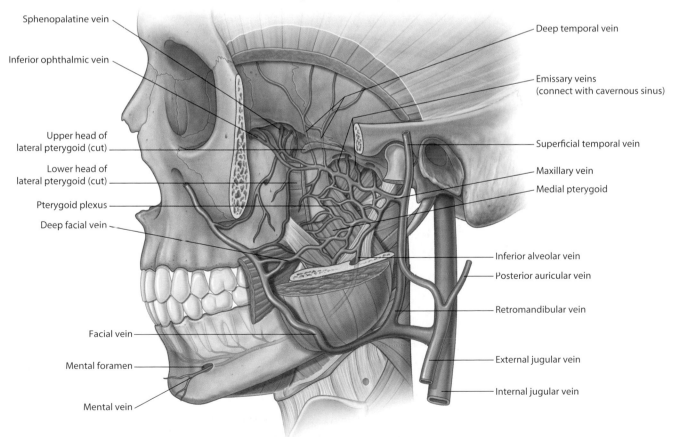

Sphenopalatine vein
Inferior ophthalmic vein
Upper head of lateral pterygoid (cut)
Lower head of lateral pterygoid (cut)
Pterygoid plexus
Deep facial vein
Facial vein
Mental foramen
Mental vein

Deep temporal vein
Emissary veins (connect with cavernous sinus)
Superficial temporal vein
Maxillary vein
Medial pterygoid
Inferior alveolar vein
Posterior auricular vein
Retromandibular vein
External jugular vein
Internal jugular vein

Veins of the temporal and infratemporal fossae

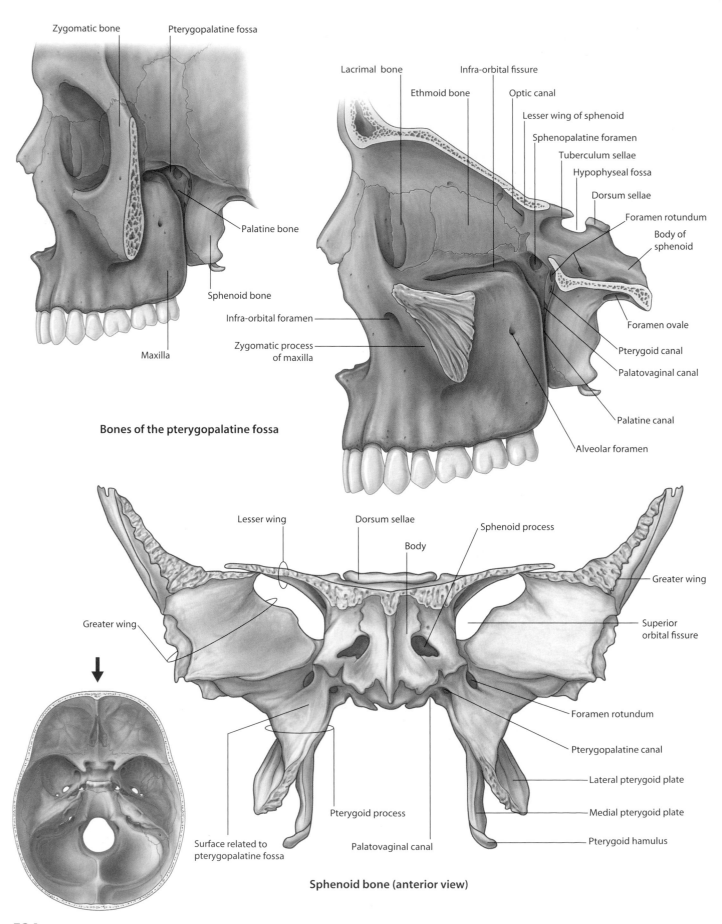

Zygomatic bone

Pterygopalatine fossa

Palatine bone

Sphenoid bone

Maxilla

Bones of the pterygopalatine fossa

Lacrimal bone

Ethmoid bone

Infra-orbital fissure

Optic canal

Lesser wing of sphenoid

Sphenopalatine foramen

Tuberculum sellae

Hypophyseal fossa

Dorsum sellae

Foramen rotundum

Body of sphenoid

Foramen ovale

Pterygoid canal

Palatovaginal canal

Palatine canal

Alveolar foramen

Infra-orbital foramen

Zygomatic process of maxilla

Lesser wing

Dorsum sellae

Body

Sphenoid process

Greater wing

Greater wing

Superior orbital fissure

Foramen rotundum

Pterygopalatine canal

Lateral pterygoid plate

Medial pterygoid plate

Pterygoid hamulus

Surface related to pterygopalatine fossa

Pterygoid process

Palatovaginal canal

Sphenoid bone (anterior view)

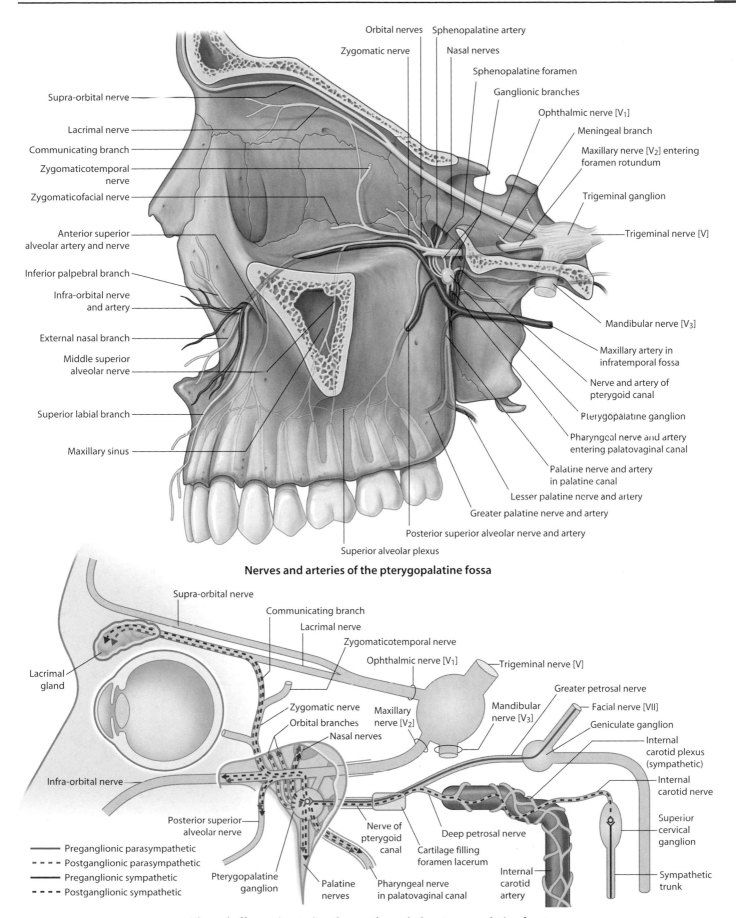

Nerves and arteries of the pterygopalatine fossa

Orbital nerves

Zygomatic nerve

Sphenopalatine artery

Nasal nerves

Sphenopalatine foramen

Ganglionic branches

Ophthalmic nerve [V₁]

Meningeal branch

Maxillary nerve [V₂] entering foramen rotundum

Trigeminal ganglion

Trigeminal nerve [V]

Supra-orbital nerve

Lacrimal nerve

Communicating branch

Zygomaticotemporal nerve

Zygomaticofacial nerve

Anterior superior alveolar artery and nerve

Inferior palpebral branch

Infra-orbital nerve and artery

External nasal branch

Middle superior alveolar nerve

Superior labial branch

Maxillary sinus

Mandibular nerve [V₃]

Maxillary artery in infratemporal fossa

Nerve and artery of pterygoid canal

Pterygopalatine ganglion

Pharyngeal nerve and artery entering palatovaginal canal

Palatine nerve and artery in palatine canal

Lesser palatine nerve and artery

Greater palatine nerve and artery

Posterior superior alveolar nerve and artery

Superior alveolar plexus

Visceral efferent (motor) pathways through the pterygopalatine fossa

Supra-orbital nerve

Communicating branch

Lacrimal nerve

Zygomaticotemporal nerve

Ophthalmic nerve [V₁]

Trigeminal nerve [V]

Greater petrosal nerve

Facial nerve [VII]

Geniculate ganglion

Internal carotid plexus (sympathetic)

Internal carotid nerve

Superior cervical ganglion

Sympathetic trunk

Lacrimal gland

Zygomatic nerve

Orbital branches

Nasal nerves

Maxillary nerve [V₂]

Mandibular nerve [V₃]

Infra-orbital nerve

Posterior superior alveolar nerve

Nerve of pterygoid canal

Cartilage filling foramen lacerum

Deep petrosal nerve

Internal carotid artery

Pterygopalatine ganglion

Palatine nerves

Pharyngeal nerve in palatovaginal canal

— Preganglionic parasympathetic
--- Postganglionic parasympathetic
— Preganglionic sympathetic
--- Postganglionic sympathetic

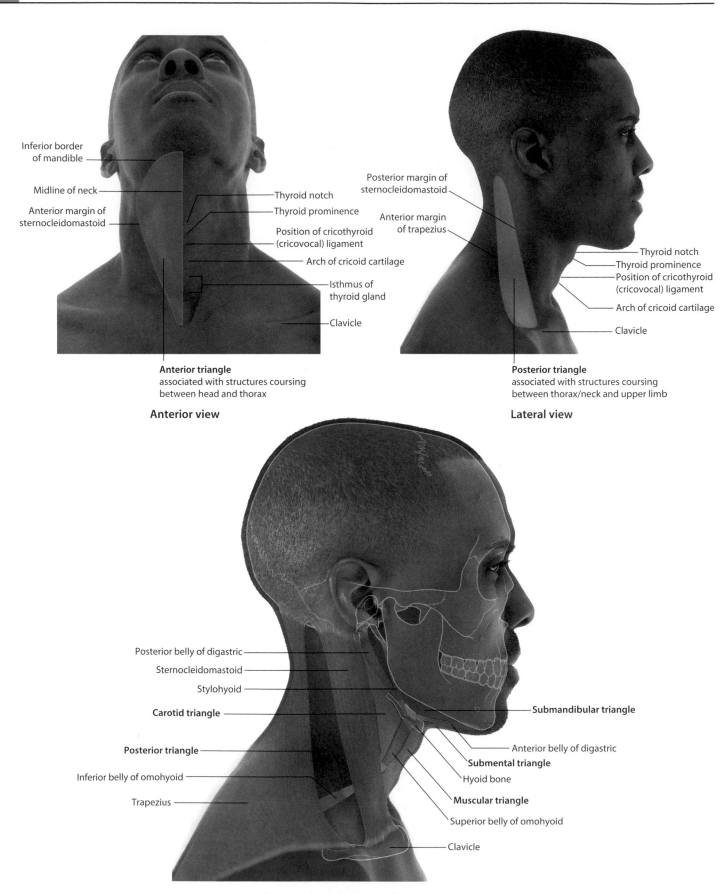

Inferior border of mandible

Midline of neck

Anterior margin of sternocleidomastoid

Thyroid notch

Thyroid prominence

Position of cricothyroid (cricovocal) ligament

Arch of cricoid cartilage

Isthmus of thyroid gland

Clavicle

Anterior triangle
associated with structures coursing between head and thorax

Anterior view

Posterior margin of sternocleidomastoid

Anterior margin of trapezius

Thyroid notch

Thyroid prominence

Position of cricothyroid (cricovocal) ligament

Arch of cricoid cartilage

Clavicle

Posterior triangle
associated with structures coursing between thorax/neck and upper limb

Lateral view

Posterior belly of digastric

Sternocleidomastoid

Stylohyoid

Carotid triangle

Posterior triangle

Inferior belly of omohyoid

Trapezius

Submandibular triangle

Anterior belly of digastric

Submental triangle

Hyoid bone

Muscular triangle

Superior belly of omohyoid

Clavicle

**Boundaries and subdivisions of the anterior triangle
and boundaries of the posterior triangle**

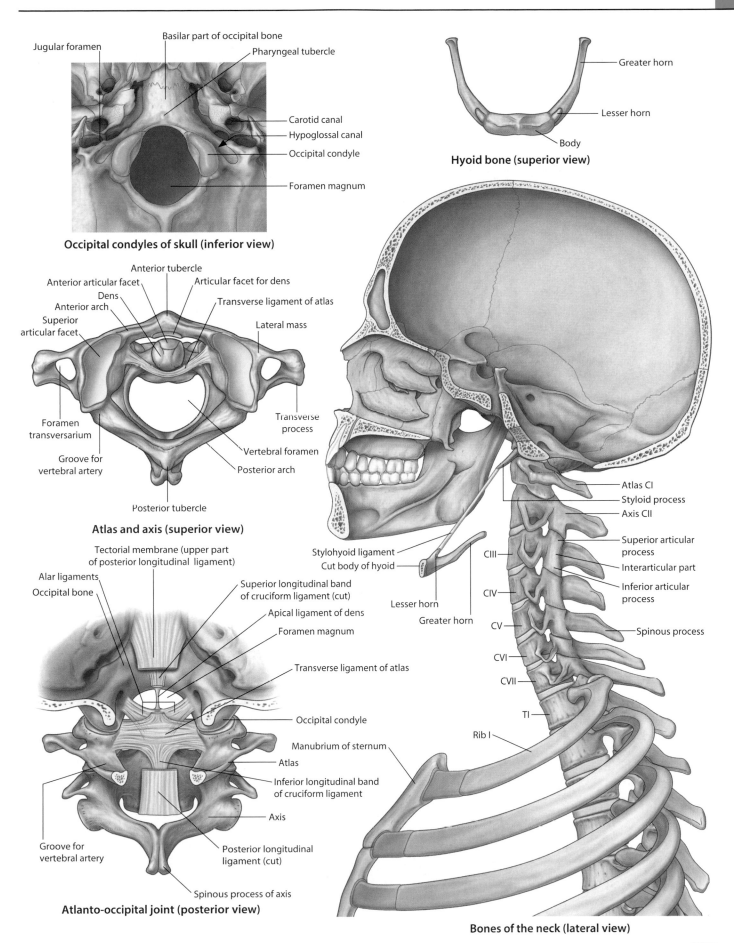

Jugular foramen

Basilar part of occipital bone

Pharyngeal tubercle

Carotid canal

Hypoglossal canal

Occipital condyle

Foramen magnum

Occipital condyles of skull (inferior view)

Greater horn

Lesser horn

Body

Hyoid bone (superior view)

Anterior tubercle

Anterior articular facet

Dens

Anterior arch

Superior articular facet

Articular facet for dens

Transverse ligament of atlas

Lateral mass

Foramen transversarium

Groove for vertebral artery

Transverse process

Vertebral foramen

Posterior arch

Posterior tubercle

Atlas and axis (superior view)

Tectorial membrane (upper part of posterior longitudinal ligament)

Alar ligaments

Occipital bone

Superior longitudinal band of cruciform ligament (cut)

Apical ligament of dens

Foramen magnum

Transverse ligament of atlas

Occipital condyle

Atlas

Inferior longitudinal band of cruciform ligament

Axis

Posterior longitudinal ligament (cut)

Groove for vertebral artery

Spinous process of axis

Atlanto-occipital joint (posterior view)

Atlas CI

Styloid process

Axis CII

Superior articular process

Interarticular part

Inferior articular process

Spinous process

Stylohyoid ligament

Cut body of hyoid

Lesser horn

Greater horn

CIII

CIV

CV

CVI

CVII

TI

Rib I

Manubrium of sternum

Bones of the neck (lateral view)

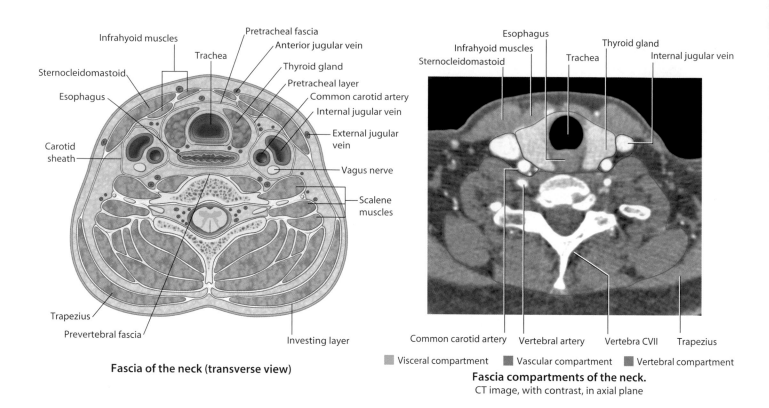

Infrahyoid muscles

Sternocleidomastoid

Esophagus

Carotid sheath

Trachea

Pretracheal fascia

Anterior jugular vein

Thyroid gland

Pretracheal layer

Common carotid artery

Internal jugular vein

External jugular vein

Vagus nerve

Scalene muscles

Trapezius

Prevertebral fascia

Investing layer

Fascia of the neck (transverse view)

Esophagus

Infrahyoid muscles

Sternocleidomastoid

Trachea

Thyroid gland

Internal jugular vein

Common carotid artery

Vertebral artery

Vertebra CVII

Trapezius

■ Visceral compartment   ■ Vascular compartment   ■ Vertebral compartment

Fascia compartments of the neck.
CT image, with contrast, in axial plane

Buccopharyngeal fascia
(posterior portion of
pretracheal layer)

Investing layer

Prevertebral layer

Trachea

Thyroid gland

Infrahyoid muscles

Pretracheal space

Suprasternal space

Pretracheal layer

Manubrium of sternum

Aorta

Investing layer

Retropharyngeal space

Esophagus

Fascial space within
prevertebral layer

Fascia of the neck (sagittal view)

538

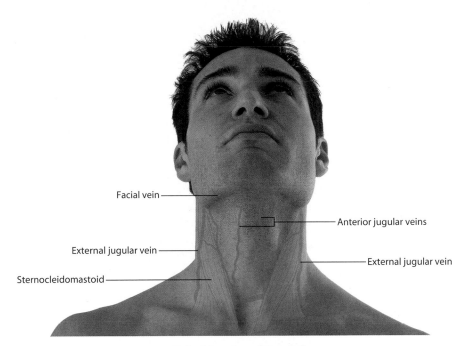

Facial vein

External jugular vein

Sternocleidomastoid

Anterior jugular veins

External jugular vein

**Palpable veins of the neck
(or visible)**

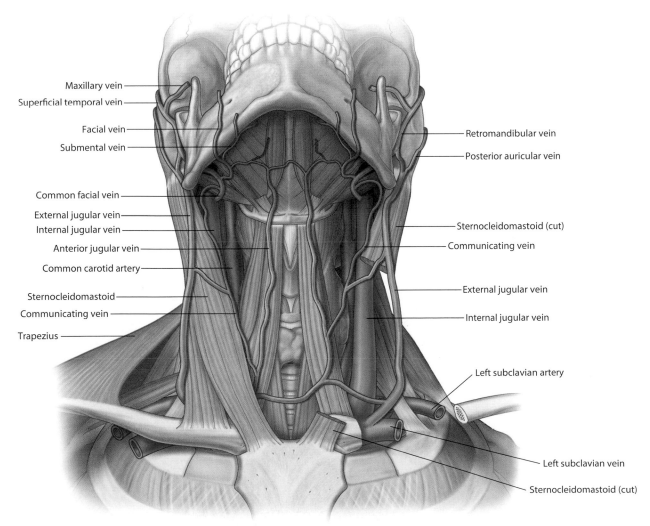

Maxillary vein

Superficial temporal vein

Facial vein

Submental vein

Common facial vein

External jugular vein

Internal jugular vein

Anterior jugular vein

Common carotid artery

Sternocleidomastoid

Communicating vein

Trapezius

Retromandibular vein

Posterior auricular vein

Sternocleidomastoid (cut)

Communicating vein

External jugular vein

Internal jugular vein

Left subclavian artery

Left subclavian vein

Sternocleidomastoid (cut)

Superficial veins of the neck

539

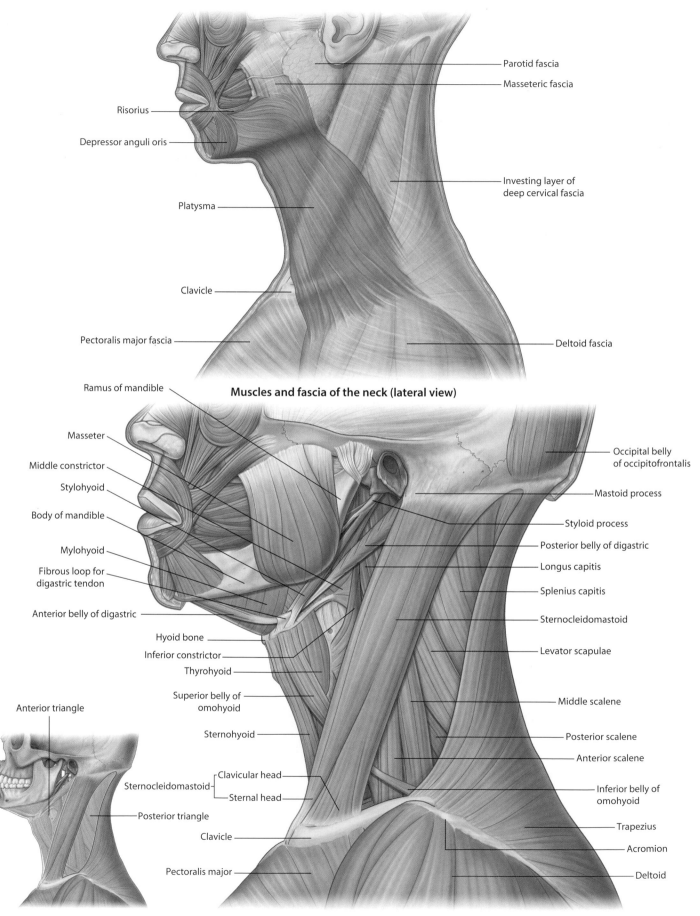

Muscles and fascia of the neck (lateral view)

Parotid fascia

Masseteric fascia

Risorius

Depressor anguli oris

Investing layer of
deep cervical fascia

Platysma

Clavicle

Pectoralis major fascia

Deltoid fascia

Ramus of mandible

Masseter

Middle constrictor

Stylohyoid

Body of mandible

Mylohyoid

Fibrous loop for
digastric tendon

Anterior belly of digastric

Hyoid bone

Inferior constrictor

Thyrohyoid

Superior belly of
omohyoid

Sternohyoid

Anterior triangle

Clavicular head

Sternocleidomastoid

Sternal head

Posterior triangle

Clavicle

Pectoralis major

Occipital belly
of occipitofrontalis

Mastoid process

Styloid process

Posterior belly of digastric

Longus capitis

Splenius capitis

Sternocleidomastoid

Levator scapulae

Middle scalene

Posterior scalene

Anterior scalene

Inferior belly of
omohyoid

Trapezius

Acromion

Deltoid

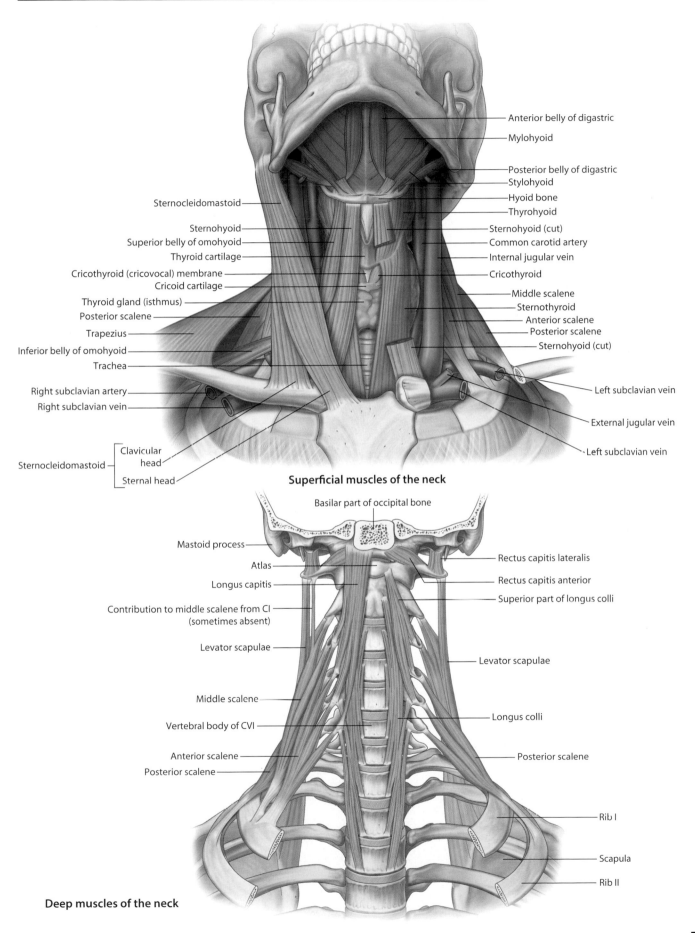

Anterior belly of digastric
Mylohyoid
Posterior belly of digastric
Stylohyoid
Hyoid bone
Thyrohyoid
Sternocleidomastoid
Sternohyoid
Superior belly of omohyoid
Thyroid cartilage
Cricothyroid (cricovocal) membrane
Cricoid cartilage
Thyroid gland (isthmus)
Posterior scalene
Trapezius
Inferior belly of omohyoid
Trachea
Right subclavian artery
Right subclavian vein
Sternohyoid (cut)
Common carotid artery
Internal jugular vein
Cricothyroid
Middle scalene
Sternothyroid
Anterior scalene
Posterior scalene
Sternohyoid (cut)
Left subclavian vein
External jugular vein
Left subclavian vein

Sternocleidomastoid — Clavicular head / Sternal head

Superficial muscles of the neck

Basilar part of occipital bone
Mastoid process
Atlas
Longus capitis
Contribution to middle scalene from CI (sometimes absent)
Levator scapulae
Middle scalene
Vertebral body of CVI
Anterior scalene
Posterior scalene
Rectus capitis lateralis
Rectus capitis anterior
Superior part of longus colli
Levator scapulae
Longus colli
Posterior scalene
Rib I
Scapula
Rib II

Deep muscles of the neck

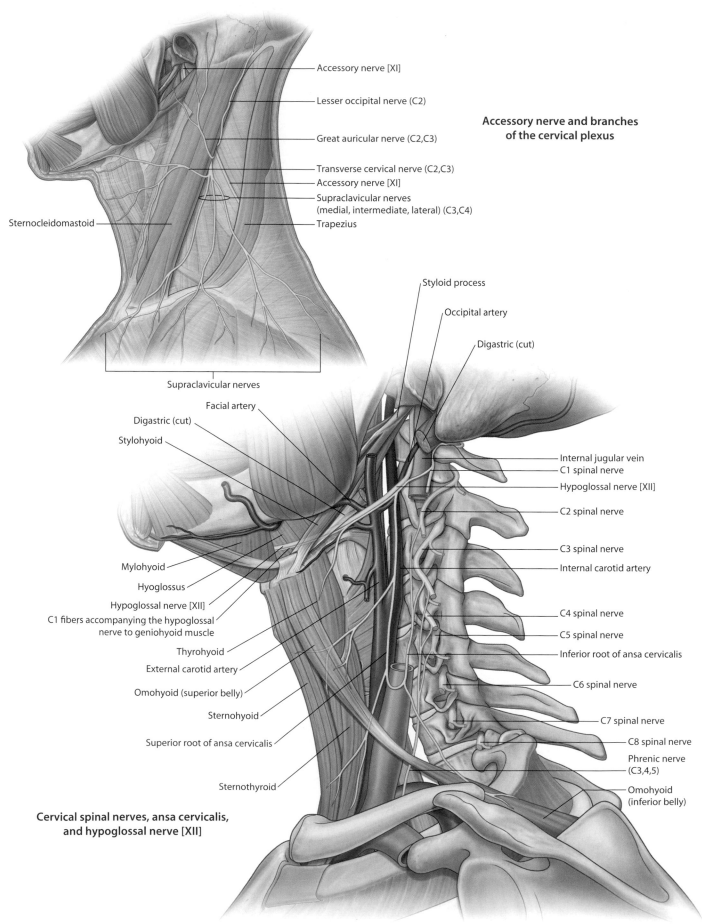

Accessory nerve [XI]

Lesser occipital nerve (C2)

Great auricular nerve (C2,C3)

Transverse cervical nerve (C2,C3)

Accessory nerve [XI]

Supraclavicular nerves
(medial, intermediate, lateral) (C3,C4)

Trapezius

Sternocleidomastoid

**Accessory nerve and branches
of the cervical plexus**

Supraclavicular nerves

Styloid process

Occipital artery

Digastric (cut)

Facial artery

Digastric (cut)

Stylohyoid

Internal jugular vein

C1 spinal nerve

Hypoglossal nerve [XII]

C2 spinal nerve

C3 spinal nerve

Internal carotid artery

Mylohyoid

Hyoglossus

Hypoglossal nerve [XII]

C1 fibers accompanying the hypoglossal
nerve to geniohyoid muscle

C4 spinal nerve

C5 spinal nerve

Thyrohyoid

Inferior root of ansa cervicalis

External carotid artery

C6 spinal nerve

Omohyoid (superior belly)

Sternohyoid

C7 spinal nerve

Superior root of ansa cervicalis

C8 spinal nerve

Phrenic nerve
(C3,4,5)

Omohyoid
(inferior belly)

Sternothyroid

**Cervical spinal nerves, ansa cervicalis,
and hypoglossal nerve [XII]**

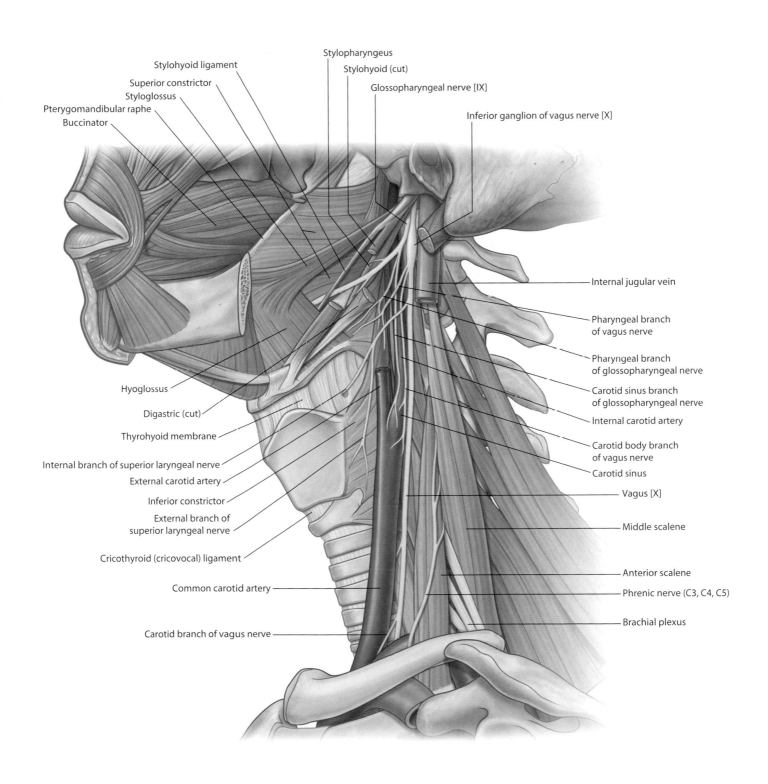

Stylohyoid ligament

Superior constrictor

Styloglossus

Pterygomandibular raphe

Buccinator

Stylopharyngeus

Stylohyoid (cut)

Glossopharyngeal nerve [IX]

Inferior ganglion of vagus nerve [X]

Internal jugular vein

Pharyngeal branch of vagus nerve

Pharyngeal branch of glossopharyngeal nerve

Carotid sinus branch of glossopharyngeal nerve

Internal carotid artery

Carotid body branch of vagus nerve

Carotid sinus

Vagus [X]

Middle scalene

Anterior scalene

Phrenic nerve (C3, C4, C5)

Brachial plexus

Hyoglossus

Digastric (cut)

Thyrohyoid membrane

Internal branch of superior laryngeal nerve

External carotid artery

Inferior constrictor

External branch of superior laryngeal nerve

Cricothyroid (cricovocal) ligament

Common carotid artery

Carotid branch of vagus nerve

Branches of glossopharyngeal [IX] and vagus nerves [X] in neck

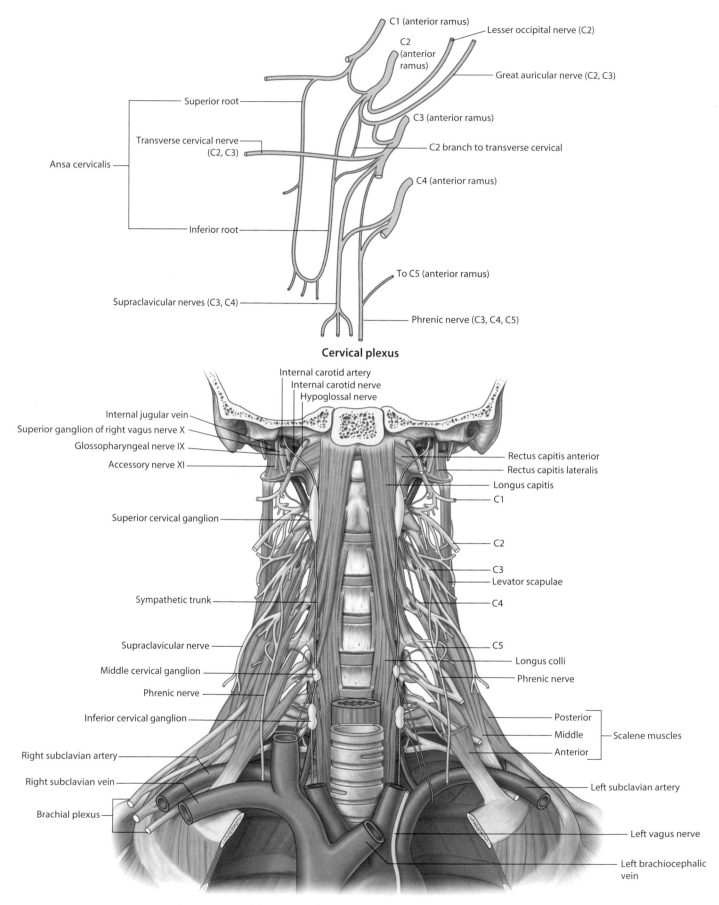

C1 (anterior ramus)

Lesser occipital nerve (C2)

C2 (anterior ramus)

Great auricular nerve (C2, C3)

Superior root

C3 (anterior ramus)

Transverse cervical nerve (C2, C3)

C2 branch to transverse cervical

Ansa cervicalis

C4 (anterior ramus)

Inferior root

To C5 (anterior ramus)

Supraclavicular nerves (C3, C4)

Phrenic nerve (C3, C4, C5)

Cervical plexus

Internal carotid artery
Internal carotid nerve
Hypoglossal nerve

Internal jugular vein

Superior ganglion of right vagus nerve X

Glossopharyngeal nerve IX

Accessory nerve XI

Rectus capitis anterior

Rectus capitis lateralis

Longus capitis

C1

Superior cervical ganglion

C2

C3

Levator scapulae

Sympathetic trunk

C4

Supraclavicular nerve

C5

Middle cervical ganglion

Longus colli

Phrenic nerve

Phrenic nerve

Inferior cervical ganglion

Posterior

Middle

Scalene muscles

Right subclavian artery

Anterior

Right subclavian vein

Left subclavian artery

Brachial plexus

Left vagus nerve

Left brachiocephalic vein

Components of the sympathetic nervous system in the root of the neck

544

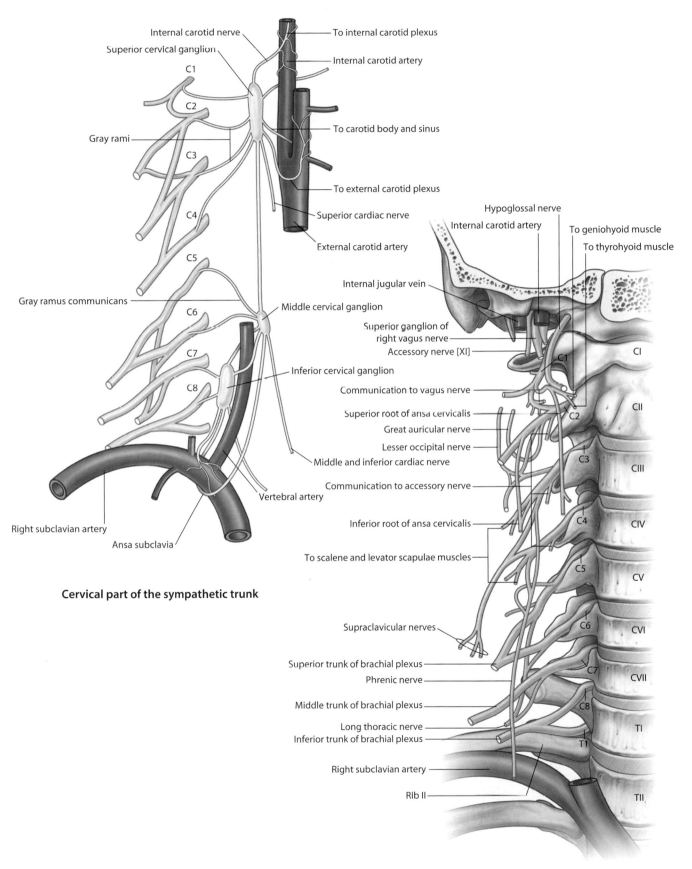

Cervical part of the sympathetic trunk

Internal carotid nerve
Superior cervical ganglion
C1
C2
Gray rami
C3
C4
C5
Gray ramus communicans
C6
C7
C8
Right subclavian artery
Ansa subclavia

To internal carotid plexus
Internal carotid artery
To carotid body and sinus
To external carotid plexus
Superior cardiac nerve
External carotid artery
Middle cervical ganglion
Inferior cervical ganglion
Middle and inferior cardiac nerve
Vertebral artery

Hypoglossal nerve
Internal carotid artery
To geniohyoid muscle
To thyrohyoid muscle
Internal jugular vein
Superior ganglion of right vagus nerve
Accessory nerve [XI]
Communication to vagus nerve
Superior root of ansa cervicalis
Great auricular nerve
Lesser occipital nerve
Communication to accessory nerve
Inferior root of ansa cervicalis
To scalene and levator scapulae muscles
Supraclavicular nerves
Superior trunk of brachial plexus
Phrenic nerve
Middle trunk of brachial plexus
Long thoracic nerve
Inferior trunk of brachial plexus
Right subclavian artery
Rib II

C1
C2
C3
C4
C5
C6
C7
C8
T1

CI
CII
CIII
CIV
CV
CVI
CVII
TI
TII

**Branches of the cervical plexus
(rib I removed)**

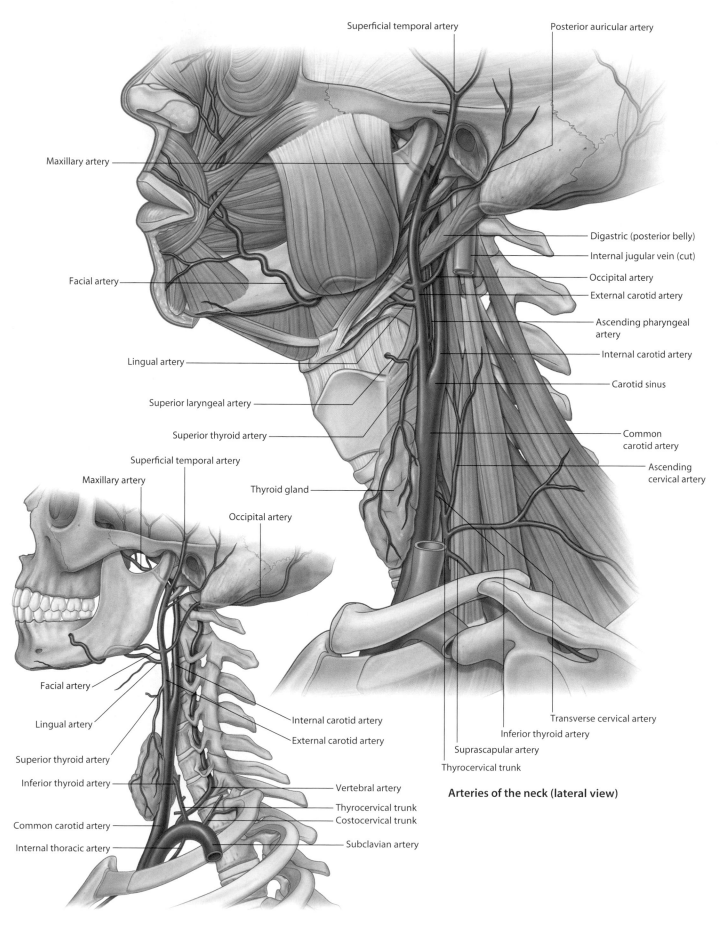

Superficial temporal artery

Posterior auricular artery

Maxillary artery

Facial artery

Lingual artery

Superior laryngeal artery

Superior thyroid artery

Superficial temporal artery

Maxillary artery

Occipital artery

Thyroid gland

Facial artery

Lingual artery

Superior thyroid artery

Inferior thyroid artery

Common carotid artery

Internal thoracic artery

Digastric (posterior belly)

Internal jugular vein (cut)

Occipital artery

External carotid artery

Ascending pharyngeal artery

Internal carotid artery

Carotid sinus

Common carotid artery

Ascending cervical artery

Transverse cervical artery

Inferior thyroid artery

Suprascapular artery

Thyrocervical trunk

Arteries of the neck (lateral view)

Internal carotid artery

External carotid artery

Vertebral artery

Thyrocervical trunk

Costocervical trunk

Subclavian artery

Facial artery   Maxillary artery   Superficial temporal artery   Occipital artery

Vertebral artery

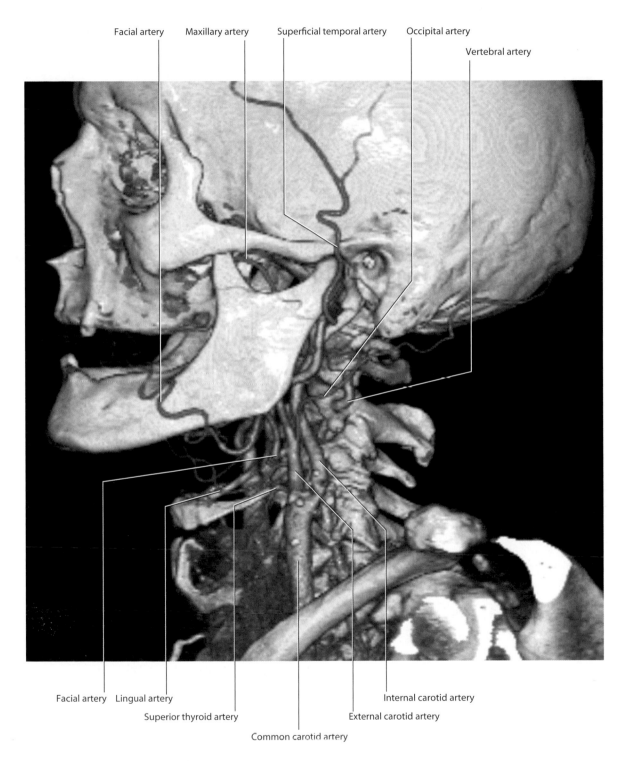

Facial artery   Lingual artery

Superior thyroid artery

Common carotid artery

Internal carotid artery

External carotid artery

Lateral view of the branches of the external carotid artery.
Volume-rendered angiographic image, with contrast, using multidetector CT

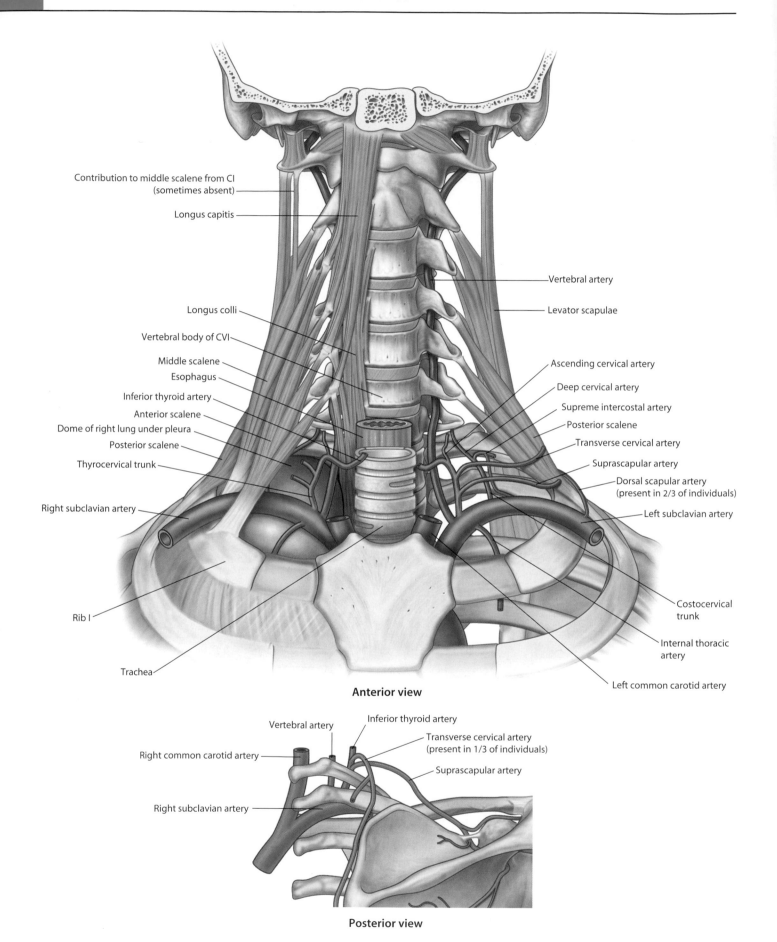

Contribution to middle scalene from CI (sometimes absent)

Longus capitis

Vertebral artery

Levator scapulae

Longus colli

Vertebral body of CVI

Ascending cervical artery

Middle scalene

Deep cervical artery

Esophagus

Supreme intercostal artery

Inferior thyroid artery

Posterior scalene

Anterior scalene

Transverse cervical artery

Dome of right lung under pleura

Suprascapular artery

Posterior scalene

Dorsal scapular artery (present in 2/3 of individuals)

Thyrocervical trunk

Left subclavian artery

Right subclavian artery

Costocervical trunk

Rib I

Internal thoracic artery

Trachea

Left common carotid artery

Anterior view

Vertebral artery

Inferior thyroid artery

Right common carotid artery

Transverse cervical artery (present in 1/3 of individuals)

Suprascapular artery

Right subclavian artery

Posterior view

548

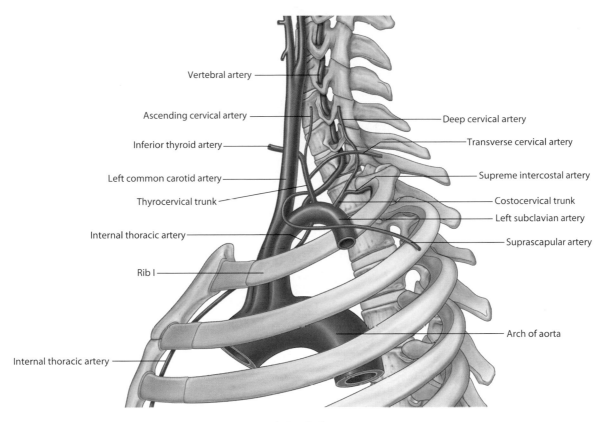

Vertebral artery

Ascending cervical artery

Inferior thyroid artery

Left common carotid artery

Thyrocervical trunk

Internal thoracic artery

Rib I

Internal thoracic artery

Deep cervical artery

Transverse cervical artery

Supreme intercostal artery

Costocervical trunk

Left subclavian artery

Suprascapular artery

Arch of aorta

Lateral view

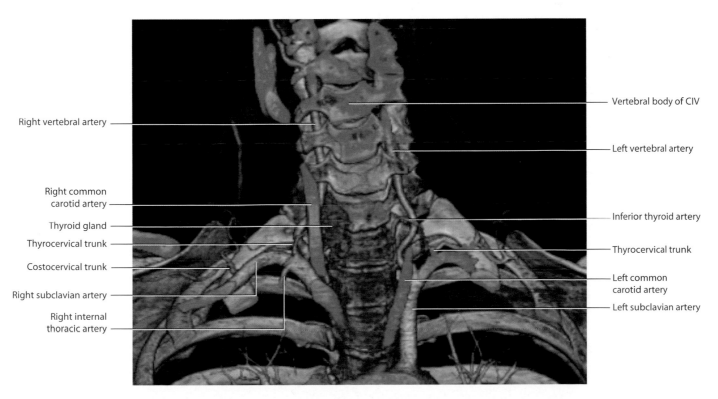

Right vertebral artery

Right common carotid artery

Thyroid gland

Thyrocervical trunk

Costocervical trunk

Right subclavian artery

Right internal thoracic artery

Vertebral body of CIV

Left vertebral artery

Inferior thyroid artery

Thyrocervical trunk

Left common carotid artery

Left subclavian artery

Anterior view of the root of the neck showing the branches of the subclavian arteries.
Volume-rendered angiographic image, with contrast, using multidetector CT

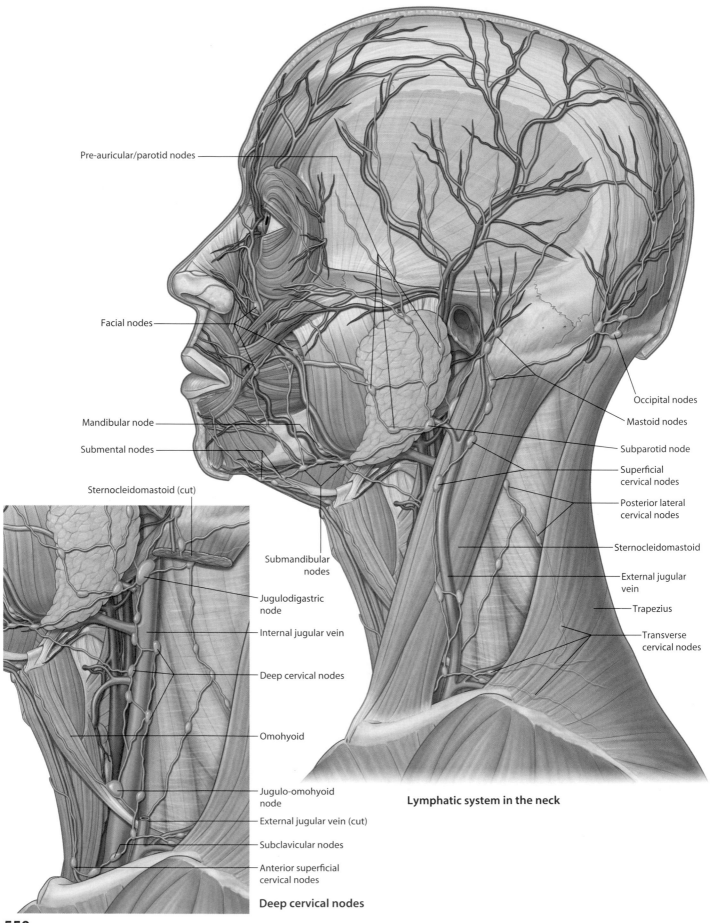

Pre-auricular/parotid nodes

Facial nodes

Mandibular node

Submental nodes

Sternocleidomastoid (cut)

Submandibular nodes

Jugulodigastric node

Internal jugular vein

Deep cervical nodes

Omohyoid

Jugulo-omohyoid node

External jugular vein (cut)

Subclavicular nodes

Anterior superficial cervical nodes

Deep cervical nodes

Occipital nodes

Mastoid nodes

Subparotid node

Superficial cervical nodes

Posterior lateral cervical nodes

Sternocleidomastoid

External jugular vein

Trapezius

Transverse cervical nodes

Lymphatic system in the neck

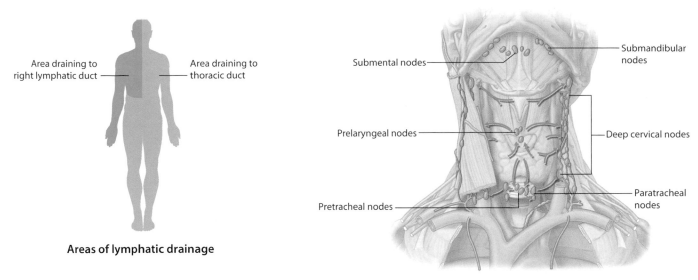

Areas of lymphatic drainage

Area draining to right lymphatic duct

Area draining to thoracic duct

Submental nodes

Submandibular nodes

Prelaryngeal nodes

Deep cervical nodes

Pretracheal nodes

Paratracheal nodes

Lymphatic drainage of the thyroid gland, larynx, and trachea

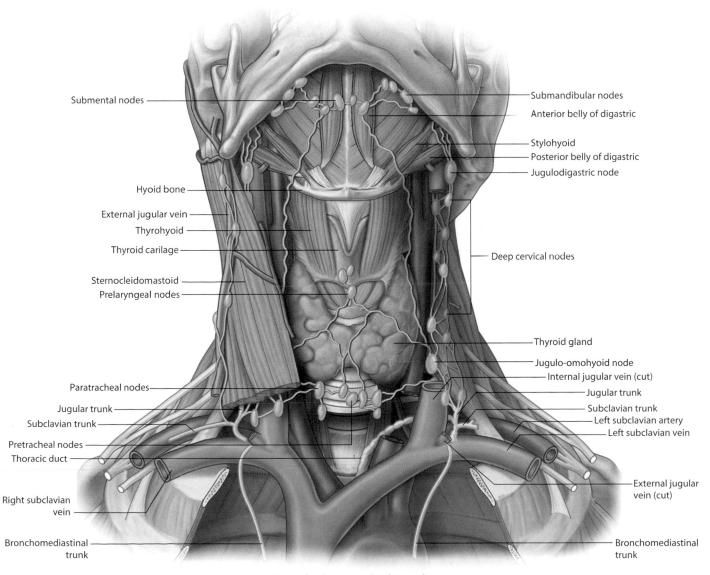

Submental nodes

Submandibular nodes
Anterior belly of digastric
Stylohyoid
Posterior belly of digastric
Jugulodigastric node

Hyoid bone
External jugular vein
Thyrohyoid
Thyroid carilage
Sternocleidomastoid
Prelaryngeal nodes

Deep cervical nodes

Thyroid gland
Jugulo-omohyoid node
Internal jugular vein (cut)
Jugular trunk
Subclavian trunk
Left subclavian artery
Left subclavian vein

Paratracheal nodes
Jugular trunk
Subclavian trunk
Pretracheal nodes
Thoracic duct

Right subclavian vein

External jugular vein (cut)

Bronchomediastinal trunk

Bronchomediastinal trunk

Lymphatic system in the neck

551

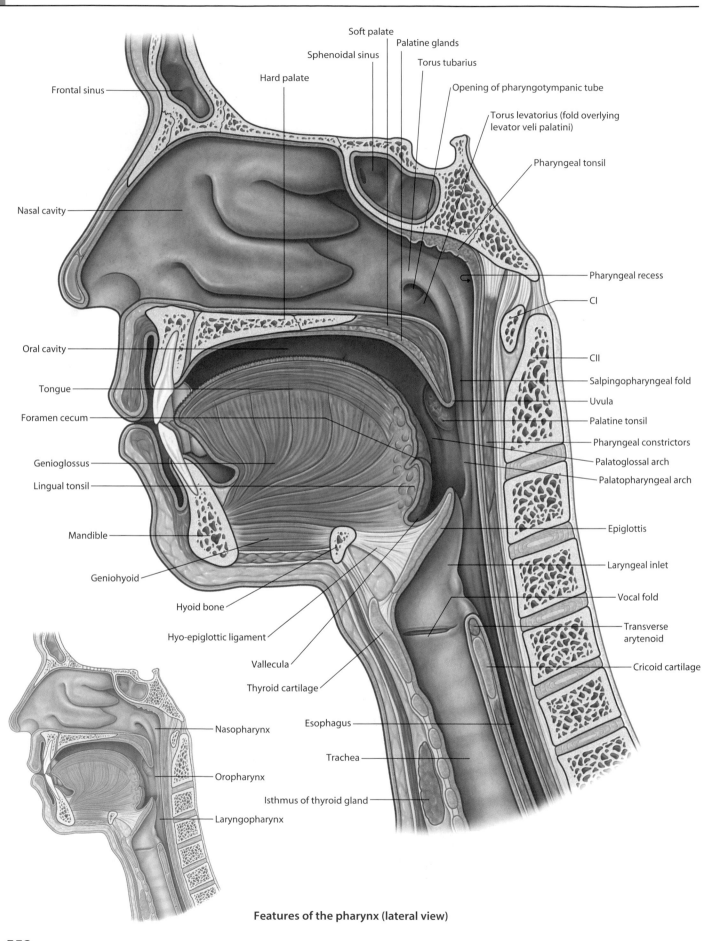

Soft palate

Sphenoidal sinus

Palatine glands

Torus tubarius

Hard palate

Opening of pharyngotympanic tube

Frontal sinus

Torus levatorius (fold overlying levator veli palatini)

Pharyngeal tonsil

Nasal cavity

Pharyngeal recess

CI

Oral cavity

CII

Tongue

Salpingopharyngeal fold

Foramen cecum

Uvula

Palatine tonsil

Genioglossus

Pharyngeal constrictors

Lingual tonsil

Palatoglossal arch

Palatopharyngeal arch

Mandible

Epiglottis

Geniohyoid

Laryngeal inlet

Vocal fold

Hyoid bone

Transverse arytenoid

Hyo-epiglottic ligament

Cricoid cartilage

Vallecula

Thyroid cartilage

Nasopharynx

Esophagus

Trachea

Oropharynx

Isthmus of thyroid gland

Laryngopharynx

Features of the pharynx (lateral view)

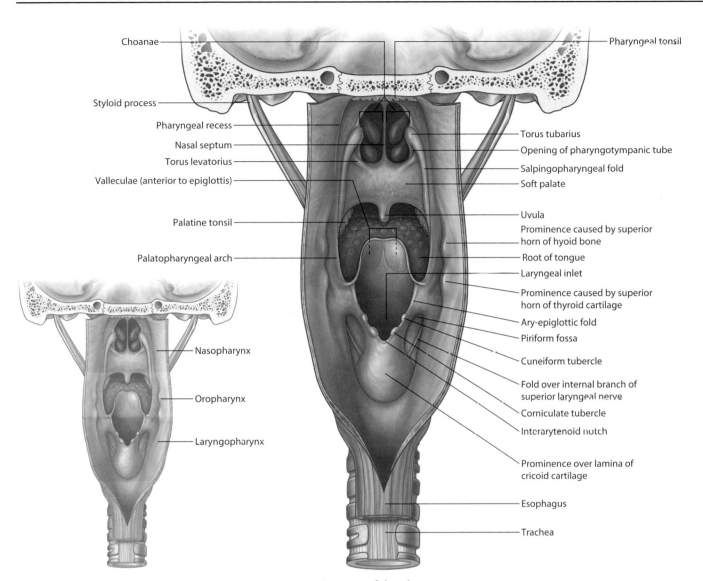

Choanae — — Pharyngeal tonsil

Styloid process —

Pharyngeal recess — — Torus tubarius

Nasal septum — — Opening of pharyngotympanic tube

Torus levatorius — — Salpingopharyngeal fold

Valleculae (anterior to epiglottis) — — Soft palate

— Uvula

Palatine tonsil — — Prominence caused by superior horn of hyoid bone

— Root of tongue

Palatopharyngeal arch — — Laryngeal inlet

— Prominence caused by superior horn of thyroid cartilage

— Ary-epiglottic fold

— Piriform fossa

— Cuneiform tubercle

— Fold over internal branch of superior laryngeal nerve

— Corniculate tubercle

— Interarytenoid notch

— Prominence over lamina of cricoid cartilage

— Esophagus

— Trachea

Nasopharynx

Oropharynx

Laryngopharynx

Features of the pharynx
(posterior view with the pharyngeal wall opened)

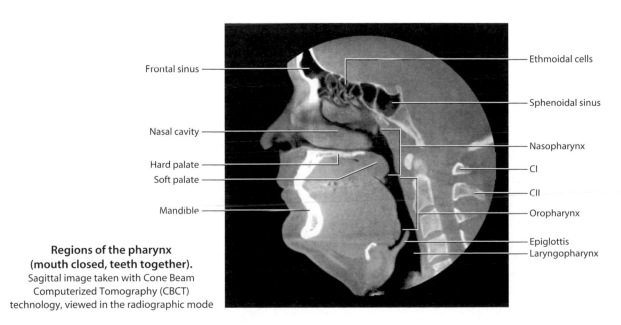

Frontal sinus — — Ethmoidal cells

— Sphenoidal sinus

Nasal cavity — — Nasopharynx

Hard palate — — CI

Soft palate — — CII

Mandible — — Oropharynx

— Epiglottis
— Laryngopharynx

Regions of the pharynx
(mouth closed, teeth together).
Sagittal image taken with Cone Beam
Computerized Tomography (CBCT)
technology, viewed in the radiographic mode

553

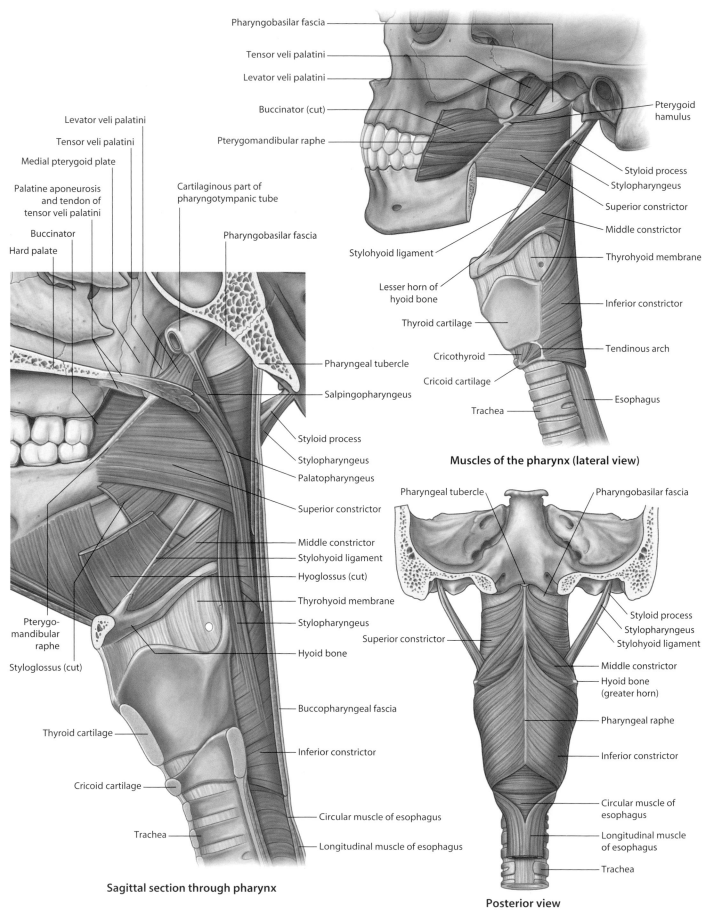

Pharyngobasilar fascia

Tensor veli palatini

Levator veli palatini

Buccinator (cut)

Pterygomandibular raphe

Pterygoid hamulus

Styloid process

Stylopharyngeus

Superior constrictor

Middle constrictor

Stylohyoid ligament

Thyrohyoid membrane

Lesser horn of hyoid bone

Inferior constrictor

Thyroid cartilage

Tendinous arch

Cricothyroid

Cricoid cartilage

Esophagus

Trachea

Muscles of the pharynx (lateral view)

Levator veli palatini

Tensor veli palatini

Medial pterygoid plate

Palatine aponeurosis and tendon of tensor veli palatini

Buccinator

Hard palate

Cartilaginous part of pharyngotympanic tube

Pharyngobasilar fascia

Pharyngeal tubercle

Salpingopharyngeus

Styloid process

Stylopharyngeus

Palatopharyngeus

Superior constrictor

Middle constrictor

Stylohyoid ligament

Hyoglossus (cut)

Thyrohyoid membrane

Stylopharyngeus

Hyoid bone

Pterygo-mandibular raphe

Styloglossus (cut)

Buccopharyngeal fascia

Thyroid cartilage

Inferior constrictor

Cricoid cartilage

Circular muscle of esophagus

Trachea

Longitudinal muscle of esophagus

Sagittal section through pharynx

Pharyngeal tubercle

Pharyngobasilar fascia

Styloid process

Stylopharyngeus

Stylohyoid ligament

Superior constrictor

Middle constrictor

Hyoid bone (greater horn)

Pharyngeal raphe

Inferior constrictor

Circular muscle of esophagus

Longitudinal muscle of esophagus

Trachea

Posterior view

554

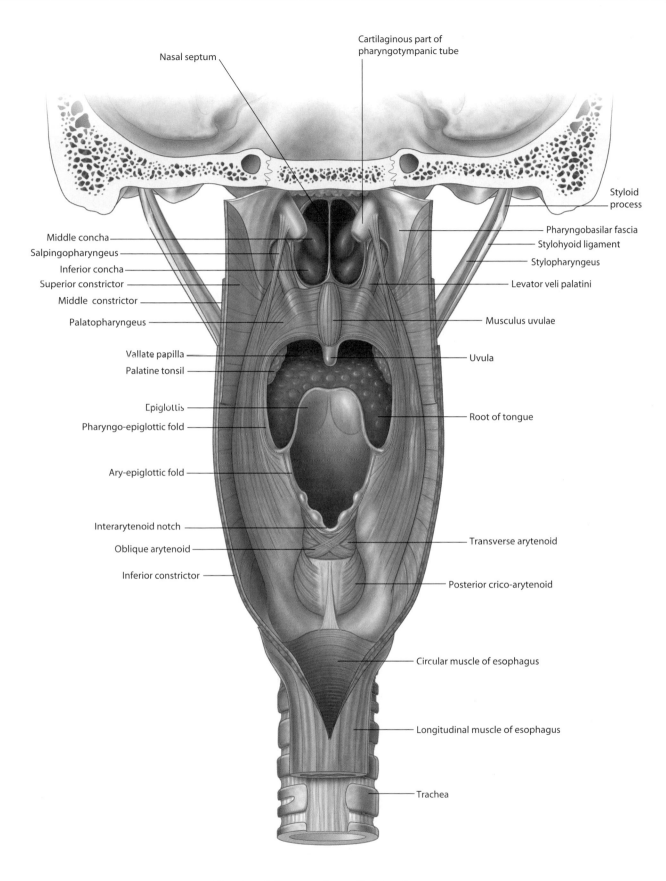

Nasal septum

Cartilaginous part of pharyngotympanic tube

Styloid process

Middle concha

Salpingopharyngeus

Inferior concha

Superior constrictor

Middle constrictor

Palatopharyngeus

Vallate papilla

Palatine tonsil

Epiglottis

Pharyngo-epiglottic fold

Ary-epiglottic fold

Interarytenoid notch

Oblique arytenoid

Inferior constrictor

Pharyngobasilar fascia

Stylohyoid ligament

Stylopharyngeus

Levator veli palatini

Musculus uvulae

Uvula

Root of tongue

Transverse arytenoid

Posterior crico-arytenoid

Circular muscle of esophagus

Longitudinal muscle of esophagus

Trachea

Muscles of the posterior wall of the pharynx

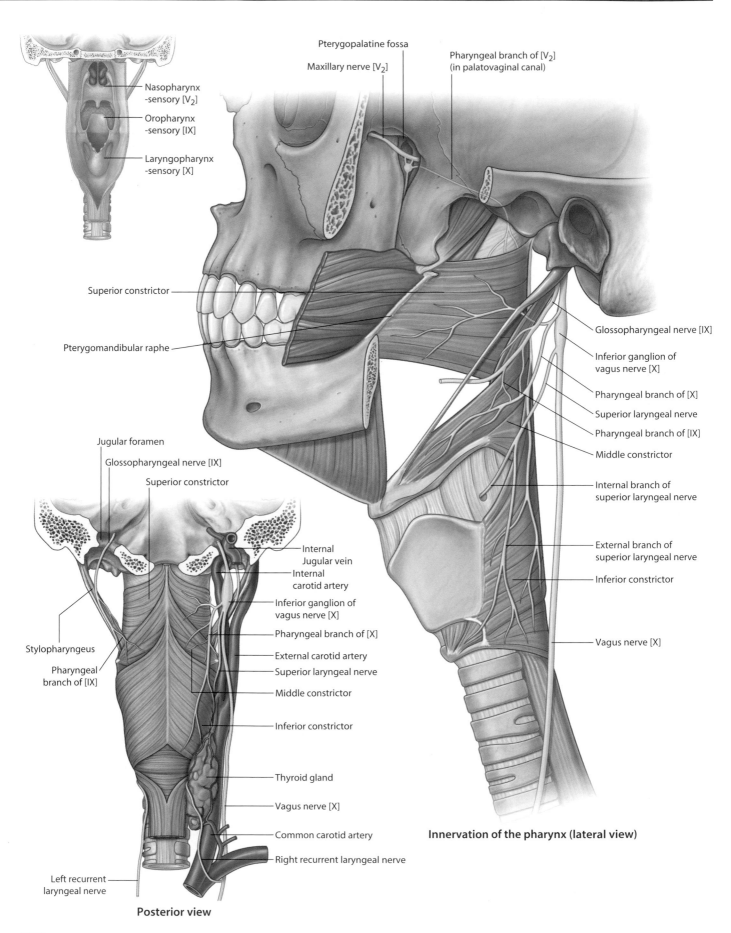

Nasopharynx -sensory [V$_2$]

Oropharynx -sensory [IX]

Laryngopharynx -sensory [X]

Pterygopalatine fossa

Maxillary nerve [V$_2$]

Pharyngeal branch of [V$_2$] (in palatovaginal canal)

Superior constrictor

Pterygomandibular raphe

Glossopharyngeal nerve [IX]

Inferior ganglion of vagus nerve [X]

Pharyngeal branch of [X]

Superior laryngeal nerve

Pharyngeal branch of [IX]

Middle constrictor

Internal branch of superior laryngeal nerve

External branch of superior laryngeal nerve

Inferior constrictor

Vagus nerve [X]

Jugular foramen

Glossopharyngeal nerve [IX]

Superior constrictor

Internal Jugular vein

Internal carotid artery

Inferior ganglion of vagus nerve [X]

Pharyngeal branch of [X]

External carotid artery

Superior laryngeal nerve

Middle constrictor

Stylopharyngeus

Pharyngeal branch of [IX]

Inferior constrictor

Thyroid gland

Vagus nerve [X]

Common carotid artery

Right recurrent laryngeal nerve

Left recurrent laryngeal nerve

Posterior view

Innervation of the pharynx (lateral view)

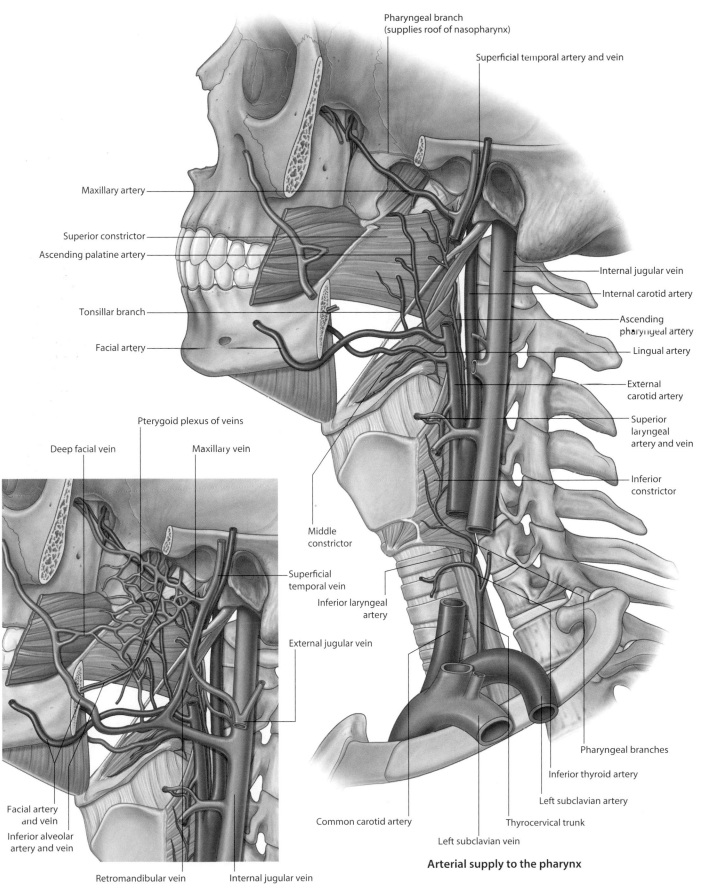

Pharyngeal branch (supplies roof of nasopharynx)

Superficial temporal artery and vein

Maxillary artery

Superior constrictor

Ascending palatine artery

Tonsillar branch

Facial artery

Internal jugular vein

Internal carotid artery

Ascending pharyngeal artery

Lingual artery

External carotid artery

Superior laryngeal artery and vein

Inferior constrictor

Pterygoid plexus of veins

Deep facial vein

Maxillary vein

Middle constrictor

Superficial temporal vein

Inferior laryngeal artery

External jugular vein

Facial artery and vein

Inferior alveolar artery and vein

Retromandibular vein

Internal jugular vein

Venous drainage of the pharynx

Common carotid artery

Left subclavian vein

Thyrocervical trunk

Inferior thyroid artery

Left subclavian artery

Pharyngeal branches

Arterial supply to the pharynx

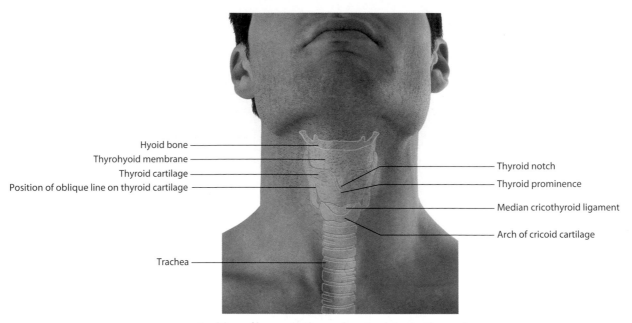

Position of larynx in the neck as it relates to the surface

Hyoid bone
Thyrohyoid membrane
Thyroid cartilage
Position of oblique line on thyroid cartilage
Thyroid notch
Thyroid prominence
Median cricothyroid ligament
Arch of cricoid cartilage
Trachea

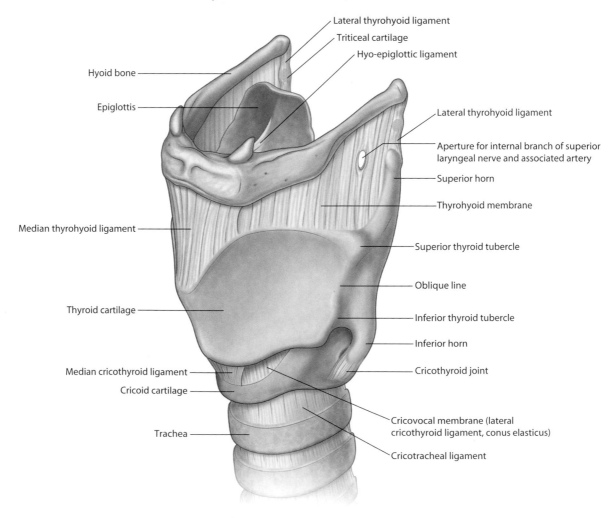

External features of the larynx (anterolateral view)

Lateral thyrohyoid ligament
Triticeal cartilage
Hyo-epiglottic ligament
Hyoid bone
Epiglottis
Lateral thyrohyoid ligament
Aperture for internal branch of superior laryngeal nerve and associated artery
Superior horn
Thyrohyoid membrane
Median thyrohyoid ligament
Superior thyroid tubercle
Oblique line
Inferior thyroid tubercle
Thyroid cartilage
Inferior horn
Cricothyroid joint
Median cricothyroid ligament
Cricoid cartilage
Cricovocal membrane (lateral cricothyroid ligament, conus elasticus)
Trachea
Cricotracheal ligament

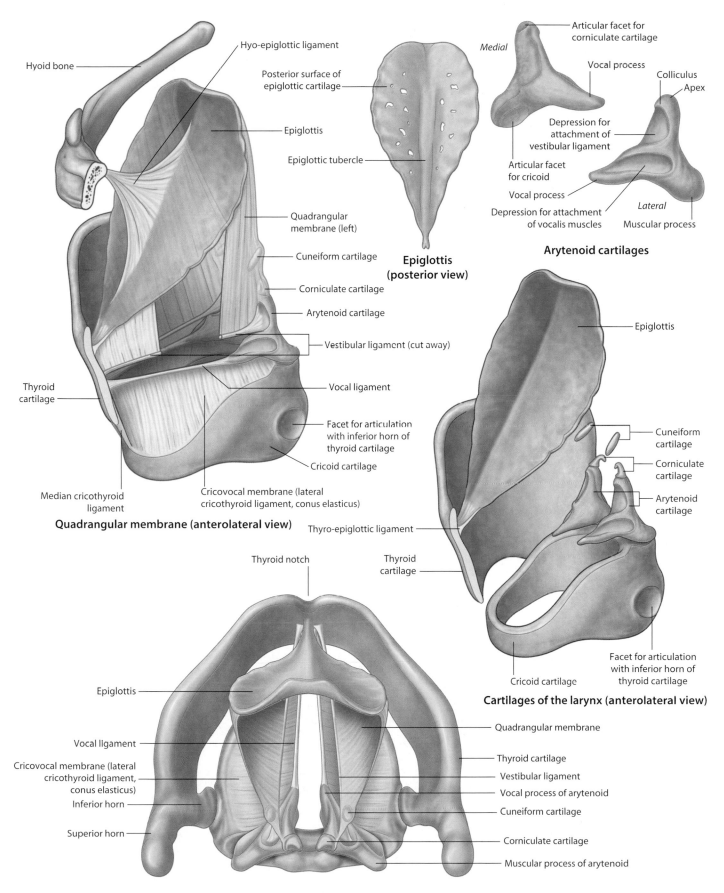

Hyoid bone

Hyo-epiglottic ligament

Posterior surface of epiglottic cartilage

Epiglottis

Epiglottic tubercle

Quadrangular membrane (left)

Cuneiform cartilage

Corniculate cartilage

Arytenoid cartilage

Vestibular ligament (cut away)

Vocal ligament

Facet for articulation with inferior horn of thyroid cartilage

Cricoid cartilage

Thyroid cartilage

Median cricothyroid ligament

Cricovocal membrane (lateral cricothyroid ligament, conus elasticus)

Quadrangular membrane (anterolateral view)

Epiglottis (posterior view)

Medial

Articular facet for corniculate cartilage

Vocal process

Colliculus

Apex

Depression for attachment of vestibular ligament

Articular facet for cricoid

Vocal process

Depression for attachment of vocalis muscles

Lateral

Muscular process

Arytenoid cartilages

Epiglottis

Cuneiform cartilage

Corniculate cartilage

Arytenoid cartilage

Thyro-epiglottic ligament

Thyroid cartilage

Cricoid cartilage

Facet for articulation with inferior horn of thyroid cartilage

Cartilages of the larynx (anterolateral view)

Thyroid notch

Epiglottis

Vocal ligament

Cricovocal membrane (lateral cricothyroid ligament, conus elasticus)

Inferior horn

Superior horn

Quadrangular membrane

Thyroid cartilage

Vestibular ligament

Vocal process of arytenoid

Cuneiform cartilage

Corniculate cartilage

Muscular process of arytenoid

Fibro-elastic membrane of the larynx (superior view)

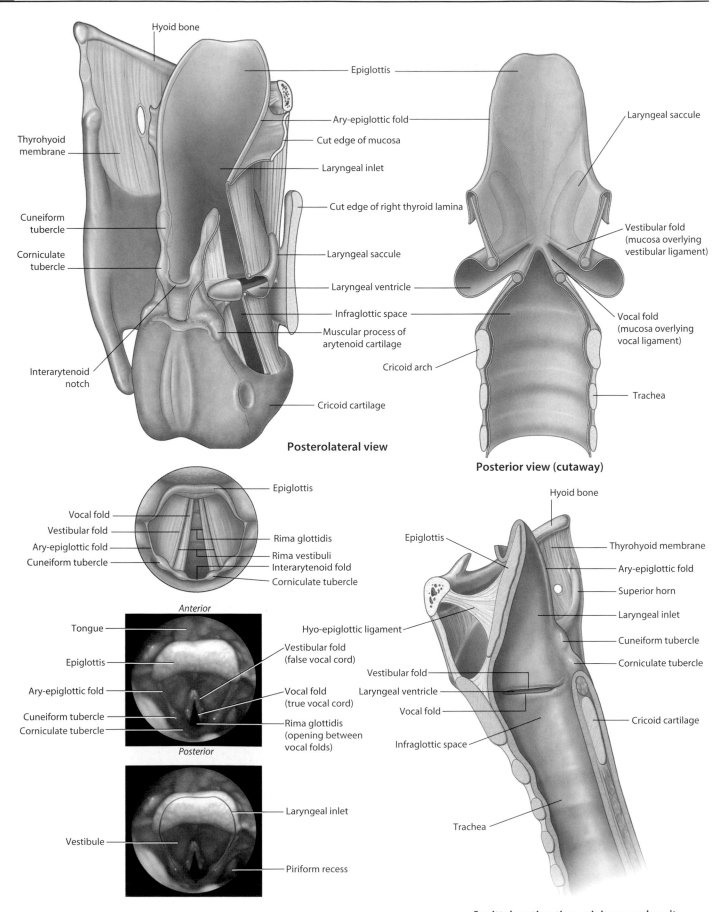

Hyoid bone

Epiglottis

Ary-epiglottic fold

Cut edge of mucosa

Thyrohyoid membrane

Laryngeal inlet

Cut edge of right thyroid lamina

Cuneiform tubercle

Corniculate tubercle

Laryngeal saccule

Laryngeal ventricle

Infraglottic space

Muscular process of arytenoid cartilage

Interarytenoid notch

Cricoid cartilage

Posterolateral view

Laryngeal saccule

Vestibular fold (mucosa overlying vestibular ligament)

Vocal fold (mucosa overlying vocal ligament)

Cricoid arch

Trachea

Posterior view (cutaway)

Epiglottis

Vocal fold

Vestibular fold

Ary-epiglottic fold

Cuneiform tubercle

Rima glottidis

Rima vestibuli

Interarytenoid fold

Corniculate tubercle

Anterior

Tongue

Epiglottis

Ary-epiglottic fold

Cuneiform tubercle

Corniculate tubercle

Vestibular fold (false vocal cord)

Vocal fold (true vocal cord)

Rima glottidis (opening between vocal folds)

Posterior

Vestibule

Laryngeal inlet

Piriform recess

Superior view through the laryngeal inlet

Hyoid bone

Epiglottis

Thyrohyoid membrane

Ary-epiglottic fold

Superior horn

Laryngeal inlet

Cuneiform tubercle

Corniculate tubercle

Hyo-epiglottic ligament

Vestibular fold

Laryngeal ventricle

Vocal fold

Infraglottic space

Cricoid cartilage

Trachea

Sagittal section through laryngeal cavity

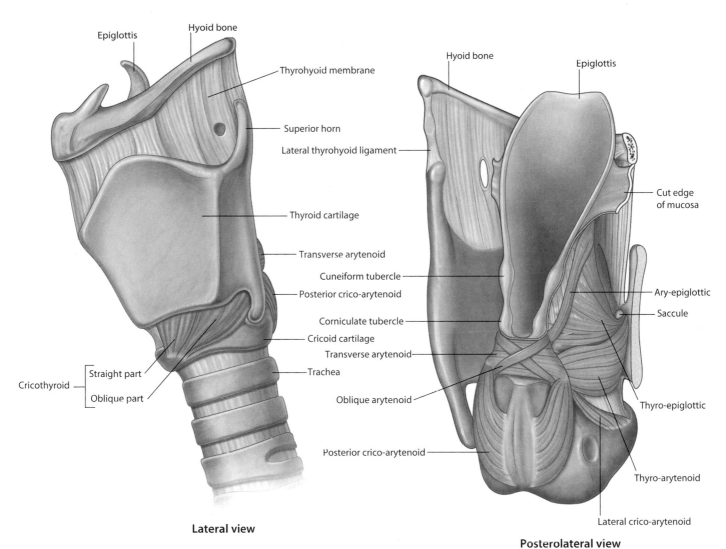

Epiglottis

Hyoid bone

Thyrohyoid membrane

Superior horn

Lateral thyrohyoid ligament

Thyroid cartilage

Transverse arytenoid

Cuneiform tubercle

Posterior crico-arytenoid

Corniculate tubercle

Cricoid cartilage

Transverse arytenoid

Trachea

Oblique arytenoid

Posterior crico-arytenoid

Cricothyroid
Straight part
Oblique part

Lateral view

Hyoid bone

Epiglottis

Cut edge of mucosa

Ary-epiglottic

Saccule

Thyro-epiglottic

Thyro-arytenoid

Lateral crico-arytenoid

Posterolateral view

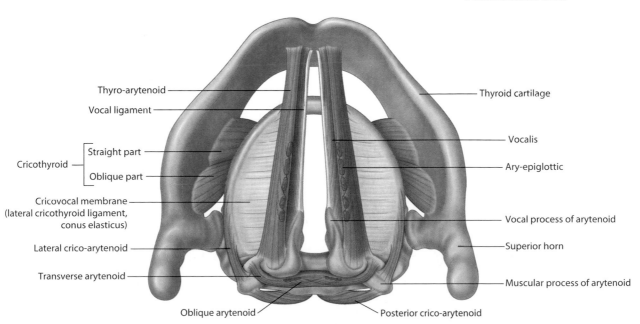

Thyro-arytenoid

Vocal ligament

Cricothyroid
Straight part
Oblique part

Cricovocal membrane
(lateral cricothyroid ligament,
conus elasticus)

Lateral crico-arytenoid

Transverse arytenoid

Oblique arytenoid

Posterior crico-arytenoid

Thyroid cartilage

Vocalis

Ary-epiglottic

Vocal process of arytenoid

Superior horn

Muscular process of arytenoid

Superior view

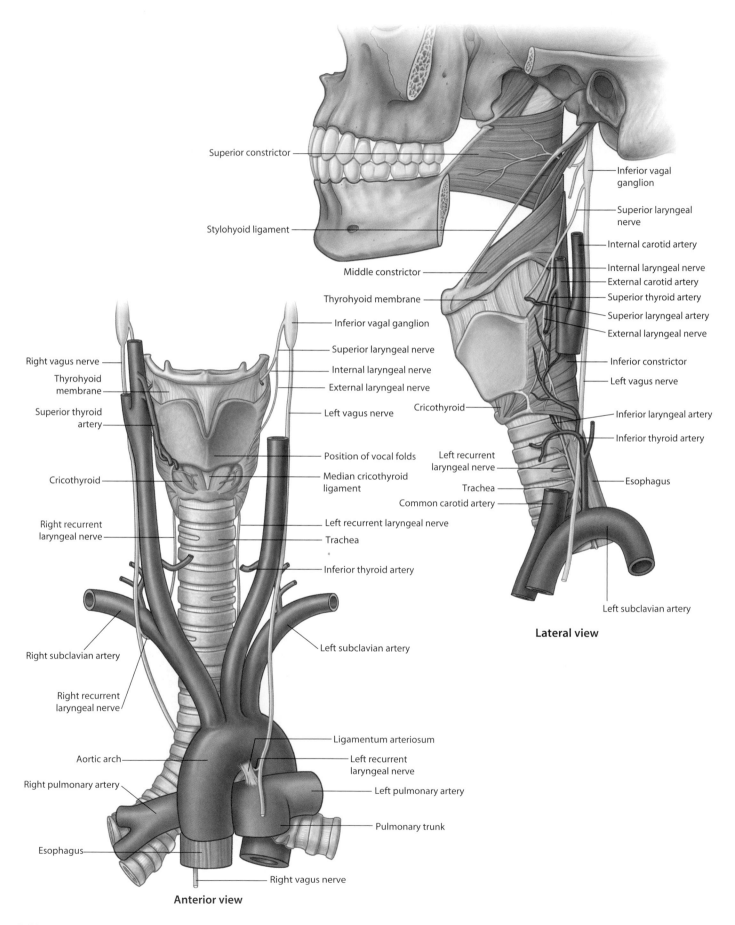

Superior constrictor

Stylohyoid ligament

Middle constrictor

Thyrohyoid membrane

Inferior vagal ganglion

Superior laryngeal nerve

Internal laryngeal nerve

External laryngeal nerve

Left vagus nerve

Position of vocal folds

Median cricothyroid ligament

Left recurrent laryngeal nerve

Trachea

Inferior thyroid artery

Inferior vagal ganglion

Superior laryngeal nerve

Internal carotid artery

Internal laryngeal nerve

External carotid artery

Superior thyroid artery

Superior laryngeal artery

External laryngeal nerve

Inferior constrictor

Left vagus nerve

Inferior laryngeal artery

Inferior thyroid artery

Esophagus

Cricothyroid

Left recurrent laryngeal nerve

Trachea

Common carotid artery

Left subclavian artery

Lateral view

Right vagus nerve

Thyrohyoid membrane

Superior thyroid artery

Cricothyroid

Right recurrent laryngeal nerve

Right subclavian artery

Right recurrent laryngeal nerve

Aortic arch

Right pulmonary artery

Esophagus

Left subclavian artery

Ligamentum arteriosum

Left recurrent laryngeal nerve

Left pulmonary artery

Pulmonary trunk

Right vagus nerve

Anterior view

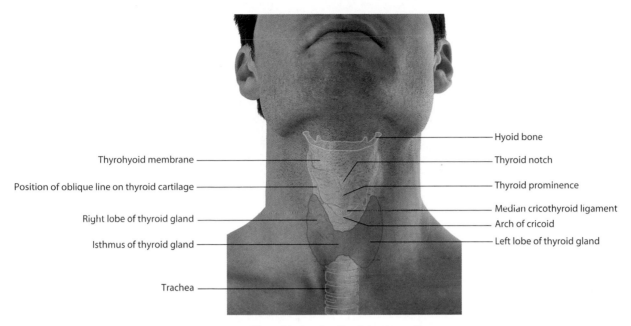

Hyoid bone

Thyrohyoid membrane

Thyroid notch

Position of oblique line on thyroid cartilage

Thyroid prominence

Median cricothyroid ligament

Right lobe of thyroid gland

Arch of cricoid

Isthmus of thyroid gland

Left lobe of thyroid gland

Trachea

Thyroid gland as it relates to surface

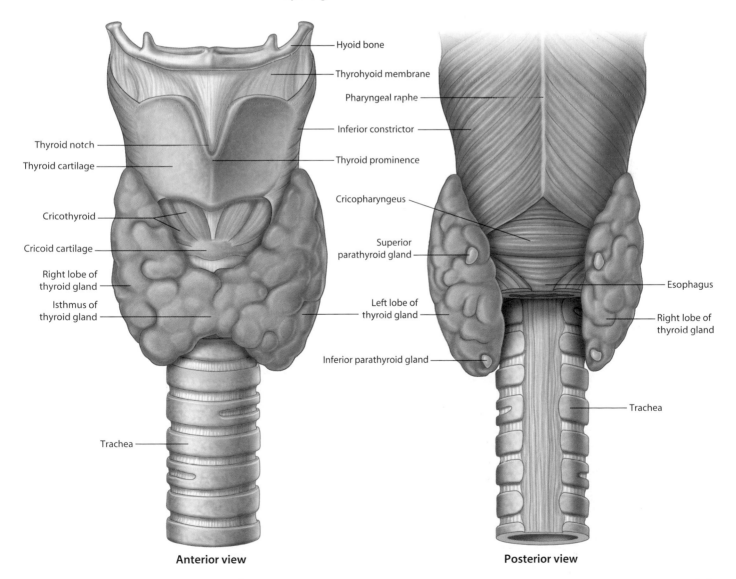

Hyoid bone

Thyrohyoid membrane

Pharyngeal raphe

Inferior constrictor

Thyroid notch

Thyroid cartilage

Thyroid prominence

Cricothyroid

Cricopharyngeus

Cricoid cartilage

Superior parathyroid gland

Right lobe of thyroid gland

Esophagus

Isthmus of thyroid gland

Left lobe of thyroid gland

Right lobe of thyroid gland

Trachea

Inferior parathyroid gland

Trachea

Anterior view

Posterior view

563

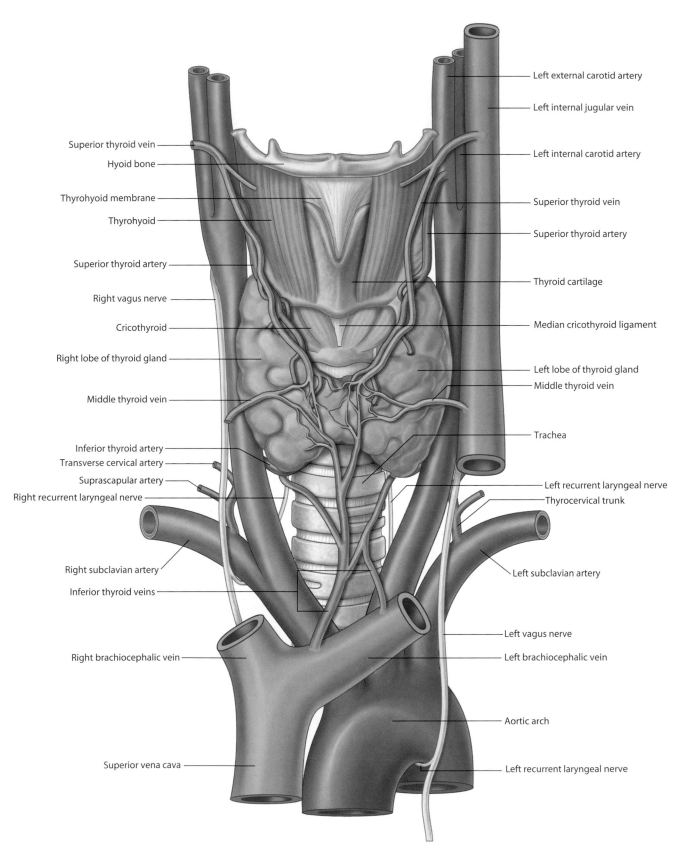

Superior thyroid vein

Hyoid bone

Thyrohyoid membrane

Thyrohyoid

Superior thyroid artery

Right vagus nerve

Cricothyroid

Right lobe of thyroid gland

Middle thyroid vein

Inferior thyroid artery

Transverse cervical artery

Suprascapular artery

Right recurrent laryngeal nerve

Right subclavian artery

Inferior thyroid veins

Right brachiocephalic vein

Superior vena cava

Left external carotid artery

Left internal jugular vein

Left internal carotid artery

Superior thyroid vein

Superior thyroid artery

Thyroid cartilage

Median cricothyroid ligament

Left lobe of thyroid gland

Middle thyroid vein

Trachea

Left recurrent laryngeal nerve

Thyrocervical trunk

Left subclavian artery

Left vagus nerve

Left brachiocephalic vein

Aortic arch

Left recurrent laryngeal nerve

Anterior view

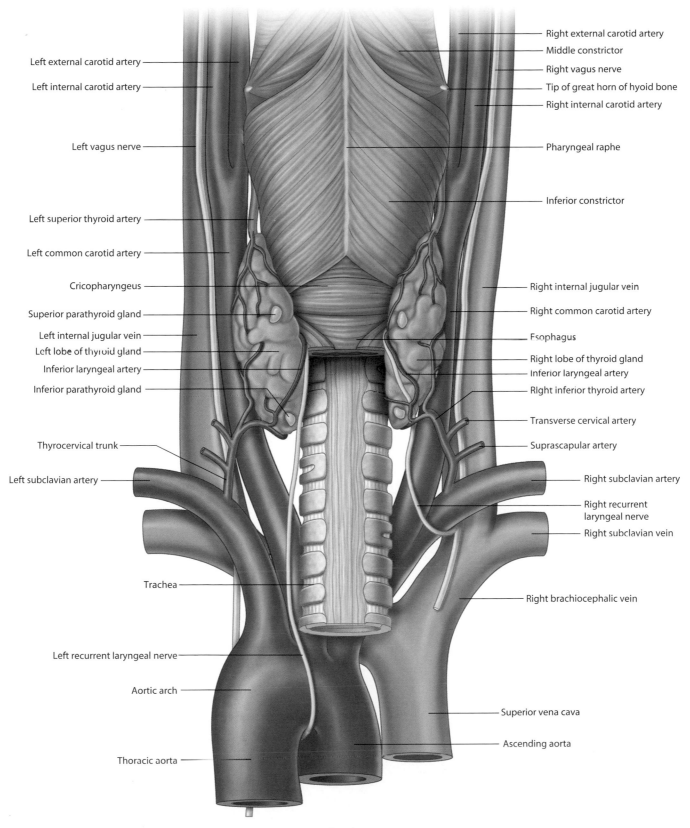

Left external carotid artery

Left internal carotid artery

Left vagus nerve

Left superior thyroid artery

Left common carotid artery

Cricopharyngeus

Superior parathyroid gland

Left internal jugular vein

Left lobe of thyroid gland

Inferior laryngeal artery

Inferior parathyroid gland

Thyrocervical trunk

Left subclavian artery

Trachea

Left recurrent laryngeal nerve

Aortic arch

Thoracic aorta

Right external carotid artery

Middle constrictor

Right vagus nerve

Tip of great horn of hyoid bone

Right internal carotid artery

Pharyngeal raphe

Inferior constrictor

Right internal jugular vein

Right common carotid artery

Esophagus

Right lobe of thyroid gland

Inferior laryngeal artery

Right inferior thyroid artery

Transverse cervical artery

Suprascapular artery

Right subclavian artery

Right recurrent laryngeal nerve

Right subclavian vein

Right brachiocephalic vein

Superior vena cava

Ascending aorta

Posterior view

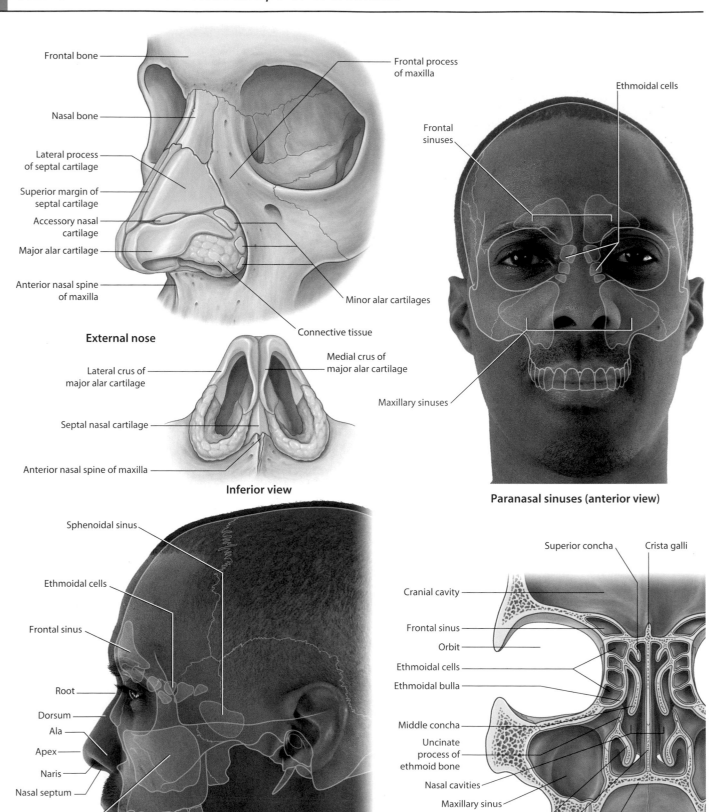

Frontal bone

Nasal bone

Lateral process of septal cartilage

Superior margin of septal cartilage

Accessory nasal cartilage

Major alar cartilage

Anterior nasal spine of maxilla

Frontal process of maxilla

Minor alar cartilages

Connective tissue

External nose

Lateral crus of major alar cartilage

Medial crus of major alar cartilage

Septal nasal cartilage

Anterior nasal spine of maxilla

Inferior view

Ethmoidal cells

Frontal sinuses

Maxillary sinuses

Paranasal sinuses (anterior view)

Sphenoidal sinus

Ethmoidal cells

Frontal sinus

Root

Dorsum

Ala

Apex

Naris

Nasal septum

Maxillary sinus

Surface anatomy of nose and paranasal sinuses (lateral view)

Superior concha

Crista galli

Cranial cavity

Frontal sinus

Orbit

Ethmoidal cells

Ethmoidal bulla

Middle concha

Uncinate process of ethmoid bone

Nasal cavities

Maxillary sinus

Inferior concha

Vomer

Palatine process of maxillary bone

Oral cavity

Coronal section through nasal cavity (posterior view)

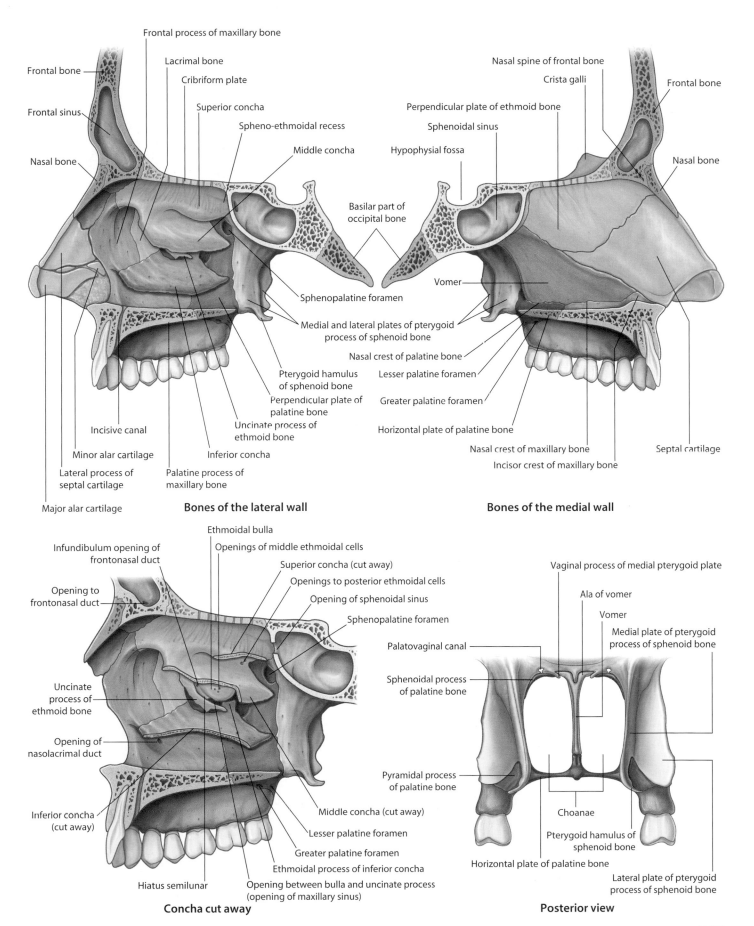

Frontal process of maxillary bone

Lacrimal bone

Frontal bone

Cribriform plate

Frontal sinus

Superior concha

Spheno-ethmoidal recess

Nasal bone

Middle concha

Nasal spine of frontal bone

Crista galli

Frontal bone

Perpendicular plate of ethmoid bone

Sphenoidal sinus

Hypophysial fossa

Nasal bone

Basilar part of occipital bone

Sphenopalatine foramen

Vomer

Medial and lateral plates of pterygoid process of sphenoid bone

Nasal crest of palatine bone

Lesser palatine foramen

Greater palatine foramen

Horizontal plate of palatine bone

Nasal crest of maxillary bone

Incisor crest of maxillary bone

Septal cartilage

Pterygoid hamulus of sphenoid bone

Perpendicular plate of palatine bone

Uncinate process of ethmoid bone

Inferior concha

Incisive canal

Minor alar cartilage

Lateral process of septal cartilage

Palatine process of maxillary bone

Major alar cartilage

Bones of the lateral wall

Bones of the medial wall

Infundibulum opening of frontonasal duct

Ethmoidal bulla

Openings of middle ethmoidal cells

Superior concha (cut away)

Opening to frontonasal duct

Openings to posterior ethmoidal cells

Opening of sphenoidal sinus

Sphenopalatine foramen

Vaginal process of medial pterygoid plate

Ala of vomer

Vomer

Medial plate of pterygoid process of sphenoid bone

Palatovaginal canal

Sphenoidal process of palatine bone

Uncinate process of ethmoid bone

Opening of nasolacrimal duct

Pyramidal process of palatine bone

Inferior concha (cut away)

Middle concha (cut away)

Lesser palatine foramen

Greater palatine foramen

Ethmoidal process of inferior concha

Opening between bulla and uncinate process (opening of maxillary sinus)

Hiatus semilunar

Choanae

Pterygoid hamulus of sphenoid bone

Horizontal plate of palatine bone

Lateral plate of pterygoid process of sphenoid bone

Concha cut away

Posterior view

567

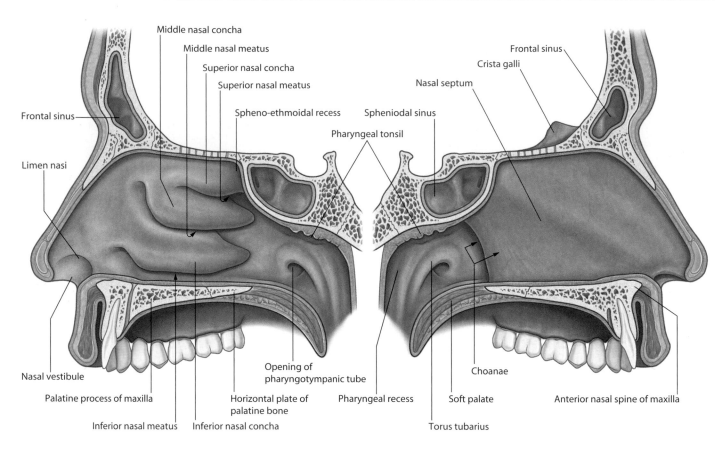

Frontal sinus

Limen nasi

Nasal vestibule

Palatine process of maxilla

Inferior nasal meatus

Middle nasal concha

Middle nasal meatus

Superior nasal concha

Superior nasal meatus

Spheno-ethmoidal recess

Spheniodal sinus

Pharyngeal tonsil

Opening of pharyngotympanic tube

Horizontal plate of palatine bone

Inferior nasal concha

Pharyngeal recess

Lateral wall of the nasal cavity

Frontal sinus

Crista galli

Nasal septum

Choanae

Soft palate

Torus tubarius

Anterior nasal spine of maxilla

Medial wall of the nasal cavity

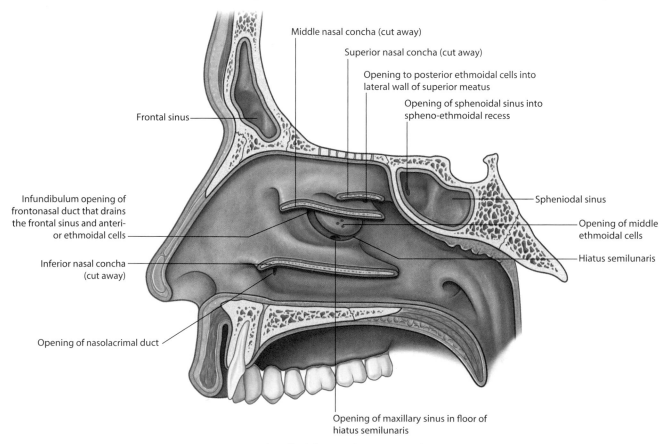

Frontal sinus

Infundibulum opening of frontonasal duct that drains the frontal sinus and anteri-or ethmoidal cells

Inferior nasal concha (cut away)

Opening of nasolacrimal duct

Middle nasal concha (cut away)

Superior nasal concha (cut away)

Opening to posterior ethmoidal cells into lateral wall of superior meatus

Opening of sphenoidal sinus into spheno-ethmoidal recess

Spheniodal sinus

Opening of middle ethmoidal cells

Hiatus semilunaris

Opening of maxillary sinus in floor of hiatus semilunaris

Lateral wall of the nasal cavity, concha cut away

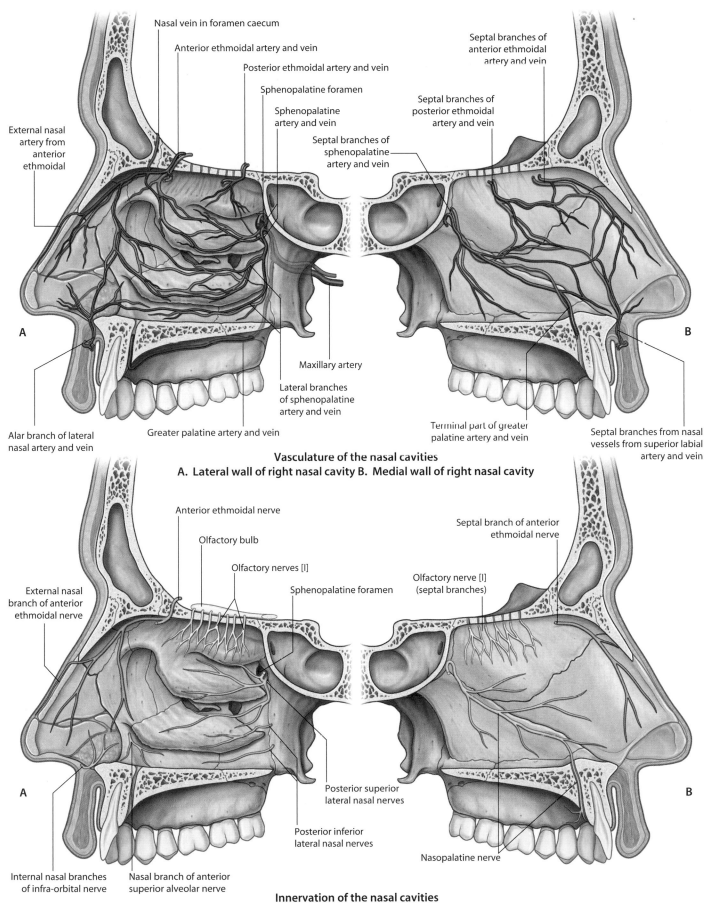

Nasal vein in foramen caecum

Anterior ethmoidal artery and vein

Posterior ethmoidal artery and vein

Sphenopalatine foramen

Sphenopalatine artery and vein

Septal branches of sphenopalatine artery and vein

Septal branches of anterior ethmoidal artery and vein

Septal branches of posterior ethmoidal artery and vein

External nasal artery from anterior ethmoidal

A

B

Maxillary artery

Lateral branches of sphenopalatine artery and vein

Greater palatine artery and vein

Terminal part of greater palatine artery and vein

Septal branches from nasal vessels from superior labial artery and vein

Alar branch of lateral nasal artery and vein

Vasculature of the nasal cavities
A. Lateral wall of right nasal cavity B. Medial wall of right nasal cavity

Anterior ethmoidal nerve

Olfactory bulb

Olfactory nerves [I]

Sphenopalatine foramen

Septal branch of anterior ethmoidal nerve

Olfactory nerve [I] (septal branches)

External nasal branch of anterior ethmoidal nerve

A

B

Posterior superior lateral nasal nerves

Posterior inferior lateral nasal nerves

Nasopalatine nerve

Internal nasal branches of infra-orbital nerve

Nasal branch of anterior superior alveolar nerve

Innervation of the nasal cavities
A. Lateral wall of right nasal cavity B. Medial wall of right nasal cavity

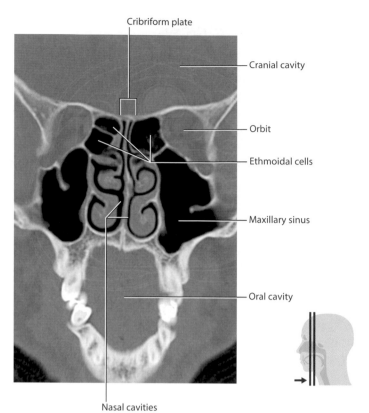

Cribriform plate

Cranial cavity

Orbit

Ethmoidal cells

Maxillary sinus

Oral cavity

Nasal cavities

Anterior view of the maxillary sinus and ethmoidal cells.
CT image in coronal plane

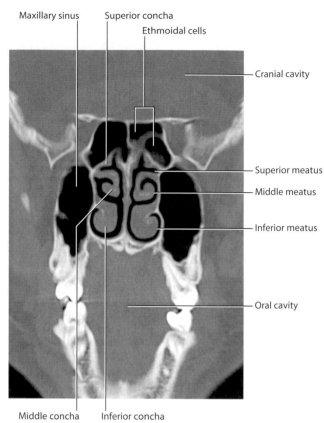

Maxillary sinus   Superior concha

Ethmoidal cells

Cranial cavity

Superior meatus

Middle meatus

Inferior meatus

Oral cavity

Middle concha   Inferior concha

**Anterior view looking into the nasal cavity showing the
relationship of various structures.**
CT image in coronal plane

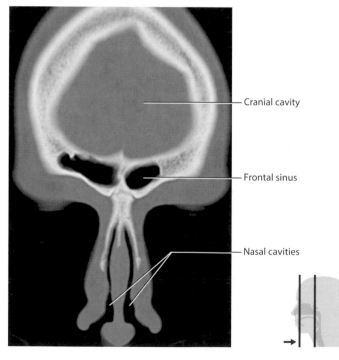

Cranial cavity

Frontal sinus

Nasal cavities

Anterior view of the frontal sinuses.
CT image in coronal plane

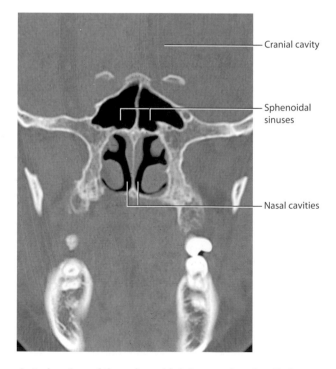

Cranial cavity

Sphenoidal sinuses

Nasal cavities

**Anterior view of the sphenoidal sinuses showing their
relationship to the nasal cavity.**
CT image in coronal plane

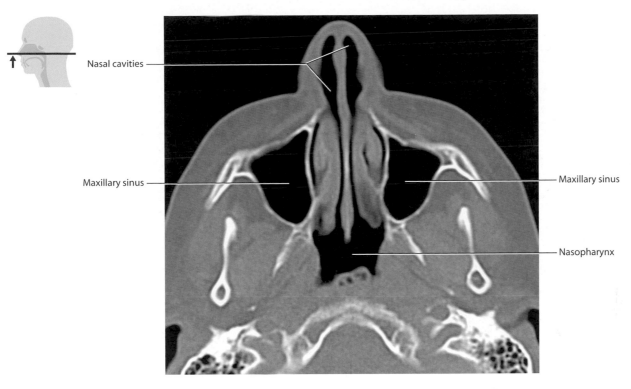

Nasal cavities

Maxillary sinus

Maxillary sinus

Nasopharynx

Axial section showing the relationship among the nasal cavity, nasopharynx, and maxillary sinuses.
CT image in axial plane

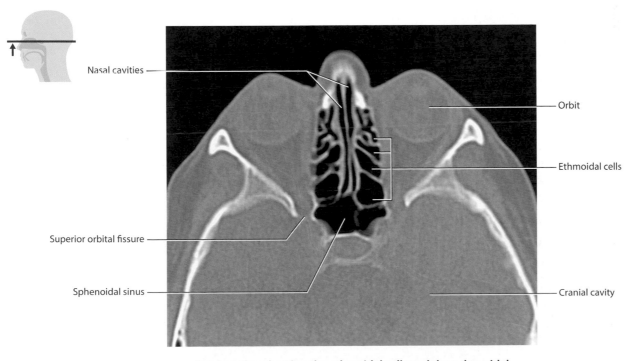

Nasal cavities

Orbit

Ethmoidal cells

Superior orbital fissure

Sphenoidal sinus

Cranial cavity

Axial section showing the ethmoidal cells and the sphenoidal sinuses and the relationship of these structures to the orbit.
CT image in axial plane

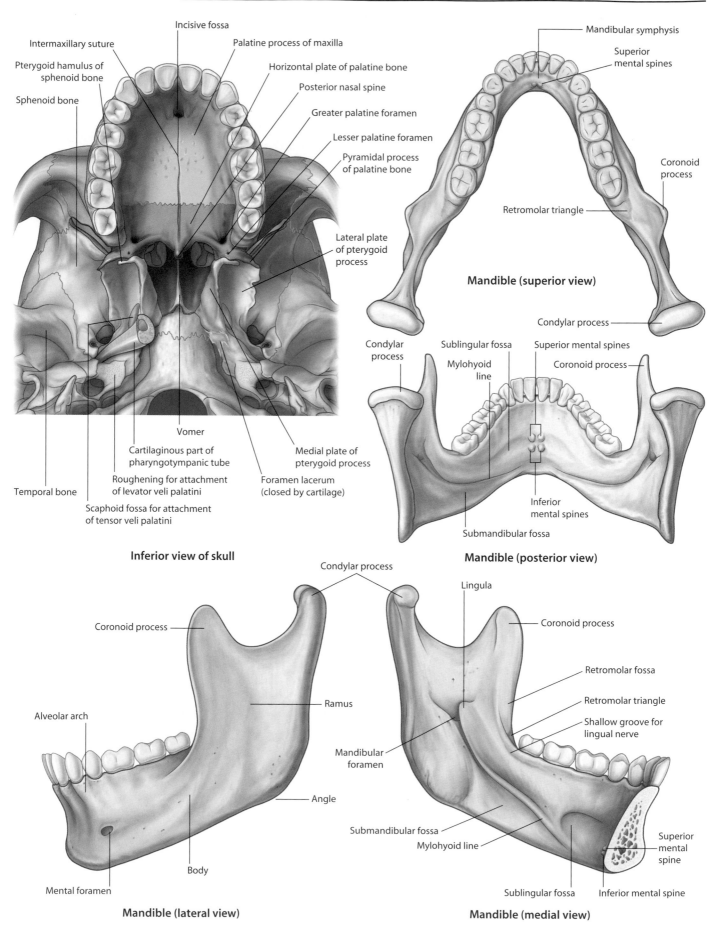

Incisive fossa

Intermaxillary suture

Pterygoid hamulus of sphenoid bone

Sphenoid bone

Palatine process of maxilla

Horizontal plate of palatine bone

Posterior nasal spine

Greater palatine foramen

Lesser palatine foramen

Pyramidal process of palatine bone

Lateral plate of pterygoid process

Vomer

Cartilaginous part of pharyngotympanic tube

Roughening for attachment of levator veli palatini

Medial plate of pterygoid process

Foramen lacerum (closed by cartilage)

Temporal bone

Scaphoid fossa for attachment of tensor veli palatini

Inferior view of skull

Mandibular symphysis

Superior mental spines

Coronoid process

Retromolar triangle

Mandible (superior view)

Condylar process

Condylar process

Sublingular fossa

Mylohyoid line

Superior mental spines

Coronoid process

Inferior mental spines

Submandibular fossa

Mandible (posterior view)

Condylar process

Coronoid process

Lingula

Coronoid process

Retromolar fossa

Retromolar triangle

Shallow groove for lingual nerve

Ramus

Alveolar arch

Mandibular foramen

Angle

Submandibular fossa

Mylohyoid line

Superior mental spine

Body

Inferior mental spine

Mental foramen

Sublingular fossa

Mandible (lateral view)

Mandible (medial view)

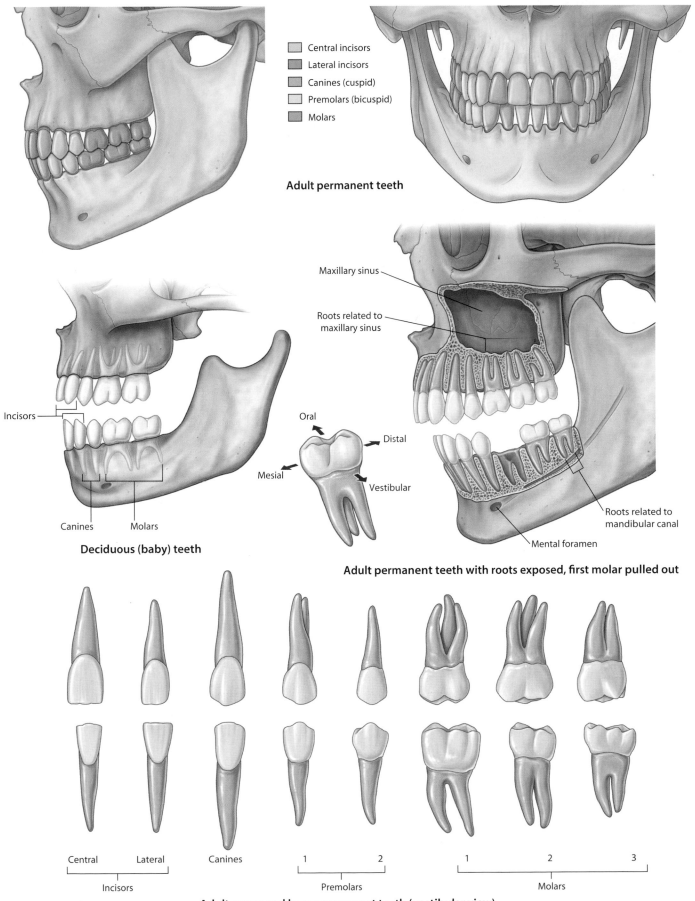

Central incisors
Lateral incisors
Canines (cuspid)
Premolars (bicuspid)
Molars

Adult permanent teeth

Maxillary sinus

Roots related to maxillary sinus

Incisors

Oral

Distal

Mesial

Vestibular

Canines   Molars

Roots related to mandibular canal

Mental foramen

Deciduous (baby) teeth

Adult permanent teeth with roots exposed, first molar pulled out

Central   Lateral   Canines   1   2   1   2   3

Incisors   Premolars   Molars

Adult upper and lower permanent teeth (vestibular view)

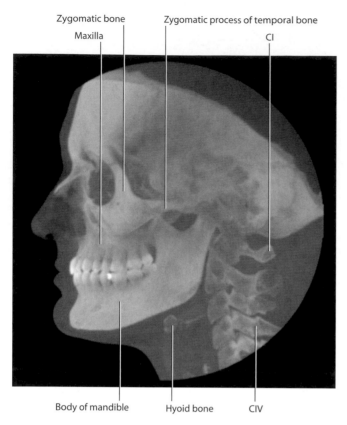

Zygomatic bone
Maxilla
Zygomatic process of temporal bone
CI

Body of mandible
Hyoid bone
CIV

View of the left side of the face showing the craniofacial structures including the teeth.
Image taken with Cone Beam Computerized Tomography (CBCT) technology, viewed in the Maximum Intensity Projection (MIP) mode, which combines a radiographic view with a view of surface structures

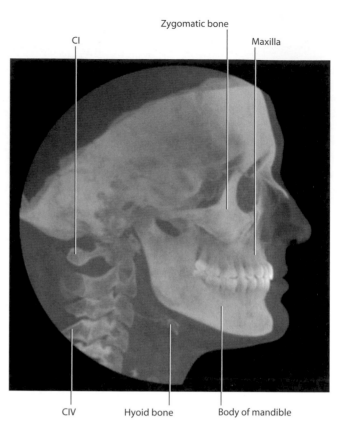

CI
Zygomatic bone
Maxilla

CIV
Hyoid bone
Body of mandible

View of the right side of the face showing the craniofacial structures including the teeth.
Image taken with Cone Beam Computerized Tomography (CBCT) technology, viewed in the Maximum Intensity Projection (MIP) mode, which combines a radiographic view with a view of surface structures

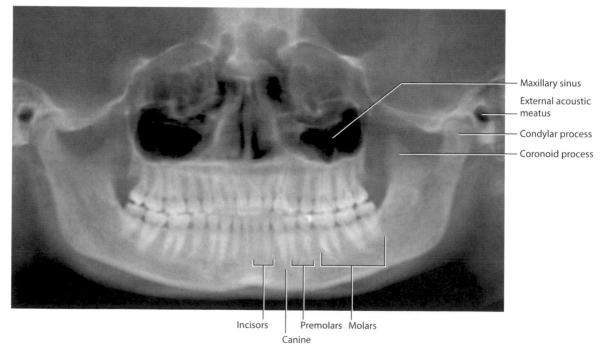

Maxillary sinus
External acoustic meatus
Condylar process
Coronoid process

Incisors
Canine
Premolars
Molars

Panoramic view of the teeth (dentition), which also shows the maxillary sinuses and mandibular condylar processes.
Image taken with Cone Beam Computerized Tomography (CBCT) technology

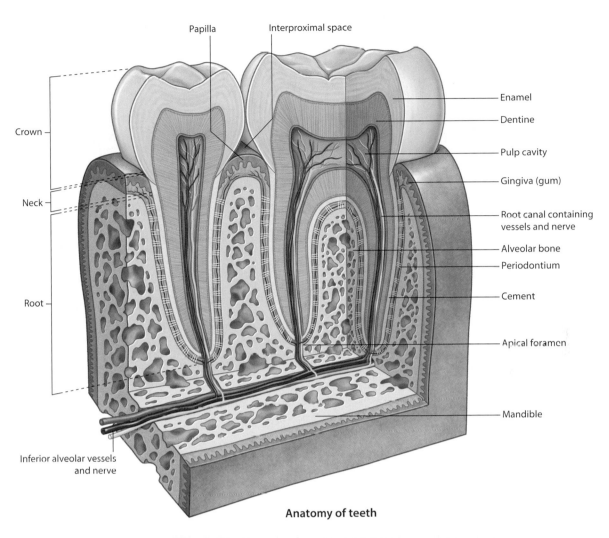

Papilla

Interproximal space

Crown

Neck

Root

Enamel

Dentine

Pulp cavity

Gingiva (gum)

Root canal containing
vessels and nerve

Alveolar bone

Periodontium

Cement

Apical foramen

Mandible

Inferior alveolar vessels
and nerve

Anatomy of teeth

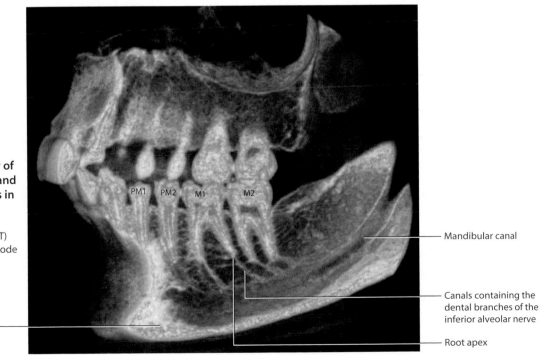

**Inside, lingual or sagittal view of
the right side of the maxillary and
mandibular alveolar processes in
occlusion (teeth together).**
Image taken with Cone Beam
Computerized Tomography (CBCT)
technology viewed in the surface mode

PM1 PM2 M1 M2

Mandibular canal

Canals containing the
dental branches of the
inferior alveolar nerve

Root apex

Mandible

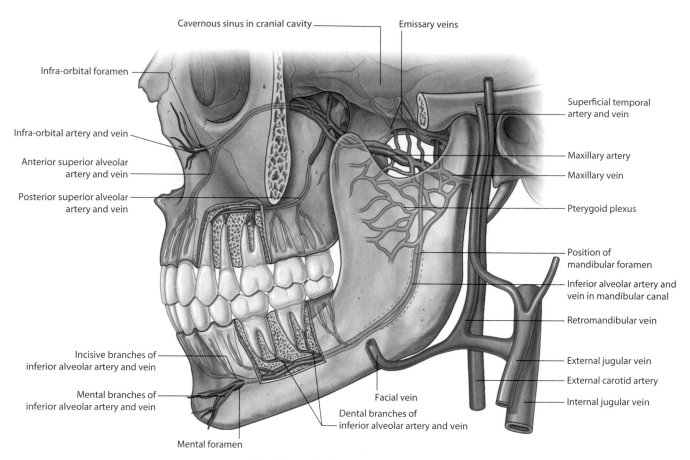

Cavernous sinus in cranial cavity

Emissary veins

Infra-orbital foramen

Infra-orbital artery and vein

Anterior superior alveolar artery and vein

Posterior superior alveolar artery and vein

Superficial temporal artery and vein

Maxillary artery

Maxillary vein

Pterygoid plexus

Position of mandibular foramen

Inferior alveolar artery and vein in mandibular canal

Retromandibular vein

Incisive branches of inferior alveolar artery and vein

External jugular vein

External carotid artery

Mental branches of inferior alveolar artery and vein

Facial vein

Internal jugular vein

Dental branches of inferior alveolar artery and vein

Mental foramen

Arteries and veins supplying teeth

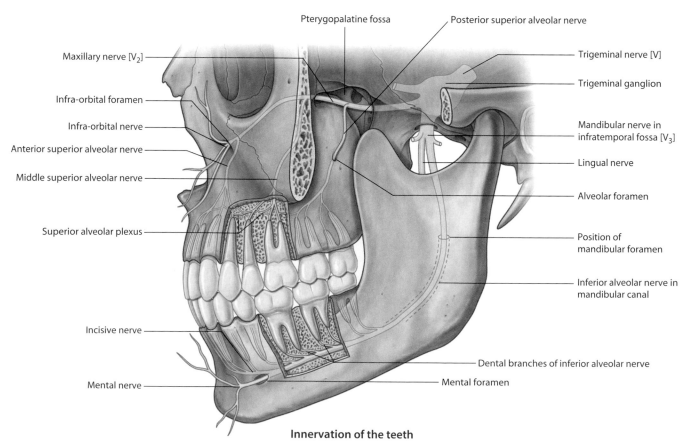

Pterygopalatine fossa

Posterior superior alveolar nerve

Maxillary nerve [V$_2$]

Trigeminal nerve [V]

Infra-orbital foramen

Trigeminal ganglion

Infra-orbital nerve

Anterior superior alveolar nerve

Mandibular nerve in infratemporal fossa [V$_3$]

Middle superior alveolar nerve

Lingual nerve

Alveolar foramen

Superior alveolar plexus

Position of mandibular foramen

Inferior alveolar nerve in mandibular canal

Incisive nerve

Dental branches of inferior alveolar nerve

Mental nerve

Mental foramen

Innervation of the teeth

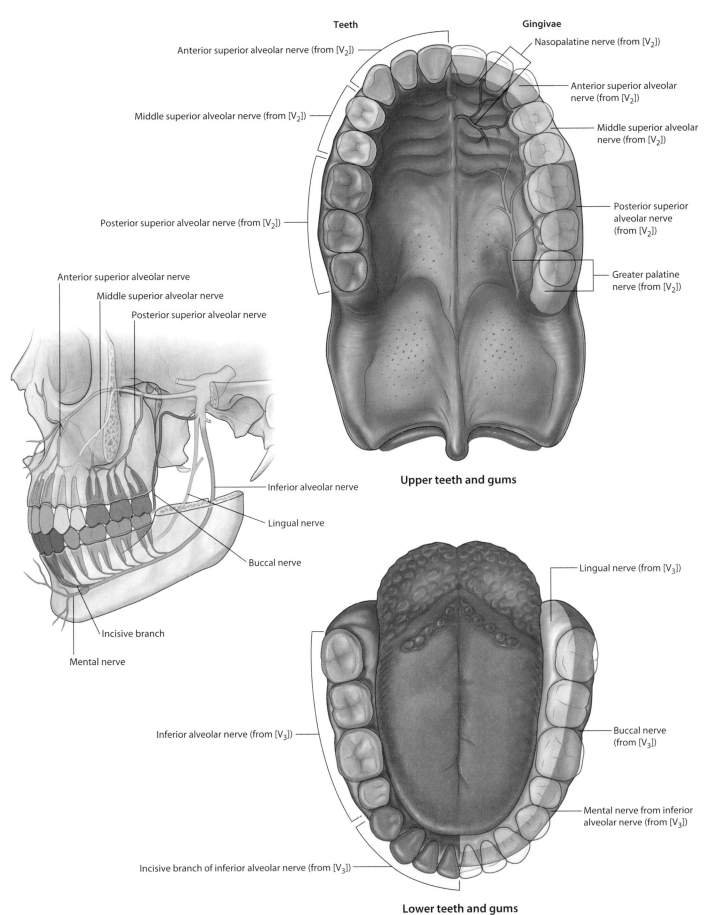

Teeth

Gingivae

Anterior superior alveolar nerve (from [V₂])

Nasopalatine nerve (from [V₂])

Anterior superior alveolar nerve (from [V₂])

Middle superior alveolar nerve (from [V₂])

Middle superior alveolar nerve (from [V₂])

Posterior superior alveolar nerve (from [V₂])

Posterior superior alveolar nerve (from [V₂])

Greater palatine nerve (from [V₂])

Upper teeth and gums

Anterior superior alveolar nerve

Middle superior alveolar nerve

Posterior superior alveolar nerve

Inferior alveolar nerve

Lingual nerve

Buccal nerve

Incisive branch

Mental nerve

Lingual nerve (from [V₃])

Inferior alveolar nerve (from [V₃])

Buccal nerve (from [V₃])

Mental nerve from inferior alveolar nerve (from [V₃])

Incisive branch of inferior alveolar nerve (from [V₃])

Lower teeth and gums

577

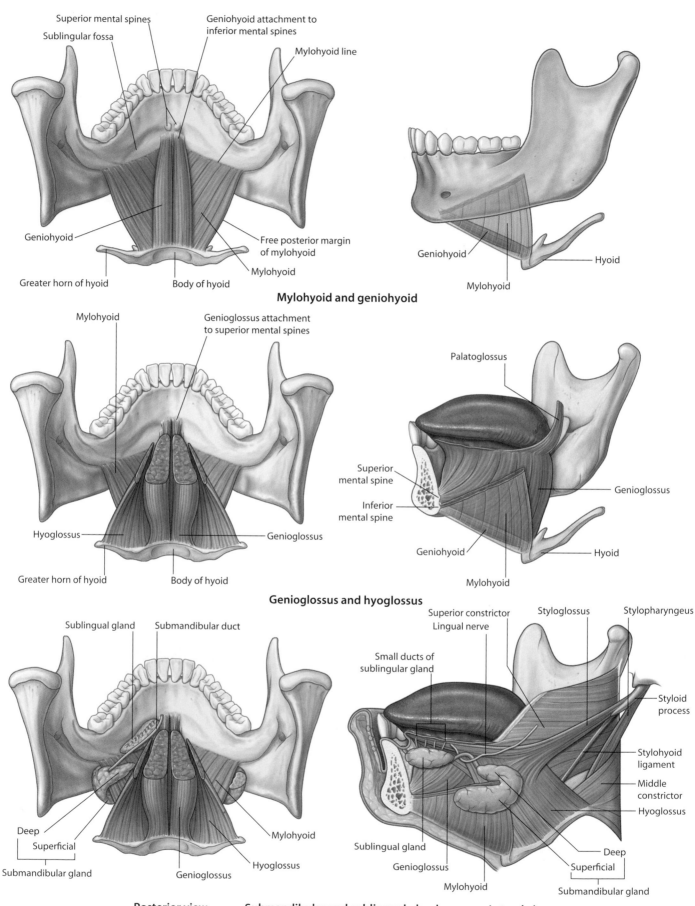

Superior mental spines
Sublingular fossa
Geniohyoid attachment to inferior mental spines
Mylohyoid line

Geniohyoid
Greater horn of hyoid
Body of hyoid
Free posterior margin of mylohyoid
Mylohyoid

Geniohyoid
Mylohyoid
Hyoid

Mylohyoid and geniohyoid

Mylohyoid
Genioglossus attachment to superior mental spines

Hyoglossus
Genioglossus
Greater horn of hyoid
Body of hyoid

Palatoglossus
Superior mental spine
Inferior mental spine
Geniohyoid
Mylohyoid
Genioglossus
Hyoid

Genioglossus and hyoglossus

Sublingual gland
Submandibular duct

Deep
Superficial
Submandibular gland
Genioglossus
Hyoglossus
Mylohyoid

Superior constrictor
Lingual nerve
Styloglossus
Stylopharyngeus
Small ducts of sublingular gland
Styloid process
Stylohyoid ligament
Middle constrictor
Hyoglossus
Sublingual gland
Genioglossus
Mylohyoid
Deep
Superficial
Submandibular gland

Posterior view   **Submandibular and sublingual glands**   **Lateral view**

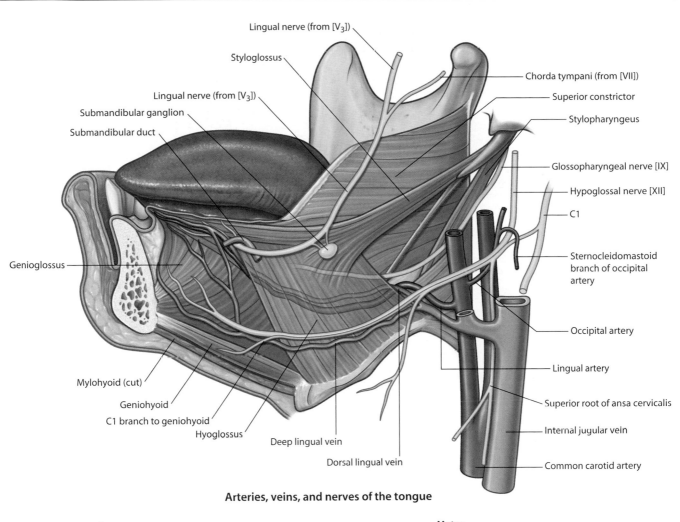

Arteries, veins, and nerves of the tongue

Lingual nerve (from [V₃])

Styloglossus

Lingual nerve (from [V₃])

Submandibular ganglion

Submandibular duct

Genioglossus

Mylohyoid (cut)

Geniohyoid

C1 branch to geniohyoid

Hyoglossus

Deep lingual vein

Dorsal lingual vein

Chorda tympani (from [VII])

Superior constrictor

Stylopharyngeus

Glossopharyngeal nerve [IX]

Hypoglossal nerve [XII]

C1

Sternocleidomastoid branch of occipital artery

Occipital artery

Lingual artery

Superior root of ansa cervicalis

Internal jugular vein

Common carotid artery

Sensory

Anterior two-thirds (oral)
• general sensation
  Mandibular nerve [V₃] via lingual nerve
• special sensation (taste)
  Facial nerve [VII] via chorda tympani

Posterior one-third (pharyngeal)
• general and special sensation (taste)
  Glossopharyngeal nerve [IX]

Motor

Palatoglossus – vagus nerve [X]

Styloglossus – hyoglossal nerve [XII]

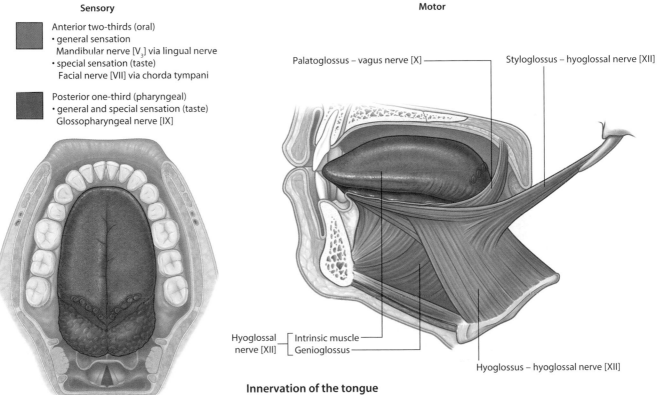

Hyoglossal nerve [XII]

Intrinsic muscle
Genioglossus

Hyoglossus – hyoglossal nerve [XII]

Innervation of the tongue

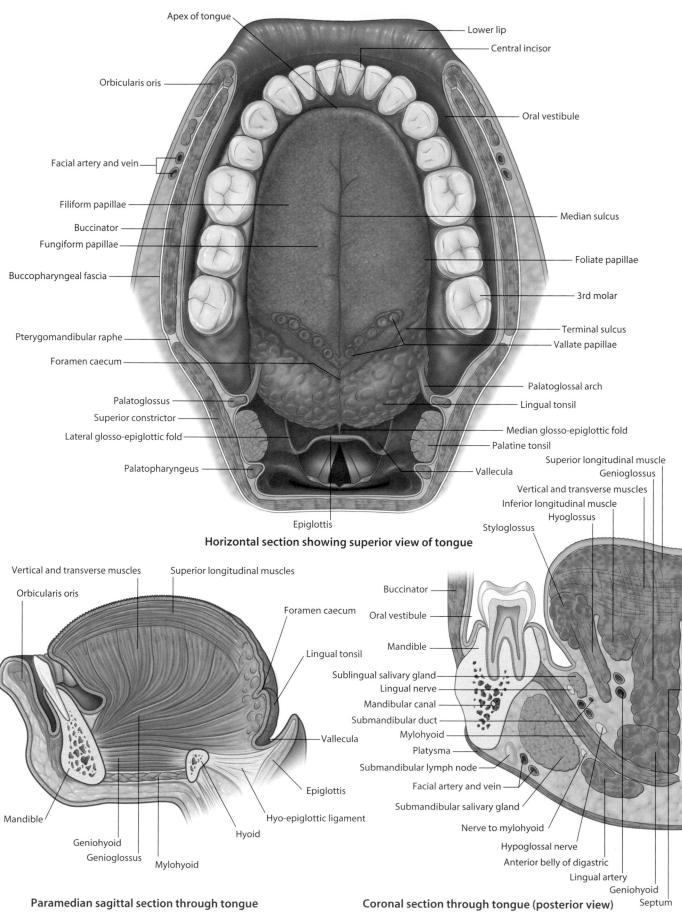

Apex of tongue

Lower lip

Central incisor

Orbicularis oris

Oral vestibule

Facial artery and vein

Filiform papillae

Median sulcus

Buccinator

Fungiform papillae

Foliate papillae

Buccopharyngeal fascia

3rd molar

Pterygomandibular raphe

Terminal sulcus

Foramen caecum

Vallate papillae

Palatoglossal arch

Palatoglossus

Lingual tonsil

Superior constrictor

Median glosso-epiglottic fold

Lateral glosso-epiglottic fold

Palatine tonsil

Palatopharyngeus

Vallecula

Epiglottis

Horizontal section showing superior view of tongue

Vertical and transverse muscles

Superior longitudinal muscles

Orbicularis oris

Foramen caecum

Lingual tonsil

Vallecula

Epiglottis

Mandible

Hyo-epiglottic ligament

Geniohyoid

Hyoid

Genioglossus

Mylohyoid

Paramedian sagittal section through tongue

Superior longitudinal muscle

Genioglossus

Vertical and transverse muscles

Inferior longitudinal muscle

Hyoglossus

Styloglossus

Buccinator

Oral vestibule

Mandible

Sublingual salivary gland

Lingual nerve

Mandibular canal

Submandibular duct

Mylohyoid

Platysma

Submandibular lymph node

Facial artery and vein

Submandibular salivary gland

Nerve to mylohyoid

Hypoglossal nerve

Anterior belly of digastric

Lingual artery

Geniohyoid

Septum

Coronal section through tongue (posterior view)

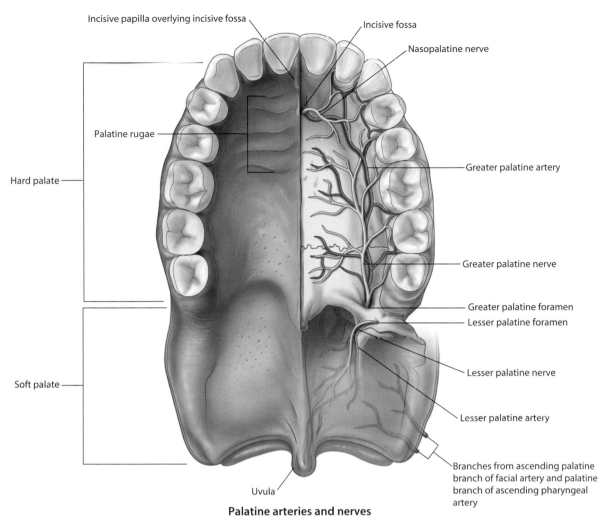

Incisive papilla overlying incisive fossa

Incisive fossa

Nasopalatine nerve

Palatine rugae

Hard palate

Greater palatine artery

Greater palatine nerve

Greater palatine foramen

Lesser palatine foramen

Soft palate

Lesser palatine nerve

Lesser palatine artery

Branches from ascending palatine branch of facial artery and palatine branch of ascending pharyngeal artery

Uvula

Palatine arteries and nerves

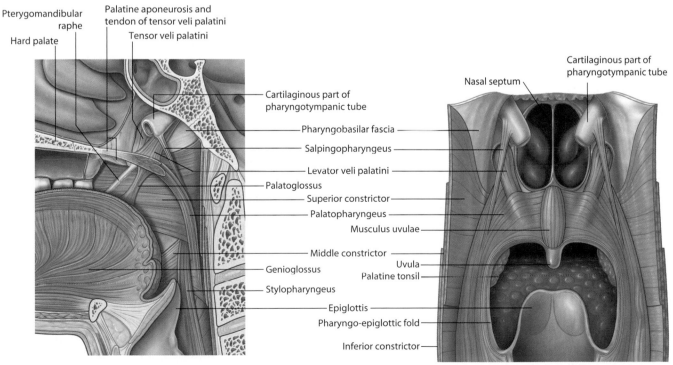

Pterygomandibular raphe

Palatine aponeurosis and tendon of tensor veli palatini

Tensor veli palatini

Hard palate

Cartilaginous part of pharyngotympanic tube

Nasal septum

Cartilaginous part of pharyngotympanic tube

Pharyngobasilar fascia

Salpingopharyngeus

Levator veli palatini

Palatoglossus

Superior constrictor

Palatopharyngeus

Musculus uvulae

Middle constrictor

Genioglossus

Uvula

Palatine tonsil

Stylopharyngeus

Epiglottis

Pharyngo-epiglottic fold

Inferior constrictor

Muscles of the soft palate (sagittal section)

Muscles of the soft palate (posterior view)

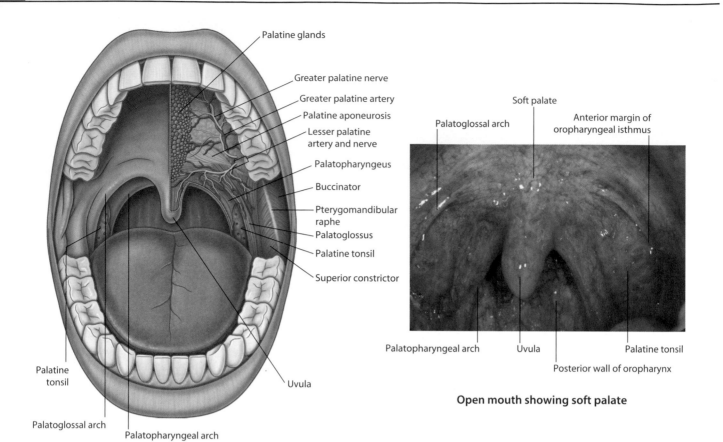

Roof of oral cavity

Palatine glands

Greater palatine nerve

Greater palatine artery

Palatine aponeurosis

Lesser palatine artery and nerve

Palatopharyngeus

Buccinator

Pterygomandibular raphe

Palatoglossus

Palatine tonsil

Superior constrictor

Uvula

Palatine tonsil

Palatoglossal arch

Palatopharyngeal arch

Open mouth showing soft palate

Soft palate

Palatoglossal arch

Anterior margin of oropharyngeal isthmus

Palatopharyngeal arch

Uvula

Palatine tonsil

Posterior wall of oropharynx

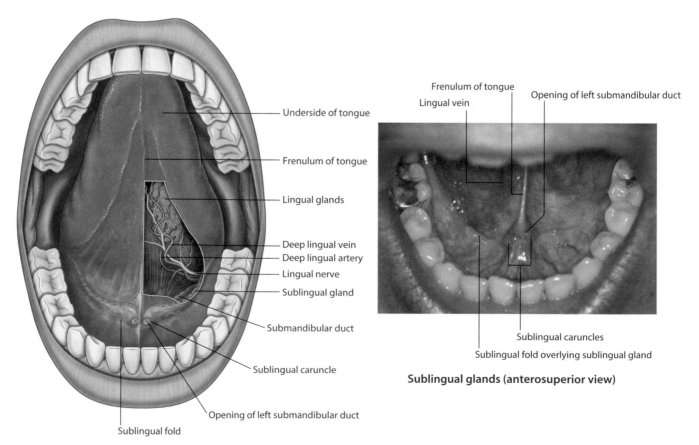

Inferior surface of tongue and floor of oral cavity

Underside of tongue

Frenulum of tongue

Lingual glands

Deep lingual vein

Deep lingual artery

Lingual nerve

Sublingual gland

Submandibular duct

Sublingual caruncle

Opening of left submandibular duct

Sublingual fold

Sublingual glands (anterosuperior view)

Frenulum of tongue

Lingual vein

Opening of left submandibular duct

Sublingual caruncles

Sublingual fold overlying sublingual gland

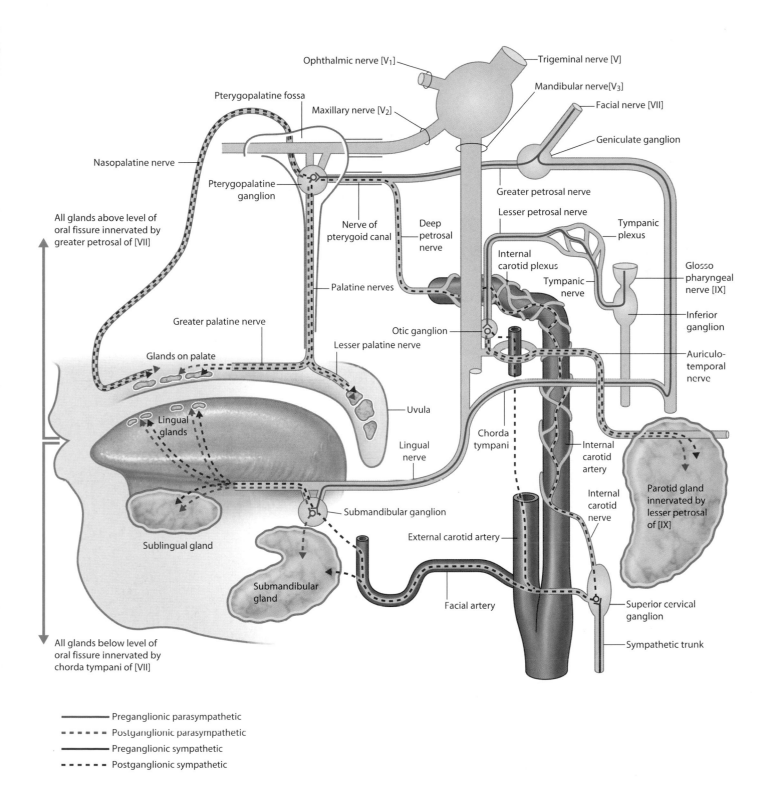

Ophthalmic nerve [V₁]

Trigeminal nerve [V]

Pterygopalatine fossa

Mandibular nerve[V₃]

Maxillary nerve [V₂]

Facial nerve [VII]

Geniculate ganglion

Nasopalatine nerve

Pterygopalatine ganglion

Greater petrosal nerve

All glands above level of oral fissure innervated by greater petrosal of [VII]

Nerve of pterygoid canal

Deep petrosal nerve

Lesser petrosal nerve

Tympanic plexus

Internal carotid plexus

Tympanic nerve

Glosso pharyngeal nerve [IX]

Palatine nerves

Greater palatine nerve

Otic ganglion

Inferior ganglion

Glands on palate

Lesser palatine nerve

Auriculo-temporal nerve

Lingual glands

Uvula

Lingual nerve

Chorda tympani

Internal carotid artery

Parotid gland innervated by lesser petrosal of [IX]

Sublingual gland

Submandibular ganglion

Internal carotid nerve

Submandibular gland

External carotid artery

Superior cervical ganglion

All glands below level of oral fissure innervated by chorda tympani of [VII]

Facial artery

Sympathetic trunk

————— Preganglionic parasympathetic

- - - - - Postganglionic parasympathetic

————— Preganglionic sympathetic

- - - - - Postganglionic sympathetic

Visceral efferent (motor) innervation of glands related to the oral cavity

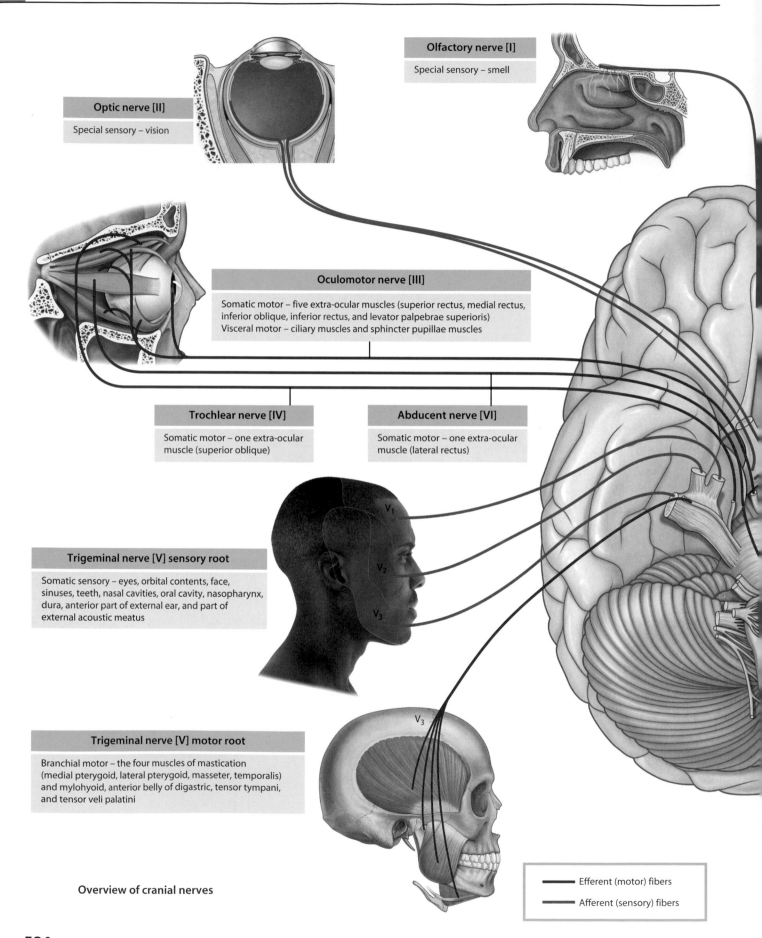

Olfactory nerve [I]

Special sensory – smell

Optic nerve [II]

Special sensory – vision

Oculomotor nerve [III]

Somatic motor – five extra-ocular muscles (superior rectus, medial rectus, inferior oblique, inferior rectus, and levator palpebrae superioris)
Visceral motor – ciliary muscles and sphincter pupillae muscles

Trochlear nerve [IV]

Somatic motor – one extra-ocular muscle (superior oblique)

Abducent nerve [VI]

Somatic motor – one extra-ocular muscle (lateral rectus)

V₁
V₂
V₃

Trigeminal nerve [V] sensory root

Somatic sensory – eyes, orbital contents, face, sinuses, teeth, nasal cavities, oral cavity, nasopharynx, dura, anterior part of external ear, and part of external acoustic meatus

Trigeminal nerve [V] motor root

Branchial motor – the four muscles of mastication (medial pterygoid, lateral pterygoid, masseter, temporalis) and mylohyoid, anterior belly of digastric, tensor tympani, and tensor veli palatini

V₃

Efferent (motor) fibers
Afferent (sensory) fibers

Overview of cranial nerves

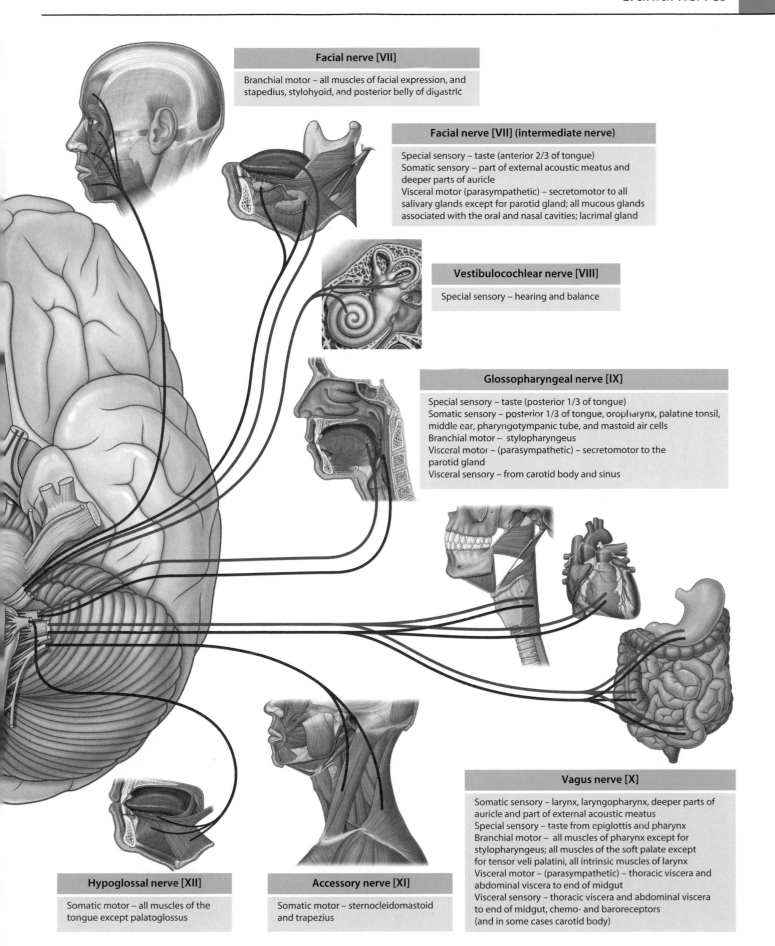

Facial nerve [VII]

Branchial motor – all muscles of facial expression, and stapedius, stylohyoid, and posterior belly of digastric

Facial nerve [VII] (intermediate nerve)

Special sensory – taste (anterior 2/3 of tongue)
Somatic sensory – part of external acoustic meatus and deeper parts of auricle
Visceral motor (parasympathetic) – secretomotor to all salivary glands except for parotid gland; all mucous glands associated with the oral and nasal cavities; lacrimal gland

Vestibulocochlear nerve [VIII]

Special sensory – hearing and balance

Glossopharyngeal nerve [IX]

Special sensory – taste (posterior 1/3 of tongue)
Somatic sensory – posterior 1/3 of tongue, oropharynx, palatine tonsil, middle ear, pharyngotympanic tube, and mastoid air cells
Branchial motor – stylopharyngeus
Visceral motor – (parasympathetic) – secretomotor to the parotid gland
Visceral sensory – from carotid body and sinus

Vagus nerve [X]

Somatic sensory – larynx, laryngopharynx, deeper parts of auricle and part of external acoustic meatus
Special sensory – taste from epiglottis and pharynx
Branchial motor – all muscles of pharynx except for stylopharyngeus; all muscles of the soft palate except for tensor veli palatini, all intrinsic muscles of larynx
Visceral motor – (parasympathetic) – thoracic viscera and abdominal viscera to end of midgut
Visceral sensory – thoracic viscera and abdominal viscera to end of midgut, chemo- and baroreceptors (and in some cases carotid body)

Hypoglossal nerve [XII]

Somatic motor – all muscles of the tongue except palatoglossus

Accessory nerve [XI]

Somatic motor – sternocleidomastoid and trapezius

585

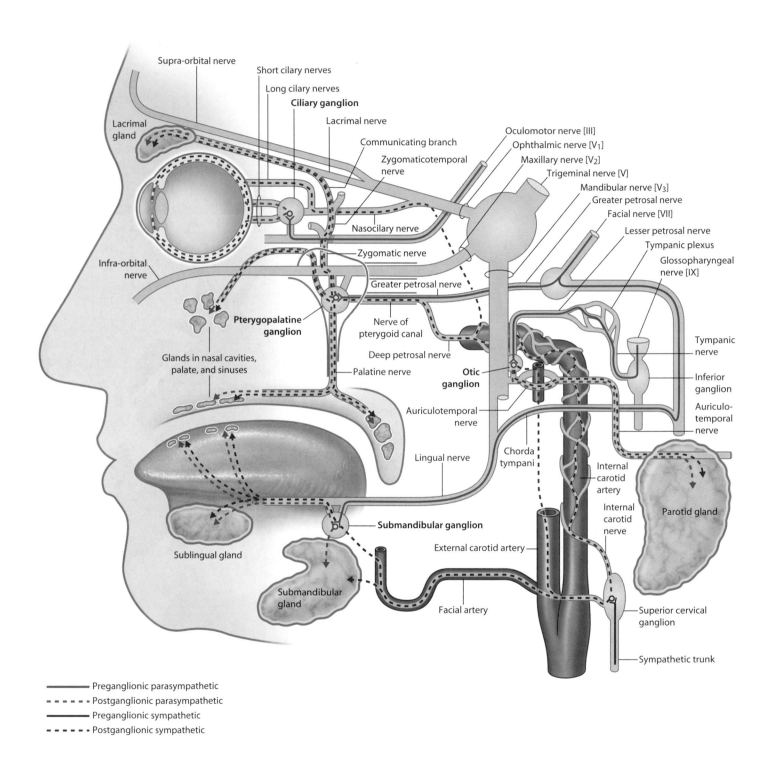

Supra-orbital nerve

Short cilary nerves

Long cilary nerves

Ciliary ganglion

Lacrimal nerve

Communicating branch

Zygomaticotemporal nerve

Oculomotor nerve [III]

Ophthalmic nerve [V₁]

Maxillary nerve [V₂]

Trigeminal nerve [V]

Mandibular nerve [V₃]

Greater petrosal nerve

Facial nerve [VII]

Lesser petrosal nerve

Tympanic plexus

Glossopharyngeal nerve [IX]

Lacrimal gland

Nasocilary nerve

Zygomatic nerve

Greater petrosal nerve

Infra-orbital nerve

Nerve of pterygoid canal

Deep petrosal nerve

Tympanic nerve

Inferior ganglion

Pterygopalatine ganglion

Palatine nerve

Otic ganglion

Auriculo-temporal nerve

Glands in nasal cavities, palate, and sinuses

Auriculotemporal nerve

Lingual nerve

Chorda tympani

Internal carotid artery

Internal carotid nerve

Parotid gland

Sublingual gland

Submandibular ganglion

External carotid artery

Submandibular gland

Facial artery

Superior cervical ganglion

Sympathetic trunk

—— Preganglionic parasympathetic

- - - - Postganglionic parasympathetic

—— Preganglionic sympathetic

- - - - Postganglionic sympathetic

Summary of visceral efferent (motor) pathways in the head

External foramina of the skull

Foramen		Structures passing through foramen
Anterior view		
Supra-orbital foramen	1	Supra-orbital nerve and vessels
Infra-orbital foramen	2	Infra-orbital nerve and vessels
Mental foramen	3	Mental nerve and vessels
Lateral view		
Zygomaticofacial foramen	4	Zygomaticofacial nerve
Superior view		
Parietal foramen	5	Emissary veins

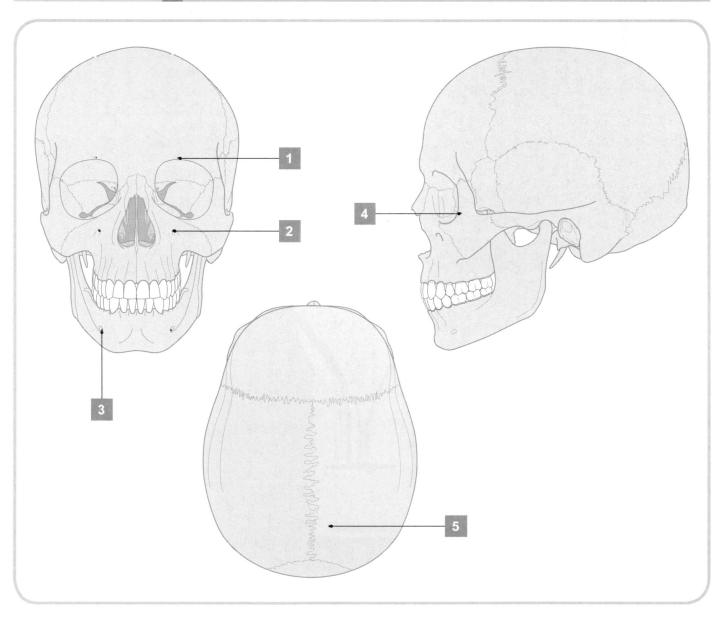

External foramina of the skull

Foramen		Structures passing through foramen
Inferior view		
Incisive foramina	1	Nasopalatine nerve; sphenopalatine vessels
Greater palatine foramen	2	Greater palatine nerve and vessels
Lesser palatine foramina	3	Lesser palatine nerves and vessels
Pterygoid canal	4	Pterygoid nerve and vessels
Foramen ovale	5	Mandibular nerve [V$_3$]; lesser petrosal nerve
Foramen spinosum	6	Middle meningeal artery
Foramen lacerum	7	Filled with cartilage
Carotid canal	8	Internal carotid artery and nerve plexus
Foramen magnum	9	Continuation of brain and spinal cord; vertebral arteries and nerve plexuses; anterior spinal artery; posterior spinal arteries; roots of accessory nerve [XI]; meninges
Condylar canal	10	Emissary veins
Hypoglossal canal	11	Hypoglossal nerve [XII] and vessels
Jugular foramen	12	Internal jugular vein; inferior petrosal sinus; glossopharyngeal nerve [IX]; vagus nerve [X]; accessory nerve [XI]
Stylomastoid foramen	13	Facial nerve [VII]

Internal foramina of the skull

Foramen		Structures passing through foramen
Anterior cranial fossa		
Foramen caecum	1	Emissary veins to nasal cavity
Olfactory foramina in cribriform plate	2	Olfactory nerves [I]
Middle cranial fossa		
Optic canal	3	Optic nerve [II]; ophthalmic artery
Superior orbital fissure	4	Oculomotor nerve [III]; trochlear nerve [IV]; ophthalmic division of the trigeminal nerve [V$_1$]; abducent nerve [VI]; ophthalmic veins
Foramen rotundum	5	Maxillary division of the trigeminal nerve [V$_2$]
Foramen ovale	6	Mandibular division of the trigeminal nerve [V$_3$]; lesser petrosal nerve
Foramen spinosum	7	Middle meningeal artery
Hiatus for the greater petrosal nerve	8	Greater petrosal nerve
Hiatus for the lesser petrosal nerve	9	Lesser petrosal nerve
Posterior cranial fossa		
Foramen magnum	10	End of brainstem/beginning of spinal cord; vertebral arteries; spinal roots of the accessory nerve; meninges
Internal acoustic meatus	11	Facial nerve [VII]; vestibulocochlear nerve [VIII]; labyrinthine artery
Jugular foramen	12	Glossopharyngeal nerve [IX]; vagus nerve [X]; accessory nerve [XI]; inferior petrosal sinus, sigmoid sinus (forming internal jugular vein)
Hypoglossal canal	13	Hypoglossal nerve [XII]; meningeal branch of the ascending pharyngeal artery
Condylar canal	14	Emissary vein

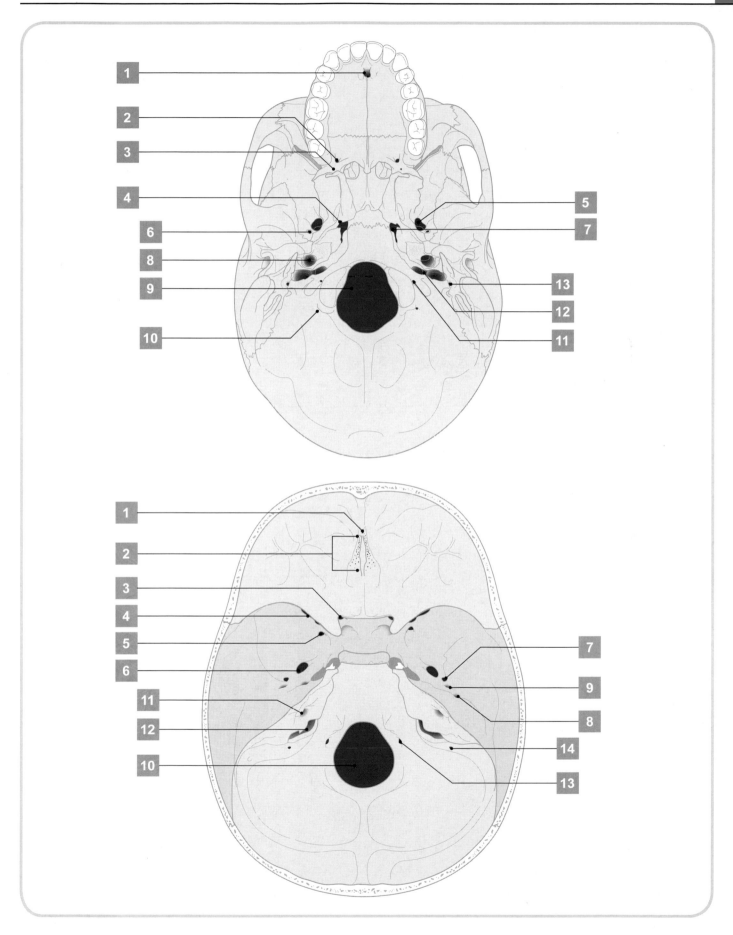

Muscles of the face

Muscle		Origin	Insertion	Innervation	Function
Orbital group					
Orbicularis oculi —Palpebral part	1	Medial palpebral ligament	Lateral palpebral raphe	Facial nerve [VII]	Closes the eyelids gently
—Orbital part	2	Nasal part of frontal bone; frontal process of maxilla; medial palpebral ligament	Fibers form an uninterrupted ellipse around orbit	Facial nerve [VII]	Closes the eyelids forcefully
Corrugator supercilii	3	Medial end of the superciliary arch	Skin of the medial half of eyebrow	Facial nerve [VII]	Draws the eyebrows medially and downward
Nasal group					
Nasalis —Transverse part	4	Maxilla just lateral to nose	Aponeurosis across dorsum of nose with muscle fibers from the other side	Facial nerve [VII]	Compresses nasal aperture
—Alar part	5	Maxilla over lateral incisor	Alar cartilage of nose	Facial nerve [VII]	Draws cartilage downward and laterally opening nostril
Procerus	6	Nasal bone and upper part of lateral nasal cartilage	Skin of lower forehead between eyebrows	Facial nerve [VII]	Draws down medial angle of eyebrows producing transverse wrinkles over bridge of nose
Depressor septi	7	Maxilla above medial incisor	Mobile part of the nasal septum	Facial nerve [VII]	Pulls nose inferiorly

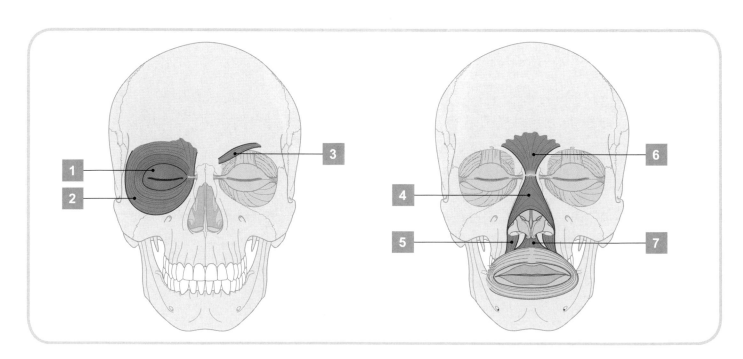

Muscles of the face

Muscle		Origin	Insertion	Innervation	Function
Oral group					
Depressor anguli oris	1	Oblique line of mandible below canine, premolar, and first molar teeth	Skin at the corner of mouth and blending with orbicularis oris	Facial nerve [VII]	Draws corner of mouth down and laterally
Depressor labii inferioris	2	Anterior part of oblique line of mandible	Lower lip at midline; blends with muscle from opposite side	Facial nerve [VII]	Draws lower lip downward and laterally
Mentalis	3	Mandible inferior to incisor teeth	Skin of chin	Facial nerve [VII]	Raises and protrudes lower lip as it wrinkles skin on chin
Risorius	4	Fascia over masseter muscle	Skin at the corner of the mouth	Facial nerve [VII]	Retracts corner of mouth
Zygomaticus major	5	Posterior part of lateral surface of zygomatic bone	Skin at the corner of the mouth	Facial nerve [VII]	Draws the corner of the mouth upward and laterally
Zygomaticus minor	6	Anterior part of lateral surface of zygomatic bone	Upper lip just medial to corner of mouth	Facial nerve [VII]	Draws the upper lip upward
Levator labii superioris	7	Infra-orbital margin of maxilla	Skin of upper lateral half of upper lip	Facial nerve [VII]	Raises upper lip; helps form nasolabial furrow
Levator labii superioris alaeque nasi	8	Frontal process of maxilla	Alar cartilage of nose and upper lip	Facial nerve [VII]	Raises upper lip and opens nostril
Levator anguli oris	9	Maxilla below infra-orbital foramen	Skin at the corner of mouth	Facial nerve [VII]	Raises corner of mouth; helps form nasolabial furrow
Orbicularis oris	10	From muscles in area; maxilla and mandible in midline	Forms ellipse around mouth	Facial nerve [VII]	Closes lips; protrudes lips
Buccinator	11	Posterior parts of maxilla and mandible; pterygomandibular raphe	Blends with orbicularis oris and into lips	Facial nerve [VII]	Presses the cheek against teeth; compresses distended cheeks

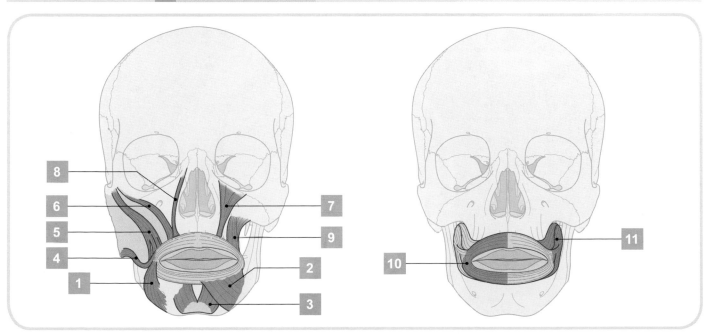

Muscles of the face

Muscle		Origin	Insertion	Innervation	Function
Other muscles or groups					
Anterior auricular	1	Anterior part of temporal fascia	Into helix of ear	Facial nerve [VII]	Draws ear upward and forward
Superior auricular	2	Epicranial aponeurosis on side of head	Upper part of auricle	Facial nerve [VII]	Elevates ear
Posterior auricular	3	Mastoid process of temporal bone	Convexity of concha of ear	Facial nerve [VII]	Draws ear upward and backward
Occipitofrontalis —Frontal belly	4	Skin of eyebrows	Into galea aponeurotica	Facial nerve [VII]	Wrinkles forehead; raises eyebrows
—Occipital belly	5	Lateral part of superior nuchal line of occipital bone and mastoid process of temporal bone	Into galea aponeurotica	Facial nerve [VII]	Draws scalp backward

Extrinsic (extra-ocular) muscles

Muscle		Origin	Insertion	Innervation	Function
Levator palpebrae superioris	1	Lesser wing of sphenoid anterior to optic canal	Anterior surface of tarsal plate; a few fibers to skin and superior conjunctival fornix	Oculomotor nerve [III]—superior branch	Elevation of upper eyelid
Superior rectus	2	Superior part of common tendinous ring	Anterior half of eyeball superiorly	Oculomotor nerve [III]—superior branch	Elevation, adduction, medial rotation of eyeball
Inferior rectus	3	Inferior part of common tendinous ring	Anterior half of eyeball inferiorly	Oculomotor nerve [III]—inferior branch	Depression, adduction, lateral rotation of eyeball
Medial rectus	4	Medial part of common tendinous ring	Anterior half of eyeball medially	Oculomotor nerve [III]—inferior branch	Adduction of eyeball
Lateral rectus	5	Lateral part of common tendinous ring	Anterior half of eyeball laterally	Abducent nerve [VI]	Abduction of eyeball
Superior oblique	6	Body of sphenoid, superior and medial to optic canal	Outer posterior quadrant of eyeball (superior surface)	Trochlear nerve [IV]	Depression, abduction, medial rotation of eyeball
Inferior oblique	7	Medial floor of orbit posterior to rim; maxilla lateral to nasolacrimal groove	Outer posterior quadrant of eyeball (inferior surface)	Oculomotor nerve [III]—inferior branch	Elevation, abduction, lateral rotation of eyeball

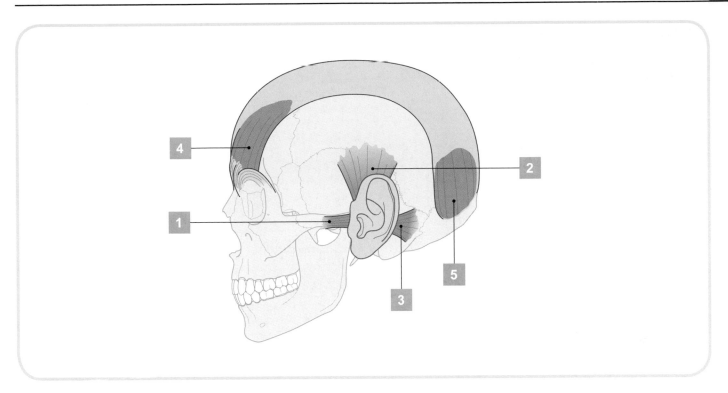

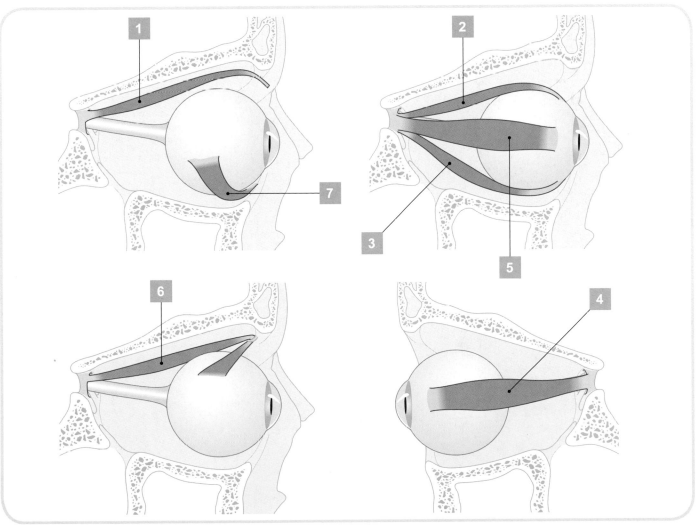

Intrinsic muscles of the eye

Muscle		Location	Innervation	Function
Ciliary	1	Muscle fibers in the ciliary body	Parasympathetics from the oculomotor nerve [III]	Constricts ciliary body, relaxes tension on lens, lens become more rounded
Sphincter pupillae	2	Circularly arranged fibers in the iris	Parasympathetics from the oculomotor nerve [III]	Constricts pupil
Dilator pupillae	3	Radially arranged fibers in the iris	Sympathetics from the superior cervical ganglion (T1)	Dilates pupil

Muscles of the middle ear

Muscle		Origin	Insertion	Innervation	Function
Tensor tympani	1	Cartilaginous part of pharyngotympanic tube, greater wing of sphenoid, its own bony canal	Upper part of handle of malleus	Branch from mandibular nerve [V₃]	Contraction pulls handle of malleus medially, tensing tympanic membrane
Stapedius	2	Attached to inside of pyramidal eminence	Neck of stapes	Branch of facial nerve [VII]	Contraction pulls stapes posteriorly, preventing excessive oscillation

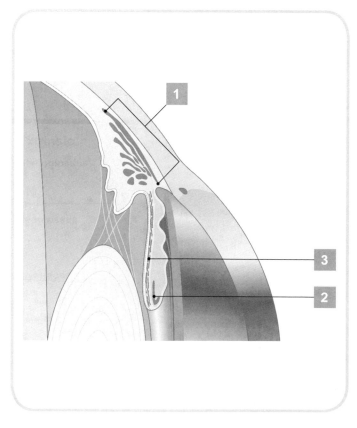

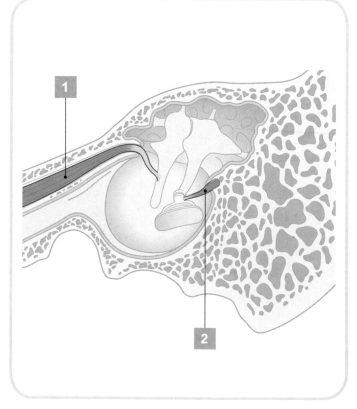

Muscles of mastication

Muscle		Origin	Insertion	Innervation	Function
Masseter	1	Zygomatic arch and maxillary process of the zygomatic bone	Lateral surface of ramus of mandible	Masseteric nerve from the anterior trunk of the mandibular nerve [V$_3$]	Elevation of mandible
Temporalis	2	Bone of temporal fossa and temporal fascia	Coronoid process of mandible and anterior margin of ramus of mandible almost to last molar tooth	Deep temporal nerves from the anterior trunk of the mandibular nerve [V$_3$]	Elevation and retraction of mandible
Medial pterygoid	3	Deep head—medial surface of lateral plate of pterygoid process and pyramidal process of palatine bone; superficial head—tuberosity of the maxilla and pyramidal process of palatine bone	Medial surface of mandible near angle	Nerve to medial pterygoid from the mandibular nerve [V$_3$].	Elevation and side-to-side movements of the mandible
Lateral pterygoid	4	Upper head—roof of infratemporal fossa; lower head—lateral surface of lateral plate of the pterygoid process	Capsule of temporomandibular joint in the region of attachment to the articular disc and to the pterygoid fovea on the neck of mandible	Nerve to lateral pterygoid directly from the anterior trunk of the mandibular nerve [V$_3$] or from the buccal branch	Protrusion and side-to-side movements of the mandible

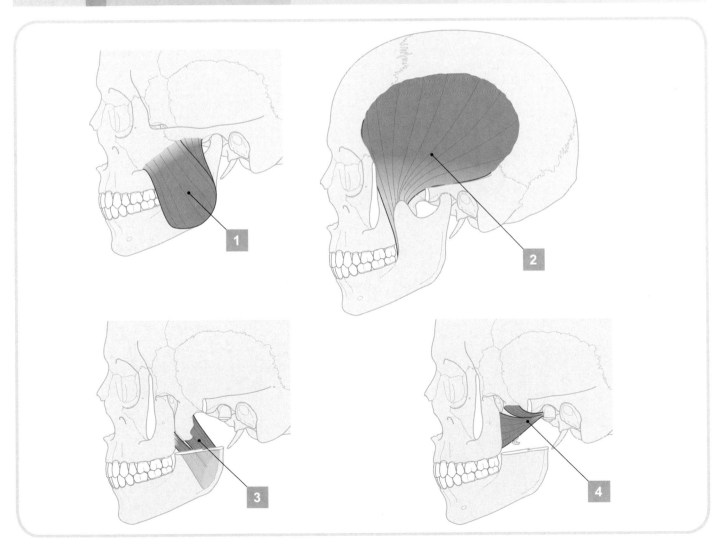

Anterior triangle of neck (suprahyoid and infrahyoid muscles)

Muscle		Origin	Insertion	Innervation	Function
Stylohyoid	1	Base of styloid process	Lateral area of body of hyoid bone	Facial nerve [VII]	Pulls hyoid bone upward in a posterosuperior direction
Digastric —Anterior belly	2	Digastric fossa on lower inside of mandible	Attachment of tendon between two bellies to body of hyoid bone	Mylohyoid nerve from inferior alveolar branch of mandibular nerve [V_3]	Opens mouth by lowering mandible; raises hyoid bone
—Posterior belly	3	Mastoid notch on medial side of mastoid process of temporal bone		Facial nerve [VII]	Pulls hyoid bone upward and back
Mylohyoid	4	Mylohyoid line on mandible	Body of hyoid bone and fibers from muscle on opposite side	Mylohyoid nerve from inferior alveolar branch of mandibular nerve [V_3]	Support and elevation of floor of mouth; elevation of hyoid
Geniohyoid	5	Inferior mental spine on inner surface of mandible	Anterior surface of body of hyoid bone	Branch from anterior ramus of C1 (carried along the hypoglossal nerve [XII])	Fixed mandible elevates and pulls hyoid bone forward; fixed hyoid bone pulls mandible downward and inward
Sternohyoid	6	Posterior aspect of sternoclavicular joint and adjacent manubrium of sternum	Body of hyoid bone medial to attachment of omohyoid muscle	Anterior rami of C1 to C3 through the ansa cervicalis	Depresses hyoid bone after swallowing
Omohyoid	7	Superior border of scapula medial to suprascapular notch	Lower border of body of hyoid bone just lateral to attachment of sternohyoid	Anterior rami of C1 to C3 through the ansa cervicalis	Depresses and fixes hyoid bone
Thyrohyoid	8	Oblique line on lamina of thyroid cartilage	Greater horn and adjacent aspect of body of hyoid bone	Fibers from anterior ramus of C1 carried along hypoglossal nerve [XII]	Depresses hyoid bone, but when hyoid bone is fixed raises larynx
Sternothyroid	9	Posterior surface of manubrium of sternum	Oblique line on lamina of thyroid cartilage	Anterior rami of C1 to C3 through the ansa cervicalis	Draws larynx (thyroid cartilage) downward

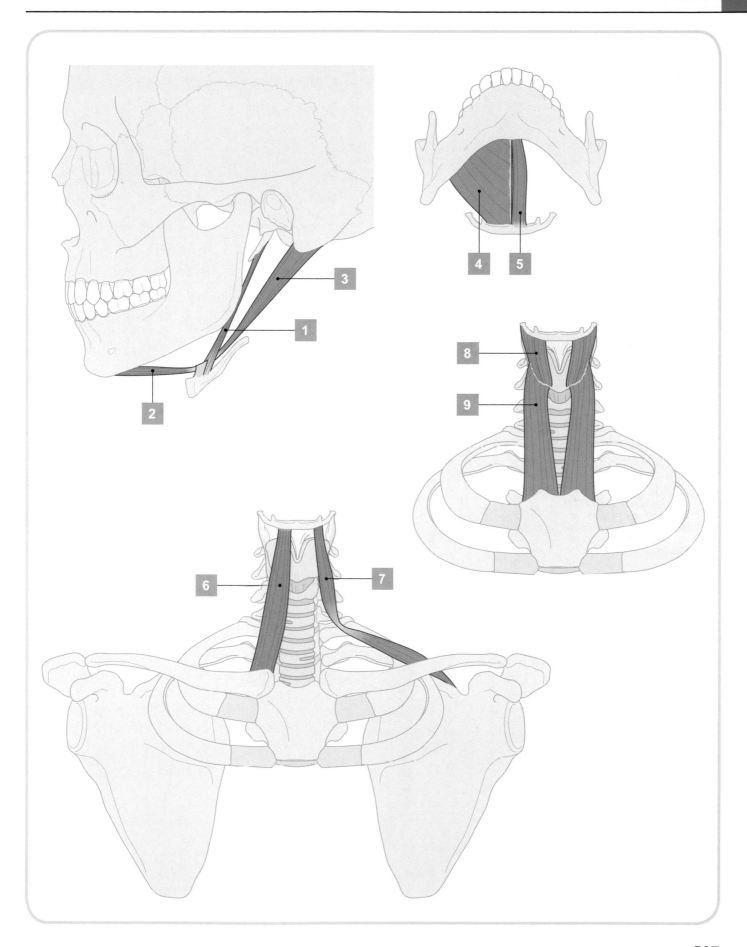

Branches of the external carotid artery

Artery		Parts supplied
Superior thyroid artery	1	Thyrohyoid muscle, internal structures of the larynx, sternocleidomastoid and cricothyroid muscles, thyroid gland
Ascending pharyngeal artery	2	Pharyngeal constrictors and stylopharyngeus muscle, palate, tonsil, pharyngotympanic tube, meninges in posterior cranial fossa
Lingual artery	3	Muscles of the tongue, palatine tonsil, soft palate, epiglottis, floor of mouth, sublingual gland
Facial artery	4	All structures in the face from the inferior border of the mandible anterior to the masseter muscle to the medial corner of the eye, the soft palate, palatine tonsil, pharyngotympanic tube, submandibular gland
Occipital artery	5	Sternocleidomastoid muscle, meninges in posterior cranial fossa, mastoid cells, deep muscles of the back, posterior scalp
Posterior auricular artery	6	Parotid gland and nearby muscles, external ear and scalp posterior to ear, middle and inner ear structures
Superficial temporal artery	7	Parotid gland and duct, masseter muscle, lateral face, anterior part of external ear, temporalis muscle, parietal and temporal fossae
Maxillary artery	8	External acoustic meatus, lateral and medial surface of tympanic membrane, temporomandibular joint, dura mater on lateral wall of skull and inner table of cranial bones, trigeminal ganglion and dura in vicinity, mylohyoid muscle, mandibular teeth, skin on chin, temporalis muscle, outer table of bones of skull in temporal fossa, structures in infratemporal fossa, maxillary sinus, upper teeth and gingivae, infra-orbital skin, palate, roof of pharynx, nasal cavity

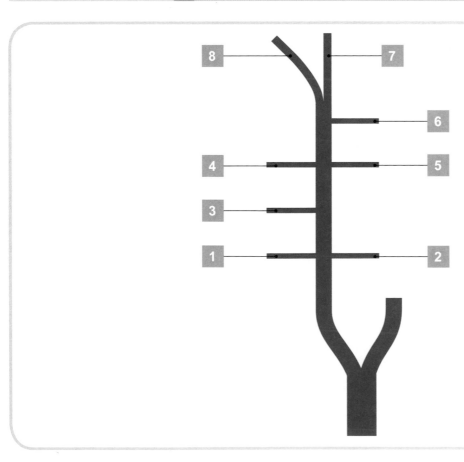

Subdivisions of the anterior triangle of the neck—a regional approach

Subdivision		Boundaries	Contents
Submental triangle (unpaired)	1	Mandibular symphysis; anterior belly of digastric muscle; body of hyoid bone	Submental lymph nodes; tributaries forming the anterior jugular vein
Submandibular triangle (paired)	2	Lower border of mandible; anterior belly of digastric muscle; posterior belly of digastric muscle	Submandibular gland; submandibular lymph nodes; hypoglossal nerve [XII]; mylohyoid nerve; facial artery and vein
Carotid triangle (paired)	3	Posterior belly of digastric muscle; superior belly of omohyoid muscle; anterior border of sternocleido-mastoid muscle	Tributaries to common facial vein; cervical branch of facial nerve [VII]; common carotid artery; external and internal carotid arteries; superior thyroid; ascending pharyngeal; lingual, facial, and occipital arteries; internal jugular vein; vagus [X], accessory [XI], and hypoglossal [XII] nerves; superior and inferior roots of ansa cervicalis; transverse cervical nerve
Muscular triangle (paired)	4	Midline of neck; superior belly of omohyoid muscle; anterior border of sternocleidomastoid muscle	Sternohyoid, omohyoid, sternohyoid, and thyrohyoid muscles; thyroid and parathyroid glands; pharynx

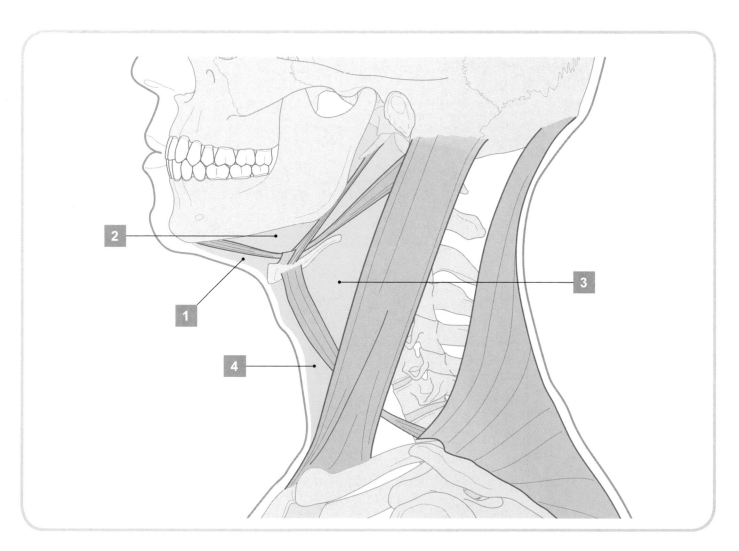

Muscles associated with the posterior triangle of the neck

Parentheses indicate possible involvement

Muscle		Origin	Insertion	Innervation	Function
Sternocleidomastoid —Sternal head	1	Upper part of anterior surface of manubrium of sternum	Lateral one half of superior nuchal line	Accessory nerve [XI] and branches from anterior rami of C2 to C3 (C4)	Individually, will tilt head toward shoulder on same side rotating head to turn face to opposite side; acting together, draw head forward
—Clavicular head	2	Superior surface of medial one third of clavicle	Lateral surface of mastoid process		
Trapezius	3	Superior nuchal line; external occipital protuberance; ligamentum nuchae; spinous processes of vertebrae CVII to TXII	Lateral one third of clavicle; acromion; spine of scapula	Motor—accessory nerve [XI]; proprioception—C3 and C4	Assists in rotating the scapula during abduction of humerus above horizontal; upper fibers—elevate, middle fibers—adduct, lower fibers—depress scapula
Splenius capitis	4	Lower half of ligamentum nuchae; spinous processes of vertebrae CVII to TIV	Mastoid process, skull below lateral one third of superior nuchal line	Posterior rami of middle cervical nerves	Together, draw head backward; individually, draw and rotate head to one side (turn face to same side)
Levator scapulae	5	Transverse processes of CI to CIV	Upper part of medial border of scapula	C3, C4; and dorsal scapular nerve (C4, C5)	Elevates scapula
Posterior scalene	6	Posterior tubercles of transverse processes of vertebrae CIV to CVI	Upper surface of rib II	Anterior rami of C5 to C7	Elevation of rib II
Middle scalene	7	Transverse processes of vertebrae CII to CVII	Upper surface of rib I posterior to the groove for the subclavian artery	Anterior rami of C3 to C7	Elevation of rib I
Anterior scalene	8	Anterior tubercles of the transverse processes of vertebrae CIII to CVI	Scalene tubercle and upper surface of rib I	Anterior rami of C4 to C7	Elevation of rib I
Omohyoid	9	Superior border of scapula medial to scapular notch	Inferior border of body of hyoid bone	Ansa cervicalis; anterior rami of C1 to C3	Depress the hyoid bone

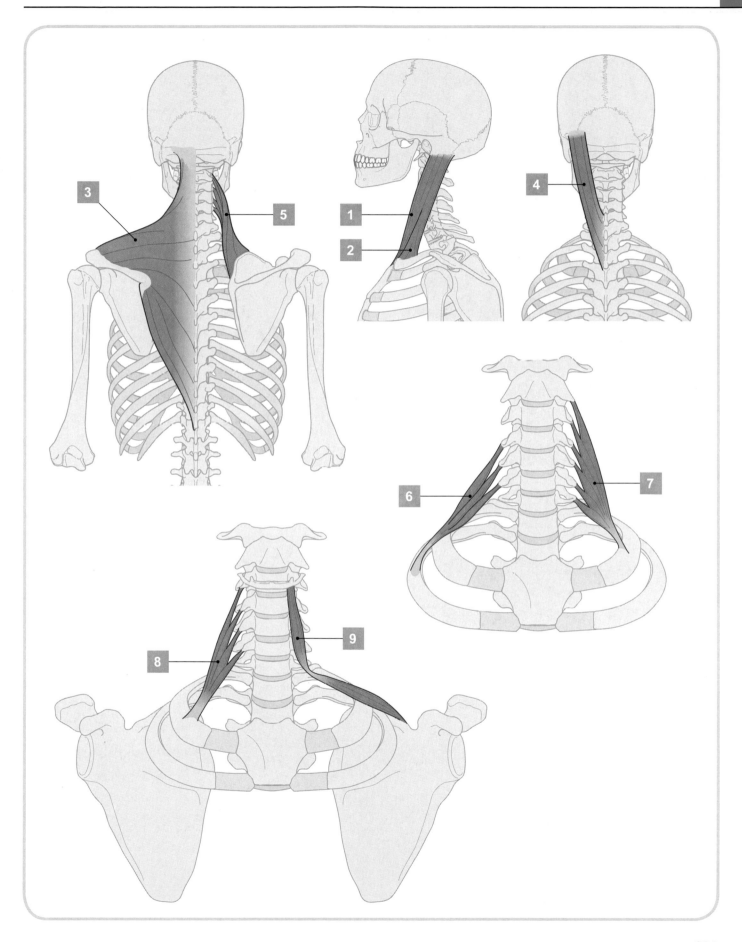

Prevertebral and lateral muscles

Muscle		Origin	Insertion	Innervation	Function
Rectus capitis anterior	1	Anterior surface of lateral part of atlas and its transverse process	Inferior surface of basilar part of occipital bone	Branches from anterior rami of C1, C2	Flexes head at atlanto-occipital joint
Rectus capitis lateralis	2	Superior surface of transverse process of atlas	Inferior surface of jugular process of occipital bone	Branches from anterior rami of C1, C2	Flexes head laterally to same side
Longus colli —Superior oblique part	3	Anterior tubercles of transverse processes of vertebrae CIII to CV	Tubercle of anterior arch of atlas	Branches from anterior rami of C2 to C6	Flexes neck anteriorly and laterally and slight rotation to opposite side
—Inferior oblique part	4	Anterior surface of bodies of vertebrae TI, TII, and maybe TIII	Anterior tubercles of transverse processes of vertebrae CV and CVI		
—Vertical part	5	Anterior surface of bodies of TI to TIII and CV to CVII	Anterior surface of bodies of vertebrae CII to CIV		
Longus capitis	6	Tendinous slips to transverse processes of vertebrae CIII to CVI	Inferior surface of basilar part of occipital bone	Branches from anterior rami of C1 to C3	Flexes the head

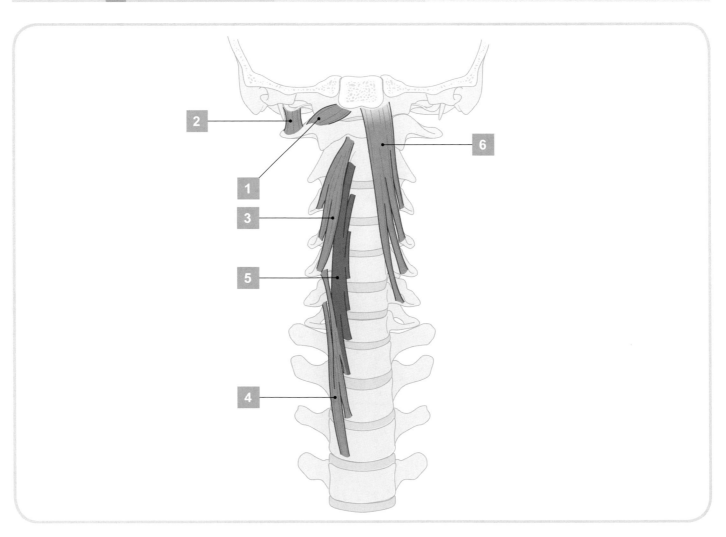

Constrictor muscles of the pharynx

Muscle		Posterior attachment	Anterior attachment	Innervation	Function
Superior constrictor	1	Pharyngeal raphe	Pterygomandibular raphe and adjacent bone on the mandible and pterygoid hamulus	Vagus nerve [X]	Constriction of pharynx
Middle constrictor	2	Pharyngeal raphe	Upper margin of greater horn of hyoid bone and adjacent margins of lesser horn and stylohyoid ligament	Vagus nerve [X]	Constriction of pharynx
Inferior constrictor	3	Pharyngeal raphe	Cricoid cartilage, oblique line of thyroid cartilage, and a ligament that spans between these attachments and crosses the cricothyroid muscle	Vagus nerve [X]	Constriction of pharynx

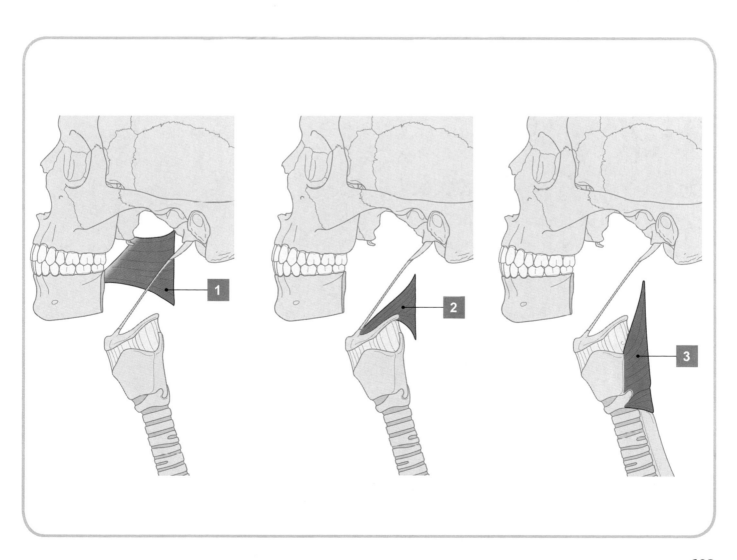

Longitudinal muscles of the pharynx

Muscle		Origin	Insertion	Innervation	Function
Stylopharyngeus	1	Medial side of base of styloid process	Pharyngeal wall	Glossopharyngeal nerve [IX]	Elevation of the pharynx
Salpingopharyngeus	2	Inferior aspect of pharyngeal end of pharyngotympanic tube	Pharyngeal wall	Vagus nerve [X]	Elevation of the pharynx
Palatopharyngeus	3	Upper surface of palatine aponeurosis	Pharyngeal wall	Vagus nerve [X]	Elevation of the pharynx; closure of the oropharyngeal isthmus

Intrinsic muscles of the larynx

Muscle		Origin	Insertion	Innervation	Function
Cricothyroid	1	Anterolateral aspect of arch of cricoid cartilage	Oblique part—inferior horn of the thyroid cartilage; straight part—inferior margin of thyroid cartilage	External branch of superior laryngeal nerve from the vagus nerve [X]	Forward and downward rotation of the thyroid cartilage at the cricothyroid joint
Posterior crico-arytenoid	2	Oval depression on posterior surface of lamina of cricoid cartilage	Posterior surface of muscular process of arytenoid cartilage	Recurrent laryngeal branch of the vagus nerve [X]	Abduction and external rotation of the arytenoid cartilage. The posterior crico-arytenoid muscles are the primary abductors of the vocal folds. In other words, they are the primary openers of the rima glottidis.
Lateral crico-arytenoid	3	Superior surface of arch of cricoid cartilage	Anterior surface of muscular process of arytenoid cartilage	Recurrent laryngeal branch of the vagus nerve [X]	Internal rotation of the arytenoid cartilage and adduction of vocal folds
Transverse arytenoid	4	Lateral border of posterior surface of arytenoid cartilage	Lateral border of posterior surface of opposite arytenoid cartilage	Recurrent laryngeal branch of the vagus nerve [X]	Adduction of arytenoid cartilages
Oblique arytenoid	5	Posterior surface of muscular process of arytenoid cartilage	Posterior surface of apex of adjacent arytenoid cartilage; extends into ary-epiglottic fold	Recurrent laryngeal branch of the vagus nerve [X]	Sphincter of the laryngeal inlet
Thyro-arytenoid	6	Thyroid angle and adjacent cricothyroid ligament	Anterolateral surface of arytenoid cartilage; some fibers continue in ary-epiglottic folds to the lateral margin of the epiglottis	Recurrent laryngeal branch of the vagus nerve [X]	Sphincter of vestibule and of laryngeal inlet
Vocalis	7	Lateral surface of vocal process of arytenoid cartilage	Vocal ligament and thyroid angle	Recurrent laryngeal branch of the vagus nerve [X]	Adjusts tension in vocal folds

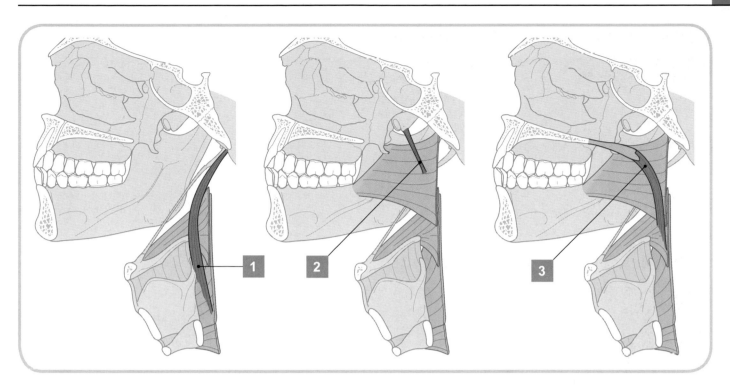

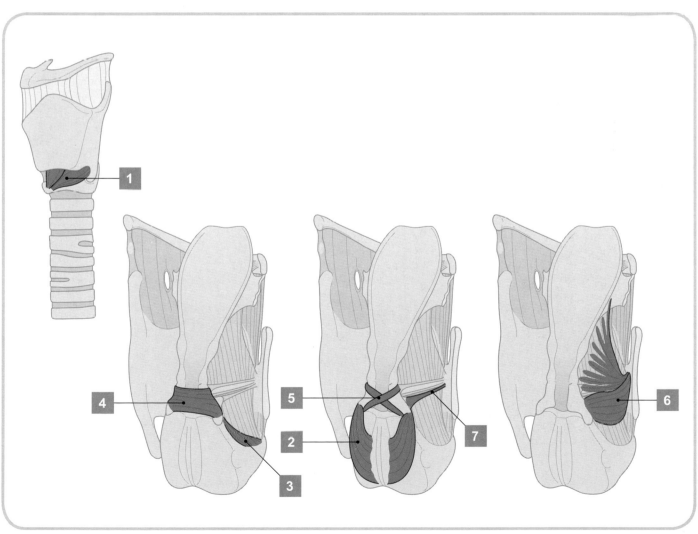

Muscles in the floor of the oral cavity

Muscle		Origin	Insertion	Innervation	Function
Mylohyoid	1	Mylohyoid line of mandible	Median fibrous raphe and adjacent part of hyoid bone	Nerve to mylohyoid from the inferior alveolar branch of mandibular nerve [V_3]	
Geniohyoid	2	Inferior mental spines of mandible	Body of hyoid bone	C1	Supports and elevates floor of oral cavity; depresses mandible when hyoid is fixed; elevates and pulls hyoid forward when mandible is fixed

Muscles of the tongue

Muscle		Origin	Insertion	Innervation	Function
Intrinsic					
Superior longitudinal (just deep to surface of tongue)	1	Submucosal connective tissue at the back of the tongue and from the median septum of the tongue	Muscle fibers pass forward and obliquely to submucosal connective tissue and mucosa on margins of tongue	Hypoglossal nerve [XII]	Shortens tongue; curls apex and sides of tongue
Inferior longitudinal (between genioglossus and hyoglossus muscles)	2	Root of tongue (some fibers from hyoid)	Apex of tongue	Hypoglossal nerve [XII]	Shortens tongue; uncurls apex and turns it downward
Transverse	3	Median septum of the tongue	Submucosal connective tissue on lateral margins of tongue	Hypoglossal nerve [XII]	Narrows and elongates tongue
Vertical	4	Submucosal connective tissue on dorsum of tongue	Connective tissue in more ventral regions of tongue	Hypoglossal nerve [XII]	Flattens and widens tongue
Extrinsic					
Genioglossus	5	Superior mental spines	Body of hyoid; entire length of tongue	Hypoglossal nerve [XII]	Protrudes tongue; depresses center of tongue
Hyoglossus	6	Greater horn and adjacent part of body of hyoid bone	Lateral surface of tongue	Hypoglossal nerve [XII]	Depresses tongue
Styloglossus	7	Styloid process (anterolateral surface)	Lateral surface of tongue	Hypoglossal nerve [XII]	Elevates and retracts tongue
Palatoglossus	8	Inferior surface of palatine aponeurosis	Lateral margin of tongue	Vagus nerve [X] (via pharyngeal branch to pharyngeal plexus)	Depresses palate; moves palatoglossal fold toward midline; elevates back of the tongue

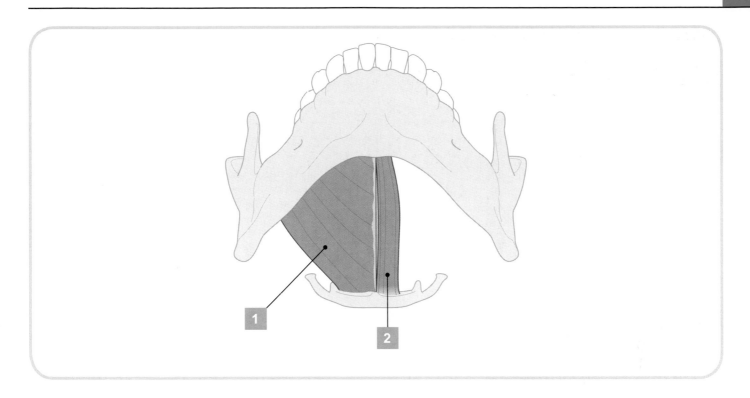

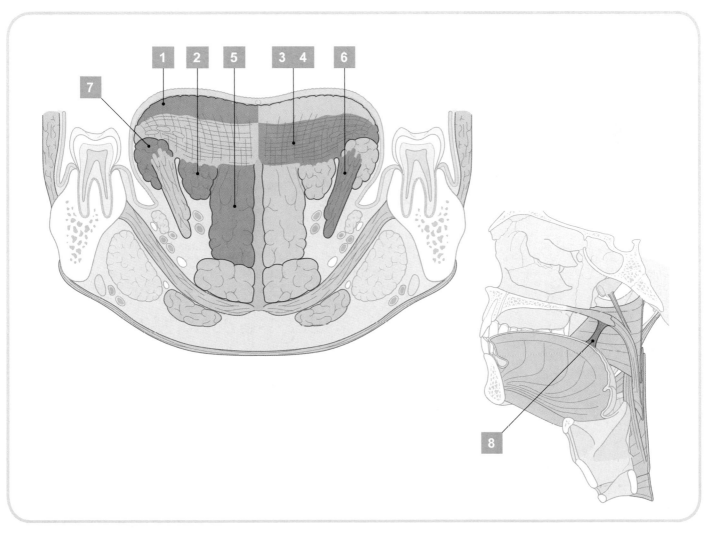

Muscles of the soft palate

Muscle		Origin	Insertion	Innervation	Function
Tensor veli palatini	1	Scaphoid fossa of sphenoid bone; fibrous part of pharyngotympanic tube; spine of sphenoid	Palatine aponeurosis	Mandibular nerve [V$_3$] via the branch to medial pterygoid muscle	Tenses the soft palate; opens the pharyngotympanic tube
Levator veli palatini	2	Petrous part of temporal bone anterior to opening for carotid canal	Superior surface of palatine aponeurosis	Vagus nerve [X] via pharyngeal branch to pharyngeal plexus	Only muscle to elevate the soft palate above the neutral position
Palatopharyngeus	3	Superior surface of palatine aponeurosis	Pharyngeal wall	Vagus nerve [X] via pharyngeal branch to pharyngeal plexus	Depresses soft palate; moves palatopharyngeal arch toward midline; elevates pharynx
Palatoglossus	4	Inferior surface of palatine aponeurosis	Lateral margin of tongue	Vagus nerve [X] via pharyngeal branch to pharyngeal plexus	Depresses palate; moves palatoglossal arch toward midline; elevates back of the tongue
Musculus uvulae	5	Posterior nasal spine of hard palate	Connective tissue of uvula	Vagus nerve [X] via pharyngeal branch to pharyngeal plexus	Elevates and retracts uvula; thickens central region of soft palate

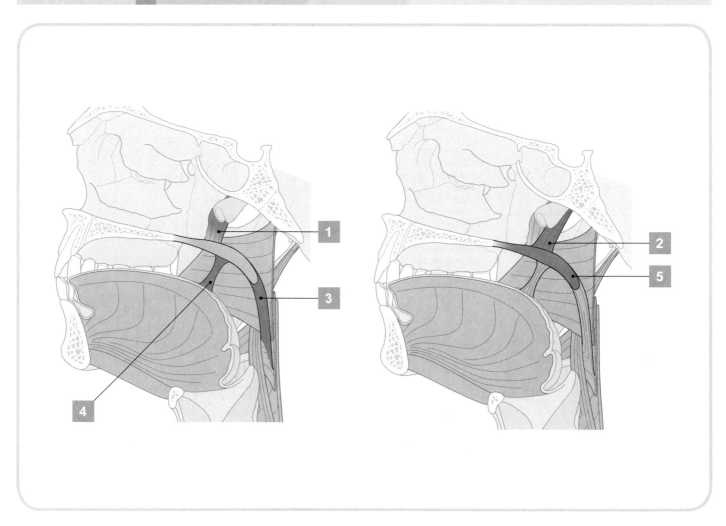